# AUTOPSY PATHOLOGY

## A MANUAL AND ATLAS

# AUTOPSY PATHOLOGY

## A MANUAL AND ATLAS

## 2nd Edition

### Walter E. Finkbeiner, MD, PhD

Professor and Vice Chair, Department of Pathology, University of California, San Francisco;
Chief, Department of Pathology, San Francisco General Hospital, San Francisco, California

### Philip C. Ursell, MD

Professor, Department of Pathology, University of California, San Francisco;
Director, Autopsy Service, Moffitt-Long Hospital, San Francisco, California

### Richard L. Davis, MD

Professor Emeritus, Department of Pathology, University of California, San Francisco, California

*Contributor:*
### Andrew J. Connolly, MD, PhD

Associate Professor, Department of Pathology, Stanford University Medical Center, Stanford, California

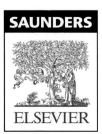

SAUNDERS

ELSEVIER

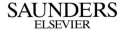

1600 John F. Kennedy Blvd.
Ste 1800
Philadelphia, PA 19103-2899

AUTOPSY PATHOLOGY: A MANUAL AND ATLAS, SECOND EDITION          ISBN: 978-1-4160-5453-5

**Library of Congress Cataloging-in-Publication Data**
Finkbeiner, Walter E.
  Autopsy pathology : a manual and atlas / Walter E. Finkbeiner, Philip
C. Ursell, Richard L. Davis ; contributor, Andrew J. Connolly—2nd ed.
    p. ; cm.
  Includes bibliographical references and index.
  ISBN 978-1-4160-5453-5
1. Autopsy—Handbooks, manuals, etc. 2. Autopsy—Atlases. I. Ursell,
Philip C. II. Davis, Richard L., M.D. III. Title.
  [DNLM: 1. Autopsy—methods. 2. Death Certificates. 3. Quality
Control. QZ 35 F499a 2009]
  RA1063.4.F566 2009
  616.07'59—dc22
                                                    2008034764

*Acquisitions Editor:* Bill Schmitt
*Developmental Editor:* Andrea Vosburgh
*Project Manager:* Mary Stermel
*Designer:* Gene Harris
*Marketing Manager:* Brenna Christensen

Printed in China

Last digit is the print number:   9  8  7  6  5  4  3  2  1

*To our students*

# Preface

The authors are gratified that the first edition of *Autopsy Pathology* was well received. Our objective in publishing a second edition remains the same as before, namely to provide a resource for those learning the art and science of postmortem examinations. Though the book is designed with the pathologist-in-training in mind, we hope that practicing pathologists, pathology assistants, and others involved in various fields of death investigation will also find it useful. The format used in the first edition remains; however, we have strived to improve each chapter. We have added illustrations to the atlas (Chapter 15), including a new section on forensic pathology. Dr. Andrew J. Connolly of Stanford University has contributed a succinct new chapter that covers autopsy practice in cases of sepsis and multiorgan failure, a much needed addition to a modern autopsy text.

A number of individuals require acknowledgment. The support and encouragement of Dr. Abul K. Abbas, chair of the UCSF Department of Pathology, is sincerely appreciated. Special thanks are owed to Dr. Connolly for his participation in this edition. We are indebted to Dr. Mark A. Super of the Sacramento County Coroner's Office and Drs. Robert Anthony and Gregory Reiber of Northern California Forensic Pathology for donating key forensic images. We thank Dr. Jonathan L. Hecht of the Beth Israel Deaconess Medical Center and Harvard Medical School for allowing us to use a slightly modified version of his template for fetal examinations. Our gratitude also goes to the Elsevier staff. Here, we must single out Ms. Andrea M. Vosburgh, developmental editor, for her singular attention to detail and many insightful suggestions that turned a manuscript into a book. Without her help, the task of revising this work would certainly have been much more difficult. Our thanks go also to our executive editor, Mr. William Schmitt, who provided guidance through each phase of the project. We are also indebted to Megan Greiner, production editor at Graphic World Inc. for her excellent work during final production. Finally, the authors thank their families for their enduring love and support.

Walter E. Finkbeiner, MD, PhD
Philip C. Ursell, MD
Richard L. Davis, MD

# Contents

# 1

# The Autopsy—Past and Present

*"Despite the disparagement of the ignorant and the patronizing smiles of the sophisticated, the necropsy still moves along at its time-honored, steady pace, maintaining standards, contributing to knowledge and even, on occasion, stimulating the sluggard."*

Edward A. Gall[1]

## THE AUTOPSY IN ANTIQUITY

The history of the autopsy is intimately connected with that of anatomy and medicine in general. According to the Egyptian historian Manetho, the king-physician Athotis (about 4000 BC) wrote books on medicine, the first of which contained some anatomic descriptions.[2] However, most scholars believe that early anatomic descriptions came primarily from the observations of animal anatomy made by early hunters, butchers, and cooks.[3,4] King and Meehan,[5] in their excellent discourse on the origins of the autopsy, trace human knowledge of anatomy to the practice of haruspicy—the inspection of animal entrails, particularly the liver, to predict the future. This form of divination was widespread in the ancient world, performed at least as early as the fourth century BC in Babylonia. Later, the ancient Hebrews contributed more practical observations. Following the Talmudic law "Thou shalt not eat anything that dyeth of itself," rabbis examined slaughtered animals for evidence of disease, especially in the lungs, meninges, and pericardium.[5]

Anatomic study of human disease evolved slowly, however. In ancient Egypt, there was considerable interest in the relationship of wounds and fractures to anatomy but little concern with the effects of nontraumatic disease. The embalmers of ancient Egypt removed the internal organs through small incisions, but their observations were neither recorded nor related to diseases. Egyptian records dating from the seventeeth (Edwin Smith Papyrus) and sixteenth (Papyrus Ebers) centuries BC dealt with surgical and medical diseases but related changes to magic rather than pathologic anatomy.[2] Similar beliefs were held by the Assyrians and Babylonians.[6] In ancient India, Susruta (circa 600 BC) advocated human dissections, but despite relatively sophisticated contemporary surgical techniques, anatomic studies (with the exception of osteology) were rather limited.[7] Practice of medicine in China and Japan was generally based on philosophy and religion rather than science, though during the Warring States Period

(457-421 BC) and in ancient texts there are references to examination of injuries.[8-10] However, dissection was forbidden, and anatomic knowledge remained largely speculative, based on rare dissected bodies.[2] The first recorded anatomic dissection of a human body in China occurred in 16 AD.[11] The first known dissection in Japan was in 456 AD when an autopsy done on the body of Princess Takukete following her suicide revealed fluid in the abdomen with a "stone."[12]

The humoral theories of disease that dominated ancient Greek medicine provided an atmosphere that discouraged investigation to correlate anatomy with disease. The Hippocratic physicians described external manifestations of disease—infections, abscesses, and ulcerating and even infiltrating cancers—but were content to observe human anatomy only through wounds. It is likely that no human dissections were performed in Greece until the third century BC.[13] Nevertheless, Aristotle (384-322 BC) inspired the study of animal anatomy and development. Aristotle's sphere of influence expanded following the battlefield success of his pupil, Alexander the Great. It was Alexander's able comrade Ptolemy of Macedonia (367-282 BC), who became Ptolemy I Soter, king of Egypt, who created the environment in which pathologic anatomy first flourished. Ptolemy established the great university and library in Alexandria at the mouth of the Nile river. For 4 centuries, Alexandria attracted the best students of medicine. Here, scholars dissected the human body at least throughout the third century BC, aided by Ptolemy's policy of making the bodies of executed criminals available.[5,14]

According to Pliny, Herophilos (335-280 BC) was the first who "searched into the cause of disease."[15] He performed dissections of humans and wrote a treatise on human anatomy. It was his contemporary Erasistratus (circa 310-250 BC), however, who broke from the humoral theories popular at the time and associated disease with changes in the organs.[4] He believed in two circulations, one that carried the nutritive substance "parenchyma" (blood) from the heart to the organs through the veins and one that carried air from the lungs through the arteries. Failure of an organ to digest the nutrient substance caused plethora or overfilling of the organ. Thus, he explained inflammation as overfilling of the veins with blood and fever as overfilling of the arteries with air. However, he correctly correlated excessive accumulation of fluid within the abdominal cavity with hardness of the liver. Although the great library of Alexandria was destroyed by the army of Julius Caesar in 48 BC, copies of some of the manuscripts had already made their way to Rome. Celsus (circa 30 BC-38 AD), a Roman patrician and not a physician, compiled much of the medical knowledge in his eight-volume *De Re Medicina*. Here are described the cardinal symptoms of inflammation ("rubor, tumor, dolor, calor, et functio laesa"), splenomegaly in what presumably were cases of malaria, and inflammation of the cecum in what later was understood as appendicitis, along with descriptions of clinical findings in what were certainly cases of rabies, meningitis, gout, hernia, gonorrhea, scrofula, and urinary calculi.[4,16]

The impressive compilation of Celsus was not influential on the physicians of the period, however, for it was unread and soon lost. Its impact came only in the Renaissance after it was discovered among stored documents in the church of St. Ambrose in Milan by Thomas of Sarzan (later Pope Nicholas V). The physicians of Rome followed the teachings of Galen (129-201 AD). Although Galen performed anatomic dissections on animals, including primates, and made many original observations, his theories on pathophysiology were worthless because they were based on the old humoral doctrine.[17] Unfortunately, his influence persisted until the late Middle Ages. Even during this generally unproductive period, however, there were some advances. In the Byzantine world, the physicians Oribasius (325-403), Aetius (502-575), Alexander of Tralles (525-605), and Paul of Aegina (625-690) preserved the teachings of others, as well as their own, through their writings. During this era, physical diagnosis and its basis in pathologic anatomy became more firmly rooted, and according to Procopius, as early as 543 physicians opened dead bodies searching for the cause of a plague epidemic in Byzantium.[18]

A small sect of Christians, probably of the Semitic or Aramean race, who eventually became known as the Nestorians, migrated from the Arabian peninsula into Syria.[19] At Edessa in Syria, the Nestorian bishop Rabboula had founded a hospital and medical school in 372 AD. Instruction was grounded in Hippocratic and Galenic teachings, and the faculty was composed of Christian and Jewish physicians. Opposed to the "heresy" of the Nestorian church, Emperor Zeno ordered the school closed in 489. The faculty fled to the town of Juní Shápúr in South Persia—a safe haven because it was administered by a Nestorian bishop. Neo-Platonist exiles from Athens arrived in 529. Instruction was given in Syriac, Greek, and Persian.[18] Scientific expeditions into India brought back the works of the great Indian doctors Susruta and Charaka (circa first century BC to circa first century AD), whose teachings were added to the Talmudic-influenced Greek medicine practiced at Juní Shápúr.[20]

Beginning in the seventh century, the Arabs pushed westward across Persia, Byzantine Asia Minor, Syria, Egypt, and northern Africa and into Spain until their advance was stopped at the Pyrenees at the battle of Poitiers by Charles Martel in 732. The Arabian armies spared Juní Shápúr from destruction, and its medical school soon became the center of medical teaching for the Islamic world until late in the ninth century, when Baghdad gained greater prominence. During the next 3 centuries, the most important works in medicine sprang from the Caliphate empire and included those of Arabic and Jewish physicians such as Rhazes (860-932), Avicenna (980-1037), and Avenzoar (1070-1162). However, the greatest advances were in pharmacology rather than pathology, for the Koran condemned dissection as mutilation of the dead.

In China, human dissections were performed occasionally during the Sung dynasty.[12] In 1045 AD, over a 2-day period, dissections of the bodies of 56 members of a band of rebels were recorded in an atlas. Between 1102 and 1106, Li Yee Siung, a government official, assembled physicians and artists to dissect a criminal and record the anatomic findings. Around 1250, there appeared a handbook, *His Yuan Lu* (*Washing Away of Wrongs*), perhaps based on earlier works that may have have originated as early as the sixth century. This text described simple autopsy techniques and guidelines, as well as the first recorded text dealing with forensic issues, such as poisoning, decomposition, wounds from various weapons, strangulation, fake wounds, and difficulties in determining causes of death when bodies are recovered in water or after fires.[21]

During this Arabic period, science was practically nonexistent in the developing European cultures. The collision of the two cultures would change that, however.[22] The Saracens, who arrived in Spain during the eighth century, intermittently raided and invaded Sicily and southern Italy and soon established colonies in the region. Jewish groups educated in Arabic thought also settled here. The town of Salerno on the Campanian coast, where a medical school had been founded as early as the ninth century, became the focal point. In 1076, the Normans took Salerno. At the same time, the monk-physician Constantine the African (?-1087), who had traveled for nearly 4 decades through Mesopotamia, India, Ethiopia, and Egypt studying medicine, arrived at the Benedictine abbey of Monte Cassino near Salerno, where a hospital had been established as early as 539.[23] Here, he and his pupils began translating medical works from Arabic into Latin. The significance of the works was quickly appreciated by the physicians at the Salerno school. The influence of the medical school grew, and it received official state sanction from Frederick II in 1231. Flourishing well into the 13th century, it attracted students widely, and its courses of instruction were adopted by the great universities that existed in Naples, Bologna, Padua, Montpellier, and Paris.[24] At the University of Bologna, Taddeo di Alderotto (1206?-1295) apparently made dissections of the human body a regular part of university teaching, and his students, such as Mondino (1265-circa 1326) and Mondeville (circa 1250-1320), followed this example.[4]

The first law authorizing human dissection (1231) is credited to Frederick II (1194-1250), Holy Roman Emperor. During the 13th and 14th centuries, restriction against opening the human body after death eased (Fig. 1-1). According to Chiari, a physician of Cremona performed autopsies on victims of the plague of 1286.[15] The Pope apparently authorized opening of bodies during the "Black Death" (1347-1350) to determine the cause of the disease.[25] Autopsies were performed in Siena in 1348 and authorized at Montpellier (Fig. 1-2) around 1376.[26] However, initially bodies were more likely opened for legal rather than educational purposes. Records indicate that William of Saliceto (about 1201-1280), a Bolognese surgeon, performed at least one medicolegal necropsy. Another early forensic autopsy was ordered by the court as part of the investigation of the death of Azzolino, an Italian nobleman who died suddenly in 1302, presumably from poisoning. Although the final judgment is unclear, the report describes an internal examination of the body.[4]

With the Renaissance, medicine and medical education were transformed. Public human dissections spread through the universities from Italy north across the Alps.[27] Professors sitting in raised chairs supervised assistants, commonly barber-surgeons, in formal dissections that lasted for several days and were attended by as many as 100 onlookers.[22] The long-held doctrines of Galen began to break down. Leonardo da Vinci (1452-1519) made drawings from some 30 human dissections.[28] Antonio Benivieni (circa 1443-1502), a Florentine physician, requested permission from relatives to perform postmortem examinations in enigmatic cases (Fig. 1-3).[25] He kept careful case records, and these were published by his brother in 1507 as *The Hidden Causes of Disease*.[29] Included in the 111 short chapters of this treatise are descriptions of 20 postmortem examinations. However, Benivieni only incised rather than dissected the bodies, and the findings reported are superficial. The first recorded autopsy in North America was an examination of conjoined twins performed in 1533 in Santo Domingo. Authorized by the clergy, its goal was not to establish cause of death but rather to determine whether there were two souls or one.[22] The records of the

second voyage (circa 1536) of Jacques Cartier up the St. Lawrence River described an internal examination of a sailor who died of a strange disease (scurvy), performed in the hope of identifying its cause and preventing its spread to other members of the crew.[25] As early as 1576 in Mexico City, Francisco Hernandez and Alonzo Lopez performed limited postmortem examinations.

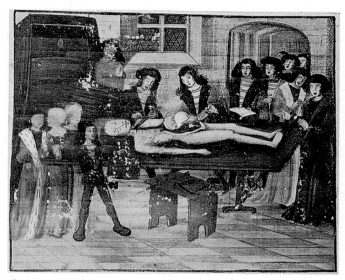

**Figure 1-2** Miniature from the Guy de Chauliac manuscript Chirurgia (1363) depicting an anatomic dissection or autopsy at Montpellier.
(From Holländer E: *Die Medizin in der Klassischen Malerei*, Stuttgart, Germany, 1913, Ferdinand Enke.)

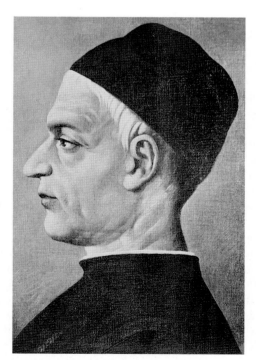

**Figure 1-3** Antonio Benivieni (from a portrait).
(From Benivieni A: *De regimine sanitotis ad laurentium medicem*, Belloni L, editor, Torino, Italy, 1951, Societa Italiana Di Patologia.)

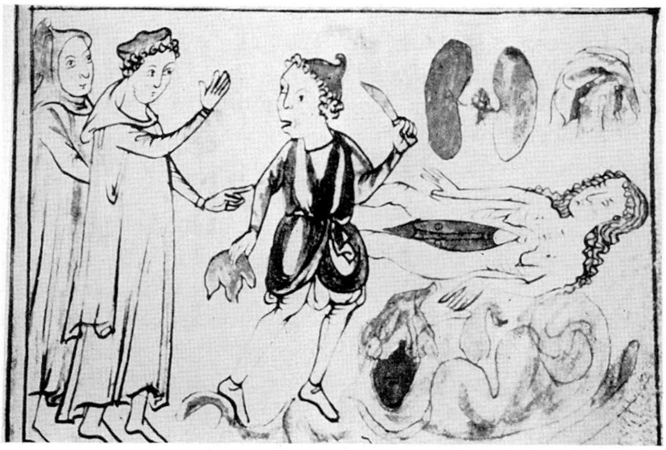

**Figure 1-1** This miniature from a thirteenth-century English manuscript did not have a caption but may represent an autopsy scene.
(From MacKinney L: *Medical illustration in medieval manuscripts*, London, 1965, Wellcome Historical Medical Library Publications; Bodleian Library, University of Oxford, Miss, Ashmole 339, fol. 34r.)

In the sixteenth century, Andreas Vesalius (1514-1564) from Brussels ushered in the modern era of studying anatomy. After completing his studies at Padua, he was appointed professor of surgery there and given the duty of conducting the public dissections. However, Vesalius did his own dissections using his students as assistants. Vesalius' pupils spread throughout Europe, advancing the anatomic concept of disease as they recognized the abnormal. In Germany, Johann Schenck von Grafenburg (1530-1598) performed postmortem examinations and recorded the findings as part of his practice as town physician for Freiburg and Strassbourg.[30] In Germany and France, by the end of the sixteenth century, death investigations that included autopsies became more common and were bolstered by laws such as the Constitutio Criminalis Carolina enacted by Holy Roman Emperor Charles V (1500-1558), which sanctioned forensic autopsies, thereby encouraging the growth of legal medicine as an academic discipline. At the University of Paris, Jean Fernel (1497-1558) supplemented his studies of medicine, and particularly tuberculosis, with postmortem examinations.[30] His chapter on pathology in his book *Medicina* (1554) was the first treatise to consider the pathogenesis of disease and contained the first clear description of what Reginald Fitz would later identify as appendicitis.[31] Following an autopsy on a 7-year-old boy who died during the Paris diphtheria epidemic of 1576, Guillaume de Baillou (1538-1616) described the false membrane covering the airway that characterizes the disease.[32] A London physician, George Thomson (1619-1677), remained in that city during the Great Plague of 1665 and attempted to determine its cause through postmortem examinations.[33] In 1666 he published his studies in *Loimotomia,* or *The Pest Anatomized,* which included an engraving of an autopsy dissection of a plague victim as its frontispiece (Fig. 1-4). In Italy, Fortunatas Fidelis (1551-1630) and the papal physician Paulo Zacchias (1584-1659) published *De Relationibus Medicorum* and *Questiones Medico-Legales,* respectively, influential textbooks of legal medicine. By the mid-seventeenth century formal lectures in forensic medicine were given in Germany by Johann Michaelis (1607-1667) and, thereafter, by Johannes Bohn (1640-1718), both of the University of Leipzig.[21] Bohn published a book on wounds *(De renunciatione vulnerum seu vulnerum lethalium examen)* in 1689 and followed it with a more extensive treatise, *De Officio Medici Duplici Clinici Nimirum ac Forensis,* in 1704. A number of professorships in forensic medicine were established at the German universities during the seventeeth century, and professorial chairs in legal medicine were in place in France by 1794 and Great Britain (Edinburgh) by 1803. By this time, additional legal medicine books or collections of cases that included forensic methods for solving them were available. In 1804, James Stringham (1775-1817) of New York gave the first lecture on legal medicine in the United States. In 1813, Stringham became the first American professor of the discipline.[34]

With William Harvey's (1578-1657) description of the circulation in 1628, the stage was set for the physiologic interpretations of pathologic findings. A pathologic anatomy museum was established by Riva (1627-1677). Marcello Malpighi (1628-1694), Francis Glisson (1597-1677), and Franciscus

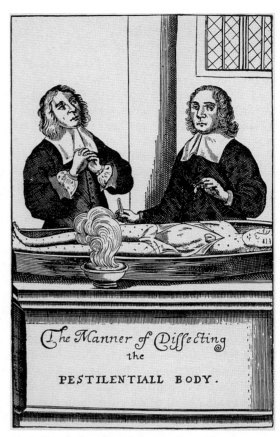

**Figure 1-4**  Frontispiece from Loimotomia, or The Pest Anatomized, by George Thomson.

Sylvius (1614-1672) routinely performed autopsies. The findings of many of these autopsies were compiled by Theophile Bonet and published in 1769 as the *Sepulchretum sive Anatomica Practica.* However, he made no attempt to correlate pathologic findings with clinical symptoms except for occasional references to the humoral doctrine. In contrast, Giovanni Morgagni (1682-1771) was among the first to correlate clinical symptoms with organic changes (Fig. 1-5). His autopsy reports, published in 1761 as *De Sedibus et Causis Morborum per Anatomen Indagatis (The Seats and Causes of Diseases Investigated by Anatomy),* numbered more than 700 and included descriptions of coronary artery atherosclerosis, aneurysms, endocarditis, lobar pneumonia, hepatic cirrhosis, fatty liver, renal calculi, hydronephrosis related to ureteral stricture, and various cancers.[35] Although Bonet's *Sepulchretum* is largely forgotten, Morgagni's work stands as one of the most influential in the history of medicine, for it convinced the physicians of its day that advancement of medicine rests in sound clinical-pathologic correlation.[36]

In France, Marie-François-Xavier Bichat (1771-1802) was perhaps the first experimental pathophysiologist and, along with his countrymen Jean-Nicolas Corvisart (1755-1821) and Réné-Théophile-Hyacinthe Laënnec (1781-1826), advocated the correlation of pathologic findings with physical diagnosis (Fig. 1-6). Bichat's career, cut short by tuberculosis, was notable for another reason, however. By subjecting organs to heat, air, water, acids, alkalis, salts, and so forth, and

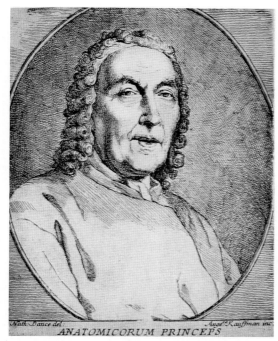

**Figure 1-5** Giovanni Battista Morgagni (from an engraving). (From Krumbhaar EB: *Pathology*, New York, 1937, Paul B Hoeber.)

without a microscope, he determined that organs were composed of tissues (from the French *tissu*, or cloth). He distinguished 21 kinds of tissues. Furthermore, he recognized that disease weakened tissues and that this effect of disease was the same no matter what organ was affected.[15]

At roughly the same time, great strides were also made in Scotland and England. William Hunter (1718-1783) and John Hunter (1728-1793) established the first English museum for the teaching of pathology. Matthew Baillie (1761-1823) published the first atlas of pathology in 1793; he described situs inversus, hydrosalpinx, dermoid ovarian cysts, and "hepatization" of the lungs in pneumonia and further clarified cirrhosis of the liver (Fig. 1-7).[37] Postmortem examinations were a regular event at Guy's Hospital in London, performed by the likes of Sir Astley Cooper (1768-1841), Richard Bright (1789-1859), Thomas Addison (1793-1860), and Thomas Hodgkin (1798-1866), who used their findings to advance the field of medicine.[17]

At the beginning of the nineteenth century, the wealth of information available from the autopsy was still largely untapped. Autopsies were usually confined to one organ, which was generally chosen by the clinician on the basis of medical judgment.[5] Autopsies begun without a specific direction were often concluded when the prosector, usually an untrained surgical assistant, determined the seat of disease, leaving many organs unexamined or at best given a cursory evaluation.

While this state of affairs persisted in Paris, Edinburgh, and London, there were new developments in Vienna and Berlin.

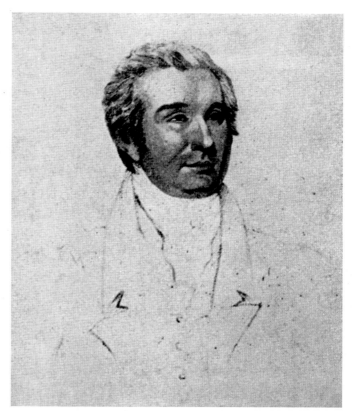

**Figure 1-6** Marie-François-Xavier Bichat (from an engraving). (From Krumbhaar EB: *Pathology*, New York, 1937, Paul B Hoeber.)

**Figure 1-7** Matthew Baillie (from an unfinished engraving). (From Krumbhaar EB: *Pathology*, New York, 1937, Paul B Hoeber.)

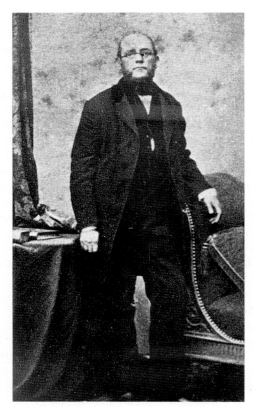

**Figure 1-8** Karl Rokitansky (from a photograph). (From Krumbhaar EB: *Pathology*, New York, 1937, Paul B Hoeber.)

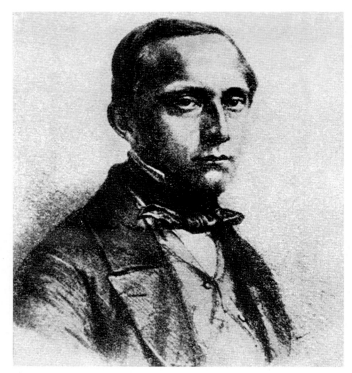

**Figure 1-9** Rudolph Virchow as a young professor. (From Krumbhaar EB: *Pathology*, New York, 1937, Paul B Hoeber.)

At the Allgemeines Krankenhaus at Vienna, Karl Rokitansky (1804-1878) performed more than 30,000 autopsies (Fig. 1-8). Through the influence of the editions of his manual *Handbook of Pathological Anatomy,* the autopsy became an important and integral part of medicine during the first half of the nineteenth century. However, Rudolph Virchow (1821-1902), by applying microscopic examination to diseased tissues and recognizing cellular alterations, became known as the founder of modern pathology (Fig. 1-9). To be sure, Virchow stood upon the shoulders of the early histologists, his mentor Johannes Müller (1801-1858) and two previous students of Müller, Theodor Schwann (1810-1882) and particularly Jacob Henle (1809-1885). Nevertheless, it was the publication in 1858 of 20 of Virchow's lectures in *Cellular Pathology as Based upon Physiological and Pathological Histology*[38,39] that ushered in the modern age of pathology.

To Rokitansky and Virchow, we can trace systematic examination of organs. In 1876, Virchow published a book on autopsy technique in which he introduced a detailed postmortem technique designed to identify abnormalities in organs and retain important anatomic relationships when necessary for demonstrations.[40] After examination of the organs and their relationships in situ, Virchow removed them one at a time. Following their removal, he performed further dissection outside the body. Moreover, he preserved regional organ relationships if indicated. This contrasts with the technique developed earlier by Rokitansky, as described by his student Chiari in a book first published in 1894.[41] Rokitansky examined and opened all organs in situ, preserving all abnormal

relationships. Friedrich Albert von Zenker (1825-1898) developed a technique similar to Rokitansky's in that it emphasized preservation of topographic anatomy, and two of his students, Heller and Hauser, each described their own versions in publications.[25] In their modifications, physiologically related organs were removed together and connections were maintained unless the pathologic process could not be demonstrated. The first substantial American works on autopsy technique were published by Delafield in 1872[42] and Thomas in 1873.[43] Joined by coauthor Prudden in 1885[44] and eventually revised by Wood,[45] the Delafield work evolved into a complete textbook of pathology but continued to include a description of autopsy technique through numerous editions.

Books by Nauwerck,[46] Woodhead,[47] Hektoen,[48] Clarke,[49] Warthin,[50,51] Cattell,[52] Mallory,[53] Box,[54] Beattie,[55] and Miller[56] described modifications of or improvements on the autopsy technique of Virchow. Versions based on all of these are in practice today. In France, Maurice Letulle (1853-1929) described a technique based on en bloc removal of the thoracic and abdominal organs.[57] With variations, it remains a popular alternative to the organ-by-organ approach that descended from Virchow. A four-volume work, *Medical Jurisprudence, Forensic Medicine and Toxicology,* edited by Witthaus and Becker with many contributors, was published in 1894 to 1896 and incorporated various burgeoning disciplines of forensic medicine and science.[58]

## THE AUTOPSY IN THE TWENTIETH CENTURY

The first half of the twentieth century saw, in addition to standardization of postmortem dissection procedures, improvements in tissue embedding, microtomy, and histochemistry. In North America, leaders of medicine, including Sir William Osler (1849-1919), stressed the importance of the autopsy in both undergraduate and postgraduate medical education (Fig. 1-10). As a student at McGill University, Osler was actively involved with autopsies. For his graduation thesis, which consisted of reports of 50 postmortem examinations and included 33 specimens, he received a special prize from the faculty. Following postgraduate study at University College in London (1872-1873), Osler spent 3 months in Berlin under Virchow and 5 months in Vienna, primarily with Rokitansky.[59,60] On his return to Montreal in 1874, Osler began a decade-long service at McGill University and its associated Montreal General Hospital, where he performed nearly 800 autopsies in addition to his clinical and teaching duties.[61] These cases formed the basis for numerous presentations and case reports and ultimately became the foundation of his textbook, *The Principles and Practice of Medicine* (1892).

Flexner's report on medical education in Canada and the United States advocated the autopsy as an important tool for ensuring hospital quality, and accrediting agencies defined acceptable autopsy rates.[62,63] In 1936 the newly formed American Board of Pathology began certifying pathologists. This raised the standards for the training of pathologists, and training centered largely around the autopsy table.[5] Forensic pathology burgeoned, becoming a subspecialty of pathology, and the medical examiner system began to replace the coroner

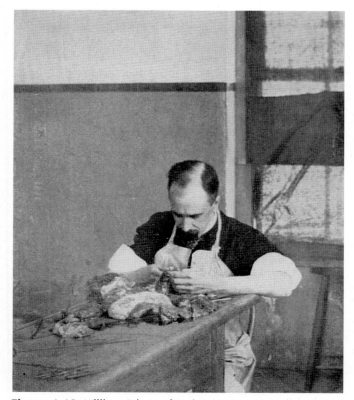

**Figure 1-10** William Osler performing a postmortem dissection at the Blockley Mortuary, Philadelphia, around 1886.
(From the Sir William Osler Memorial Number, International Association of Medical Museums, Bulletin 9, 1926.)

system.[64] In the United States, the autopsy rate, which was about 12% in 1910,[65] climbed to about 50% by the late 1940s.[66]

In an editorial that appeared in the *Journal of the American Medical Association* in 1956, Starr[67] questioned the value of the "classical" autopsy. Although his premise generated a lively rebuttal, the fact remains that after a century, the autopsy was moving from its place in the center of the medical stage. Autopsy rates declined. In 1971 the Joint Commission for the Accreditation of Hospitals (JCAH) dropped its recommendation for a 20% to 25% autopsy rate in accredited hospitals.[68] Although the numbers of hospital autopsies were decreasing before this change in policy, the JCAH decision lent tacit acceptance to this state of affairs. Rigorous objections to the decision appeared in print[69-71] but failed to sway the policy makers.

Why was there such a precipitous drop in autopsy rate? At the height of autopsy activity, new demands diverted pathologists' attentions. The role of clinical pathologists grew as physicians relied on newer, more sophisticated laboratory tests. Operations and endoscopies increased surgical pathology specimen numbers and the demands on pathologists' time. The value of cytologic examinations in disease prevention and recognition led to their expanded use and consequently increased pathologists' workload. All these endeavors provide direct remuneration for pathologists. In contrast, U.S. pathologists' compensation for autopsy practice generally remains hidden in the hospital budget and daily room rate, where it is essentially considered overhead.[72] For the pathologist practicing in the community, the morgue became a place to avoid. At the medical schools, pathology departments invested in experimental pathologists, not autopsy prosectors. Too frequently, the inexperienced house officer was left on his or her own while performing a postmortem examination. A generation of pathologists was trained in an environment that devalued the autopsy.

The responsibility for the decline of the autopsy does not rest on the shoulders of pathologists alone. Clinicians, who along with hospitals and health care organizations are the prime "consumers" of the autopsy, have requested fewer. A number of reasons for this have been suggested, the following most frequently: (1) greater confidence in modern diagnostic techniques, (2) unwillingness to dwell on clinical "failures," (3) fear that autopsy results will increase malpractice risks, (4) difficulty in obtaining autopsy authorization from the grieving family, and (5) dissatisfaction with the quality or timeliness, or both, of autopsy reports.[73-75] The shift in care of patients from a general practitioner to multiple specialists and the concomitant lack of rapport between physician, patient, and family made it easier for relatives to refuse an autopsy request from a physician with whom they had no long-term relationship.[76] Families of the deceased have resisted autopsies for numerous reasons, including being poorly informed about the value of the autopsy, fear that they might be billed for the service, anxiety about delays in funeral arrangements, concern that the deceased had suffered enough, religious convictions, or cultural beliefs.[77-81] Although funeral directors often believe in the value of autopsies, delays in receiving the remains, increased difficulties in embalming, and concern of the family about possible disfigurement of their relatives after autopsy have led morticians to counsel families against authorizing autopsies.[82] Increasing numbers of patients with chronic diseases are dying outside the hospital—at home or in nursing homes or hospices—in sites where there is often little interest in postmortem examination.

Near the end of the twentieth century, the autopsy rate in the United States, including medical examiner/coroner cases, fell below 10% and to nearly 5% if deaths caused by accidents, homicide, and suicide are excluded.[83] The autopsy rate at academic medical centers continues to decline (Figs. 1-11 and 1-12).[84] In some cases, the shift of terminal care away from the hospitals (and pathology departments) has resulted in a reduction in the total number of postmortem examinations, though autopsy rates remain relatively constant. In other cases, the decrease in numbers of autopsies performed is due primarily to a decrease in the autopsy rate. More alarming, the rate of postmortem examinations performed at some community hospitals is at or near zero.[85] As a consequence, the autopsy rates for certain groups (e.g., elderly people) and diseases (e.g., cerebrovascular) are particularly low.[86,87] From 1980 to 1984, the autopsy rate in New York state nursing homes was less than 1%, although 20% of all deaths in the state occurred in these institutions.[88] In fact, this represents the current situation nationwide, in which old age and death in a nursing home both have a statistically negative relationship with whether an autopsy is performed.[89] Similar data come from Australia,[90] Denmark,[91] Japan,[92] Sweden,[93] and the United Kingdom.[94]

## THE AUTOPSY TODAY

Have the nonforensic autopsy rate and the autopsy as a relevant medical procedure reached their nadir? If anything,

health care cost containment policies will exert additional restraints. In the past, autopsy costs in the United States have been recovered through both insurance and Medicare Part A reimbursements.[95] However, as payers switch to different methods such as capitation, cost recovery for autopsy services is essentially lost. The College of American Pathologists[96] has strongly advocated for a method of direct reimbursement for autopsy; however, its voice has fallen on deaf ears. As the United States moves slowly but inevitably toward a single payer form of universal health coverage, perhaps new resources and interest will be directed to the postmortem examination. Of note, a survey of Swedish citizens indicated that declining autopsy rates are apparently not a consequence of negative attitudes toward the procedure.[97] And in the United States, some entrepreneurs have found commercial success providing private autopsy services to a receptive public. Thus, it seems the major challenge in preserving the autopsy rests not on convincing the public of the merits of autopsies but rather on reengaging the medical professions—including pathologists.

## THE OBJECTIVES OF THE AUTOPSY

Despite the decline in autopsy rates, the procedure still has its champions. The autopsy—its place in medicine, role in society, and future—has been the subject of numerous symposia,[98-106] editorials,[76,84,107-122] and books.[123,124] Proponents laud the autopsy for its role in establishing public trust in medicine. Detractors question the risk and cost effectiveness of the autopsy. For others, the autopsy needs no justification—it remains a focal point for the integration of medical knowledge. Most would agree, however, that the autopsy benefits physicians, patients, and society and therein demonstrates its value. These benefits fall into seven broad categories.

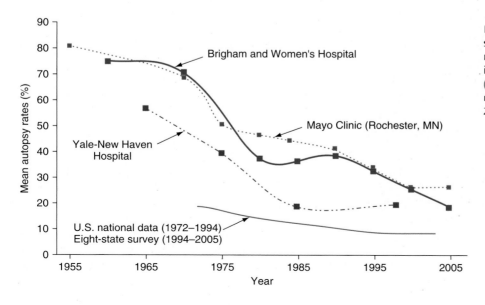

**Figure 1-11** Trends in U.S. autopsy rates and several academic medical centers. Autopsy rates at many institutions are inflated by the inclusion of forensic cases and stillbirths. (Data from Shojania KG, Burton EC: The vanishing nonforensic autopsy, *N Engl J Med* 358:873-875, 2008.)

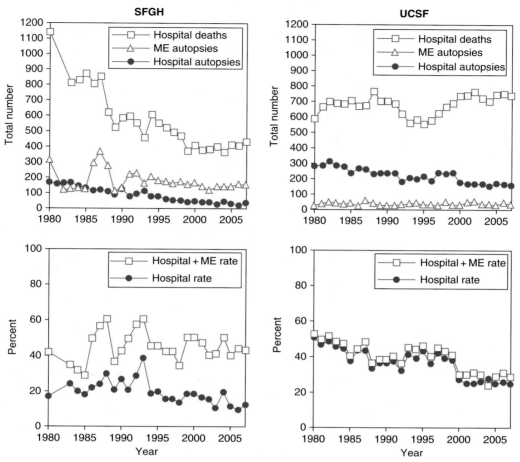

**Figure 1-12** Number of autopsies and autopsy rates at two hospitals affiliated with the same medical school. San Fancisco General Hospital (SFGH) is a public hospital and trauma center. The University of California (UCSF) Hospital is an academic medical center. Upper panels show total hospital deaths, medical examiner (ME), and nonforensic (hospital) autopsies from 1980 to 2007. Lower panels show hospital and total (hospital autopsies plus medical examiner) autopsy rates. At SFGH, the autopsy rate has fluctuated slightly, but the main factor that has led to fewer hospital autopsies has been a drop in the number of in-hospital deaths. At UCSF, the decrease in autopsies since 1980 has been mainly due to a decrease in the hospital autopsy rate.

## Benefits to Physicians and Health Care Organizations

Two of the major objectives of the autopsy are the establishment of final diagnoses and determination, whenever possible, of the cause of death. Autopsy cases provide a unique opportunity for physicians to correlate their physical and laboratory findings with the pathologic changes of disease. In essence, the autopsy is a "gold standard" for evaluating the accuracy of diagnosis and the outcome of therapy. Through autopsy findings, pathologists alert hospital infection control committees of possible contagion. Thus the autopsy provides critical data for medical quality assurance and, ultimately, quality improvement (see Chapter 14).

Autopsies may also reduce hospital and physician malpractice risk. Valaske[125] surveyed 183 hospitals and 39 malpractice liability companies and from their responses concluded that autopsies (1) eliminate suspicion, (2) provide reassurance to families, (3) substitute facts for conjecture, (4) construct a better defense, (5) reduce the number of claims, and (6) improve the quality of care. In a small, biased sample of autopsies performed after families filed a malpractice suit,

postmortem findings clarified the cause of death in 10 of 15 cases, contributing to the resolution of conflicts and safety of future patients.[126] In a retrospective analysis of outcomes of medical malpractice cases, Bove and colleagues[127] concluded that a finding of medical negligence was based on standard-of-care issues rather than accuracy of clinical diagnosis even when a major discrepancy was discovered at autopsy. In fact, major discrepancies in diagnosis identified by autopsy were relatively uncommon in suits in which a physician was found to be negligent; however, in about 20% of cases, autopsy findings were helpful to defendant physicians.

One of the most overlooked benefits of the autopsy may be its contribution to accurate billing. Under the Diagnosis-Related Group (DRG) system of Medicare reimbursement, autopsy data increased allowable billing by 6.6%.[128]

## Benefits to the Family of the Deceased

The therapeutic value of the autopsy for surviving family is often overlooked.[129] At autopsy, pathologists can identify or define hereditary or contagious diseases. This information not only provides the basis for genetic counseling but also may indicate preventive care for relatives. In a study of the value of autopsies performed in cases of death during the perinatal period, Faye-Petersen and colleagues[130] determined that autopsy findings altered parental counseling or recurrence risk estimates in 26% of cases. Autopsies help families with the grieving process, especially by removing guilt on the part of the immediate family for believing that they may have contributed to death.[131,132] This is particularly true after sudden death. In the setting of a postautopsy conference, the clinician or pathologist can console the family by reporting the cause of death, provide information about the disease process, answer any lingering questions about the terminal events, and alleviate irrational guilt.[133,134] Finally, the autopsy provides accurate data for determination of insurance benefits or workers' compensation. McPhee and coauthors,[135] in a survey of family members who had consented to an autopsy of their relatives, found that 88% considered the postmortem examination beneficial. Reasons given, in order of frequency, included consolation through contributing to the advancement of medical knowledge, comfort in knowing the cause of death, reassurance that the therapy was complete and appropriate, identification of genetic or contagious diseases, and settlement of insurance claims. Despite the autopsy's proven value to families, one study indicates that physicians and pathologists can still do a better job of communicating autopsy findings to the families of decedents.[136]

## Benefits to Public Health

The autopsy contributes to public health surveillance through detection of contagious diseases, identification of environmental hazards, and contribution of accurate vital statistics. Direct benefits accrue when an autopsy pathologist alerts public health officials about a communicable disease or an environmental hazard. In the age of global terrorism, the autopsy may help in the early identification of bioterrorism.[137] Indirectly, the autopsy contributes to population health planning and disease prevention by providing reliable data. Unfortunately, as the autopsy rate declines, so does the accuracy of vital statistics. Numerous studies document serious discrepancies in the underlying cause of death as recorded on death certificates when determined clinically rather than from autopsies.[124,138-140] Major inaccuracies reach levels of approximately 30%.[138,141] The discordance crosses national boundaries,[138,142-144] diseases,[145-156] and age of the deceased[157] (although errors are magnified in the geriatric population).[158-160] Furthermore, because the practice of amending death certificates after autopsy is sporadic at best, mortality statistics based on these documents are probably too inaccurate for meaningful use. With this concern in mind, a committee of the College of American Pathologists proposed the creation of a National Autopsy Data Bank.[161,162] This has never been fully realized, but a publicly accessible autopsy database has been established on the Internet.[163]

## Benefits to Medical Education

The majority of medical students,[164,165] house officers,[166-168] pathology residents,[168] physicians and medical educators,[169-172] and nurses[173] agree on the usefulness of the autopsy in medical practice and education. However, surveys of medical students and faculty suggest that the educational value of the autopsy is not fully realized.[174,175] The autopsy aids in the education of students in medicine and other health-related disciplines by providing teaching material for anatomy, histology, and pathology. Direct exposure of medical students as participants offers opportunities not just in the instruction of pathology but also in that of anatomy.[176] In the arena of medical school education, the autopsy is a focal point for integration and correlation of basic and clinical medical knowledge.[177,178] Medical students and hospital residents and fellows learn from observing or discussing at conferences the postmortem findings of patients whom they treated. The autopsy also provides an opportunity for pathologists-in-training to improve their knowledge of normal and abnormal gross and microscopic anatomy.

## Benefits to Medical Discovery and Applied Clinical Research

Despite the decline in autopsy numbers, autopsy data continue to embellish the medical literature and figure most prominently in neuroscience, cardiovascular, oncology, hematology, and respiratory fields.[179] Modern molecular techniques coupled with and supplementing postmortem examinations have identified diseases related to emerging and reemerging infectious agents.[180] Hill and Anderson,[124] compiling the data of others,[1,181-184] identified 87 diseases that were discovered or critically clarified through the autopsy between 1950 and 1988. Regarding this list, one can conclude two things: First, it is an underestimate, and second, it continues to grow. In addition to discovering new diseases, the autopsy pathologist may uncover changing patterns of diseases.[185-187] However, the value of the autopsy lies not just in documenting disease processes. It is the autopsy pathologist who helps evaluate the toxic effects of the latest drugs, the accuracy of imaging techniques, and the efficacy of new therapies.

## Benefits to Basic Biomedical Research

The autopsy provides investigators with normal and diseased human tissues for research. Tissues obtained at autopsies are useful for establishing cell and organ cultures, xenotransplantation, biochemical analysis, and morphologic studies despite the often lengthy interval between death and examination.[188,189] Cooperation between families (who are frequently interested in the study of an inherited disease), clinicians, pathologists, and basic scientists often provides an opportunity for donations of organs or tissues shortly after death.[190] Many human organs such as those of the central nervous system are not available by other means, accounting for the importance of the autopsy in research in the fields of neuropathology and neuroscience.[191-193] An immediate autopsy program,[194] in addition to supplying well-preserved normal tissues for study, allows investigators the opportunity to examine pathologic processes at the molecular and cellular levels. However, a fountain of knowledge also comes from autopsies performed after the usual time intervals.[5,188] Tissues collected and banked by institutions and research societies around the world provide investigators with normal and diseased tissues.[195-197] As large-scale efforts have revealed the human genome,[198,199] the importance of stored tissue expressing specific disease phenotypes increases.

## Benefits to Law Enforcement and Jurisprudence

The medicolegal investigation of death is a key component of a crime investigation. The forensic autopsy is focused on establishing the cause, time, and manner of death, including the circumstances preceding and surrounding death. Thus, in addition to the postmortem examination, the medicolegal investigation may involve inspection of the site where the body was found. Anticipating the potential for legal action, the forensic pathologist must collect and preserve evidence obtained at the scene and from the autopsy.

## REFERENCES

1. Gall EA: The necropsy as a tool in medical progress, *Bull N Y Acad Med* 44:808-829, 1968.
2. Gordon BL: *Medicine throughout antiquity.* Philadelphia, 1949, FA Davis.
3. Dawson WR: Egypt's place in medical history. In Underwood EA, editor: *Science, medicine and history; essays on the evolution of scientific thought and medical practice written in honour of Charles Singer,* vol 1, London, 1953, Oxford University Press, pp 47-60.
4. Long ER: *A history of pathology,* New York, 1965, Dover.
5. King LS, Meehan MC: A history of the autopsy. A review, *Am J Pathol* 73:514-544, 1973.
6. Dawson WR: *The beginnings: Egypt and Assyria.* New York, 1930, Paul B Hoeber.
7. Hoernle AFR: *Studies in the medicine of ancient India, Part I: Osteology or the bones of the human body.* Oxford, 1907, Clarendon.
8. Morse WR: *Chinese medicine,* New York, 1934, Paul B Hoeber.
9. Fujikawa Y: *Japanese medicine,* New York, 1934, Paul B Hoeber.
10. Peng Z, Pounder DJ: Forensic medicine in China, *Am J Forensic Med Pathol* 19:368-371, 1998.
11. Mori O: *Anatomy,* vol 1, Tokyo, 1964, Kanahara.
12. Nickey WM Jr, Dill RE, Vendrell DD: Autopsy pathology and neuropathology. In Race GJ, editor: *Laboratory medicine,* Hagerstown, Md, 1980, Harper & Row, pp 1-29.
13. Edelstein L: The history of anatomy in antiquity. In Temkin O, Temkin CL, editors: *Ancient medicine: selected papers,* Baltimore, 1967, The Johns Hopkins Press, pp 247-301.
14. Diamandopoulos AA, Goudas PC: The late Greco-Roman and Byzantine contribution towards the evolution of laboratory examinations of bodily excrement. Part 2: Sputum, vomit, blood, sweat, autopsies, *Clin Chem Lab Med* 43:90-96, 2005.
15. Krumbhaar EB: *Pathology,* New York, 1937, Paul B Hoeber.
16. Lund FB: *Greek medicine,* New York, 1936, Paul B Hoeber.
17. Malkin HM: *Out of the mist. The foundation of modern pathology and medicine during the nineteenth century.* Berkeley, Calif, 1993, Vesalius Books.
18. Klemperer P: Introduction. In Morgagni JB: *The seats and causes of diseases investigated by anatomy,* vol 1, Mount Kisco, NY, 1980, Futura, pp III-VIII.
19. Elgood C: *A medical history of Persia and the Eastern Caliphate.* Cambridge, 1951, Cambridge University Press.
20. Elgood C: *Medicine in Persia.* New York, 1934, Paul B Hoeber.
21. Smith S: History and development of legal medicine. In Gradwohl RBH, editor: *Legal medicine.* St. Louis, 1954, Mosby, pp 1-19.
22. Corner GW: *Anatomy,* New York, 1930, Paul B Hoeber.
23. Castiglioni A: *Italian medicine,* New York, 1932, Paul B Hoeber.
24. Venzmer G: *Five thousand years of medicine,* New York, 1972, Taplinger (Translated by M Koenig M).
25. Farber SB: *The postmortem examination.* Springfield, Ill, 1937, Charles C Thomas.
26. Garrison FH: *An introduction to the history of medicine,* ed 4, Philadelphia, 1929, WB Saunders.
27. Baker F: The two Sylviuses. An historical study, *Bull Johns Hopkins Hosp* 20:329-339, 1909.
28. Florey HW: The history and scope of pathology. In Florey L, editor: *General pathology,* Philadelphia, 1970, WB Saunders, pp 1-21.
29. Benivieni A: *The hidden causes of disease.* Singer C, trans. Springfield, Ill: Charles C Thomas, 1954.
30. Spiro RK: A backward glance at the study of postmortem anatomy. *Int Surg* 56:27-40, 101-112, 1971.
31. Fitz RH: Perforating inflammation of the vermiform appendix, with special reference to its early diagnosis and treatment. *Bost Med Surg J* 15:13-14, 1886.
32. Major RH: *Classic descriptions of disease,* Springfield, Ill, 1945, Charles C Thomas.
33. Guthrie D: *A history of medicine,* Philadelphia, 1946, JB Lippincott.
34. Myers RO, Brittain R: The history of legal medicine. In Camps FE, editor: *Gradwhohl's legal medicine,* ed 2, Bristol, UK, 1968, John Wright & Sons, pp 1-14.
35. Morgagni JB: *The seats and causes of diseases investigated by anatomy,* Mount Kisco, NY, 1980, Futura (Translated by B Alexander).
36. Tedeschi CG: The pathology of Bonet and Morgagni: A historical introduction to the autopsy, *Hum Pathol* 5:601-603, 1974.
37. Baillie M: *The morbid anatomy of some of the most important parts of the human body,* Albany, NY, 1795, Barbeer & Southwick (First American edition based on the London edition of 1793).
38. Virchow R: *Die Cellularpathologie in ihre Begründung auf Physiologische und Pathologische Gwebelehre,* Berlin, 1858, A Hirschwald.
39. Virchow RLK: *Cellular pathology as based upon physiological and pathological histology,* New York, 1971, Dover (Translated from the second German edition).
40. Virchow RLK: *Description and explanation of the method of performing post-mortem examinations in the dead house of the Berlin Charite Hospital, with especial reference to medico-legal practice,* London, 1880, Churchill (Translated from the second German edition by TP Smith).
41. Chiari H: *Pathologisch-Anatomische Sektionstechnik,* Berlin, 1894, H Kornfeld.
42. Delafield F: *A hand-book of post-mortem examinations and of morbid anatomy,* New York, 1872, William Wood.
43. Thomas AR: *A practical guide for making post-mortem examinations, and for the study of morbid anatomy, with directions for embalming the dead, and for the preservation of specimens of morbid anatomy,* New York, 1873, Boericke & Tafel.
44. Delafield F, Prudden TM: *A handbook of pathological anatomy and histology,* New York, 1885, William Wood.
45. Wood FC: *Delafield and Prudden's text-book of pathology,* ed 16, Baltimore, 1936, William Wood.
46. Nauwerck C: *Sectionstechnik für Studirende und Aerzte,* Jena, Germany, 1891, Gustav Fischer.
47. Woodhead GS: *Practical pathology: A manual for students and practitioners,* ed 3, Philadelphia, 1892, JB Lippincott.
48. Hektoen L: *The technique of post-mortem examination,* Chicago, 1893, Chicago Medical Book.

49. Clarke JJ: *Post-mortem examinations in medico-legal and ordinary cases*, London, 1896, Longmans, Green.

50. Warthin AS: *Practical pathology for students and physicians*, ed 1, Ann Arbor, Mich, 1897, George Wahr.

51. Warthin AS: *Practical pathology: A manual of autopsy and laboratory technique for students and physicians*, ed 2, Ann Arbor, Mich, 1928, George Wahr.

52. Cattell HM: *Post-mortem pathology*, Philadelphia, 1903, JB Lippincott.

53. Mallory FB: *Pathological technique: A practical manual for workers in pathological histology and bacteriology including directions for the performance of autopsies and for clinical diagnosis by laboratory methods*, Philadelphia, 1908, WB Saunders.

54. Box CR: *Post-mortem manual: A handbook of morbid anatomy and post-mortem technique*, ed 1, London, 1910, J & A Churchill.

55. Beattie JM: *Post-mortem methods*, Cambridge, UK, 1915, Cambridge University Press.

56. Miller J: *Practical pathology including morbid anatomy and post-mortem technique*, New York, 1914, Macmillan.

57. Letulle MEJL: *La pratique des autopsies*, Paris, 1903, C Naud.

58. Witthaus RA, Becker TC: *Medical jurisprudence, forensic medicine and toxicology*, New York, 1894 (vols 1 and 2), 1896 (vols 3 and 4), W.Wood & Co.

59. Osler W: Berlin correspondence, *Can Med Surg J* 2:308-315, 1874.

60. Osler W: Vienna correspondence, *Can Med Surg J* 2:451-456, 1874.

61. Rodin AE: *Oslerian pathology. An assessment and annotated atlas of museum specimens*, Lawrence, Kan, 1981, Coronado Press.

62. Flexner A: *Medical education in the United States and Canada: A report to the Carnegie Foundation for the Advancement of Teaching, Bulletin 4*, New York, 1910, The Carnegie Foundation.

63. Council on Scientific Affairs: Autopsy: A comprehensive review of current issues, *JAMA* 258:364-369, 1987.

64. Fisher RS, Platt MS: History of forensic pathology and related laboratory sciences. In Spitz WU, editor: *Medicolegal investigation of death*, Springfield, Ill, 1993, Charles C Thomas, pp 3-13.

65. Oertal H, Lewinski-Corwin EH: Report on post-mortem examinations in the United States, *JAMA* 60:1784-1791, 1913.

66. Roberts WC: The autopsy: Its decline and a suggestion for its revival, *N Engl J Med* 299:332-338, 1978.

67. Starr I: Potential values of the autopsy today, *JAMA* 160:1144-1145, 1956.

68. Joint Commission on Accreditation of Hospitals: *Accreditation manual for hospitals*, Chicago, 1971, JCAH.

69. Prutting J: Abolition of percentage requirement for accreditation of hospital: Et tu brute, *N Y State J Med* 72:2507-2509, 1972.

70. Ebert RV, Porterfield JD, Trump BF, et al: Open forum: A debate on the autopsy: Its quality control function in medicine, *Hum Pathol* 5:605-618, 1974.

71. Wagner BW: The JCAH and the autopsy, *Hum Pathol* 16:1-2, 1985.

72. Pontius EE: Financing mechanisms for autopsy, *Am J Clin Pathol* 69(Suppl 2):245-247, 1977.

73. Goodale F: Future of the autopsy, *Am J Clin Pathol* 69(Suppl 2):260-262, 1978.

74. Kaplan RA: The autopsy—to be or not to be, *Hum Pathol* 9:127-129, 1978.

75. Wheeler MS: One resident's view of the autopsy, *Arch Pathol Lab Med* 106:311-313, 1982.

76. Caplan AL: Morality dissected: A plea for reform of current policies with respect to autopsy, *Hum Pathol* 15:1105-1106, 1984.

77. Lundberg GD: Medicine without the autopsy, *Arch Pathol Lab Med* 108:449-454, 1984.

78. Brown HG: Lay perceptions of autopsy, *Arch Pathol Lab Med* 108:446-448, 1984.

79. Brown HG: Perceptions of the autopsy: Views from the lay public and program proposals, *Hum Pathol* 21:154-158, 1990.

80. Perkins HS: Cultural differences and ethical issues in the problem of autopsy requests, *Tex Med* 87:72-77, 1991.

81. González-Villalpando C: The influence of culture in the authorization of an autopsy, *J Clin Ethics* 4:192-194, 1993.

82. Heckerling PS, Williams MJ: Attitudes of funeral directors and embalmers toward autopsy, *Arch Pathol Lab Med* 116:1147-1151, 1992.

83. Sinard JH: Factors affecting autopsy rates, autopsy request rates, and autopsy findings at a large academic medical center, *Exp Mol Pathol* 70:333-343, 2001.

84. Shojania KG, Burton EC: The vanishing nonforensic autopsy, *N Engl J Med* 358:873-875, 2008.

85. Lundberg GD: Low-tech autopsies in the era of high-tech medicine, *JAMA* 280:1273-1274, 1998.

86. Ahronheim JC, Bernholc AS, Clark WD: Age trends in autopsy rates: Striking decline in late life, *JAMA* 250:1182-1186, 1983.

87. Lanska DJ: Decline in autopsies for deaths attributed to cerebrovascular disease, *Stroke* 24:71-75, 1993.

88. Katz PR, Seidel G: Nursing home autopsies: Survey of physician attitudes and practice patterns, *Arch Pathol Lab Med* 114:145-147, 1990.

89. Nemetz PN, Leibson C, Naessens JM, et al: Determinants of the autopsy decision: A statistical analysis, *Am J Clin Pathol* 108:175-183, 1997.

90. McKelvie PA, Rode J: Autopsy rate and a clinicopathological audit in an Australian metropolitan hospital—cause for concern? *Med J Aust* 156:456-462, 1992.

91. Petri CN: Decrease in the frequency of autopsies in Denmark after the introduction of a new autopsy act, *Qual Assur Health Care* 5:315-318, 1993.

92. Sugiyama T, Fujiimori T, Maeda S: Autopsy rates in medical schools and hospitals in Japan. In Riboli E, Delendi M, editors: *Autopsy in epidemiology and medical research*, Lyon, France, 1991, IARC Scientific Publications, pp 245-252.

93. Eriksson L, Sundstrom C: Decreasing autopsy rate in Sweden reflects changing attitudes among clinicians, *Qual Assur Health Care* 5:319-323, 1993.

94. Start RD, McCulloch TA, Benbow EW, et al: Clinical necropsy rates during the 1980s: The continued decline, *J Pathol* 171:63-66, 1993.

95. Shapiro MJ: Reimbursement for autopsies: A personal view, *Arch Pathol Lab Med* 108:473-475, 1984.

96. Carey K: Board takes stance on autopsy service pay, *CAP Today* 14:5, 11, 2000.

97. Sanner MA: In perspective of the declining autopsy rate: Attitudes of the public, *Arch Pathol Lab Med* 118:878-883, 1994.

98. Hazard JB: The autopsy, *JAMA* 193:805-806, 1965.

99. Prutting JM: Symposium on medical progress and the post-mortem, *Bull N Y Acad Med* 44:793-798, 1968.

100. Williams MJ, Peery TM: The autopsy, a beginning, not an end, *Am J Clin Pathol* 69(Suppl 2):215-216, 1977.

101. Bowman HE, Williams MJ: Revitalizing the ultimate medical consultation, *Arch Pathol Lab Med* 108:437-438, 1984.

102. Yesner R, Robinson MJ, Goldman L, et al: A symposium on the autopsy, *Pathol Annu* 20:441-477, 1985.

103. Cameron HM, McGoogan E, Lowe J, Cardesa A: Summary of the symposium on "the hospital autopsy: its contribution to medical audit," *Pathol Res Pract* 181:480-481, 1986.

104. Hill RB, Anderson RE, Vance RP: The autopsy: A professional obligation dissected, *Hum Pathol* 21:127, 1990.

105. Sundström C: The impact of autopsies on the quality of care, *Qual Assur Health Care* 5:279, 1993.

106. Hutchins GM: College of American Pathologists Conference XXIX on Restructuring Autopsy Practice for Health Care Reform: Introduction, *Arch Pathol Lab Med* 120:733, 1996.

107. Edwards JE: The autopsy: Do we still need it? *Mayo Clin Proc* 56:457-458, 1981.

108. Cameron HM: The autopsy as a clinical investigation, *J R Soc Med* 74:713-715, 1981.

109. Robinson MJ: The autopsy, 1983: Can it be revived? *Hum Pathol* 14:566-568, 1983.

110. Lundberg GD: Medical students, truth, and autopsies, *JAMA* 250:1199-1200, 1983.

111. Hill RB, Anderson RE: The autopsy and affairs of health, *Arch Pathol Lab Med* 113:1111-1113, 1989.

112. Vance RP: Autopsies and attitudes: Where do we go from here? *Arch Pathol Lab Med* 116:1111-1112, 1992.

113. McManus BM: The autopsy and the public need: Can medicine respond? *Arch Pathol Lab Med* 118:870-872, 1994.

114. Diamond I: New approach needed to revive the autopsy, *Arch Pathol Lab Med* 120:713, 1996.

115. Haber SL: Whither the autopsy? *Arch Pathol Lab Med* 120:714-717, 1996.

116. Hutchins GM: Whither the autopsy?...To regional autopsy centers, *Arch Pathol Lab Med* 120:718, 1996.

117. Seckinger DL: Our two-day exploration of the autopsy, *Arch Pathol Lab Med* 120:719, 1996.

118. King LSK: Of autopsies, *JAMA* 191:1078-1079, 1965.

119. Jeganathan VS, Walker SR, Lawrence C: Resuscitating the autopsy in Australian hospitals, *ANZ J Surg* 76:205-207, 2006.

120. Burton JL, Underwood J: Clinical, educational, and epidemiological value of autopsy, *Lancet* 369:1471-1480, 2007.

121. Horowitz RE, Naritoku WY: The autopsy as a performance measure and teaching tool, *Hum Patholol* 38:688-695, 2007.

122. Aiello VD, Debich-Spicer D, Anderson RH: Is there still a role for cardiac autopsy in 2007? *Cardio Young* 17(Suppl 2):97-103, 2007.

123. Waldron HA, Vickerstaff L: *Intimations of quality: Ante-mortem and post-mortem diagnoses*, London, 1977, Nuffield Provincial Hospitals Trust.

124. Hill RB, Anderson RE: *The autopsy—medical practice and public policy*, Boston, 1988, Butterworths.

125. Valaske MJ: Loss control/risk management. A survey of the contribution of autopsy examination, *Arch Pathol Lab Med* 108:462-468, 1984.

126. Juvin P, Teissière F, Brion F, et al: Postoperative death and malpractice suits: Is autopsy useful? *Anesth Analg* 91:344-346, 2000.

127. Bove KE, Iery C, Autopsy Committee, College of American Pathologist: The role of autopsy in medical malpractice cases, I, *Arch Pathol Lab Med* 126:1023-1031, 2002.

128. Guariglia P, Abrahams C: The impact of autopsy data on DRG reimbursement, *Hum Pathol* 16:1184-1186, 1985.

129. Roberts ME, Fody EP: The therapeutic value in the autopsy request, *J Relig Health* 25:161-166, 1986.

130. Faye-Petersen OM, Guinn DA, Wenstrom KD: Value of perinatal autopsy, *Obstet Gynecol* 94:915-920, 1999.

131. Reynolds RC: Autopsies—benefits to the family, *Am J Clin Pathol* 69(Suppl 2):220-222, 1978.

132. Oppewal F, Mayboom-de Jong B: Family members' experience of autopsy, *Fam Pract* 18:304-308, 2001.

133. Hirsch CS: Talking to the family after an autopsy, *Arch Pathol Lab Med* 108:513-514, 1984.

134. Valdés-Dapena M: The postautopsy conference with families, *Arch Pathol Lab Med* 108:497-498, 1984.

135. McPhee SJ, Bottles K, Lo B, et al: To redeem them from death, *Am J Med* 80:665-671, 1986.

136. Keys E, Brownlee C, Ruff M, et al, : How well do we communicate autopsy findings to next of kin? *Arch Pathol Lab Med* 132:66-71, 2008.

137. Nolte KB, Lathrop SL, Nashelsky MB, et al: "Med-X": A medical examiner surveillance model for bioterrorism and infectious disease mortality, *Hum Pathol* 38:718-725, 2007.

138. Kircher T, Nelson J, Burdo H: The autopsy as a measure of accuracy of the death certificate, *N Engl J Med* 313:1263-1269, 1985.

139. Carter JR: The problematic death certificate, *N Engl J Med* 313:1285-1286, 1985.

140. Kircher T: The autopsy and vital statistics, *Hum Pathol* 21:166-173, 1990.

141. Nielsen GP, Björnsson J, Jonasson JG: The accuracy of death certificates. Implications for health statistics, *Virchows Arch A Pathol Anat Histopathol* 419:143-146, 1991.

142. Doyle YG, Harrison M, O'Malley F: A study of selected death certificates from three Dublin teaching hospitals, *J Public Health Med* 12:118-123, 1990.

143. Maclaine GD, Macarthur EB, Heathcote CR: A comparison of death certificates and autopsies in the Australian Capital Territory, *Med J Aust* 156:462-463, 466-468, 1992.

144. Modelmog D, Rahlenbeck S, Trichopoulos D: Accuracy of death certificates: A population-based, complete-coverage, one-year autopsy study in East Germany, *Cancer Causes Control* 3:541-546, 1992.

145. Beadenkopf WG, Abrams M, Daoud A, Marks RU: An assessment of certain medical aspects of death certificate data for epidemiologic study of arteriosclerotic heart disease, *J Chron Dis* 16:249-262, 1963.

146. Barclay THC, Phillips AJ: The accuracy of cancer diagnosis on death certificates, *Cancer* 15:5-9, 1962.

147. Kuller LH, Bolker A, Saslaw MS, et al: Nationwide cerebrovascular disease mortality study. II. Comparison of clinical records and death certificates, *Am J Epidemiol* 90:545-555, 1969.

148. Mitchell RS, Maisel JC, Dart GA, Silvers GW: The accuracy of the death certificate in reporting cause of death in adults, *Am Rev Respir Dis* 104:844-850, 1971.

149. Bauer F, Robbins SL: An autopsy study of cancer patients. I. Accuracy of the clinical diagnosis (1955 to 1965) Boston City Hospital, *JAMA* 221:1471-1474, 1972.

150. Gobbato F, Vecchiet F, Barbierato D, et al: Inaccuracy of death certificate diagnoses in malignancy: An analysis of 1,405 autopsies cases, *Hum Pathol* 13 : 1036-1038, 1982.

151. Burns A, Jacoby R, Luthert P, Levy R: Cause of death in Alzheimer's disease, *Age Ageing* 19:341-344, 1990.

152. Di Bonito L, Stanta G, Delendi M, et al: Comparison between diagnoses on death certificates and autopsy reports in Trieste: Gynaecological cancers. In Riboli E, Delendi M, editors: *Autopsy in epidemiology and medical research*, vol 112, Lyon, France, 1991, IARC Scientific Publications, pp 63-71.

153. Selikoff IJ: Use of death certificates in epidemiological studies, including occupational hazards: Discordance with clinical and autopsy findings, *Am J Ind Med* 22:469-480, 1992.

154. Hunt LW Jr, Silverstein MD, Reed CE, et al: Accuracy of the death certificate in a population-based study of asthmatic patients, *JAMA* 269:1947-1952, 1993.

155. Hoel DG, Ron E, Carter R, Mabuchi K: Influence of death certificate errors on cancer mortality trends, *J Natl Cancer Inst* 85:1063-1068, 1993.

156. Lee PN: Comparison of autopsy, clinical and death certificate diagnosis with particular reference to lung cancer. A review of the published data, *APMIS* 102(Suppl 45):1-42, 1994.

157. Valdés-Dapena M, Arey JB: The causes of neonatal mortality: An analysis of 501 autopsies on newborn infants, *J Pediatr* 77:366-375, 1970.

158. Dean G: The need for accurate certification of cause of death and for more autopsies, *J Ir Med Assoc* 62:273-278, 1969.

159. Rossman I, Rodstein M, Bornstein A: Undiagnosed disease in an aging population: Pulmonary embolism and bronchopneumonia, *Arch Intern Med* 133:366-369, 1974.

160. Puxty JAH, Horan MA, Fox RA: Necropsies in the elderly, *Lancet* 1:1262-1264, 1983.

161. Peery TM: The Autopsy Data Bank. A proposal for pathologists to contribute to the health care of the nation, *Am J Clin Pathol* 69:258-259, 1978.

162. Carter JR, Nash NP, Cechner RL, Platt RD: Proposal for a national autopsy data bank: A potential major contribution of pathologists to the health care of the nation, *Am J Clin Pathol* 76(Suppl 4):597-617, 1981.

163. Moore GW, Berman JJ, Hanzlick RL, et al: A prototype internet autopsy database: 1625 consecutive fetal and neonatal autopsy facesheets spanning 20 years, *Arch Pathol Lab Med* 120:782-785, 1996.

164. Benbow EW: Medical students' views on necropsies, *J Clin Pathol* 43:969-976, 1990.

165. Galloway M: The role of the autopsy in medical education, *Hosp Med* 60:756-758, 1999.

166. Wilkes MS, Link RN, Jacobs TA, et al: Attitudes of house officers toward the autopsy, *J Gen Intern Med* 5:122-125, 1990.

167. Lund JN, Tierney GM: Hospital autopsy: Standardised questionnaire survey to determine junior doctors' perceptions, *Br Med J* 323:21-22, 2001.

168. Hull JM, Nazarian RM, Wheeler AM, Black-Schaffer, WS, Mark EJ: Resident physician opinions on autopsy importance and procurement, *Hum Pathol* 38:342-350, 2007.

169. Wilkes MS, Fortin AH, Jacobs TA: Physicians' attitudes toward the autopsy of patients with AIDS, *N Y State J Med* 91:386-389, 1991.

170. Durning S, Cation L: The educational value of autopsy in a residency training program, *Arch Intern Med* 160:997-999, 2000.

171. Burton JL: The autopsy in modern undergraduate medical education: A qualitative study of uses and curriculum considerations, *Med Educ* 37:1073-1081, 2003.

172. Hooper JE, Geller SA: Relevance of the autopsy as a medical tool: A large database of physician attitudes, *Arch Pathol Lab Med* 131:268-274, 2007.

173. Dziobon MD, Roberts ISD, Benbow EW: Attitudes of nursing staff to the autopsy, *J Adv Nurs* 32:969-974, 2000.

174. DeRoy AK: The autopsy as a teaching-learning tool for medical undergraduates, *J Med Educ* 51:1016-1018, 1976.

175. Inanici MA, Sözen MS, Alkan N, et al: The attitudes of medical students to autopsy, *Forensic Sci Int* 113:303-308, 2000.

176. Hartmann WH: Contributions of the autopsy to medical education, *Am J Clin Pathol* 69(Suppl 2):228-229, 1978.

177. Angrist AA: Effective use of autopsy in medical education: Its role in correlation and integration, *JAMA* 161:303-309, 1956.

178. Sánchez H, Ursell P: Use of autopsy cases for integrating and applying the first two years of medical education, *Acad Med* 76:530-531, 2001.

179. Start RD, Firth JA, Macgillivray F, Cross SS: Have declining clinical necropsy rates reduced the contribution of necropsy to medical research? *J Clin Pathol* 48:402-404, 1995.

180. Schwartz DA, Herman C: The importance of the autopsy in emerging and reemerging infectious diseases, *Clin Infect Dis* 23:248-254, 1996.

181. Angrist A: Breaking the postmortem barrier, *Bull N Y Acad Med* 44:830-842, 1968.

182. Cannon PR: Clinical lessons learned in the morgue, *JAMA* 161:730-732, 1956.

183. Garcia JH, Wilmes FJ: Autopsy: The path to progress, *Pathologist* 37:793-797, 1983.

184. Geller SA: Autopsy, *Sci Am* 248:124-129, 132, 135-136, 1983.

185. Klatt EC, Nichols L, Noguchi TT: Evolving trends revealed by autopsies of patients with the acquired immunodeficiency syndrome: 565 autopsies in adults with the acquired immunodeficiency syndrome, Los Angeles, Calif, 1982-1993, *Arch Pathol Lab Med* 118:884-890, 1994.

186. Zaki SR, Khan AS, Goodman RA, et al: Retrospective diagnosis of hantavirus pulmonary syndrome, 1978-1993. Implications for emerging infectious diseases, *Arch Pathol Lab Med* 120:134-139, 1996.

187. Sehonanda A, Choi YJ, Blum S: Changing patterns of autopsy findings among persons with acquired immunodeficiency syndrome in an inner-city population. A 12-year retrospective study, *Arch Pathol Lab Med* 120:459-464, 1996.

188. Carter JR: A renascence role of anatomic pathology in modern medicine, *Hum Pathol* 8:237-241, 1977.

189. Trump BF, Mergner WJ, Jones RT, Cowley RA: The use and application of autopsy in research, *Am J Clin Pathol* 69(Suppl 2):230-234, 1978.

190. Lindell KO, Erien JA, Kaminski N: Lessons for our patients: Development of a warm autopsy program. *PLoS Med* 3:e234, 2006. (http://journal.pmed.0030234; http://medicine.plosjournals.org/perlserv/?request=get-document=10.1371/journal.pmed.0030234 [accessed October 1, 2008])

191. Hulette C, Welsh-Bohmer KA, Crain B, et al: Rapid brain autopsy: The Joseph and Kathleen Bryan Alzheimer's Disease Research Center experience, *Arch Pathol Lab Med* 121:615-618, 1997.

192. McKee AC: Brain banking: Basic science methods, *Alzheimer Dis Assoc Disord* 13(Suppl 1):S39-S44, 1999.

193. Chariot P, Witt K, Pautot V, et al: Declining autopsy rate in a French hospital: Physicians' attitudes to the autopsy and use of autopsy material in research publications, *Arch Pathol Lab Med* 124:739-745, 2000.

194. Trump B, Valigorsky JM, Dees JH, et al: Cellular change in human disease: A new method of pathological analysis, *Hum Pathol* 4:89-109, 1973.

195. Newcombe J, Cuzner ML: Organization and research applications of the U.K. Multiple Sclerosis Society Tissue Bank, *J Neural Transm* 39(Suppl):155-163, 1993.

196. Kemper FH: Human organ specimen banking—15 years of experience, *Sci Total Environ* 139-140:13-25, 1993.

197. Ravid R, Swaab DF: The Netherlands brain bank—a clinico-pathological link in aging and dementia research, *J Neural Transm* 39(Suppl):143-153, 1993.

198. Lander ES, Linton LM, Birren B, et al: Initial sequencing and analysis of the human genome, *Nature* 409:860-921, 2001.

199. Venter JC, Adams MD, Myers EW, et al: The sequence of the human genome, *Science* 291:1304-1351, 2001.

# 2

# Legal, Social, and Ethical Issues

*"The autopsy is uniquely suited to study individual illness, provided the pathologist is aware of the broad interrelations between physiologic, pathologic and even social factors."*

Milton G. Bohrod[1]

## DEATH NOTIFICATION

Notifying family of the death of a relative is clearly one of the more difficult and stressful duties of medical personnel.[2] Although the hospital-based pathologist is not likely to be called on to perform this function, the medical examiner almost certainly is.[3] Police or other law enforcement officers may make the initial notification in cases of suspected homicide. Emergency personnel or physicians may inform relatives arriving at the scene or hospital. However, in most cases of sudden or violent death in which death is determined at the scene and the family is not present, the medical examiner traditionally notifies the next of kin, although this responsibility is usually not spelled out legally.[3]

Death notification initiates bereavement, and the manner in which notification is performed may worsen or attenuate grief.[4,5] Death notification should be prompt to avoid having the family learn of a death from an unofficial, uninformed source. Unless the distance is prohibitive, notification should be in person. However, when telephone notification is necessary and the next of kin is alone or elderly, one must consider arranging support in the person of a friend, relative, or member of Clergy Chaplain Corps (volunteers recruited from the local community or municipal law enforcement or fire districts).[3] The International Red Cross assists with notification of family members serving in the armed forces. Contact is made through local Red Cross duty officers.[3] In many jurisdictions, local law enforcement makes death notification on an "as time permits" basis, which could lead to delayed notification of next of kin.

The individual notifying next of kin should provide an accurate and informative account of events leading up to and including the death, as well as any rescue or emergency efforts. He or she should expect reactions including despair, disbelief, denial, helplessness, guilt, anger, and acceptance and must be prepared to provide or arrange for emotional support. Box 2-1 provides brief guidelines for death notification. When the family's initial needs have been met, any issues related to a medicolegal autopsy should be discussed.

Because a distraught family may have difficulty remembering complicated information or may have additional questions, it is useful to provide a telephone number and a written explanation of procedures related to the body and the family's responsibilities.[3]

## AUTOPSY AUTHORIZATION

The laws pertaining to authorization for autopsy vary among the states. Local jurisdictions may establish policies or procedures for compliance, and it behooves the practicing pathologist to know the relevant statutes in his or her region. In the United States, statutes pertaining to human remains stem from Old English common law.[6] Thus, at death, possession or custody of the remains passes to a surviving spouse or legal next of kin. The legal custodian of the deceased has the duty to arrange proper disposition of the remains. Although this individual does not have ordinary property rights to the corpse, he or she may authorize an autopsy; donate tissues, organs, or the entire body for therapeutic or educational purposes; or, following appropriate legal statutes, have the remains cremated or embalmed and moved to a final resting place. The next of kin may place restrictions on the extent and manner in which an autopsy is performed. Any unauthorized dissection may be considered mutilation and is tortious or even criminal.[7] Tissue and organ retention is regulated in the United States under state rather than federal law; other countries such as Australia and the United Kingdom have enacted specific legislation with respect to retention of organs.[8]

Svendsen and Hill[9] surveyed autopsy law in a number of industrialized countries. Although there has been a tendency for countries to enact laws requiring next-of-kin authorization for autopsy, there are still a number of nations (Italy, Austria, and many of the countries of Eastern Europe) that give the authority to perform postmortem examinations to the medical or legal community, or both. In some countries (Denmark,

**Box 2-1    Important guidelines for death notification by medical examiners**

1. Notification at the residence of a family member is ideal. If notification occurs in a public setting, seek a private area.
2. Introduce yourself. Speak slowly and calmly.
3. Briefly describe the events leading to death, but tell the family that their relative is dead early in the conversation. Fill in details after this or in response to questions.
4. Use the word "dead" or "died," not confusing terms such as "passed on," "expired," or "gone." Refer to the deceased by name, and do not refer to the "body."
5. Avoid medical jargon and graphic terms.
6. If you can honestly tell them that the deceased did not suffer, do so. This may help their grieving process.
7. If this is a medical examiner's case, advise the family. Explain issues related to release of the body.
8. Discuss how the deceased's belongings will be returned to the family. Explain whether clothing and other belongings may be retained as evidence.
9. After the family's immediate needs are met, discuss any issues related to autopsy. Provide them with written information detailing their responsibilities and a telephone number they may call with any questions.
10. Help them call other relatives or friends, and arrange for any necessary support.
11. Allow them the opportunity to view the deceased, but prepare them for his or her appearance. Accompany them initially, but permit them time alone with their relative.

France, Iceland, Norway), objections from members of the decedent's family may prevent autopsies authorized by the medical community.

Not all jurisdictions in the United States specify a strict order of preference for the person from whom permission for autopsy should be obtained. However, many establish a specific priority or rely on the code of common law or the order specified in the probate code (Box 2-2). Variations,

**Box 2-2    Example of order of priority for consenting for autopsy**

1. Consent from the deceased prior to death*
2. An "attorney-in-fact" appointed as a result of the decedent's execution of a durable power of attorney for health care and authorized to consent to an autopsy
3. Spouse (not legally separated or divorced unless he or she has custody of eldest child who is a minor)
4. Adult child age 18 or older
5. Adult grandchild
6. Parent
7. Adult sibling
8. Grandparents
9. Adult uncles and aunts
10. Other adult relative
11. Friend accepting responsibility for disposition of the body†
12. Public official acting within his or her legal authority‡

*Accepted in some jurisdictions. In some jurisdictions may be nullified by objection of next of kin after death of the deceased.
†Not accepted in all jurisdictions.
‡For unclaimed bodies.

restrictions, or exceptions may exist. For example, a legally separated spouse cannot authorize an autopsy unless he or she has custody of an eldest child who is a minor. Minor emancipated children have full right with respect to their deceased spouse or children and, even if not emancipated, may have custody and the right to authorize autopsy for their children.

States vary in how they legally define stillbirths.[10] In the state of California, stillborn fetuses of less than 20 weeks' gestation do not require authorization for autopsy but rather are handled according to the rules covering organs and tissues removed surgically. However, the law does not establish a standard for determining whether a fetus has advanced to 20 weeks' gestation. Unless there is an obvious discrepancy, we rely on the clinician's assessment of gestational age as determined by medical history, examination, and testing. In ambiguous cases, it is advisable to seek parental consent before the examination. A parent may object to postmortem examination of a stillborn fetus of less than 20 weeks' gestation. Our approach to such a situation would include counseling the family about the value of examination. However, the parents maintain ultimate jurisdiction, and their instructions would be honored. Stillbirths of 20 weeks' gestation and beyond require a standard death certificate and authorization for autopsy, and the usual laws related to disposition of the body pertain.

In cases in which the dead are unclaimed and without a will or other instructions concerning disposition of remains, designated public officials are usually given jurisdiction. If the next of kin are not identified following a thorough search of a length specified by law, the responsible official may authorize an autopsy at the request of the decedent's physician. An individual of legal age who is an acquaintance of the deceased and is assuming responsibility for burial may be allowed to authorize autopsy under the laws of some states.[11]

The enactment of anatomic gifts acts and related laws provides a living person with the authority to will his or her body or its parts for transplantation, anatomic instruction, or research. Included in the statutes of many states are provisions for allowing individuals to authorize specific disposition of their remains, including postmortem examination. However, in a majority of these states, an individual's directives regarding autopsy or interment, or both, may be nullified by the objection of the legal next of kin.[12] Before death, the decedent may indicate objection, and in some jurisdictions this is sufficient to prevent routine postmortem examination.[13] Some statutes include provisions stating that consent from only one of several persons with custody of the remains is sufficient. In such cases, the wishes of the relative accepting responsibility for burial are often given preference.[11] Because disposition of a dead body requires timely action, failure of an individual to assert these rights constitutes a waiver of the right.[14] When a party waives these rights, he or she cannot also allege wrongful autopsy. However, some statutes clearly indicate that objection by another person with equal right of custody may preclude an autopsy. Thus, it seems that a pathologist should seek local legal guidance before proceeding with a postmortem examination in which he or she is aware of conflicts among equal next of kin.

Acceptable methods of documenting consent also vary. Some jurisdictions require an original signed and witnessed written document, whereas others also accept consent in the form of a telegram or facsimile transmission. In certain circumstances, some states accept witnessed telephone authorization.[13] For example, Florida accepts witnessed telephone consent when written permission would cause undue delay in the examination. In Indiana, witnessed telephone consent may replace written authorization when the legal next of kin is outside the county where death occurred. In other states (e.g., California), telephone consents must be recorded on tape or other recording device. However, given the ease and ready availability of authorization obtained through facsimile when the consent cannot be obtained in person, our institution accepts authorization only on an approved institutional consent form.

Unlike the consent obtained by a physician before performing a medical procedure on a living patient, the consent for postmortem examination is not usually obtained by the individual responsible for the autopsy. Why is this so? First, it is the decedent's clinician who has the closest rapport with family members and is best positioned to approach the next of kin with the sensitivity that the situation requires. Second, the clinician is probably present at the time of death; she or he notifies the family of the event and helps the family begin dealing with the legal responsibilities that accompany the death of a relative. Finally, except in situations in which the family actively requests a postmortem examination, the clinician is usually most persuasive because he or she is interested in the answers to unresolved clinical questions. Although all these reasons explain the situation of consent through proxy, the pathologist is potentially vulnerable to an improperly obtained informed consent. For these reasons, institutions may elect to require stricter criteria for autopsy consent than required by state law.

Some institutions have sought to improve the autopsy consent process by establishing offices of decedent affairs composed of individuals trained to support the family and discuss issues surrounding death, including not only postmortem examinations but also organ and tissue donations and interment.[15,16] Rarely, pathologists have provided preautopsy consultations to the next of kin in order to discuss the autopsy procedure, removal and retention (or return) of organs, and other questions that family members might have about the examination.[17]

Regardless of whether physicians or other health care workers obtain the authorization, the autopsy consent form should include an adequate description of the procedure and provisions for retention of fluids, tissues, organs, and prosthetic and implantable devices as deemed necessary by the pathologist for diagnostic, scientific, educational, or therapeutic purposes. The autopsy consent should state and the individual consenting to autopsy should be informed of the eventual appropriate disposition of these materials by the pathologist or hospital. The College of American Pathologists has provided a sample autopsy consent form (Fig. 2-1).[18]

Hospitals serving large numbers of patients who do not speak English should provide written translations of the autopsy consent form. We find it helpful to provide these on the back side of our consent form. In an age of increasingly powerful methods of genetic analysis, autopsy consent forms may need modification to ensure that the pathologists, the guardians of human tissues removed for diagnostic purposes, maintain strict confidentiality not just for the patient but also for his or her descendants, who may have inherited similar genetic risks for disease.[19]

## IDENTIFICATION OF THE DECEASED

Before beginning a legally authorized autopsy, the pathologist must ensure that the body is correctly identified. Typically, dead bodies are identified by means of a tag on the great toe that lists the deceased's full name and perhaps other information. Deceased hospital patients may be identified by bracelets placed around their wrists or ankles that contain both their name and a unique hospital identification number. Before beginning the prosection, it is our practice to have both the pathologist and the assistant initial the bracelet after matching it to the appropriate consent form. This also serves to remind both individuals of any restrictions placed on the examination. A photocopy of the consent form should be kept in the pathology department. We keep this permanently as an attachment to the final report held in our departmental archives.

## MEDICAL EXAMINER/CORONER CASES

By statute, a medical examiner or coroner may perform or authorize others to perform a postmortem examination without liability if the procedure is performed in good faith, without negligence, and does not wantonly disfigure the body. Although all states sanction autopsy in suspected criminal cases, they vary on authorization for other circumstances or situations. Box 2-3 lists death circumstances that should be reported to the medical examiner or coroner.[20]

It is our hospital's policy that at the time of a patient's death, a member of the team of physicians who cared for the patient report the case to the medical examiner's office or certify that the medical examiner need not be consulted. Sometimes authorization for autopsy is obtained without appropriate notification of the legal authorities. In such situations, the pathologist assumes equal responsibility for properly notifying the medical examiner. This has particular legal consequence for the pathologist. A study by Start and colleagues[21] indicated that clinicians have considerable difficulty recognizing the full range of cases that require notification of a medical examiner or coroner. Therefore, at any stage of an autopsy—review of the medical history, prosection, or microscopic examination—at which a pathologist recognizes issues or findings that indicate that the case should be reported, it is the pathologist's obligation to notify the medical examiner or coroner. This applies equally in cases previously released by the authorities if new discoveries might place the case within their purview. Finally, notification should be made immediately at the time of discovery, not after completion of the dissection or autopsy report. As a

## Consent and Authorization for Autopsy

Addressograph
or Patient Name / Hospital Number
*The College recommends that each pathology group develop its own specific consent form tailored to applicable law, institutional policies, and local practice. This autopsy consent form is offered as a starting point. Prior to adopting a specific form, the pathology group should have the form reviewed by an attorney knowledgeable about applicable law and sensitive to local practice. The group should also have the form reviewed by appropriate individuals within any institution in which autopsies will be performed.*

Service

Attending physician

Date of death            Time of death

I, (printed name) _____, the (relationship to the deceased) _____ of the deceased, _____, being entitled by law to control the disposition of the remains, hereby request the pathologists of (name of hospital)_____ to perform an autopsy on the body of said deceased. I understand that any diagnostic information gained from the autopsy will become part of the deceased's medical record and will be subject to applicable disclosure laws.

Retention of Organs/Tissues:
I authorize the removal, examination, and retention of organs, tissues, prosthetic and implantable devices, and fluids as the pathologists deem proper for diagnostic, education, quality improvement and research purposes. I further agree to the eventual disposition of these materials as the pathologists or the hospital determine or as required by law. This consent does not extend to removal or use of any of these materials for transplantation or similar purposes. I understand that organs and tissues not needed for diagnostic, education, quality improvement, or research purposes will be sent to the funeral home or disposed of appropriately.
I understand that I may place limitations on both the extent of the autopsy and on the retention of organs, tissue, and devices. I understand that any limitations may compromise the diagnostic value of the autopsy and may limit the usefulness of the autopsy for education, quality improvement, or research purposes. I have been given the opportunity to ask any questions that I may have regarding the scope or purpose of the autopsy.

Limitations: ☐ None. Permission is granted for a complete autopsy, with removal, examination, and retention of material as the pathologists deem proper for the purposes set forth above, and for disposition of such material as the pathologists or the hospital determine.

☐ Permission is granted for an autopsy with the following limitations and conditions (specify):

_____

_____

Signature of person authorizing the autopsy          Date          Time

Signature of person obtaining permission          Printed name of person obtaining permission

Signature of witness          Printed name of witness

☐ Permission was obtained by telephone.
The above statements were read by the person obtaining permission to the person granting permission. The person granting permission was provided the opportunity to ask questions regarding the scope and purpose of the autopsy. The undersigned listened to the conversation with the permission of the parties and affirms that the person granting permission gave consent to the autopsy as indicated above.

Signature of Witness          Printed name of Witness

Date          Time

INSTRUCTIONS: To be valid, this document 1) must be dated, 2) must be signed by the person obtaining permission, AND 3) must be signed either by the person granting permission or the witness monitoring the phone call in which permission was given.

**Figure 2-1** Consent and authorization form for autopsy.
(From Collins KA, Hutchins GM: *Autopsy performance & reporting,* ed 2, Northfield, Ill, 2003, College of American Pathologists, p 41. Used with permssion.)

common courtesy, the responsible pathologist should inform the physician and family of the deceased of any changes in circumstances.

## PUBLIC HEALTH, PUBLIC RECORDS, AND PATIENTS' CONFIDENTIALITY

Health care institutions and employees must protect a patient's right to privacy and confidentiality unless excepted by law. Exceptions occur with communicable diseases because the responsible physician or health care worker has a legal or ethical obligation to notify public health authorities, warn endangered third parties such as sexual partners or other close contacts, advise health personnel involved with the care of the patient, and alert funeral directors or others who might have contact with infectious tissues or fluids. In the United States, state laws stipulate which diseases physicians must report to public health agencies. Thus, the pathologist has a legal obligation to report

**Box 2-3**     Brief guide to deaths reportable to the medical examiner

*Violent deaths by:*
Homicide
Suicide
Accident/injury (primarily or only contributory to death, whether immediate or at a remote time)

*Deaths associated with possible public health risks:*
Poisoning
Occupational disease
Contagious disease constituting a public health hazard

*Physician cannot sign the death certificate because:*
No physician in attendance
Not under physician's care for previous 20 days
Physician in attendance for less than 24 hours
Physician unable to state cause of death

*Other:*
Under such circumstances as to afford a reasonable ground to suspect that death was caused by the criminal act of another
Operating room deaths (even if expected)
Postanesthesia death where patient does not fully recover from anesthesia
Solitary deaths
Patient comatose for entire period of medical evaluation
Death of an unidentified person
Sudden death of an infant
Deaths of prisoners
Deaths of patients in hospitals for mentally or developmentally disabled
Deaths where questions of civil liability exist

Adapted from Stephens BG, Newman C: *Digest of rules and regulations, San Francisco Medical Examiner,* City and County of San Francisco, 2001.

cases when certain infectious diseases come to light at autopsy. Diseases that are deemed notifiable vary slightly from state to state. However, state laws are influenced by input from the Centers for Disease Control and Prevention (CDC), which makes annual recommendations for the list of nationally notifiable diseases (Box 2-4).[22] Most state public health agencies voluntarily report nationally notifiable diseases to the CDC.

Among patients, physicians, public health officials, and the courts, acquired immunodeficiency syndrome (AIDS) raises significant questions and concerns regarding rights to privacy and confidentiality of patients and patients' relatives and has been the subject of specific legislation.[23,24] These laws vary widely among states, and the pathologist performing autopsies should be familiar with the specific local statutes. In general, two documents are of concern for the autopsy pathologist: the autopsy report and the death certificate. Autopsy reports prepared in the setting of a hospital practice are legally protected as part of the confidential medical record. However, in some states, autopsies reported by a medical examiner become part of the public record. Likewise, the public may gain access to causes of death listed on death certificates.[25] For these reasons, the Council on Ethical and Judicial Affairs of the American Medical Association recommends that infection with human immunodeficiency virus or AIDS appear in the autopsy report only when it is relevant

**Box 2-4**     Infectious diseases designated as notifiable to the Centers for Disease Control and Prevention during 2008

Acquired immunodeficiency syndrome (AIDS)
Anthrax
Arboviral neuroinvasive and non-neuroinvasive diseases
   California serogroup virus disease
   Eastern equine encephalitis virus disease
   Powassan virus disease
   St. Louis encephalitis virus disease
   West Nile virus disease
   Western equine encephalitis virus disease
Botulism
   Botulism, foodborne
   Botulism, infant
   Botulism, other (wound and unspecified)
Brucellosis
Chancroid
*Chlamydia trachomatis* (genital infections)
Cholera
Coccidioidomycosis
Cryptosporidiosis
Cyclosporiasis
Diphtheria
Ehrlichiosis/anaplasmosis
   Ehrlichiosis chaffeensis
   Ehrlichia ewingii
   Anaplasma phagocytophilum
   Undetermined
Giardiasis
Gonorrhea
*Haemophilus influenzae,* invasive disease
Hansen disease (leprosy)
Hantavirus pulmonary syndrome
Hemolytic-uremic syndrome, post-diarrheal
Hepatitis, viral, acute
   Hepatitis A, acute
   Hepatitis B, acute
   Hepatitis B virus, perinatal infection
   Hepatitis C, acute
Hepatitis, viral, chronic
   Chronic hepatitis B
   Hepatitis C virus infection (past or present)
HIV infection
   HIV infection, adult ($\geq$13 years)
   HIV infection, pediatric (<13 years)
Influenza-associated pediatric mortality
Legionellosis
Listeriosis
Lyme disease
Malaria
Measles
Meningococcal disease
Mumps
Novel influenza A virus infections
Pertussis
Plague
Poliomyelitis, paralytic
Poliovirus infection, nonparalytic
Psittacosis
Q fever

*box continues*

**Box 2-4** *(continued)*

Rabies
    Rabies, animal
    Rabies, human
Rocky Mountain spotted fever
Rubella
    Rubella, congenital syndrome
Salmonellosis
Severe acute respiratory syndrome–associated Coronavirus
    (SARS-CoV) disease
Shiga toxin-producing *Escherichia coli* (STEC)
Shigellosis
Smallpox
Streptococcal disease, invasive, Group A
Streptococcal toxic-shock syndrome
*Streptococcus pneumoniae*, drug-resistant, invasive disease
*Streptococcus pneumoniae*, invasive disease non–drug resistant, in
    children <5 years of age
Syphilis
    Syphilis, primary
    Syphilis, secondary
    Syphilis, latent
    Syphilis, early latent
    Syphilis, late latent
    Syphilis, latent unknown duration
    Neurosyphilis
    Syphilis, late, non-neurological
Syphilitic stillbirth
    Syphilis, congenital
Tetanus
Toxic shock syndrome (other than streptococcal)
Trichinellosis (trichinosis)
Tuberculosis
Tularemia
Typhoid fever
Vancomycin-intermediate *Staphylococcus aureus* (VISA)
Vancomycin-resistant *Staphylococcus aureus* (VRSA)
Varicella (morbidity)
Varicella (deaths only)
Vibriosis
Yellow fever

From Centers for Disease Control and Prevention (CDC): *Nationally notifiable infectious diseases, United States 2008,* http://www.cdc.gov/ncphi/disss/nndss/phs/infdis2008.htm (accessed October 1, 2008).

to the patient's cause of death.[25] Others suggest that government offices adopt a two-part death certificate that includes one part for interment and immediate legal purposes and another for medical certification.[26,27] This would provide greater privacy to the family of the deceased.

## ORGAN AND TISSUE DONATION

In the past, American pathologists donated pituitary glands removed at autopsy to the National Pituitary Agency, which extracted human growth hormone for therapeutic use. Although recombinant DNA technology has rendered such harvesting of pituitary glands obsolete, other human organs and tissues removed after death are used in transplantation and reconstructive surgery. A procedure separate from the autopsy, tissue and organ donation does not usually involve the pathologist other than in a cooperative role. In cases in which there is consent for both autopsy and organ donation, procurement of viable organs must take place before any postmortem examination. An exception to this occurs in medicolegal cases in which the medical examiner or coroner must determine whether organ donation would interfere with a forensic examination. The usual regulations for reporting cases to the medical examiner or coroner are still in effect; in fact, organ harvesting from a "brain-dead" individual cannot occur legally without prior consent from the medical examiner or coroner.

The National Association of Medical Examiners[28] has published a position paper on medical examiner release of organs and tissues for transplantation stating that procurement of organs and/or tissues for transplantation can be accomplished in virtually all cases. However, supplemental imaging or laboratory tests may be needed to determine injury or disease in organs prior to harvesting. Davis and Wright[29] recommended that the surgeon harvesting donated organs be required to provide a detailed note of the surgical dissection for inclusion in the medical examiner's record. Findings such as injured organs or blood within body cavities must be documented accurately. Surgeons and others procuring organs must agree to testify at no expense to the taxpayers.[28]

A small number of states allow medical examiners to remove corneas if they are unaware of any objection from the next of kin; however, they may still be liable if a plaintiff can show that the pathologist removed the tissue on the basis of "intentional ignorance" of the family's wishes.[30]

## REQUEST FOR HUMAN TISSUE FOR RESEARCH

Requests for human tissue from biomedical scientists reach pathologists, particularly those affiliated with research institutions. Providing investigators with tissue for research is a noble endeavor. However, the pathologist must ensure that appropriate informed consent (usually but not necessarily part of the autopsy consent) has been received and that investigators' research protocols have been granted authorization from the appropriate regulatory committee (e.g., in the United States, institutional review boards). Approval safeguards the patient's and family's privacy and confidentiality. Some advocates of patients' privacy believe that patients or their next of kin must be informed on an ongoing basis regarding the use of archival tissue to prevent genetic testing that could have deleterious effects on a patient's well-being or ability to obtain employment or insurance.[31] Debates about genetic or tissue-based research with respect to informed consent and patients' confidentiality or anonymity are likely to continue before regulatory agencies attain guidelines that protect patients yet leave scientists sufficiently unencumbered.[32] Pathologists should consult with their institutions review boards if questions arise.

## RELIGIOUS AND CULTURAL ISSUES

A number of states have enacted specific statutes limiting or even preventing forensic examination in cases in which

---

**Box 2-5    Procedures that may alleviate the need to perform a complete autopsy in the presence of religious objections**

1. In-depth investigation of the scene, environment, terminal circumstances, and social and medical history of the deceased
2. Careful exclusion of criminal act suspicion
3. External examination
4. Radiographs or other imaging studies
5. Toxicology or other analysis performed on blood, urine, gastric samples, or cerebrospinal fluid obtained percutaneously
6. Endoscopic examination
7. In situ or minimal procedure examinations

---

religious beliefs are the basis for a family's objection to autopsy.[33] In such cases, the forensic pathologist should not proceed until it has been determined that there is a compelling legal reason for autopsy and the nature of the family's objection has been clarified.[30] Understanding of and sensitivity to cultural or religious beliefs with respect to the deceased may aid in reaching an acceptable solution to conflicts. Mittelman and colleagues[34] provided a number of alternatives to autopsy in such situations, and Box 2-5 lists these. A brief summary of attitudes of specific religions or cultural groups toward the autopsy follows.

## Judaism

Interpretations of Jewish religious law as it relates to autopsy vary from the traditional Orthodox to more liberal points of view. Discussion centers around two main issues: sanctity of the human body, which must remain inviolate even after death, and the prospect that a postmortem examination might save a life.[35,36] The Orthodox view stems primarily from the 18th-century attitude that the benefit of an autopsy must be readily apparent; that is, the knowledge obtained from an autopsy must help save another human life in immediate danger.[37] Its benefit cannot be exclusively experimental or theoretical. In the modern world, in which communication in effect establishes a single great parish and the autopsy has a greater influence on the treatment of disease, others express the opinion that postmortem examinations may honor the dead through service to humanity.[36,38] Consistent with this more liberal attitude, a formal agreement between the Chief Rabbinate of the State of Israel and the Hadassah Hospital and Medical School in Jerusalem permitted autopsies in cases required by law, when in the opinion of three physicians the cause of death cannot otherwise be established; in cases involving hereditary diseases when necessary to guide medical care for a family; or when an autopsy may save the lives of others with a similar disease.[39,40] However, more recently enacted laws have had the effect of limiting the number of autopsies performed in Israeli hospitals.[41]

## Christianity

The Roman Catholic faith has no ecclesiastical law forbidding autopsies, although it does hold that the dignity of the human body must be recognized even in death.[12] During the early years of Christianity, the general attitude of Catholic church leaders toward autopsy and dissection was unfavorable; however, this was based more on aesthetic or humanitarian grounds than on theological opinion.[42] The attitude of the church changed as the physicians of the late Middle Ages and Renaissance performed dissections. In 1410, Pietro D'Argelata performed an autopsy on Pope Alexander V after his sudden death. In the late fifteenth century, Pope Sixtus IV issued a decree allowing the medical students at Bologna and Padua to study human remains.[42] The acceptance of autopsies by the church was well established when, in 1556, the autopsy of Ignatius Loyola revealed stones in the kidneys, bladder, and gallbladder.[43]

Recognizing an autopsy as a legitimate method for extending medical knowledge and thereby improving the health of the living, the modern Protestant attitude holds that through an autopsy the deceased still serves God by contributing to the well-being of others.[12] However, in earlier times, the opinion of anatomic dissection in Protestant countries was often unfavorable.[44] For example, in England, from the Middle Ages until the end of the 19th century when the first English anatomic law was passed, the major source of human bodies for anatomic study was executed criminals. This tradition produced an association of postmortem dissection with crime and contributed to the public's negative attitude toward autopsies.[12] The limited numbers of bodies available for dissection in nations under Protestant rule led to the practice of grave robbing and clandestine anatomic studies, resulting in additional adverse public reaction to dissection.[38]

The Eastern Orthodox churches (Greek Orthodox Church, Russian Orthodox Church, and others) do not forbid autopsy in the belief that it may lead to knowledge for physicians that could help them treat others in the future.[45] The Church of Christ, Scientist (Christian Scientist) forbids autopsy except in cases of sudden death.[46] Jehovah's Witnesses forbid autopsy except under specific circumstances.[33]

## Native Americans

Although many Native Americans follow Christian practices, some maintain traditional tenets. Death rituals and burial practices vary among tribes. Traditionally, Native Americans believe in the integrity of the body and consider postmortem examinations a violation of that integrity.[46]

## Islam

There has been and continues to be debate among Islamic scholars regarding topics such as postmortem examination and organ transplantation.[47] Although the issues surrounding organ donation and transplantation are not settled, both occur in some Muslim sects.[48,49] However, unless required by law, postmortem examinations are not sanctioned.[50] Similarly, the Islamic beliefs prohibit dissection for medical teaching or research. Muslim bodies are not embalmed or cremated, and the religion requires that the body be buried as soon as possible after death. Following death, the head is turned toward Mecca or to the right, the arms and legs are straightened, and the mouth and eyes are closed.[50]

Preparation of the body includes ritual washing and draping with a simple white cloth by family or friends of the same sex.

### Eastern Religions

Autopsy rates in Eastern countries are generally low, but one cannot attribute this to religious beliefs. Hinduism, Buddhism, Shintoism, Taoism, Shamanism, and Confucianism do not prohibit autopsy or other postmortem procedures such as organ donation.[46] Hindus do not approve of autopsies, but those required by law are accepted.[51] The Buddhist faith allows autopsies after the soul has made its transition (3 days after death or sooner if determined by a religious teacher).[45]

## MORTICIAN AND FUNERAL ISSUES

The funeral director is often faced with responsibilities for which time may be critical. Thus, he or she is most concerned with issues (such as autopsies) that delay release of the body from the hospital and problems related to the state of the body following death that may make it more difficult to prepare the body for viewing or burial or both. Hence, it is important that both pathologist and hospital staff expedite autopsies and other decedent affairs with concern for subsequent funeral arrangements.

Following death and unless prohibited by religious faith, bodies should be placed in the supine position with the head straight and slightly elevated. The arms may be folded over the abdomen. If restraints are used, they should be soft and tied only lightly and above the elbow to ensure that the skin of the hands or arms does not become deformed. Restraints of any kind should not be used on decedents under the jurisdiction of the medical examiner or coroner to avoid causing any misleading external markings. Intravenous and other medical tubing should generally not be removed; however, it can be capped or clamped and then clipped close to the clamp. Excess tubing may be coiled, covered with gauze and taped (paper tape only) to the skin. Remains are covered with a clean white sheet and stored in zippered plastic body pouches that are resistant to leakage. A plastic bag loosely secured over the head reduces the possibility of problems from purges of respiratory and gastric contents. Absorbable pads should be placed wherever there is persistent drainage. An identification tag should be placed on the body and on the outside of the bag.

Properly protecting individuals handling decedents is a legal requirement. Therefore, alert the funeral director to any biohazard, such as radioactivity or infection, by noting it on an exterior label. To delay postmortem staining and lividity, the body should be removed to a refrigerated area as soon as reasonably possible. Before performing dissections that might interfere with embalming, the pathologist should alert the mortuary. In some instances, embalming prior to autopsy may be appropriate.

## OBLIGATIONS OF THE AUTOPSY PATHOLOGIST

The pathologist incurs certain moral responsibilities if the autopsy is an important element in (1) the welfare of patients, families, and society; (2) quality control and improvement of care provided by health care organizations and providers; and (3) education of tomorrow's physicians.[52] The pathologist must always perform autopsies with proper respect for the dead, the feelings of relatives, and the patient's physicians. He or she should evaluate the quality of the autopsy consent and ensure that it is valid. Permission obtained through deception or coercion is morally invalid. If the pathologist suspects such, he or she must ensure that the next of kin understands and consents knowingly and willingly before the autopsy is begun. Next, the pathologist has a professional obligation to perform a competent postmortem examination and report the autopsy results accurately and promptly.

The pathologist must communicate and consult with clinicians to avoid misinterpretations of clinical information and, ultimately, diagnostic errors.[53,54] Except under unusual circumstances that might prevent the pathologist from performing a competent examination, the pathologist has an obligation not only to allow the clinicians responsible for the patient's care the opportunity to observe the autopsy but also to encourage their attendance at the procedure. Therefore, whenever possible and with consideration of the families' need for timely funeral arrangements, the pathologist should accommodate the schedules of the clinicians. If the clinician's obligations to other patients prevent his or her attendance at an autopsy, the pathologist should communicate the findings by conversation, as well as by the usual report. The pathologist should be readily available to present autopsy findings at hospital conferences or at quality improvement meetings. In complicated cases, the pathologist also has an obligation to seek consultation from his or her pathology colleagues or, when necessary, from expert consultants.[55]

In the United States, the laws covering confidential postmortem medical information vary. Autopsy reports of medical examiners' and coroners' offices are part of the public record in a number of states. In the hospital setting, the pathologist must protect the patient's confidentiality unless withholding information results in probable harm to others.[56] This includes protecting sensitive information made available electronically on the Internet.[57]

Although the autopsy has inherent teaching value for other health care professionals and students, these individuals are allowed in the autopsy suite only at the discretion of the pathologist. The pathologist must provide protective clothing and so on to any observers because she or he assumes legal liability for any injury or exposure. Generally, the pathologist has the right to exclude physicians hired by the next of kin to view the autopsy except in cases of workers' compensation where state statutes allow such representation.[12] There is no place at an autopsy for members of the lay public or curiosity seekers.

As already discussed, the pathologist has an obligation to report the autopsy findings to the physician or physicians of the deceased. The primary obligation to inform the relatives of the patient lies with the clinician. However, in the event that the legal next of kin requests (in writing) the autopsy report, it is our practice to send it along with a letter encouraging the family to approach the patient's physician for clarification or counseling. At the time of such a request, we routinely notify clinicians of the request and our action so that they may offer their service to the family in answering questions or in discussing any unresolved issues. Because even in the best of possible worlds this may not occur, the cover letter from our office also offers the assistance of the director of the autopsy service regarding any questions or concerns about the autopsy report. In our experience, calls from family members occur in four well-defined settings: (1) when the family has not identified the primary physician among the many physicians in a complex medical center; (2) when the physician with the closest relationship to the family and the one they may wish to reach is a member of the house staff and difficult to reach because he or she may have rotated to a different hospital or completed his or her training; (3) when the family has no established relationship with their relative's physician; or (4) when the family had reservations about the patient's medical care.

When choosing the specialty of pathology, a physician must accept the obligation to clinicians, families, and society to perform autopsies despite potential dangers. However, pathologists have the right to demand adequate protection from biologic and physical hazards for themselves and their assistants so that the examination can be performed safely and efficiently. Chapter 3 contains a discussion of safe autopsy practice.

## REFERENCES

1. Bohrod MG: Uses of the autopsy, *JAMA* 193:154-156, 1965.
2. Swisher LA, Nieman LZ, Nilsen DJ, Spivey WH: Death notification in the emergency department: A survey of residents and attending physicians, *Ann Emerg Med* 22:1319-1323, 1993.
3. Haglund WD, Reay DT, Fligner C: Death notification, *Am J Forensic Med Pathol* 11:342-347, 1990.
4. Robinson MA: Informing the family of sudden death, *Am Fam Pract* 23:115-118, 1981.
5. Schmidt TA, Norton RL, Tolle SW: Sudden death in the ED: Educating residents to compassionately inform families, *J Emerg Med* 10:643-647, 1992.
6. Lind CJ Jr: Caveat prosecutor. The pathologist and autopsy law, *Am J Clin Pathol* 69(Suppl 2):263-265, 1978.
7. Waltz JR: Legal liability for unauthorized autopsies and related procedures, *J Forensic Sci* 16:1-14, 1971.
8. Klaiman MH: Whose brain is it anyway? The comparative law of post-mortem retention, *J Legal Med* 26:475-490, 2005.
9. Svendsen E, Hill RB: Autopsy legislation and practice in various countries, *Arch Pathol Lab Med* 111:846-850, 1987.
10. Schultz OT: The law of the dead human body, *Arch Pathol* 9:1220-1221, 1930.
11. Chayet NL: Consent for autopsy, *N Engl J Med* 274:268-269, 1966.
12. American Hospital Association: *Postmortem procedures*, Chicago, 1970, American Hospital Association.
13. Schmidt S: Consent for autopsies, *JAMA* 250:1161-1164, 1983.
14. Stump A, Emswiller B: The law pertaining to autopsies, *J Indiana State Med Assoc* 49:761-765, 1956.
15. Haque AK, Cowan WT, Smith JH: The Decedent Affairs Office: A unique centralized service, *JAMA* 266:1397-1399, 1991.
16. Haque AK, Patterson RC, Grafe MR: High autopsy rates at a university medical center. What has gone right? *Arch Pathol Lab Med* 120:727-732, 1996.
17. McDermott MB: Obtaining consent for autopsy, *Br Med J* 327:804-806, 2003.
18. Collins KA, Hutchins GM: Autopsy performance & reporting, Northfield, Ill, 2003, College of American Pathologists, p 41.
19. Clayton EW, Steinberg KK, Khoury M, et al: Informed consent for genetic research on stored tissue samples, *JAMA* 274:1786-1792, 1995.
20. Stephens BG, Newman C: *Digest of rules and regulations, San Francisco Medical Examiner*, City and County of San Francisco, 2001.
21. Start RD, Delargy-Aziz Y, Dorries CP, et al: Clinicians and the coronial system: Ability of clinicians to recognise reportable deaths, *Br Med J* 306:1038-1041, 1993.
22. Centers for Disease Control and Prevention (CDC): *Nationally notifiable infectious diseases, United States 2008*, http://www.cdc.gov/ncphi/disss/nndss/phs/infdis2008.htm (accessed October 1, 2008).
23. Mills M, Wofsy CB, Mills J: The acquired immunodeficiency syndrome. Infection control and public health law, *N Engl J Med* 314:931-936, 1986.
24. Lentz SL: Confidentiality and informed consent and the acquired immunodeficiency syndrome epidemic, *Arch Pathol Lab Med* 114:304-308, 1990.
25. Council on Ethical and Judicial Affairs, American Medical Association: Confidentiality of human immunodeficiency virus status on autopsy reports, *Arch Pathol Lab Med* 116:1120-1123, 1992.
26. Carter JR: The problematic death certificate, *N Engl J Med* 313:1285-1286, 1985.
27. King MB: AIDS on the death certificate: The final stigma, *Br Med J* 298:734-736, 1989.
28. Pinckard JK, Wetli CV, Graham MA: National Association of Medical Examiners position paper on the medical examiner release of organs and tissues for transplantation, *Am J Forensic Pathol* 28:202-207, 2007.
29. Davis JH, Wright RK: Influence of the medical examiner on cadaver organ procurement, *J Forensic Sci* 22:824-826, 1977.
30. Bierig JR: A potpourri of legal issues relating to the autopsy, *Arch Pathol Lab Med* 120:759-762, 1996.
31. Marshall E: Policy on DNA research troubles tissue bankers, *Science* 271:440, 1996.
32. Stephenson J: Pathologists enter debate on consent for genetic research on stored tissue, *JAMA* 275:503-504, 1996.
33. Boglioli LR, Taff ML: Religious objection to autopsy. An ethical dilemma for medical examiners, *Am J Forensic Med Pathol* 11:1-8, 1990.
34. Mittelman RE, Davis JH, Kasztl W, Graves WM Jr: Practical approach to investigative ethics and religious objections to the autopsy, *J Forensic Sci* 37:824-829, 1991.
35. Spivak CD: Post mortem examinations among the Jews. An historical sketch and a plea to Jewish physicians, *N Y Med J* 99:1185-1189, 1914.
36. Plotz M: The Jewish attitude toward autopsies, *Mod Hosp* 45:67-68, 1935.
37. Geller SA: Autopsy, *Mt Sinai J Med* 51:77, 1984.
38. Geller SA: Religious attitudes and the autopsy, *Arch Pathol Lab Med* 108:494-496, 1984.
39. Kottler A: The Jewish attitude on autopsy, *N Y State J Med* 57:1649-1650, 1957.
40. Dorff EN: End-of-life: Jewish perspectives, *Lancet* 366:862-865, 2005.
41. Meyers N: Medicine confronts Jewish law, *Nature* 318:97, 1985.
42. King LS, Meehan MC: A history of the autopsy, *Am J Pathol* 73:514-544, 1973.

43. Ullman WH: Obduziert wurder Ignatius von Loyola, *Med Welt* 35:1758-1763, 1963.

44. Jarcho S: Problems of the autopsy in 1670 A.D, *Bull N Y Acad Med* 47:792-796, 1971.

45. Gordijn S, Erwich JJHM, Khong TY: The perinatal autopsy: Pertinent issues in multicultural Western Europe, *Eur J Obstet Gynecol Reprod Biol* 132:3-7, 2007.

46. McQuay JE: Cross-cultural customs and beliefs related to health crises, death, and organ donation/transplantation: A guide to assist health care professionals understand different responses and provide cross-cultural assistance, *Crit Care Nurs Clin North Am* 7:581-594, 1995.

47. Rispler-Chaim V: The ethics of postmortem examinations in contemporary Islam, *J Med Ethics* 19:164-168, 1993.

48. Rasheed HZA: Organ donation and transplantation—a Muslim viewpoint, *Transplant Proc* 24:2116-2117, 1992.

49. Sellami MM: Islamic position on organ donation and transplantation, *Transplant Proc* 25:2307-2309, 1993.

50. Gatrad AR: Muslim customs surrounding death, bereavement, postmortem examinations, and organ transplants, *Br Med J* 309:521-523, 1994.

51. Black J: Broaden your mind about death and bereavement in certain ethnic groups in Britain, *Br Med J* 295:536-539, 1987.

52. Pellegrino ED: The autopsy. Some ethical reflections on the obligations of pathologists, hospitals, families, and society, *Arch Pathol Lab Med* 120:739-742, 1996.

53. Legg MA: What role for the diagnostic pathologist? *N Engl J Med* 305:950-951, 1981.

54. Stempsey WE: The virtuous pathologist. An ethical basis for laboratory medicine, *Am J Clin Pathol* 91:730-738, 1989.

55. Baron DN: Ethical issues and clinical pathology, *Am J Clin Pathol* 46:385-387, 1993.

56. Maixner AH, Morin K: Confidentiality of health information postmortem, *Arch Pathol Lab Med* 125:1189-1192, 2001.

57. Stewart P: Legal trends in E-health care, *Group Pract J* 51:11-22, 2002.

# 3

# Autopsy Biosafety

*"The danger to the operator can be eliminated in the most simple and complete manner without in the least degree impairing the efficacy of the examination."*

J. Jackson Clarke[1]

During the course of work, the autopsy pathologist and staff members encounter a number of potential biohazards. By adhering to strict safety precautions, practicing proper autopsy technique, and using proper instruments and equipment, the pathologist can limit the risk of injury to individuals working at the autopsy table. This chapter provides an overview of important autopsy biosafety recommendations for usual hospital-based practice. Many points cannot be discussed in sufficient detail, however. Pathologists must work with their local infection control and occupational health and safety departments to implement a complete biosafety plan that includes ongoing review of all safety concerns and a continuing program of safety education.

In the current age of global travel and bioterrorism threats, there is heightened awareness of the possibility of epidemics of severe disease caused by highly transmissible agents. The experience with severe acute respiratory syndrome (SARS) due to coronavirus in which a high percentage of health care workers were infected offered many lessons in biosafety.[2] The precautions required for such specialized lethal diseases are beyond the scope of this chapter. Suspected cases of these conditions should be referred to the Centers for Disease Control and Prevention (CDC) as soon as possible and hopefully before postmortem examination. Local medical examiners or offices and public health laboratories may provide guidance.[3] The CDC, in association with other federal, state, and local agencies, has designated regional laboratories (Laboratory Response Network) to aid in the diagnosis and containment of lethal transmissible conditions.[4,5]

## AUTOPSY INFECTION CONTROL PRECAUTIONS

### General Autopsy Biosafety Practices

Historically, most physicians and other healthcare workers have accepted the moral responsibility of caring for patients with contagious disease.[5] The occupational exposure, however, places them at risk for developing communicable diseases. Infective agents such as viruses, bacteria, fungi, parasites, and prions are capable of causing disease in healthcare workers exposed to sufficient inocula, especially when usual body defensive barriers are either disrupted or bypassed. In general, infective material is introduced through accidental puncture wounds from needles or other sharps, splashes into mucous membranes, inhalation, or the passage of the infective agent through preexistent wounds. To minimize the risk of infection, adequate barriers should be in place.

It is the policy of our department to perform as complete a postmortem examination, including brain and spinal cord, as the signed autopsy permit allows. Because it is difficult to ascertain which cases harbor infective agents, it is prudent to consider *all* autopsies as a potential infective source. The cornerstone of any autopsy biosafety program, therefore, is the practice of standard (universal) infection control precautions as established by the U.S. Centers for Disease Control and Prevention, the National Institutes of Health,[6] or the World Health Organization.[7] This approach includes proper attire, barrier protection, care while using sharp instruments, tissue fixation, decontamination of equipment and work surfaces, and hand washing (Box 3-1). It also demands containment and treatment, proper cleaning of spills, immediate treatment of any injuries, and notification of the proper authorities (e.g., Infection Control, Environmental Health and Safety).

### General Rules

All autopsies or fresh autopsy tissues must be handled as if they contain an infective agent (standard precautions). The entire autopsy area and its contents are designated a biohazard area and posted with appropriate warning signs. The ideal autopsy suite is well ventilated with a negative airflow exhaust system and contains a separate low-traffic isolation room. Whenever possible, postmortem examinations are carried out during normal working hours by adequate, well-trained staff. It is helpful to have a second autopsy assistant who remains "clean" to record weights, measurements, and other observations, as well as to circulate for any needed supplies. If multiple autopsies are to be performed sequentially, those with the greatest infective risk should be done first, before the staff becomes fatigued. All procedures are carried out in a way that reduces the risk of splashes, spills, droplets, or aerosols. All contaminated equipment, instruments, containers, and so forth should be confined to designated areas (autopsy table, instrument table, dissection area, sink). Paperwork leaving the autopsy suite must not be contaminated.

### Attire

For all autopsies, personal protective equipment (PPE) includes scrub suits, gowns, waterproof sleeves, plastic disposable aprons, caps, N95 particulate masks, eye protection (goggles or face shields), shoe covers or footwear restricted to contaminated areas, and double sets of gloves. Cut-resistant and puncture-resistant hand protection (plastic or steel gloves) is also available and certainly recommended for high-risk procedures. A retrospective study has demonstrated their effectiveness in reducing injuries.[8]

### Use of Sharp Instruments

One should exercise extraordinary care to minimize the risk of injury from sharp instruments and needles. Whenever possible, the use of needles should be avoided. Needlestick injuries occurring during routine autopsy procedures are entirely preventable; blunt needles and bulb syringes should be used to aspirate fluids in most situations. Because many needlestick accidents occur during disposal of needles, needles should *never* be recapped after use. Needles and other sharps should be disposed of directly into the approved receptacle; they should not be left lying around the work area.

Accidental self-inflicted cuts, particularly to the distal thumb and index and middle fingers, are the most frequent injuries sustained by pathologists.[9] This type of injury usually occurs during dissection or trimming of tissues for microscopy. The frequency of hand injuries sustained while performing autopsy procedures can be reduced by several simple practices (Box 3-2). A pair of scissors can adequately substitute for a scalpel during most autopsy procedures, including evisceration. The use of blunt-tipped, rather than pointed, scissors for almost all autopsy tissue dissection is advisable. When dissecting with a sharp implement in one hand, one should apply countertraction on tissues by using a long-handled tissue forceps held in the opposite hand; do *not* hold tissues with the fingers of the noncutting hand. For high-risk cases or dissections, steel-link gloves or some other scalpel-resistant material can be used. Plastic or Kevlar cut-

resistant gloves provide protection while still allowing relative dexterity, and we encourage their use whenever possible.

Rib cutters or shears are used to cut the costal cartilage near the costochondral junction during removal of the sternum. Surgical towels should be placed over the cut edges of the ribs to protect against a scrape injury. When making slices of large organs with a long knife, the prosector should use a thick (3-inch) sponge to stabilize the organ with the noncutting hand. When suturing the body wall at the end of the autopsy, hold skin flaps with a large toothed forceps or toothed clamp rather than with a hand.

### Limiting Aerosols

Aerosolization of bone dust during the removal of the calvaria or vertebral bodies can be reduced with a plastic cover or a vacuum bone dust collector, or both, on the saw. A number of systems utilizing high-efficiency particulate air (HEPA) filtering systems are commercially available. Bone surfaces should be moistened before sawing to cut down the dispersal of bone dust. To limit aerosols, screw cap containers are preferable to snap-top, rubber-stoppered, or cork-stoppered containers. When opening capped containers, cover the opening with a plastic bag to contain aerosols and splashes. Do not overfill a blood specimen vacuum tube by applying pressure through a syringe. To avoid spattering, do *not* sear tissue to sterilize it before obtaining a culture. Rather, the organ surface should be swabbed centrifugally with an iodine solution and incised centrally before a sample is removed.

### Photography

Photography of fresh specimens requires the same precautions employed for doing the autopsy, and the camera must be kept clean. In situ photographs obviate the additional risk of moving fresh tissue around the room. Photography of fixed specimens is cleaner and, in this respect, preferable, especially when an infective agent is known to be present. Whether the specimen is fresh or fixed, a pan is used for cleanliness during transport of the organ to the photographic stand. The camera should be handled with clean gloves or by a second person who stays clean. After photographs have been taken, the photostand should be cleaned with disinfectant. Cameras, lenses, and other photographic equipment may be disinfected with a variety of germicidal substances without compromising their functionality.[10] A hands-free camera system would also reduce contamination risk.

### Tissue Fixation

Adequate fixation in 10% formalin (containing 3.7% formaldehyde) requires an amount that is at least 10 times the tissue volume; this kills or inactivates all important infective agents except prions and mycobacteria. Embalming fluid containing glutaraldehyde is similarly effective. Mycobacteria remain viable in tissues for days, and these organisms are even difficult to kill with standard formalin fixatives or embalming fluids.[11-13] Mycobacterium are killed in a fixative of 10% formalin in 50% ethyl alcohol.[14] Adequate time must be allowed for fixatives to penetrate tissues before trimming blocks for histology. Fixation of tissue suspected of containing prions is discussed later in this chapter.

### Decontamination of Equipment, Work Surfaces, and Laundry

For decontamination, one should use a germicidal solution appropriate for any known or suspected agents. For routine decontamination, all instruments and autopsy devices should be immersed in an enzymatic cleaner or detergent solution for at least 10 minutes, then rinsed with water and decontaminated with disinfectant such as 5.25% sodium hypochlorite (1:10 solution of household bleach in water) for another 10 minutes. Instruments used for infective cases are immersed in an enzymatic cleaner or detergent, then rinsed and soaked in 2% aqueous glutaraldehyde or 1:10 solution of bleach for at least 10 minutes. Glutaraldehye is advantageous because, unlike bleach, it doesn't damage aluminum and steel. One should rinse work surfaces with hot water followed by a 1:10 solution of bleach. Several commercial products containing bleach are suitable. Splashing should be avoided. Floors in the autopsy work area should be cleaned with a detergent solution, decontaminated, and rinsed with water. If available, ultraviolet light provides a secondary source for decontaminating room surfaces and air. All laundry should be treated as contaminated and disinfected in a routine fashion. Any wet clothing, towels, or other reusable laundry should be placed into leakproof biohazard bags before transport.

### Remains

After autopsy, one should wash the body with a detergent solution followed by an antiseptic such as a 1:10 solution of household bleach. The body should be rinsed with water and placed in a disposable leakproof plastic body bag. By law, in many states, all bodies with known infective diseases must be labeled as such for the mortician and others who may come in contact with the remains. Usually this is indicated on the death certificate as well. Absence of this warning, however, should *not* be taken to mean there is no risk; all bodies should be handled with caution. We find it helpful to inspect bodies in storage on a daily basis to assess whether there has been any undue leakage of fluid into the body bag. Obviously, fluid accumulations should be carefully removed by aspiration or blotting. If necessary, place a warning on the outside of the body bag, alerting others to the possibility of leaking fluids.

### Storage and Transportation of Tissue and Waste

Tissue to be stored should be placed in a nonbreakable, watertight plastic container. Before transporting tissue outside the autopsy suite, the container should be placed in a plastic bag and sealed adequately. Waste for disposal should be double-bagged in specially designated biohazard waste bags, secured, and stored in metal or plastic canisters until removal.

### Handling of Spills

Spills should be cleaned up with absorbent, disposable paper towels. The contaminated area should be cleaned with detergent, then decontaminated using a 1:10 dilution of bleach. After the area has been decontaminated, wipe it dry.

### Hand Washing

After removing gloves, the pathologist should wash his or her hands with soap and water. In fact, hands should be washed immediately and thoroughly any time they become contaminated.

### Employee Health

Employees are strongly urged to be vaccinated against hepatitis B.[15] Each employee is encouraged to maintain tetanus and diphtheria immunity. Other immunizations (e.g., against rubella, measles, and polio) are also advisable. We have initiated preexposure rabies prophylaxis before performing an autopsy on a decedent infected with rabies.[16] However, if exposure as defined by the Centers for Disease Control and Prevention (i.e., potential introduction of virus through skin puncture or contact with mucous membranes) occurs, postexposure prophylaxis that includes vaccination and administration of rabies immune globulin should be undertaken. Smallpox vaccinations for healthcare workers is advisable but controversial.[15] All employees should have yearly purified protein derivative (PPD) skin tests.

Cuts and puncture wounds should be washed and irrigated *immediately* with soap and water. If conjunctival splashes occur, the eyes should be washed immediately at the nearest eye wash station in the autopsy suite. Injured employees should go to the emergency department or employee health service; the infection control nurse or appropriate employee health official can be notified from there. Most hospitals have hotlines manned by personnel trained in counseling, treatment, and follow-up for healthcare workers who suffer on-the-job injuries. The employee should always protect his or her rights by completing an incident report. Persons with uncovered wounds or dermatitis should not assist in autopsy procedures unless the injured skin can be completely covered with a waterproof dressing or other acceptable barrier.

## Isolation Procedures

Although all autopsies are performed in a manner that reduces the risk of contamination, autopsies of bodies that

---

**Box 3-3   Some infections for which postmortem examinations should be performed in a separate or "isolation" room**

Anthrax
Hantavirus
Hepatitis
Human immunodeficiency virus/acquired immunodeficiency
   syndrome
Influenza
Leprosy
Meningococcal meningitis
Multidrug-resistant bacteria (methicillin-resistant *Staphylococcus*,
   vancomycin-resistant *Enterococcus*)
Plague
Prion diseases
Rabies
Rickettsial diseases (Rocky Mountain spotted fever)
Systemic infections of unknown etiology
Tuberculosis
Typhoid fever

---

harbor a known pathogenic microorganism are best performed in a separate specially designed room to isolate and contain any infective material (Box 3-3). While performing these autopsies, personnel are limited to only those necessary—the pathologist, autopsy assistant, and possibly a circulating assistant—to accomplish the task. As usual, standard precautions are strictly enforced. Special safety and decontamination procedures are instituted as required. With proper precautions, overhead ultraviolet lights may be used for secondary decontamination. If an isolation room is nonexistent and there is more than one autopsy table in the room, the table with the least traffic should be used for the infective case. In cases in which facilities are inadequate, it is advisable to identify alternative, better-designed, safer sites for postmortem examinations. Health and safety requirements may exceed the capabilities of even the best hospital morgues in suspected cases of infection with highly contagious organisms such as arboviruses, arenaviruses, or filoviruses. In such situations, guidance should be sought from the appropriate public health agency.

## Practices to Reduce Transmission by Infective Aerosols

Even in the current age, those performing and attending autopsies are at increased risk for tuberculous infection via aerosols produced during the procedure on a patient with tuberculosis.[17-22] Other infections including rabies, plague, legionellosis, meningococcemia, rickettsioses, coccidiomycosis, and anthrax may also be acquired by aerosols such as those generated during an autopsy.[23] Thus, it is clear that the utmost care must be taken to provide adequate protection against infective aerosols. For protection against diseases transmissible by aerosols, such as tuberculosis, N95 particulate masks (masks able to filter 1-μm particles in the unloaded state with a filter efficiency of 95%, given flow rates up to 50 liters/minute) or containment hoods or suits equipped with powered, air-purifying respirators with high-efficiency particulate air (HEPA) filters are used. Collecting body cavity fluids with

a ladle or bulb syringe generates less aerosol than a hose aspirator connected to a sink faucet. Placing plastic bags over the head of the decedent during removal of the calvarium with a Stryker saw or saws equipped with HEPA filters within the vacuum system can also reduce the amount of aerosolization. Towfighi and colleagues designed a relatively simple tentlike device for reducing aerosal dispersion during brain removal.[24]

## Practices Specific to Autopsies if a Prion Disorder Is Suspected

The infective agent that transmits Creutzfeldt-Jakob disease (CJD) and related prion disorders has been termed a *prion* because it does not have the morphologic and chemical composition of a virus or other conventional infective agent. Rather, all the evidence indicates that the sole functional component of the prion is an abnormal protease-resistant isoform of a normal brain protein. The normal isoform is designated $PrP^C$ and the pathogenic isoform $PrP^{CJD}$ in humans and $PrP^{Sc}$ in animals. Some investigators refer to the pathogenic form as $PrP^{res}$ because of resistance to protease digestion.

Consistent with these characteristics, prions are resistant to inactivation by procedures that denature nucleic acids, such as ultraviolet radiation, but are inactivated by procedures that denature or hydrolyze proteins, such as exposure to some detergents or to NaOH. Because it is a protein, $PrP^{CJD}$ is not easily aerosolized by routine procedures used in the morgue or in the histology laboratory. The procedures outlined here are more than adequate to prevent aerosolization of prions. Although CJD can be transmitted to laboratory animals by intracerebral inoculation of formalin-fixed tissues, it should be noted that aldehyde fixatives cross-link proteins in a tissue block, and therefore prions are not readily transmissible from the tissue block.

The incidence of CJD among medical personnel, histotechnologists, and morgue attendants is the same as that in the general population (1 per million), and the disease in these medical personnel resembles sporadic CJD and not CJD caused by infection, such as occurred with contaminated lots of human growth hormone.[25] In contrast, many medical personnel have contracted serious illness due to tuberculosis or hepatitis acquired directly or indirectly from patients. Thus, although CJD and related disorders are transmissible, they are not contagious.

When working with prion-infected or contaminated material, caution must be taken to avoid breach of the skin. The prosector should wear cut-resistant gloves. If accidental contamination of skin occurs, swab the area with 1 N sodium hydroxide for 5 minutes and then irrigate with copious amounts of water. Boxes 3-4 through 3-6 list specific modifications to routine safety procedures for cases of suspected spongiform encephalopathies.

## EXPOSURE TO OTHER BIOHAZARDS AT AUTOPSY

### Formaldehyde

Formaldehyde is a highly toxic chemical, and exposure to formaldehyde or its vapors may cause a variety of symptoms or diseases. These include contact dermatitis; headache; eye,

**Box 3-4** Autopsies of patients with suspected prion disease (human transmissible spongiform encephalopathies)—modifications of standard precautions

1. Attendance is limited to three staff members, including at least one experienced pathologist. One of the staff avoids direct contact with the deceased but assists with handling of instruments and specimen containers.
2. Standard autopsy attire is mandatory. However, a disposable, waterproof gown is worn in place of a cloth gown. Cut-resistant gloves are worn underneath two pairs of surgical gloves, or chain mail gloves are worn between two pairs of surgical gloves.
3. Containment hoods or suits equipped with powered, air-purifying respirator with high-efficiency particulate air (HEPA) filters are worn by all staff.
4. Reduce contamination of the autopsy suite.
   a. Cover the autopsy table with an absorbent sheet that has a waterproof backing. Drape instrument trays, working surfaces, and weighing pans with plastic or disposable plastic underpads. Use clear 2-inch plastic tape to connect seams and to secure edges against the table.
   b. Because prion infectivity is retained after drying and the dried material is harder to clean from surfaces, reusable instruments should be kept wet between time of use and disinfection.
   c. Use disposable equipment (headrest, cutting board, scalpels, forceps, scissors, brain knife, plastic formalin containers) to the greatest extent possible.
   d. Dedicate a set of instruments for autopsies involving possible transmissible spongiform encephalopathies, to include Stryker saw, blade and wrench, skull breaker and hammer, 5-inch forceps, 5-inch scissors, and rib cutter.
   e. Reduce bone dust aerosol during brain removal. Place a plastic bag over the head, and tie it securely around the neck. Open the sealed end of the bag. Remove the brain within a plastic bag to reduce potential aerosol exposure.
   f. Immediately place brain into a preweighed container of 10% neutral buffered formalin. Reweighing the container provides the weight of the brain.
5. Mix liquid waste 1:1 with 2N NaOH in a waste collection bottle.

**Box 3-5** Autopsies of patients with suspected prion disease (human transmissible spongiform encephalopathies)—modifications of autopsy suite decontamination procedures

1. Place instruments (open box locks and jaws) and saw blades into a large stainless steel dish.
2. Soak instruments for 1 hour in Kleenzyme; immerse for 1 hour in 1N sodium hydroxide, and rinse for 2 to 3 minutes in water. (Collect all waste.)
3. Transfer instruments into red autoclavable biohazard waste bags, and autoclave at 134 °C (gravity displacement steam autoclaving for 1 hour; porous load steam autoclaving for one 18-minute cycle at 30 lb psi or six 3-minute cycles at 30 lb psi).
4. Clean the Stryker saw by repeated wiping with 1N sodium hydroxide solution.
5. Double bag the absorbent table cover and instrument pads, disposable clothing, and so forth in appropriate infective waste bags for incineration.
6. Decontaminate any suspected areas of contamination of the autopsy table or room by repeated wetting with 1N sodium hydroxide over 1 hour, followed by thorough rinsing and washing.

**Box 3-6** Autopsies of patients with suspected prion disease (human transmissible spongiform encephalopathies)—modifications of brain cutting procedures

1. After adequate formaldehyde fixation (at least 10 to 14 days), the brain is examined and cut on a table covered with an absorbent pad with an nonpermeable (i.e., plastic) backing.
2. Samples for histology are placed in cassettes labeled with "CJD precautions." These are placed in 95% to 100% formic acid for 1 hour, followed by fresh 10% neutral buffered formalin solution for at least 48 hours. This procedure eliminates all prion infectivity in the embedded specimen.
3. All instruments and surfaces that come in contact with the tissue are decontaminated as described in Box 3-5.
4. Tissue remnants, cutting debris, and contaminated formaldehyde solution should be discarded in a water-tight plastic container as infective hospital waste for incineration.

nose, and throat irritation; shortness of breath; wheezing; chronic cough; mucus hypersecretion; asthma; chronic airway obstruction; bronchitis; rhinitis; pharyngitis; menstrual and reproductive disorders; and sexual dysfunction.[26] Although many individuals have experienced the milder irritative disorders following acute limited formaldehyde exposure, the incidence of most of the more severe reactions is extremely low. Nonetheless, the sensitivity of individuals is highly variable. Exposure studies performed in rats have shown that formaldehyde appears to induce nasal squamous cell carcinomas[27,28]; however, implications for humans are equivocal. Studies relating the rat and human data indicate that the carcinogenic risk for humans at relevant levels of formaldehyde exposure is minimal; further, it is likely that precautions effective against noncancer toxic effects of the chemical are sufficient to protect against its carcinogenic effects.[29]

The autopsy suite should have sufficient ventilation and effective chemical fume hoods to reduce employee exposure to formaldehyde vapor. As mandated by the Occupational Health and Safety Administration (OHSA), employers must monitor formaldehyde levels in the workplace and maintain employee exposures below the legal safe limits. Institutions should provide a mandatory training program for all employees exposed to formaldehyde at or above 0.1 ppm on an 8-hour time-weighted average. Box 3-7 lists some important components of a safety training program for employees exposed to formaldehyde.

## Radioactivity

On rare occasions, the autopsy pathologist may be required to examine the body of a patient who died shortly after receiving diagnostic or therapeutic radioactive substances or after

1. Explanation of the OSHA standard and contents of the formaldehyde material safety data sheet (MSDA).
2. A description of the medical surveillance program including potential health hazards, signs and symptoms, and instructions to report the development of signs and symptoms the employee suspects are related to formaldehyde exposure.
3. A description of operations in which formaldehyde is present and explanation of safe work practices for jobs requiring the use of formaldehyde.
4. A discussion of the purpose, proper use, and limitations of personal protective equipment.
5. Instruction on the handling of spills, emergencies, and cleanups.
6. An explanation of the importance of engineering and work practice controls and instruction and, if applicable, training in how to use the controls.
7. A review of emergency procedures and the role of each employee in the event of an emergency.

OSHA, Occupational Safety and Health Administration.
Modified from Lott AL, Greenblatt M: Formaldehyde regulations: What you need to know, CAP Today 4:32-35, 1993.

accidental radioactive contamination.[30] In such circumstances, the body may contain a level of radiation that would result in a radiation exposure risk to autopsy staff. Handling of the radioactive cadaver requires special care and is best done with the assistance of personnel trained in radiation safety.[30-32]

In most cases, radioisotopes used for diagnostic studies are given in small doses (less than a millicurie) or have short half-lives, and patients who die after recent nuclear medicine examinations are usually not a radiation hazard. Patients who die after receiving therapeutic doses of radioisotopes or implanted radioactive sources may require special handling, depending on the level of radioactivity remaining (Table 3-1). Hospitals where such patients are treated will have patient treatment records available, as well as radiation safety specialists who can advise the pathologist.

The United States Atomic Energy Commission recommends that patients who have received radioisotopes remain in the hospital until the level of radioactivity falls to 30 mCi or less. Thus, most patients who die after hospital discharge present minimal hazard. However, because radioisotopes may be concentrated in tissue or body fluids, the attending physician signing the death certificate should alert the pathologist and the radiation safety officer if the body contains more than 5 mCi. The assigned mortuary should also be advised. A form identifying the isotope, the amount given, and the time of administration should be attached to the death certificate, the autopsy consent, and the medical record.

If an implanted radioactive source cannot be removed from the patient before an autopsy, if radioactive fluid is present after administration of an isotope, or if high levels of radioactivity are likely to be present in a specific organ, a radiation safety specialist should be consulted for assistance in the safe

collection and proper disposal of the radioactive source, fluid, or tissue. In consultation with the specialist, the amount of activity remaining in the body should be estimated by reference to the half-life of the isotope. If the remaining amount is less than 5 mCi, no special precautions are necessary, other than the usual wearing of gloves. An exception is cases of $^{131}$I therapy or therapy with insoluble radioisotopes, in which specific tissues (e.g., thyroid) or body cavities contain most of the activity.

When the residual activity exceeds 5 mCi, a survey of residual radioactivity before the body is opened helps establish the maximum working time allowed. A team of pathologists, each prosector performing a limited portion of the autopsy, may be required to limit individual exposures. Film badges may be required to monitor exposure. The pathologist should drain potentially contaminated body fluids carefully first and immediately shield them for assay later. For example, in cases of $^{131}$I therapy, the blood, urine, and thyroid are radioactive. Highly radioactive fluids should be stored behind appropriate shields until they can be safely removed from the autopsy suite.

After the body is opened, a second survey should be made to estimate the level of beta dose for $^{32}$P or other beta-emitting radionuclide. In cases of $^{131}$I administration, the thyroid gland may emit a sufficient gamma dose that it should not be touched by hand directly but rather removed with the aid of a long instrument.

After the autopsy, all instruments, towels, and clothing involved in the procedure should be checked for radioactivity and either stored shielded until safe or decontaminated before being returned to general use or sent to the laundry. The autopsy room should be monitored for radioactive contamination and decontaminated if necessary.

Similar to gamma rays, X-rays pass easily through fairly thick materials. X-ray machines, including the cabinet type used commonly by pathologists, have built-in shielding. The radiation safety specialist should assist the pathology department in monitoring and complying with any safety measures required for the operation of these machines.

## Implantable Cardioverter-Defibrillator

An implantable cardioverter-defibrillator (ICD), also known as an automatic implantable cardioverter-defibrillator (AICD), consists of a pulse generator, one or two sensing electrodes, and a set of anode and cathode electrodes for countershock. As in pacemakers, which they resemble, the generator is usually placed subcutaneously within the left anterior chest wall. Depending on the make and model, the electrodes reach their attachment points on the heart by a transthoracic or transvenous route.

Prahlow and colleagues[33] have reviewed the safety issues surrounding ICDs encountered at autopsy. A small but definite risk of electric shock exists when the detection lead of an ICD is broken or cut, resulting in a discharge of 25 to 40 J. Although shocks of this magnitude are unlikely to cause death, manufacturers recommend that the ICDs be deactivated before manipulation and that high-quality latex surgical gloves be used when handling the devices. In many cases, the autopsy prosector is aware of the presence of an ICD after

**Table 3-1**  Diagnostic and therapeutic procedures involving administration of radioactive substances

| Indication | Radionuclide | Physical half-life | Form of administration |
|---|---|---|---|
| **Nuclear medicine diagnostic tests** | | | |
| Bone, renal parathyroid, cerebral blood flow imaging | Tc-99 | 6.6 hours | Intravenous |
| Somatostatin receptor imaging | In-111 | 2.8 days | Intravenous |
| Neurectodermal tumor imaging | I-123 | 13.2 hours | Intravenous |
| PET tumor imaging | F-18 | 1.8 hours | Intravenous |
| **Therapeutic procedures involving administration of unsealed radioactive substances** | | | |
| Thyrotoxicosis and nontoxic goiter | I-131 | 8.04 days | Usually oral |
| Carcinoma of thyroid | I-131 | 8.04 days | Usually oral |
| Malignant disease | I-131 | 8.04 days | Intravenous |
| Arthritic conditions | Y-90 | 2.7 days | Intraarticular |
| Polycythemia vera | P-32 | 14.2 days | Intravenous or oral |
| Bone metastases | Sm-153 Sr-89 | 46.2 hours 51 days | Intravenous |
| Non-Hodgkin's lymphoma | Y-90 | 2.7 days | Intravenous |
| Liver cancer | Y-90 | 2.7 days | Hepatic arterial injection |
| Carcinoid | Y-90 | 2.7 days | Intravenous |
| **Therapeutic procedures involving administration of temporarily implanted sealed radioactive substances (brachytherapy)** | | | |
| Malignant disease | Y-90 | 2.7 days | Rods |
| Malignant disease | Cs-137 | | Tubes, wire, small diameter cylinders or pellets |
| Malignant disease | Ir-192 | 74 days | Wire, pins, or small diameter cylinders |
| Eye diseases | Sr-90 and daughter Y-90 | 28.7 years | Metal eye plaques |
| Eye diseases | Ru-106 | | Metal eye plaques |
| **Therapeutic procedures involving administration of permanently implanted sealed radioactive substances** | | | |
| Prostate cancer | I-125 | 60 days | Metal seeds |
| Prostate cancer | Pd-103 | 17 days | Seeds |
| Various sites, e.g., tongue, rectal margin | Au-198 | 2.7 days | Grains |

Modified from Singleton M, Start RD, Richardson C, Conway M: The radioactive autopsy: Safe working practices, *Histopathology* 51:289-304, 2007. Reprinted with permission from *Archives of Pathology & Laboratory Medicine,* copyright College of American Pathologists.

review of the medical history of the deceased. However, in cases in which history is incomplete or totally lacking, the pathologist encountering an implanted device during autopsy dissection should ascertain whether it is a pacemaker or an ICD before continuing with the autopsy. If an ICD is present, the pathologist should discontinue the postmortem examination until the device is properly deactivated (Box 3-8 and Table 3-2). Because ICDs may explode if incinerated, they should never be discarded without special attention. Because most ICD manufacturers request the return of the device after its removal, the manufacturer's representative usually assists in the removal and collection of an ICD.

## Foreign Bodies and Occult Medical Devices

### Bullet Recovery

Bullets may fragment on impact or may by design raise pointed edges on entering their target. In either case, the resulting deformation can produce sharp edges in shrapnel that present a risk for injury to those who remove or handle them. For autopsies of gunshot victims, Russell and coworkers[34] recommended that anteroposterior and lateral radiographs be taken to locate bullets, bullet fragments, and any sharp or irregular edges. Bullets should be handled only by personnel wearing double heavy-duty gloves. To prevent marring of the projectile surface, a rubber-tipped bullet extractor

**Box 3-8    Safety precautions for autopsies on patients with an implantable cardioverter-defibrillator (ICD)**

1. Obtain medical history.
2. Use universal precautions (gloves) and other insulating devices.
3. Locate and identify all implanted electrical devices; avoid cutting leads.
4. If ICD is present, do NOT proceed until deactivated.
5. Call dedicated local cardiologist or manufacturer's representative (see Table 3-2).
6. Wait for cardiologist or representative to deactivate ICD, or follow representative's instructions for deactivation.
7. Request manufacturer's representative to obtain information from internal memory of ICD.
8. Do NOT discard ICD.
9. Do NOT incinerate ICD.
10. Contact manufacturer representative for removal or collection of ICD.

From Prahlow JA, Guileyardo JM, Barnard JJ: The implantable cardioverter-defibrillator: A potential hazard for autopsy pathologists, *Arch Pathol Lab Med* 121:1076-1080, 1997. Reprinted with permission from Archives of Pathology & Laboratory Medicine, copyright College of American Pathologists.

fashioned from a Kelly forceps fitted with 2 cm of rubber catheter over its ends or a plastic forceps should be used to recover bullets and bullet fragments. After collection of any trace evidence on the projectile itself, the bullet should be gently rinsed to remove contaminating blood or body fluids to decrease its subsequent infective risk. Finally, the bullet or bullet fragments should be double packed in leakproof packaging with at least one of the containers composed of hard plastic to prevent injury during subsequent handling. In addition to the appropriate identifying information, the container should be labeled with a biohazard sticker.

### Needle Fragments and Other Sharp Objects

Medical devices such as surgical staples, vena-caval (Greenfield) filters, and other devices may have sharp edges or points that can be encountered unexpectedly at autopsy.[35] Needle fragments are a potential hazard to pathologists performing autopsies on drug-addicted patients. Embolized needle foreign bodies have been discovered in soft tissues of the neck and even within internal organs.[36-38] Hutchins and colleagues[38] recommended preautopsy radiographic screening, reduced tissue manipulation during prosection, and delay of autopsy in

**Table 3-2    Selected manufacturers of implantable cardioverter-defibrillators**

| Manufacturer | Toll-free telephone number | Brand name |
|---|---|---|
| Biotronik (Lake Oswego, Ore) | 1-800-547-0394 | Phylax 06<br>Phylax 03<br>Phylax XM<br>Phylax AV<br>Mycrophylax<br>Mycrophylax Plus<br>TACHos |
| ELA Medical (Plymouth, Minn) | 1-800-352-6466 | Defender I, II, III, and IV<br>Sentinel* |
| Guidant (Redmond, Wash) Division of Boston Scientific<br>Intermedics, Inc Division of Boston Scientific | 1-800-227-3422 | Metrix†<br>Res-Q |
| Medtronic Inc (Minneapolis, Minn) | 1-800-328-2518 | PCD<br>Jewel<br>Gemini |
| St. Jude's Medical Cardiac Rhythm Management Division, formerly Telectronics Pacing Systems (Sylmar, Calif) | 1-800-722-3422 | GUARDIAN<br>SENTRY |
| St. Jude's Medical Cardiac Rhythm Management Division, formerly Ventritex Incorporated (Sunnyvale, Calif) | | Cadence<br>Cadet<br>Contour<br>Ventritex<br>Angstrom<br>Profile<br>Photon |
| St. Jude's Medical Cardiac Rhythm Management Division, formerly Cardiac Pacemakers, Inc. | | AIDB<br>VENTAK |

*Device is an atrial defibrillator.
†Device manufactured by Angeion, Plymouth, Minn.
Data from Prahlow JA, Guileyardo JM, Barnard JJ: The implantable cardioverter-defibrillator: A potential hazard for autopsy pathologists, *Arch Pathol Lab Med* 121:1076-1080, 1997.

human immunodeficiency virus–positive cases, along with the standard recommendations for protection against injury from sharp instruments.

## Cyanide Exposure

Exposure to cyanide vapors during autopsy has been associated with clinical symptoms and toxic concentrations of cyanide in autopsy personnel.[39,40] Autopsies on victims of cyanide poisoning should be performed in a negative-pressure isolation room. Although cyanide may vaporize from other tissues, stomach contents containing ingested cyanide salts present the highest risk, because the gastric acid converts cyanide salts to volatile hydrocyanic gas. Therefore, the prosector should open the stomach only in a chemical fume hood or externally vented biologic safety cabinet to reduce the risk of exposure to the toxic gas. Similarly, toxicology laboratory workers handling samples possibly containing cyanide should wear gloves and face and eye protection and manipulate the specimen only in a chemical fume hood.

## CONCLUSION

This chapter has reviewed the main components of autopsy biosafety. The objective of any autopsy biosafety program must be to provide autopsy staff and any visiting personnel with an environment as free from hazardous exposure risk as possible. Achieving this goal requires a continuous program of safety education and constant diligence in enforcing safe methods of autopsy practice.

## REFERENCES

1. Clarke JJ: *Post-mortem examinations in medico-legal and ordinary cases*, London, 1896, Longmans, Green.
2. Li L, Gu J, Shi X, et al: Biosafety level 3 laboratory to autopsies of patients with severe acute respiratory syndrome: Principles, practice and prospects, *Clin Infect Dis* 41:815-821, 2005.
3. Nolte KB, Hanzlic RL, Payne DC, et al: Medical examiners, coroners, and biologic terrorism. A guidebook for surveillance and case management, *MMWR Recomm Rep* 53(RR-8):1-27, 2004.
4. Marty AM: Anatomic laboratory and forensic aspects of biological threat agents, *Clin Lab Med* 26:515-540, 2006.
5. Sharp SC: The physician's obligation to treat AIDS patients, *South Med J* 81:1282-1285, 1988.
6. Richmond JY, McKinney RW: *Biosafety in microbiological and biomedical laboratories*, ed 4, Washington, DC, 1999, U.S. Department of Health and Human Services.
7. World Health Organization: *Laboratory biosafety manual*, ed 2, Geneva, 1993, WHO.
8. Fritzsche FR, Dietel M, Weichert W, Buckendahl AC: Cut-resistant protective gloves in pathology—effective and cost-effective, *Virshows Arch* 452:313-318, 2008.
9. O'Briain DS: Patterns of occupational hand injury in pathology. The interaction of blades, needles and the dissector's digits, *Arch Pathol Lab Med* 115:610-613, 1991.
10. LeBeau LJ: Health hazards in biomedical photography. In Vetter JP, editor: *Biomedical photography*, Boston, 1992, Butterworth-Heinemann, pp 499-507.
11. Nolte KB: Survival of *Mycobacterium tuberculosis* organisms for 8 days in fresh lung tissue from an exhumed body, *Hum Pathol* 36:915-916, 2005.
12. Gerston KF, Blumberg L, Tshabalala VA, Murray J: Viability of mycobacteria in formalin-fixed lungs, *Hum Pathol* 35:571-575, 2004.
13. Meade GM, Steenken WM, Jr: Viability of tubercle bacilli in embalmed human lung tissue, *Am Rev Tuberc* 59:429-437, 1949.
14. Bauer S, Daniel A, Alpert LI, et al: *Protection of laboratory workers from instrument biohazards and infectious disease transmitted by blood, body fluids, and tissue; approved guideline*, NCCLS M29-A, December 1997, Clinical and Laboratory Standards Institute.
15. Ruef C: Immunization for hospital staff, *Curr Opin Infect Dis* 17:335-339, 2004.
16. Centers for Disease Control and Prevention (CDC): Human rabies prevention—United States, 1999. Recommendations of the Advisory Committee on Immunization Practices (ACIP), *MMWR Recomm Rep* 48:1-21, 1999.
17. Hedvall E: The incidence of tuberculosis among students at Lund University, *Am Rev Tuberc* 41:770-780, 1940.
18. Morris SI: Tuberculosis as an occupational hazard during medical training, *Am Rev Tuberc* 54:140-157, 1946.
19. Meade GM: The prevention of primary tuberculosis infections in medical students, *Am Rev Tuberc* 58:675-683, 1948.
20. Reid DD: Incidence of tuberculosis among workers in medical laboratories, *Br Med J* 2:10-14, 1957.
21. Wilkins D, Woolcock AJ, Cossart YE: Tuberculosis: Medical students at risk, *Med J Aust* 160:395-397, 1994.
22. Templeton GL, Illing LA, Young L, et al: The risk for transmission of *Mycobacterium tuberculosis* at the bedside and during autopsy, *Ann Intern Med* 122:922-925, 1995.
23. Nolte KB, Taylor DG, Richmond JY: Biosafety considerations for autopsy, *Am J Forensic Med Pathol* 23:107-122, 2002.
24. Towfighi J, Roberts AF, Foster NE, Abt AB: A protective device for performing cranial autopsies, *Hum Pathol* 20:288-289, 1989.
25. Brown P, Preece MA, Will RG: "Friendly fire" in medicine: Hormones, homografts, and Creutzfeldt-Jakob disease, *Lancet* 340:24-27, 1992.
26. Greenblatt M, Swenberg J, Kang H: Facts about formaldehyde, *Pathologist* 37:648-651, 1983.
27. Swenberg JA, Kerns WD, Mitchell RI, et al: Induction of squamous cell carcinoma of the rat nasal cavity by inhalation exposure to formaldehyde vapor, *Cancer Res* 40:3398-3402, 1980.
28. Albert RE, Sellakumar AR, Laskin S, et al: Gaseous formaldehyde and hydrogen chloride induction of nasal cancer in the rat, *J Natl Cancer Inst* 68:597-603, 1982.
29. Connolly RB, Kimbell JS, Janszen D, et al: Human respiratory tract cancer risks of inhaled formaldehyde: dose-response predictions derived from biologically-motivated computational modeling of a combined rodent and human dataset, *Toxicol Sci* 82:279-296, 2004.
30. Singleton M, Start RD, Richardson C, Conway M: The radioactive autopsy: Safe working practices, *Histopathology* 51:289-304, 2007.
31. Wallace AB, Bush V: Management and autopsy of a radioactive cadaver, *Australas Phys Eng Sci Med* 14:119-124, 1991.
32. Schraml FV, Parr LF, Ghurani S, Silverman ED: Autopsy of a cadaver containing strontium-89-chloride, *J Nucl Med* 38:380-382, 1997.
33. Prahlow JA, Guileyardo JM, Barnard JJ: The implantable cardioverter-defibrillator: A potential hazard for autopsy pathologists, *Arch Pathol Lab Med* 121:1076-1080, 1997.
34. Russell MA, Atkinson RD, Klatt EC, Noguchi TT: Safety in bullet recovery procedures: A study of the Black Talon bullet, *Am J Forensic Med Pathol* 16:120-123, 1995.
35. Burton JL: Health and safety at necropsy, *J Clin Pathol* 56:254-260, 2003.

36. Williams MF, Eisele DW, Wyatt SH: Neck needle foreign bodies in intravenous drug abuse, *Laryngoscope* 103:59-63, 1993.

37. Thorne LB, Collins KA: Speedballing with needle embolization: Case study and review of the literature, *J Forensic Sci* 43:1074-1076, 1998.

38. Hutchins KD, Williams AW, Natarajan GA. Neck needle foreign bodies: An added risk for autopsy pathologists, *Arch Pathol Lab Med* 125:790-792, 2001.

39. Andrews JM, Sweeney ES, Grey TC, Wetzel T: The biohazard potential of cyanide poisoning during postmortem examination, *J Forensic Sci* 34:1280-1284, 1989.

40. Nolte KB, Dasgupta A: Prevention of occupational cyanide exposure in autopsy prosectors, *J Forensic Sci* 41:146-147, 1996.

# 4

# Basic Postmortem Examination

*"In a systematic and scientific performance of an autopsy nothing is more difficult, and at the same time more important, than the insight into the reasons for pursuing a definite order of sequence in every detail of the examination."*

Rudolph Virchow[1]

This chapter describes and illustrates systematic dissection sequences and procedures. However, although developing a systematic approach to autopsy dissection and organ examination is efficient and generally desirable, the pathologist must be prepared to alter the examination as required for the best demonstration and diagnosis of specific diseases. Although a given method may be adequate for revealing the pathologic findings of one disease or condition, it may be entirely inadequate for identifying or best demonstrating another.

Modern autopsy techniques include modifications of the Virchow,[1,2] Ghon,[3-5] or Letulle[3-8] methods. The method attributed to Rokitansky,[3,9] characterized by in situ dissection, has not stood the test of time, although many erroneously apply his name to the method of Letulle. Using the Virchow method, the prosector removes organs one by one. In contrast, the pathologist using the Ghon or Letulle method removes the cervical, thoracic, abdominal, and genitourinary organs as separate organ blocks ("en bloc") or as a single group ("en masse"), respectively.

The Virchow method, removing organs one by one, is excellent for demonstrating pathologic changes in organs but sacrifices interorgan relationships and makes interpretation of regional disease more difficult. The advantages of the Ghon and Letulle techniques include excellent preservation of the interrelationships of the various organs, their regional lymphatic drainage, and their vasculature. The Letulle technique, removing the organs together in toto, allows the most rapid preparation of the body for removal to the mortuary and, because there is less dissection within the confines of the body cavity, probably offers greater safety to the prosector and assistant. However, the examination performed with this method takes a bit longer than that with the Virchow method and is difficult for some to perform without an assistant. The Ghon method, removing the organs in regional and functional groups, is relatively easier for one person to carry out. However, the prosector using the Ghon technique transects the esophagus and aorta at the diaphragm, a disadvantage in cases

of aortic dissection or aneurysm and esophageal varices or neoplasm. Skill in the Rokitansky technique (i.e., in situ dissection) is advantageous because it allows one to open and examine organs without removing them from the body, a condition sometimes mandated by a restrictive autopsy consent or severe time limitations.

This chapter focuses on postmortem methods based on modifications of the Virchow and Letulle methods. However, the prosector should be prepared to modify any standard autopsy technique to best demonstrate the pathologic changes and important pathologic relationships. Regardless of the method of dissection, well-maintained instruments make the work easier. A list of instruments useful in various standard and specialized postmortem procedures is presented in Box 4-1.

## EXTERNAL INSPECTION

### Identification

It is important to review the autopsy consent for specific restrictions. It is equally important to check the toe tag or other identifier of the patient, match it with the autopsy consent, and initial it before continuing. If possible, it is extremely profitable to review imaging studies with the local experts in these areas. They can offer great help in giving you the information to plan your examination to yield maximum results. Prepare for any anticipated special procedures such as angiography. Consider the need for collection of body fluids, microbiologic cultures, electron or immunofluorescence microscopy, and biochemical or molecular analysis at the beginning of the autopsy, and plan the dissection accordingly. We discuss these ancillary procedures in detail in Chapters 7, 8, and 9.

### Inspection and Palpation

Remove any bandages, and document any therapeutic devices. Remove superficial, peripheral venous catheters, but leave indwelling central lines, endotracheal tubes, feeding tubes,

**Box 4-1    Instruments and equipment useful for postmortem examinations**

Organ knife 10 inches/254 mm or 15 inches/381 mm
Scalpel knife holder and no. 22 disposable blades
Forceps, 1 × 2 teeth, 10 inches/254 mm
Forceps, 1 × 2 teeth, 6 inches/152 mm
Forceps, serrated tips, 6 inches/152 mm
Forceps, Adson 1 × 2 teeth, 4¾ inches/121 mm
Forceps, Adson, serrated tips, 4¾ inches/121 mm
Forceps, Rochester Pean, straight and curved, 8 inches/203 mm
Forceps, Halstead mosquito, straight and curved, 5 inches/127 mm
Scissors, Mayo or Doyen abdominal, straight, 9 inches/229 mm
Scissors, Mayo or Doyen abdominal curved, 9 inches/229 mm
Scissors, Metzenbaum, straight round point 5.5 inches/139 mm
Scissors, Metzenbaum, curved round point 5.5 inches/139 mm
Enterotomy (intestinal) scissors, 8 inches/203 mm
Wire cutters
Rib shears
Probe, 1 mm
Postmortem hammer/hook
Virchow skull breaker or chisel
Bone-cutting forceps
Rongeurs, double action
Self-retaining retractors[2]
Vibratory (Stryker) saw
Small rule
Meter stick
Plastic-coated measuring tape
Postmortem needles, serpentine and curved

urinary bladder catheters, and so forth in place until the internal examination confirms their proper location. Measure the body length, and if possible, weigh it. Note the anteroposterior dimension of the chest, identify any abdominal distention, and determine whether the extremities are symmetrical. Document abnormalities by measuring the circumferences of the chest (at the level of the nipples), abdomen (at the umbilicus), or extremities (bilaterally at a specific distance above or below an anatomic landmark such as the superior margin of the patella or the acromioclavicular joint).

Inspect the skin anteriorly and posteriorly. Note its color and elasticity, and characterize any cutaneous lesions. Document surgical and nonsurgical scars. Record any tattoos or other identifying features. While inspecting the dorsum, also inspect the anus. Examine the character and color of the nails. Estimate the degree of rigor mortis by flexing the joints. Note the color, length, and character of the hair. Inspect and palpate the scalp and skull. Examine the eyes, including the condition of the conjunctivae and sclerae and the color of the irides. Measure the width of the pupils. Examine the ears and their location. If necessary, use an otoscope to inspect the external ear canal. Inspect the nose, including the nasal mucosa and the integrity of the nasal septum, and note any nasal discharge. Open the mouth and inspect the buccal mucosa and the tongue. Examine the teeth and their state of repair. In the case of unidentified bodies, prepare a detailed dental chart or consult a forensic odontologist.

The illumination provided by an otoscope or penlight may be helpful in examining nasal and oral cavities. Palpate the neck, noting the position of the trachea and the size and consistency of the thyroid gland. Check for cervical, axillary, or inguinal lymphadenopathy. Examine the breasts and palpate for masses. Palpate the abdomen. Inspect the genitalia. In the male, palpate the scrotum, determining whether the testes are descended and noting any abnormalities. In the female, separate the legs and inspect the vulva. In some forensic cases, a vaginal speculum is required to complete a detailed inspection of the vagina and cervix that includes appropriate sampling of secretions. Before beginning the internal examination, consider the need to document any significant findings with photographs.

## INITIAL DISSECTION AND INTERNAL EXAMINATION

After you have completed the external examination, place a block under the shoulders to extend the neck. For fetuses or small infants, a rolled towel may provide adequate elevation of the upper torso. The incision is roughly Y-shaped and most easily made with a sharp scalpel. It begins at the shoulders, anterior to the acromial processes and sparing the top of the shoulders. The upper limbs of the incision penetrate to the ribs and meet at the level of the xiphoid process. Some prefer to extend the upper limb incisions in an arc around the inferior portion of the female breasts. We prefer to direct the upper limb incision medial to the breasts, believing that this results in less chance of fluids inadvertently leaking from the closed body after the autopsy.

The descending limb of the incision extends along the midline from the xiphoid process to the symphysis pubis, except where it diverts briefly around either side of the umbilicus, through subcutaneous tissue and muscle to the peritoneum. At the level of the umbilicus, measure the thickness of the abdominal fat. At this point, we use a scissors to enter the peritoneal cavity to reduce the likelihood of inadvertently piercing the abdominal organs (Fig. 4-1). Expose the

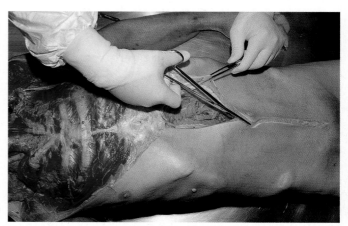

**Figure 4-1** After the initial Y-shaped incision has been made and the skin and subcutaneous tissues over the chest have been reflected, scissors are used to open the peritoneal cavity.

abdominal cavity, and prepare for removal of the sternum and anterior portions of the ribs by separating the skin and subcutaneous tissues of the lateral chest and abdominal walls from their bony attachments. Using care not to puncture or "buttonhole" the skin, reflect the skin and subcutaneous tissues of the chest and neck to the level of the hyoid bone. Examine the breasts from their posterior aspects by making parallel incisions through the pectoralis muscles and into the breast tissue.

Inspect the peritoneal lining and omentum. Survey the abdominal viscera and note the location of the organs. Characterize, aspirate, and measure any ascitic fluid. Estimate the height (rib or intercostal space) of the dome of the diaphragm, which should reach to approximately the fourth rib on the right and the fifth on the left before opening the chest (Fig. 4-2).

Check for pneumothorax (see Chapter 6). Open the thorax by cutting the sternoclavicular joint and then the ribs near the lateral margin of the costal cartilage. Retract the sternum anteriorly, freeing it from the body. In young individuals, a scalpel penetrates the cartilaginous portions of the ribs quite easily; however, in older patients rib cutters are usually necessary. In patients who have had coronary artery bypass surgery, avoid injury to the bypass grafts during removal of the sternum. Because calcified rib cartilages leave ragged edges, place towels over their cut margins for added safety (Fig. 4-3). Characterize, aspirate, and measure any pleural fluid. Then sweep your hands carefully along the pleural surfaces of the lungs, noting and lysing any fibrinous pleural adhesions. Fibrous adhesions require careful sharp dissection to avoid tearing the visceral pleura. Examine the thymus. In adults, adipose tissue normally replaces the thymic tissue, although its lobes may still be discernible. In pediatric cases, it is convenient to remove and weigh the thymus at this point. Next, open the pericardium in the midline and examine the pericardial cavity (Fig. 4-4). Characterize, aspirate, and measure any pericardial fluid or blood clot. Unless you plan to fix the heart by perfusion (e.g., in cases of congenital heart disease), open the pulmonary artery above its valve and examine for the presence of saddle or central pulmonary artery emboli by

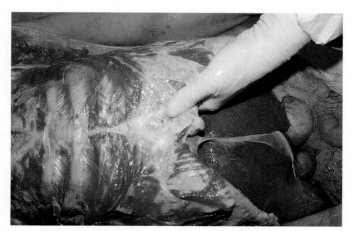

**Figure 4-2** The prosector checks the height of the dome of the diaphragm before opening the thoracic cavity.

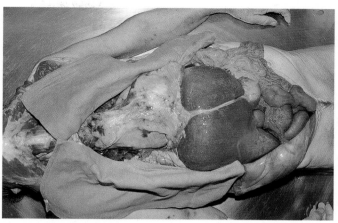

**Figure 4-3** Towels placed over the cut margins of the ribs protect against any sharp edges.

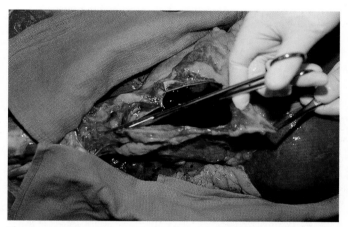

**Figure 4-4** The pericardium is opened in the midline from inferior to superior, and the pericardial cavity is inspected. In this case a ruptured myocardial infarct has led to hemopericardium.

inserting a finger into the main pulmonary artery and its right and left branches. At this time, urine can be collected from the bladder with a syringe and needle.

Are there any indications to check blood vessels or surgical anastomoses before removing the intestines? If there are no indications for leaving the intestines attached to the other viscera, remove them now. Displace the omentum and transverse colon superiorly and the small intestine to the right, exposing the ligament of Treitz. Clamp or ligate the small intestine near the ligament, and remove the intestines by cutting (with the rear portion of a large scissors) the mesentery as near its junction with the serosa as possible (Fig. 4-5). Pulling the intestines toward the scissors effects this most easily (Fig. 4-6). Collect the liberated bowel in a stainless steel basin, noting any obvious serosal lesions during the process. Identify the appendix near the ileocecal junction, and note its location and condition. Examine the external surface of the cecum and ascending colon; then remove it in continuity with the small intestine by lifting it up and cutting the ascending mesocolon and any other fibroadipose tissues securing the bowel. At the hepatic flexure, return the omentum and transverse colon back to their anatomic positions and cut through the transverse mesocolon to the splenic flexure and in turn along the

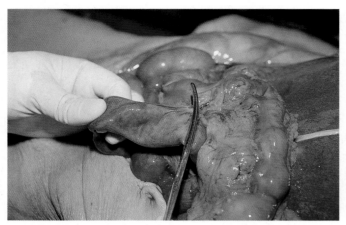

**Figure 4-5** View from the left side of the body with the head toward the right side of the figure. The colon has been flipped superiorly to expose the small intestine at the level of the ligament of Treitz. Here the small intestine is clamped before removal.

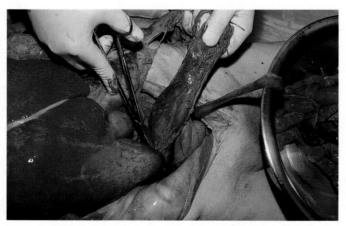

**Figure 4-6** The small intestine distal to the ligament of Treitz has been largely removed, the transverse colon is freed, and the posterior attachments of the cecum to the peritoneum are about to be transected. The intestines are collected in a basin before further examination.

descending colon. Employ double clamps or ligatures at the rectosigmoid junction and transect the bowel. Lay the intestines aside until later.

When the abdominal contents are altered by the presence of numerous adhesions (e.g., with extensive peritoneal metastasis or following peritonitis), it may be necessary to leave the intestines attached to the other abdominal organs. The Letulle autopsy method, described next, coupled with a careful layer-by-layer dissection of the abdominal contents from the posterior aspect, may demonstrate pathologic findings that would otherwise be missed.[10]

## LETULLE METHOD

### Organ Removal

After the initial inspection of the organs and body cavities and removal of the gut, prepare for removal of the remaining viscera. Identify and inspect the carotid arteries (Fig. 4-7).

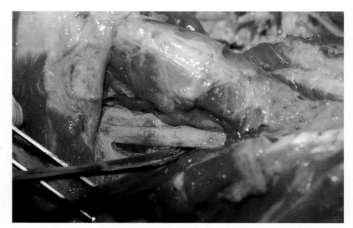

**Figure 4-7** The right carotid artery is identified and inspected.

A long ligature may be placed around each carotid artery where it enters the base of the neck. Using scissors or a scalpel, transect the laryngeal pharynx above the epiglottis through the thyrohyoid membrane or include the hyoid bone by cutting superiorly. Transect the esophagus as well, but avoid injury to the carotid arteries. Reflect the larynx inferiorly, and cut the carotid arteries below their ligatures. It is relatively easy to include the hyoid bone or the tongue and associated tissues as part of the neck dissection, and some pathologists do this routinely because it allows a much better examination of the oropharynx and superior neck. However, the facial artery, a vessel important to the embalmer, is vulnerable to injury during this dissection. Removal of the tongue is facilitated by cutting posterior to the rami of the hyoid bone. Through the neck, reach into the oral cavity, grasp the tongue, flip its tip posteriorly into the neck, and cut the anterior attachments free. More extensive neck dissections are discussed in Chapter 6.

Having readied the neck organs for removal, free any pleural and connective tissue attachments to the apical thoracic cavity. Next, cut the right and left hemidiaphragms along their lateral and posterior body walls. On each side, while the posterior aspect of the upper abdominal cavity is exposed, extend the cut through the psoas muscle to the vertebral column. This makes removal of the organ block easier.

Next, turn your attention to the pelvis. Using your hand and fingers, separate the bladder and prostate from the pelvic wall. Extend the plane of dissection posteriorly, separating the rectum along the coccyx (Fig. 4-8). Some physical exertion is necessary here to separate the pelvic organs completely along their entire circumference. Using large scissors, transect at the level of the proximal urethra (distal to the prostate in the male and through the proximal vagina in the female). Continue the cut through the rectum, generally not less than 2 cm above the anorectal junction (Fig. 4-9). Reflect the pelvic organs upward and outward, exposing in turn the iliac vessels bilaterally. Divide these, along with any connective tissue attachments, along the pelvic brim and curve of the sacrum.

At this point, the organ block is ready for removal. Lift the neck and thoracic organs anteriorly and then inferiorly, carefully separating the aorta and other posterior attachments

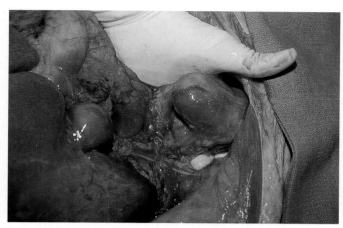

**Figure 4-8** Blunt dissection posterior to the rectosigmoid readies the pelvic organs for evisceration.

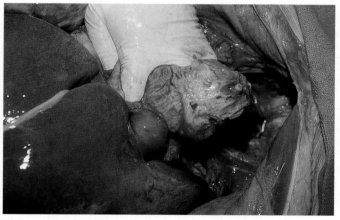

**Figure 4-9** The urethra is transected just distal to the prostate, and the cut is continued through the rectum. The pelvic organs are retracted up and out to each side, exposing in turn the right and left iliac vessels, which are then transected just above the femoral canal.

from the vertebral column. Continue applying inferior and upward traction, cutting as needed any remaining diaphragmatic or posterior abdominal wall attachments (Fig. 4-10). An assistant makes this a relatively easy maneuver. If you are working alone, it may be easier to cut posterior attachments by rotating the organ block to one side or the other before lifting it out of the body.

## Inspection of the Body Cavities and Removal of the Testes

After removal of the thoracic and abdominal viscera, make a final inspection of the body cavities and their walls. Take samples of sciatic nerve, skeletal muscle (psoas or deltoid), skin, and breasts for eventual microscopic examination. Remove the testes by entering the scrotal sac through the inguinal canal from above the pubic ramus. Push and lift the testes and spermatic cords up and out of the inguinal canal, cutting the cords to free the testes (Fig. 4-11).

## Initial Dissection and Separation of the Organ Blocks

We place the adult organ block, posterior side up, on a polypropylene or polyethylene cutting board measuring approximately 75 × 50 × 3 cm. (Placing this at a workstation that accommodates a chair or elevating the dissection to a height comfortable for a standing examiner reduces stress on one's back.) Beginning distally, open the inferior vena cava to the level of the diaphragm, carefully sparing the right renal artery. Note the appearance of the paraaortic lymph nodes, sampling them for microscopy as needed. Next, starting at the distal aortic arch, open the descending aorta and iliac and renal arteries posteriorly, and examine their intimal surfaces (Fig. 4-12). Probe the proximal portions of the other major arterial branches of the abdominal aorta for patency. Transect the aorta at the distal arch and reflect it from the posterior mediastinal tissues. We leave the abdominal aorta attached to the retroperitoneal tissues until dissection of the abdominal organs is completed. Obviously, leaving the thoracic or, for that matter, the entire descending aorta attached to the aortic arch and heart may best demonstrate dissecting hematomas, aneurysms, or acquired aortic diseases. In fetuses and infants, the aorta is initially opened only below the level of the diaphragm, at the point where it can subsequently be transected during separation of the thoracic and abdominal organs. Thus, the descending thoracic aorta is left in continuity with the aortic arch to aid in evaluation of possible arch malformations.

In cases requiring a more detailed vascular dissection— for example, when indicated by the medical history or by initial autopsy findings such as infarcts, organ atrophy or hypoplasia, primary vascular pathology such as stenosis or occlusion, or the need to demonstrate patency of surgical anastomoses—it may be best to perform the dissection of the pertinent vasculature before removing organs from the autopsy block. Those equipped for postmortem angiography might consider the use of this technique in their dissection plan (see Chapter 8).

Open the esophagus along its posterior aspect, and examine it for fistulous communications, mucosal lesions, or abnormalities in the submucosa, such as varices or neoplasms (Fig. 4-13). Reflect it to the level of the diaphragm. Next, remove the adrenal glands by exposing their bed beneath the posterior aspects of the hemidiaphragms. Identify the glands by palpation. Failing that, begin carefully dissecting away the suprarenal fat, starting at the superior pole of the kidneys. The adrenal glands may be difficult to locate in patients with excessive abdominal fat, with hypoplastic glands secondary to corticosteroid therapy, or with altered anatomy related to extensive retroperitoneal fibrosis or tumor metastasis. In such cases, the adrenal glands can be located by dissection of the venous drainage of these organs retrograde from the inferior vena cava.[11]

After locating the adrenal glands, remove them carefully, trim any adherent fat, and weigh them (Fig. 4-14). Sometimes the adrenals are so soft and friable from postmortem autolysis that it is better to remove them with their investing

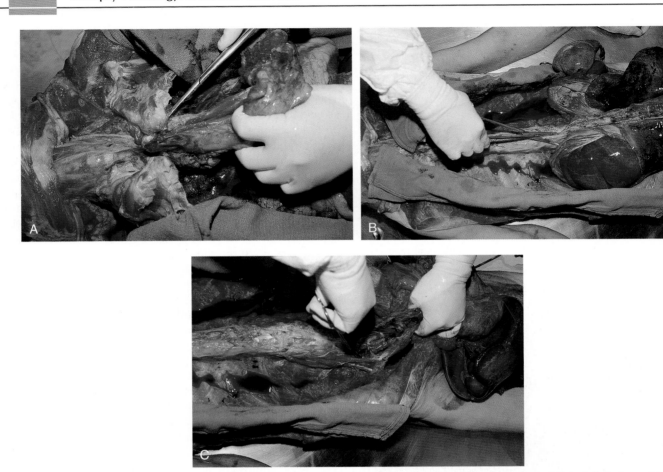

**Figure 4-10** The organ block is ready for removal. **A,** The neck and thoracic organs are lifted anteriorly and then inferiorly, and the aorta and other posterior attachments are separated from the vertebral column. **B,** The evisceration is continued by applying inferior and upward traction, cutting as needed any remaining diaphragmatic or posterior abdominal wall attachments. **C,** Finally, any posterior attachments in the pelvis are severed to free the entire organ block.

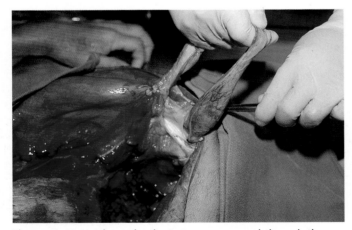

**Figure 4-11** In the male, the testes are removed through the peritoneal cavity by entering the scrotal sac through the inguinal canal from above the pubic ramus. The testis and spermatic cord are pulled up and out of the inguinal canal, and the cord is cut.

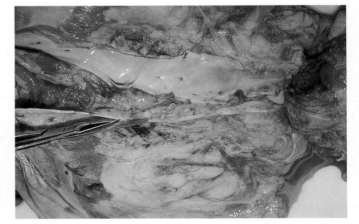

**Figure 4-12** Posterior view of the organ block with superior to the left, inferior to the right. The inferior vena cava has been opened to the level of the diaphragm, and the aorta is being opened along its posterior aspect.

adipose tissue and trim them after fixation. In any case, do not slice them until they are adequately fixed because the fragile medulla would become distorted. For identification purposes, it is helpful to know that the right adrenal gland is pyramidal in shape and the left is generally larger with a

semilunar shape. Separate the neck and thoracic organs from the abdominal organs by cutting between the inferior aspect of the pericardium and the superior aspect of the diaphragm. Take care not to transect the esophagus accidentally.

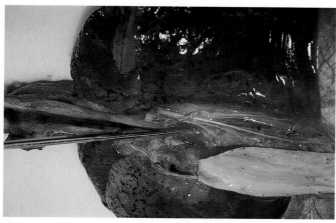

**Figure 4-13** The esophagus is opened along its posterior aspect.

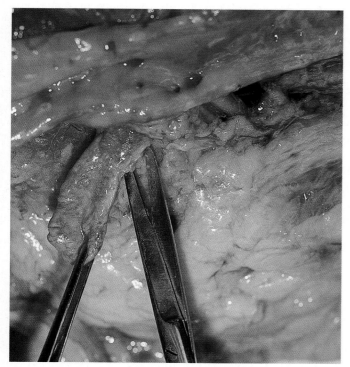

**Figure 4-14** Here the left adrenal gland is exposed and carefully removed from the surrounding adipose tissue.

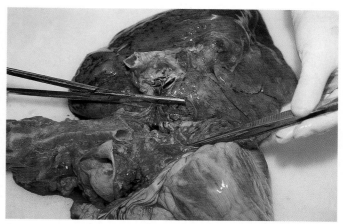

**Figure 4-15** Posterior view of the trachea, right lung, and heart. The right main stem bronchus has been transected at the carina, and the hilar attachments of the lung are then cut.

In either case, clamp the perfused orifice, add fixative to the container, and cover the lungs with a paper towel moistened with fixative to prevent drying of the pleural surfaces. Set aside the perfused lungs for at least 1 hour. Attending to the lungs early in the case allows adequate fixation before slicing and does not result in a delay in the communication of the gross pathologic findings. Many pathologists examine the lungs fresh by cutting sequentially along the arteries, airways, and veins. If you elect to do so, the method of McCulloch and Rutty[13] is best for examination of fresh lungs. Some pathologists compromise, inflating one lung and cutting one fresh. However, we feel that it is difficult to assess subtle parenchymal changes in the fresh lung.

We cut formalin-inflated lungs in 1- to 2-cm parasagittal slices. Coronal slices, including a midcoronal cut through the main stem bronchus, may demonstrate a central carcinoma to advantage. The only advantage of horizontal sections is that they correlate with modern imaging examinations. For slicing lungs, a sharp knife with a long blade is a necessity. Although one can cut the lungs freehand, an acrylic plastic (Plexiglas) cutting board with knife slots on two opposite sides permits finer control (Fig. 4-16). After slicing the lungs, the prosector examines the lung parenchyma with eyes and fingers to identify abnormalities and areas of consolidation or scarring. The larger airways and vessels are opened as needed to complete the examination.

### Neck and Anterior Mediastinal Organs

Examine the mediastinum, and sample any abnormal lymph nodes. Remove the larynx and trachea. Inspect the still-attached thyroid gland. While removing the thyroid gland from the thyroid cartilage, identify and save any tissue resembling the parathyroid glands. Normally, these small glands are tan or light brown and have a more acutely angled edge than the small lobules of fat, lymph nodes, and extraneous bits of thyroid tissue that masquerade as parathyroid glands. The superior parathyroid glands, frequently found at the level of the middle of the posterior border of each lobe of the thyroid gland, rest in a shallow groove. Unfortunately, the inferior parathyroid glands lie in various positions, including but not

## Examination of the Neck and Thoracic Organs

### Lungs

Remove the lungs, transecting the bronchi at the carinae and the pulmonary arteries and veins near the hilus of the lung unless you plan to perfuse through the artery (Fig. 4-15). Weigh the lungs, inspect their pleural surfaces, and palpate the pulmonary parenchyma. Routinely, we inflate lungs through the bronchi with formalin by simple gravity perfusion, generated by placing a container of fixative approximately 1 m above the floor and running a plastic tube from its spigot to the floor. Apparatuses for perfusion at constant, regulated pressure are also easily constructed.[12] Consider perfusing the lungs with formalin through the pulmonary arteries if mucus plugs might have contributed to the patient's death.

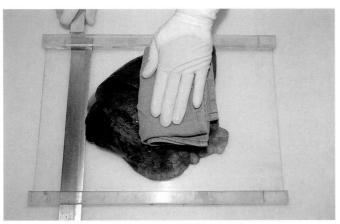

**Figure 4-16** Slicing the lungs. A Plexiglas cutting board can be used to obtain even slices. For safety, a towel has been placed under the hand.

limited to the fascial sheath of the thyroid gland near its inferior pole, behind and outside the thyroid gland immediately superior to the inferior thyroid artery, or within the substance of the lobe of the thyroid gland near its inferior posterior border. If there is a question of parathyroid disease, weigh the parathyroid glands because weight is the best criterion for hyperplasia or hypertrophy. After placing the parathyroid glands in a tissue cassette for safe keeping, continue the examination of the thyroid gland by weighing it, inspecting its surface, and then making nearly complete horizontal sections into its parenchyma. Open the larynx and trachea lengthwise along their softer posterior aspects and view their mucosal surfaces.

### Heart

Many approaches can be taken to examining the heart. Select the appropriate method on the basis of the age of the patient and any suspected abnormality. In any case, first dissect and remove pericardial tissue and fat and clean and expose the great vessels. In cases of suspected atherosclerotic cardiovascular disease, consider performing postmortem coronary angiography (see Chapter 7) before dissection. For routine examination, cut the extramural coronary arteries in cross section at 2- to 3-mm intervals or longitudinally if there is no or only minimal atherosclerosis (additional methods for examination of the coronary arteries are discussed in Chapter 8). Next, slice the heart at 1-cm intervals in the short axis (horizontal plane) at the apex and continuing to just below the inferior margin of the atrioventricular valve leaflets (Fig. 4-17). This is the best technique for inspecting the myocardium for infarcts. Because the papillary muscles are vulnerable to infarction during periods of hypotension, make longitudinal incisions along their length. Next, open the atrial and the remaining portions of the ventricular chambers as shown in Figure 4-17. The presence of artificial valves with metal valve rings makes interruptions in the usual cuts necessary. For hearts of younger patients without coronary artery disease, cardiomyopathy cases without an ischemic component, or congenitally malformed hearts, omit the short-axis cross sections and continue the ventricular cuts to and from their respective apices. Hearts cut along echocardiographic planes may make excellent teaching or demonstration pieces but detract from a thorough evaluation of cardiac structure. Weigh the heart after removal of extraneous vessels and residual postmortem blood clot.

### Examination of the Genitourinary Organs

#### Kidneys and Ureters

The ureters running along each side of the midline are identified through the translucent fat and fascia. Open these with a small pair of scissors from the renal pelvis to their entrance into the bladder (Fig. 4-18). Measure their average luminal circumference and examine their contents, if any, and the appearance of their mucosa. Remove the kidneys by blunt dissection in the plane between the renal capsule and the perinephric fat (Fig. 4-19). Clean the extracted kidneys of any

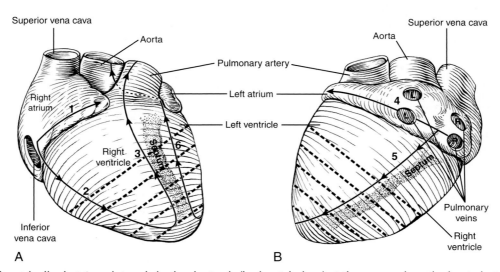

**A**                              **B**

**Figure 4-17** The heart is sliced at 1-cm intervals in the short axis (horizontal plane) at the apex and continuing to just below the inferior margin of the atrioventricular valve leaflets *(dashed lines)*. The atria and the remaining portions of the ventricular chambers are cut along the indicated lines in the sequence indicated. **A,** Anterior aspect. **B,** Posterior aspect.

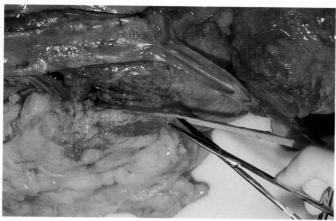

**Figure 4-18** The ureters running along each side of the midline are identified through the translucent fat and fascia. Open these with a small pair of scissors from the renal pelvis to their entrance into the bladder. Measure their average luminal circumference and examine their contents, if any, and the appearance of their mucosa.

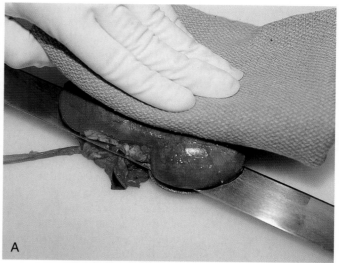

A

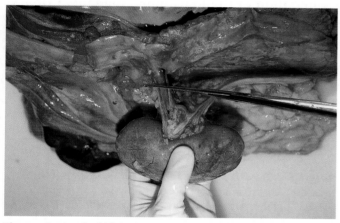

**Figure 4-19** The kidney has been dissected in the plane between the renal capsule and the perinephric fat and, after examination in situ, is ready to be detached from the organ block.

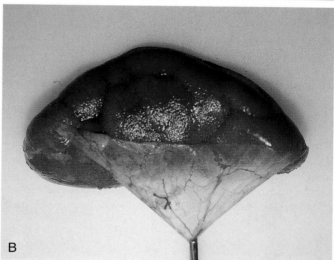

B

**Figure 4-20** Cutting the kidneys. **A,** The kidneys are sliced in half beginning from the medial aspect. **B,** After examination of renal parenchyma, the renal capsules are stripped, allowing the cortical surfaces to be inspected for lesions or irregularities.

adherent fat, weigh them, and determine the average thickness of the cortex and medulla. In most cases, we separate the kidneys from the bladder, leaving a greater length of left than right ureter attached for identification purposes. However, for demonstration of diseases such as hydronephrosis that involve the entire genitourinary system, do not separate the organs. Next, slice the kidneys completely in half through their longitudinal (coronal) axis (Fig. 4-20, *A*). Beginning from the medial aspect helps center the cut through the pelvis. Examine the cortex, medullary pyramids, and pelvis, opening individual major and minor calices as needed. Collect any calculi for possible biochemical analysis. Completely strip the renal capsule, noting the difficulty required, and then examine the cortical surfaces carefully for any lesions or irregularities (Fig. 4-20, *B*).

### Lower Genitourinary Tract (Male)

The rectum, still attached to the genitourinary organ block, is opened, inspected, and then removed from the rest of the

pelvic organs. Measure the size of the prostate in three dimensions; then cut across it at the approximate level of the seminal colliculus. The distal portion of this cut provides an excellent microscopic section at the point where the prostatic ducts enter the urethra. Additional transverse incisions into the prostate are useful for identifying any suspicious nodules. Open the proximal urethra and bladder anteriorly in the midline and inspect the urothelial mucosa. Probe the ureteral openings at the trigone. Make serial cuts into the seminal vesicles, noting the thickness of their walls and the color of any seminal fluid. Make several crosscuts along each vas deferens as well.

### Testis

Examine the previously removed testes. Knowing that the head of the epididymis is located superiorly and posteriorly and that a recess of the tunica vaginalis, the sinus of the epididymis, lies between the body of the epididymis and the lateral surface of the testis allows one to differentiate the right testis from the left. Crosscut any attached spermatic cord. Weigh the testes and then cut them in the sagittal plane and examine the parenchyma. Using a forceps, grasp a portion of the cut surface and pull, testing whether or not the seminiferous tubules string out easily. Failure of this test indicates testicular atrophy in the postpubertal male.[14]

### Lower Genitourinary Tract (Female)

Open the rectum through the midline posteriorly, inspect it, and then remove it from the pelvic organs. Introduce a scissors into the urethra at the point where it was transected during evisceration. Open the bladder anteriorly in the midline and examine it. Next, separate the bladder along its attachments along the uterus. Inspect the fallopian tubes and ovaries. Measure the ovaries in three dimensions, and cut them lengthwise to expose the parenchyma. Open the fallopian tubes longitudinally following insertion of a probe, or cut them in serial cross sections. Open the proximal vagina along its lateral surfaces, noting any abnormalities of its epithelial surface. Inspect the uterine cervix, noting any lesions, erosions, and so forth and the shape and greatest width of the os. Open the uterus along its lateral aspects (Fig. 4-21). Measure the dimensions of the uterine cavity, and note the thickness of the endometrium.

### Male and Female External Genitalia

We do not remove the male external genitalia as part of a routine autopsy examination. However, in special circumstances (e.g., for the study of urethral strictures, urethral or penile tumors, or congenital posterior urethral valves [see Chapter 5]), more extensive dissections are required. The abdominal incision is extended to the base of the penis. The midportion of the pubic arch is removed using a saw. The penis, scrotum, and anus can then be removed in continuity with the bladder, prostate, and rectum. Alternatively, the penis alone with or without its skin can be dissected from the undersurface of the symphysis pubis and pulled through the pubic arch. If the penile skin is left undisturbed, it can be filled with cotton batting to present a normal external appearance.

The female external genitalia are readily examined without their removal. However, the rare case of vulvar neoplasia or certain cases of sexual assault may necessitate the removal of the pudendum. This can be accomplished by continuing the abdominal incision over the symphysis pubis to the labia majora. The pubic arch is removed with a saw. The legs are separated to expose the urogenital triangle, an elliptical incision is made around the external genitalia and anus, and this specimen is removed in continuity with the vagina, uterus, urinary bladder, and rectum.

## Examination of the Remaining Abdominal Organs

### Spleen

Remove the spleen at its hilus, inspect its capsular surface, and weigh it (Fig. 4-22). Many pathologists make multiple slices of the spleen along its short axis. We prefer to make sections along the long axis of the spleen either parallel or perpendicular to the plane of the hilus. With any method, make sufficient sections to inspect the parenchyma fully. Note whether the follicles are visible, and examine the condition of the connective tissue trabeculae.

### Upper Gastrointestinal Organs and Biliary Tract

Turn the organ block over to expose the anterior aspect. Dissect the diaphragm away from esophagus and liver. Remove the omental fat from the greater curvature of the stomach. Open the stomach along its greater curvature and through the pylorus, anteriorly (Fig. 4-23). Continue this cut through the duodenum, exposing the ampulla of Vater and the duodenal mucosa. Rotating the liver posteriorly to reveal its inferior aspect helps expose the region of interest. Slight compression on the gallbladder usually extrudes bile from the ampulla. Cannulate the common bile duct and with fine scissors open

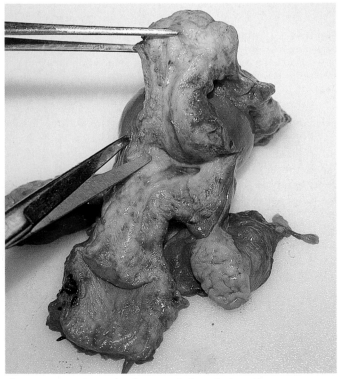

**Figure 4-21** The uterus is opened along its lateral aspects.

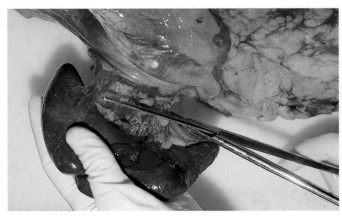

**Figure 4-22** The spleen is easily removed near its hilus.

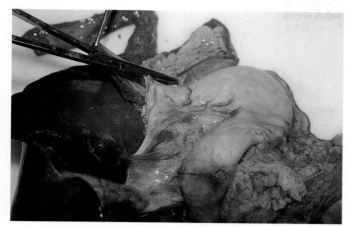

**Figure 4-23** The stomach is opened along its greater curvature, and this cut is continued through the pylorus into the duodenum.

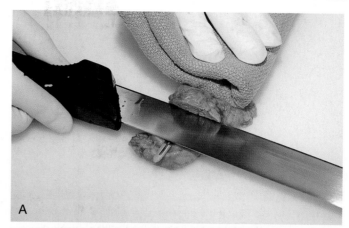

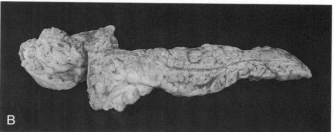

**Figure 4-25** Cutting the pancreas. **A,** Several serial transverse sections have been made through the head of the pancreas, allowing examination of the pancreatic parenchyma and the ducts. A probe has been passed into the main pancreatic duct. Then a lengthwise coronal section is made along the probe. **B,** The cut pancreas showing a considerable length of the duct.

it retrograde into the hepatic ducts, cystic duct, and gallbladder, examining for patency and looking for any calculi or mucosal abnormalities (Fig. 4-24). Note that it is quite difficult to enter the gallbladder because of the numerous spiral valves of the cystic duct. It may be necessary to open the gallbladder first and then extend this incision though the duct. Save any stones for possible biochemical analysis. Next remove the esophagus, stomach, and first portion of the duodenum in continuity, taking care to leave the head of the pancreas as intact as possible. Also, in the presence of interesting biliary tract disease, consider retaining the pancreas with this specimen.

### Pancreas

Dissect the pancreas free of any peripancreatic fat and weigh it. To examine the pancreatic parenchyma, cut by making serial transverse slices along its short axis (parasagittal sections). This allows adequate examination of the duct system. Figure 4-25 depicts a method that we favor because it yields a more interesting specimen for demonstration. We make several serial transverse sections through the head of the pancreas, allowing examination of the pancreatic parenchyma

and the main duct (Wirsung) and, if present, the accessory duct (Santorini). At the point distal to an accessory duct, a probe is inserted into the duct of Wirsung. Then we make a lengthwise coronal section along the probe that usually reveals a considerable length of the duct. The free section of the neck, body, and tail of the pancreas provides material for microscopy.

### Liver

Turn your attention to the liver. Remove any remaining adherent diaphragm and lesser omentum, and weigh the liver. Pathologists have cut the liver variously in parasagittal, coronal, and horizontal planes. Only the coronal and horizontal planes include the right and left lobes of the liver in the same section. The middle coronal sections provide the best demonstration of the hilar structures, but a horizontal section (preferred by us) includes the most parenchyma and therefore demonstrates the organ's size to best advantage.

### Aorta, Diaphragm, and Mesentery

Dissect the abdominal portion of the aorta from the remaining organ block. If the diaphragm was not removed during dissection of the liver, remove and examine it now. Finally isolate the mesentery. Palpate its tissues for enlarged lymph nodes and abnormal masses. The vessels coursing through the mesenteric fat can be examined by making a series of arcing cuts (Fig. 4-26).

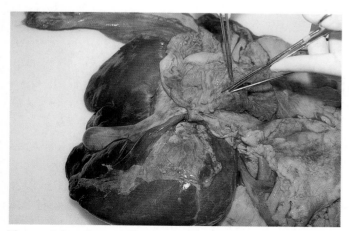

**Figure 4-24** The ampulla of Vater is identified and cannulated with a probe. Fine scissors are used to open the biliary tract.

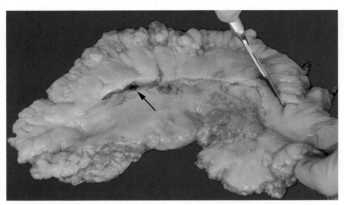

**Figure 4-26** Examining the mesentery. A series of arcing cuts exposes lymph nodes and sections vessels coursing through the mesenteric fat. The lymph node *(arrow)* identified here was affected by Hodgkin's lymphoma.

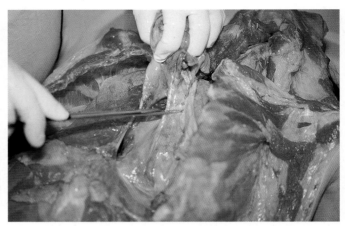

**Figure 4-27** Virchow procedure, removal of the heart. The inferior vena cava has been cut at the diaphragm. The pulmonary veins have been transected, allowing the heart to be reflected. In this photograph, the prosector is cutting the aorta distal to great vessels.

## Intestines

Using bowel (enterotome) scissors, open the small and large intestines along their antimesenteric borders, a procedure best done in a hopper or hooded sink. If you removed the gut with minimal attached mesentery, opening the intestines is a relatively quick and easy procedure. Again, it helps to pull the bowel toward the hinge of the scissors rather than try to snip through the bowel wall. Gently wash the mucosal surfaces before inspecting them. Consider pinning out regions of significant disease such as tumors on a dissection board and fixing them overnight. Inflation and fixation of segments of the intestines with formalin make for good demonstrations but are not generally performed. Examine the appendix by serial transverse cuts to its tip.

In the presence of multiple intestinal adhesions, exert extreme care to avoid transverse cuts across segments of bowel. It may be better to leave some of the bowel unopened where adhesions have rendered the organ a mass of complex loops. Of course, it is critical that the prosector establish patency or lack thereof through all these segments.

## VIRCHOW METHOD OF ORGAN REMOVAL

The Virchow method remains the autopsy technique of choice for many pathologists, particularly those doing forensic work. The body cavities are exposed and inspected as described previously.

## Thoracic Organs

If it is evident, remove and weigh the thymus. Open the pericardium, and describe and measure any fluid. Examine the ascending aorta, its arch, and the arch branches. Trace the course of the great vessels in situ. Identify the pulmonary veins, and trace them back to the heart. Open the main pulmonary artery in situ, and examine for thromboemboli. Identify the right and left pulmonary artery branches, and trace them to the lungs. Cut them near the pulmonary hila. Examine the inferior vena cava as it passes through the diaphragmatic hiatus. While holding the heart at its apex, transect

the inferior vena cava at the diaphragm and reflect the heart upward, severing the pulmonary veins near the lung and the superior vena cava. Transect the aorta distal to great vessels (Fig. 4-27). At this point, the heart is free and the prosector turns his or her attention to the lungs. In turn, reflect each lung laterally, cutting the bronchi and any remaining hilar connections (Fig. 4-28).

## Neck Organs

Identify the thyroid gland. Tracing the superior and inferior thyroid arteries to their small branches may help locate the parathyroid glands. At this time, sever the upper end of the esophagus after first placing a clamp distally to prevent loss of gastric contents (Fig. 4-29). Remove the neck organs (larynx, thyroid, trachea, upper esophagus) as a block by transecting the thyrohyoid membrane and cutting any posterior connections (Fig. 4-30). If required, include the tongue in continuity with the other neck structures.

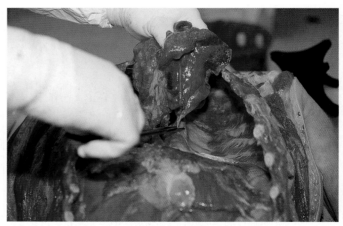

**Figure 4-28** Virchow procedure, removal of the lungs. In turn, the prosector reflects each lung laterally, cutting the bronchi and any remaining hilar connections.

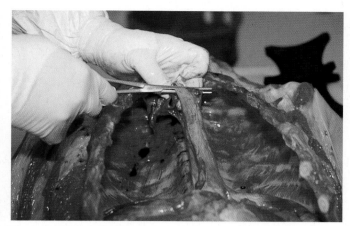

**Figure 4-29**  Virchow procedure. Before removal of the neck organs, the esophagus is clamped superiorly to prevent loss of gastric contents.

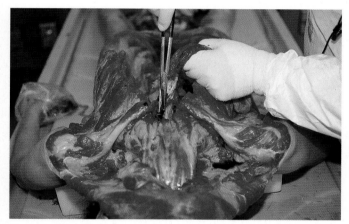

**Figure 4-30**  Virchow procedure. The neck organs (larynx, thyroid, trachea, upper esophagus) are removed as a block.

## Abdominal Organs

Cut across the hepatoduodenal connections, and lift the stomach and the first portion of the duodenum forward. Dissect them free of their inferior connective tissue and vascular connections. Advance the dissection into the chest to include the esophagus severed previously, thus removing the esophagus, stomach, and proximal duodenum in continuity (Fig. 4-31). If indicated, include the second portion of the duodenum and the pancreas with this specimen. Lift the liver to expose the gallbladder. Determine the patency of the biliary system by opening the first and second portions of the duodenum, locating the ampulla of Vater, and compressing the gallbladder. Note the exit of bile. Simple dissection exposes the lower portion of the common duct. Open it upward to the hepatic ducts, cystic duct, and gallbladder and downward to the ampulla. Alternatively, free the gallbladder from its bed in the liver and include it and the common bile duct with the duodenum for dissection later.

Locate the portal vein, and open it to the superior mesenteric and splenic veins. Examine the hepatic arteries by transverse sections. Remove the liver by lifting up the right lobe

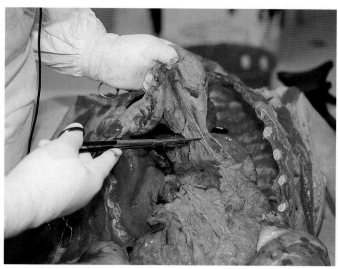

**Figure 4-31**  Virchow procedure. The esophagus, stomach, and proximal duodenum are removed in continuity and clamped at proximal and distal ends if collection of stomach contents is required.

and freeing it from any posterior attachments as far as the vertebral column. Place this lobe against the right ribs, elevate the left lobe, and free any remaining attachments. After investigating the biliary system, remove the liver by first freeing it as far as possible from the diaphragm on the right. With an assistant holding the diaphragm up, cut the falciform and coronary ligaments, including the vena cava and hepatic veins. Rotate the liver forward, down, and to the left, and isolate it from the right adrenal gland. Elevate the liver and divide its connections with the duodenum, inspecting carefully any cut vessels. Trace the splenic artery to the hilum of the spleen, noting the splenic vein and body and tail of the pancreas as well. Free the spleen by lifting it anterolaterally and dividing its hilar connections (Fig. 4-32). Removing the stomach, liver, and spleen in turn exposes the pancreas, and this organ is now completely accessible. Carefully dissect it free of the retroperitoneal fat and any other attachments (Fig. 4-33).

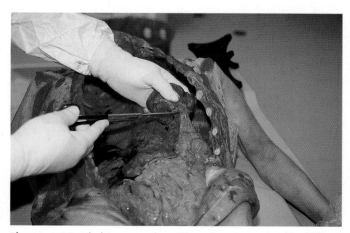

**Figure 4-32**  Virchow procedure. The spleen is removed by lifting it anterolaterally and dividing its hilar connections.

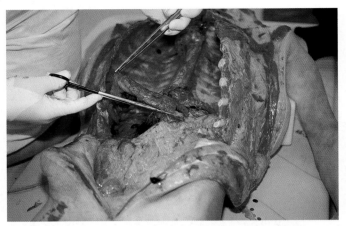

**Figure 4-33** Virchow procedure. The exposed pancreas is dissected free of the retroperitoneal fat and any other attachments.

## Aorta, Adrenal Glands, Kidneys, and Pelvic Organs

Next, open the thoracic aorta in situ along its ventral surface into the iliac arteries. Apply some superior traction on the vessel to make this easier. Open the renal arteries along their course and then cut them from the aorta. Locate the kidneys and the adrenal glands by palpation, and using a forceps and scissors separate the adrenal glands from the kidneys (Fig. 4-34). Bluntly dissect the kidneys from the perirenal fat. Lift them anteriorly, exposing the ureters (Fig. 4-35). Open the ureters along their course to the bladder. Sever them or leave them connected to the bladder. Remove the remaining pelvic organs (bladder, rectum, and prostate or uterus) as a block using the technique described in the description of the Letulle method. Finally, using sharp dissection with scissors, remove the aorta from its posterior connections.

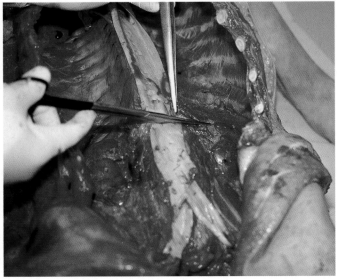

**Figure 4-34** Virchow procedure, removal of the adrenal glands. The adrenal glands are located by palpation and carefully removed.

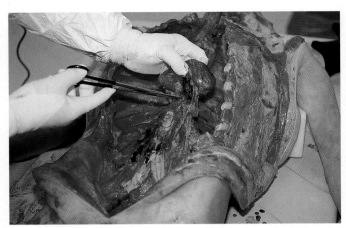

**Figure 4-35** Virchow procedure, dissection and removal of the kidneys and ureters. The kidneys are dissected free of the perirenal fat and lifted anteriorly, exposing the ureters, which are then opened to the bladder before the kidneys are removed.

Unless discussed otherwise as a specific part of the Virchow method, perform the dissection of individual organs as already described.

## REMOVING THE BRAIN AND SPINAL CORD

As with many mechanical procedures, there are various ways in which a brain and spinal cord may be successfully removed. There should usually be some difference depending upon the age of the patient, but the goal is an intact organ ready for preliminary gross examination and without or with minimal removal artifacts. Fixation methods also vary, and we describe several methods in Chapter 8. Finally, sectioning methods that have been proved over the years are explained here. Chapter 9 includes techniques for obtaining spinal fluid for culture or biochemical examination.

For removal of the adult brain, the head is held in proper position with a block, and a bitemporal incision passing near the vertex is almost universally used. Take care not to remove too much hair (Fig. 4-36). Incise the scalp down to the bone, and then peel the skin and subcutaneous tissues back to below the occipital protuberance posteriorly and to the level of the forehead anteriorly by a combination of sharp and blunt dissection. Give additional care to patients who have had craniotomies, major head trauma, or major malformations to avoid penetrating the skin or otherwise causing cosmetic problems.

Using a vibrating (Stryker) saw or comparable instrument, cut the bone in the plane a crown would have on the head. Triangular notches placed laterally in the skull cap facilitate realignment for postmortem reconstruction. Others use a "step cut" or angled cut; this is a personal or institutional preference (Fig. 4-37). Take particular care to avoid aerosolizing the bone and tissues at this time. A moistened towel is often helpful without hindering the procedure. Elaborate mechanisms to avoid aerosolizing tissue often hinder more than help and, fortunately, are largely unnecessary. Additional care is necessary to avoid penetration of the dura or at least to avoid penetration of the brain itself at this time. The

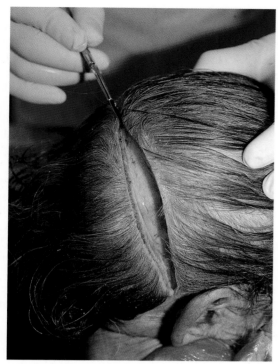

**Figure 4-36** Brain removal. The scalp is incised down to the bone, taking care not to cut the hair.

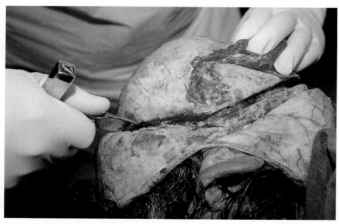

**Figure 4-37** Brain removal. The skull has been cut with a vibrating saw using an angled cut. A chisel helps separate the skull cap.

Check for and note abnormalities of the bone structures, the dura, the anterior cranial nerves, and the vessels. The olfactory bulbs are bluntly dissected from the cribriform plates, and the optic nerves, carotid arteries, and third cranial nerves are cut where they enter the skull (Fig. 4-38).

At the posterior extent of the middle cranial fossa, incise the tentorial attachment to the petrous edge, elevate the occipital tips, and free the posterior bony attachments of the dura and tentorium. The contents of the anterior basal posterior fossa can then be seen and the cranial nerves and vessels visualized and transected (Fig. 4-39). Finally, the medulla or upper cervical cord is transected (Fig. 4-40). It is usually also desirable to cut the vertebral arteries as low as possible at this point to free the brain from the cranial cavity and remove it for the final stages of preliminary examination (Fig. 4-41).

At this stage, weigh the unfixed brain (and note whether the dura is included in this weight). Survey the nerves, vessels, and gross anatomy for abnormalities. If indicated, take additional culture specimens and smears and prepare sections for rush processing. Also take tissues for electron microscopy and other special studies (e.g., RNA, DNA) now. If there is a

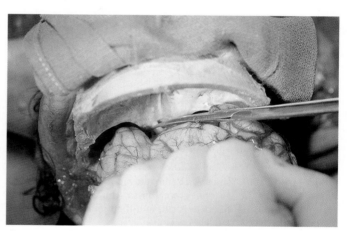

**Figure 4-38** Brain removal. The dura at the anterior attachment of the falx to the crista galli is cut and the brain is gently elevated and retracted posteriorly. The anterior fossa is examined, and the optic nerves, carotid arteries, and third cranial nerves are cut where they enter the skull.

pathologist in training should observe carefully this operation as done by an experienced person and note the variations in thickness of the bone in the different areas. Unfortunately, there are significant variations from person to person, and ongoing care during this procedure is essential.

A hook or other wedge helps separate the skull cap after completion of the bone cut (see Fig. 4-37). In adults, carefully separate the dura, which is almost always densely adherent to the inner table of the skull, if maintenance of the dura-brain relationships is desired. To remove the brain after separating the skull cap, cut the dura at the anterior attachment of the falx to the crista galli and gently elevate and retract the brain posteriorly while examining the anterior skull and brain base.

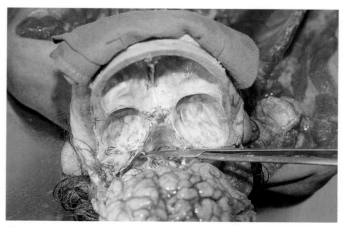

**Figure 4-39** Brain removal. The brain is supported as the cranial nerves and vessels are transected.

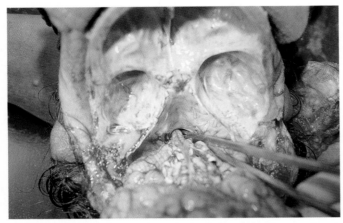

**Figure 4-40** Brain removal. As the brain is retracted upward and posteriorly, the medulla and upper cervical spinal cord are visualized. The spinal cord is cut transversely as low as possible.

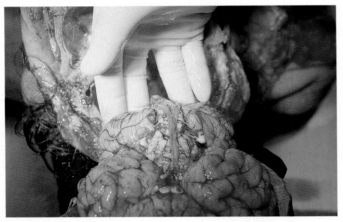

**Figure 4-41** Brain removal. The fingers aid in freeing the cerebellum from the posterior cranial fossa. The brain is supported by one hand, the falx cerebelli is cut, and the brain is removed from the cranial vault.

good deal of subarachnoid hemorrhage, especially if localized, it is often best to dissect it fresh because fixation most often hardens the mass of blood and makes later dissection quite difficult. Documentation should be done before the dissection as indicated. Then very deliberate dissection of the blood clot, taking care to identify the vessels in the area, should be performed, remembering that aneurysmal walls are often quite friable and need to be searched for and identified. A gentle stream of water as from a piece of flexible tubing can be of great assistance in this procedure, washing the dissected blood away during the operation and significantly aiding in the visualization of areas of interest.

After removal of the brain, open the dural sinuses at the base of the skull and search for any obstructions. Check for cerebral pressure markings. Perfuse the carotid and vertebral arteries with saline or water to document patency. Next, strip the basal dura from the base of the skull with a bone forceps. This allows unhindered inspection of the base of the skull in order to identify fractures or other lesions. With a chisel and hammer, fracture the dorsum sellae along its upper anterior

surface. Grasp the diaphragm of the sella with a forceps, and cut around its margins with scissors. Upward traction on the diaphragm raises the pituitary gland from its fossa, allowing the point of a scalpel or fine scissors access to the gland's inferior connections and its easy removal.

Spinal cord removal by the anterior approach is similar in adults and children. After evisceration of the neck and thoracic and abdominal organs, followed by dissection of the paravertebral muscle and soft tissues laterally, cut the lateral processes of the vertebra using a vibrating saw (but carefully avoiding penetration deep enough to damage the spinal cord) from the lower lumbar level as high as the high thoracic or lower cervical levels (Fig. 4-42). Make transverse cuts through the high and low disks and remove the block of vertebral bodies, demonstrating the spinal cord within the dural sleeve, the emerging nerves and roots, and the ganglia. Next, incise the dura longitudinally to the highest visible level, and *cut the dura circumferentially, carefully avoiding the spinal cord itself.* Examine and cut the lower nerves and transect the cord itself at the cauda level. Lift the mass of cord, dura, and nerves up toward the head, cutting the nerves and other connections (Fig. 4-43). Because the dura has been cut circumferentially at a high level, all that attaches the cervical cord to the body (as the brain has already been removed) are the cervical nerves and the dentate ligaments. Rupture these by tugging on the cord (we prefer to wrap it in a towel), and then deliver the entire cord from below. If there has been a significant postmortem interval or prolonged hypoxia before death, significant artifact often is associated with this removal, an inevitable reality.

One can also remove the spinal cord by the posterior approach (Fig. 4-44). This is more time consuming but is much less subject to artifacts than anterior removal. This approach is essential for careful review of cervical and upper thoracic cord abnormalities and bone changes at these levels (Fig. 4-45). It is sometimes required for a proper forensic assessment of these anatomic areas. It is also a useful approach in cases restricted to spinal cord or brain and spinal cord.

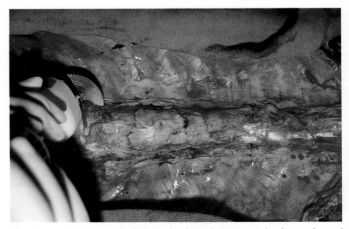

**Figure 4-42** Removal of the spinal cord. Paravertebral muscle and soft tissues have been displaced laterally, and the lateral processes of the vertebrae are cut.

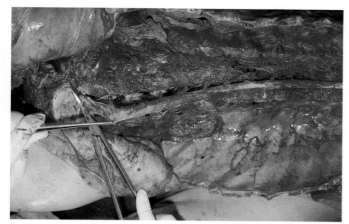

**Figure 4-43** The lower nerves are examined, and the spinal cord is picked up by its dura and cut from the inferior dural connection. The cord is elevated and the nerve roots are cut from inferior to superior.

It is important to have the appropriate tools at hand for this approach. The vibrating saw is again helpful, but double-action rongeurs of the appropriate size (adult or child sized) can be essential to this dissection. The obvious long midline incision is necessary, with dissection of the paravertebral muscle and soft tissues laterally. The posterior aspect of the arch can then be cut, again with care to avoid too deep penetration with cord damage. The rongeurs are most helpful with this. Finally, the cord is visualized and the various elements are examined. Removal, after documentation of abnormalities (or normalities, if needed), is accomplished by cutting the nerves and dissecting the dura from its attachments.

As with the brain, after removal and before fixation, final preliminary examination can be done at this time. Cut the dura longitudinally, dorsally, or ventrally according to local custom, and survey the spinal cord, roots, nerves, ganglia, vessels, and meninges for abnormalities. Document as needed, and remove sample materials for other studies before fixation.

Fixation is an extremely important step in the proper examination of the brain and spinal cord (see Chapter 8). Good quality fixation makes reasonably thin sectioning of the gross brain possible, aiding in the preparation of blocks for processing and embedding and ultimately the production of good quality sections with interpretable stains, both routine and special. Poorly fixed tissue renders all these procedures difficult or less productive.

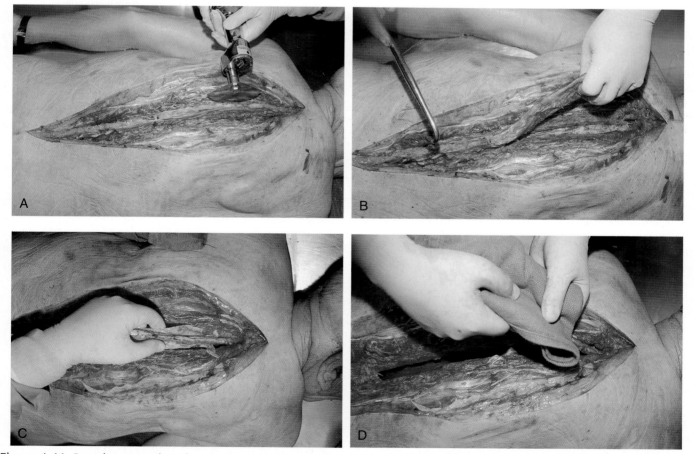

**Figure 4-44** Posterior approach to the spinal cord. **A,** A long midline incision has been made and the muscle and soft tissues dissected from the vertebral column. The posterior arch is cut with the vibrating saw. Though not shown here, this dissection can extend superiorly along the cervical vertebrae to the foramen magnum. **B,** The spinal processes and posterior portions of the laminae are removed. **C,** The dura is opened longitudinally to the uppermost part of the incision, where it is cut circumferentially. **D,** The nerves are cut and the cord is delivered by steady traction. A towel placed around the cord protects it from damage during this step.

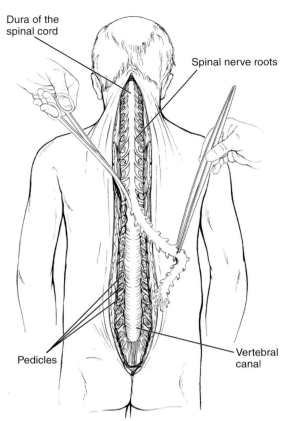

**Figure 4-45** Posterior approach to the cervical spinal cord. The skin and adjacent soft tissues can be incised up to the level of the foramen magnum. The spinal processes (at these levels) can be separated and the entire upper spinal cord examined in situ and subsequently removed as needed. Remember that the spinal dura is attached firmly to the skull at the level of the foramen magnum. (Modified from Baker RD: *Postmortem examination: specific methods and procedures,* Philadelphia, 1967, WB Saunders, as redrawn from Letulle MEJL: *La pratique des autopsies,* Paris, 1903, C Naud.)

## BRAIN CUTTING—GENERAL AND SPECIFIC

There are many "correct" ways to cut a brain after fixation. Always remember that the purpose of the cut is to recognize and demonstrate the abnormalities present, describe them with accuracy, and localize them anatomically. Ideally, another experienced person reading a description of the lesions should be able to know precisely what areas are involved and reach the same gross diagnosis or differential diagnosis. For these reasons, it is important to *describe* and *not diagnose*. This also enables learning because with the description in hand one can recall what was seen. Then, when the diagnosis is known, add it to the list if it was not originally part of the differential diagnosis.

All that being said, for most persons it is best to learn one or perhaps two methods of brain cutting, learn them well, and become experienced in using them. It is easy to become confused anatomically if you are not very experienced.

Before describing the cutting method, note that it is important to have at hand the tools needed to achieve the cut with efficiency and accuracy. We believe that brain-cutting tools should be kept separate from those used in the general

autopsy or general organ dissection and reserved for that purpose. A set of tools for each prosector is preferred. The minimum tools are listed in Box 4-2. We prefer to cut brains on a large (18 × 24 inch) wooden cutting board because wood does not dull knives as plastic does. Additionally useful are long, 8-inch to 10-inch toothless forceps to allow easy manipulation of the cut sections, a metal cooking spatula to assist in reassembly of the cut brain for storage, and a plastic salad colander that can be lined with cheesecloth and used to assemble and store the brain after cutting. All the tools should be carefully maintained to avoid rust and damage and stored carefully so that they are readily available.

Probably the most utilized and reliable method of brain cutting is the coronal cutting method. Several variations on this method exist, and the one that we use is described here. It has the added advantage of being illustrated in multiple anatomic atlases so that anatomic reference is readily available.

The fixed brain should be carefully washed in running water for at least 2 hours and preferably overnight before the cut occurs. This process minimizes eye discomfort caused by the fixing fumes for all concerned and also minimizes exposure to at least potentially hazardous materials.

The fixed brain should be carefully examined externally prior to cutting. The dura, if present, should be removed, usually by blunt dissection but using the scalpel if needed. The surfaces of the fixed brain should be carefully examined. The cranial nerves should be identified at each level bilaterally, at least as far down as the ninth. Below this the nerves are most commonly torn during brain removal. Then, using the chemical spatula, the arachnoid membrane can be dissected from the major vessels of the circle of Willis and supplying arterial system. Care should be take to avoid tearing the brain tissue itself, especially as the temporal lobes are retracted to visualize the middle cerebral artery and its branches and the frontal lobes separated to visualize the anterior cerebral arteries and the anterior communicating artery. Comparably, the posterior cerebral arteries can be dissected as they pass around the midbrain, the posterior communicators identified, and the posterior fossa arterial branches examined.

Sampling of any abnormalities seen thus far should be done at this time. Furthermore, if special studies of cerebral cortical areas are necessary, this is the best time to achieve easy identification of these areas.

| **Box 4-2    Instruments and equipment for cutting the brain** |
|---|
| Knife, straight-edged, nonserrated, at least 10 inches/254 mm, preferably 15 inches/381 mm |
| Forceps, toothless, bayonet type, slender, 8 inches/203 mm long |
| Forceps, tissue, fine point, 4½ inches/127 mm |
| Chemical spatula with rounded and squared ends for blunt dissection |
| Scissors, conjunctival or iris, 4½ inches/127 mm |
| Scissors, Mayo, straight, 5½ inches/140 mm, for blunt dissection and cutting dura and other firm tissue |
| Scalpel knife holder and no. 22 disposable blade |
| Small flexible rule, preferably transparent |

At this point, separation of the cerebrum from the brainstem is most often best achieved. Using a scalpel blade inserted lateral to one cerebral peduncle, a horizontal cut through the midbrain can be made. The midbrain section is often most easily made now, and the sections of the brainstem can also be cut. However, before cutting the brainstem, we prefer to make a cut paralleling the coronal cuts of the cerbrum vertically through the cerebellum, separating it from the brainstem structures; this cut should begin just behind the midbrain and just miss the medulla oblongata; this section demonstrates the distribution of the cerebellar arteries (Fig. 4-46 and Box 8-2, region 7). Then the brainstem is examined by cutting serial coronal sections (as used, this means horizontal sections relative to the body as a whole).

The cerebrum should be cut with the base up so that it is easily seen by the prosector. This orientation is important because all the identifying anatomic structures are on the base. A series of coronal cuts is then made; one smooth cut should be made through the entire brain, beginning with the heel of the knife and ending at the tip. If the knife is sharp, this is not difficult. "Sawing" should be avoided, as should "crushing"; the former is a back-and-forth movement of the edge of the knife, the latter pushing down on the knife blade without horizontal movement. The result should be smooth cut surfaces with usually easily identifiable anatomic landmarks.

Make the first cut at the level of the temporal tips. This marks the anterior walls of the anterior horns of the lateral ventricles, and if hydrocephalus of these structures is present, it is seen at this time. Cuts at 0.5-cm intervals in both directions can be accomplished with experience, the sections laid out, and abnormalities searched for, reviewing normal anatomy at the same time. If the brain is softened for any reason or if there is massive hemorrhage, thicker sections are necessary to avoid disrupting the anatomy and allow identification of the extent and type of abnormality.

It is most important to establish some local norm for laying out the brain so as not to have right-left confusion. Many

prefer to follow the radiologic norm and lay out the sections as if the observer were looking at the patient, with sides reversed relative to the observer. We prefer the reverse, with the brain laid out with the posterior aspect of the sections toward us so that our right and that of the cut brain are on the same side (Fig. 4-47). It is important that a local norm be set so that incorrect side identification is minimized.

At this time, the gross abnormalities should all be identified, their anatomic location and extent agreed upon, and their characteristics described. A differential diagnosis, preferably with causal relationships to the general autopsy, should be arrived at. Appropriate sections can then be cut for histologic preparation and examination (see Chapter 8). Before this, photographic documentation should be obtained as appropriate.

Other means of gross cutting may be necessary for particular purposes. It is important to do the necessary homework before such cutting to make yourself familiar with the anatomic landmarks. Such variant cutting modes may be used, for example, for correlation with computed tomographic or magnetic resonance imaging cuts of the cerebrum (but be careful; even longer knives are necessary for such horizontal cuts); for demonstration of midline abnormalities (e.g., Chiari type II [Arnold-Chiari] malformation or pineal area tumors), often better demonstrated with a midsagittal cut of the entire brain; or for special purposes such as demonstrating anatomic fiber tracts using parasagittal or steep angular cuts.

## EXAMINATION OF THE VERTEBRAL COLUMN AND BONE MARROW

The vertebral column, removed to expose the spinal cord, is sawed in half using a band saw or large meat saw. Examine the appearance of the intervertebral joints and vertebral marrow, and test the degree of ossification of the vertebral bodies by compressing them under your thumb. Using a hammer and bone knife, obtain a thin (1 cm or less) section of bone for decalcification and histology. Never use the vibrating saw because it introduces a great deal of bone dust into the specimen. Process the bone as described in Chapter 8. If the patient suffered from a hematologic disease, take samples of femoral (Fig. 4-48) or rib bone marrow, or both, because these do not require decalcification.

## A FINAL WORD ABOUT EXAMINING ORGANS

Clearly, sharp scissors and knives help the prosector in his or her task. However, several suggestions may help those who are inexperienced. When slicing organs with a knife, start at the heel of the knife blade and carry the cut as far through the organ as possible to avoid excessive saw marks. Longer blades are an advantage here, too. Inexperienced prosectors tend to compress organs downward with their nondominant hand in an attempt to stabilize the organ during the cutting process. Doing so has the added effect of compressing the knife blade as it tries to move through the tissue. Rather, direct the stabilizing force somewhat more against the direction of the knife cut. Some pathologists advocate leaving a tag or hinge of tissue at

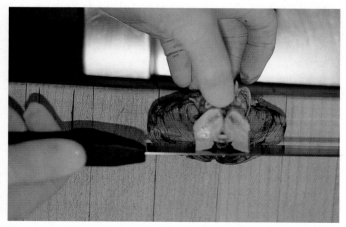

**Figure 4-46** Cutting the cerebellum and brainstem. The initial cut is vertical, made through the cerebellum just behind the midbrain and just missing the medulla oblongata so as to demonstrate the vascular distributions of the cerebellar arteries. Gentle posterior traction on the medulla oblongata and a thick cutting board help make this an easy operation.

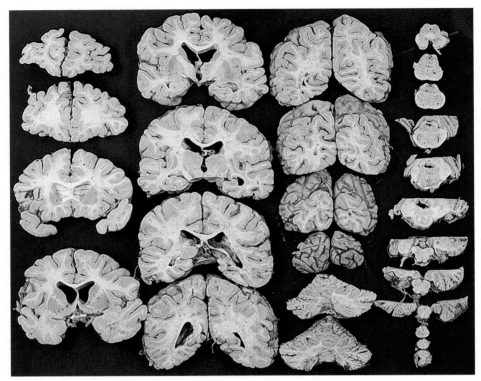

**Figure 4-47** The brain displayed for examination and microscopic sampling.

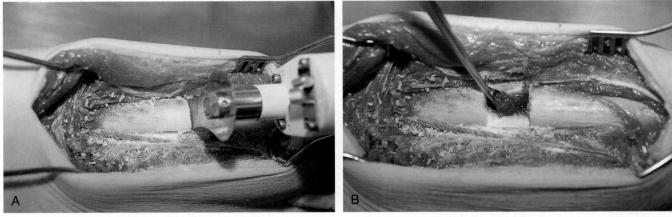

**Figure 4-48** Sampling the femoral bone marrow. **A,** The anterior aspect of the femur is exposed and the surrounding tissues are retracted with self-retaining retractors. A rectangular portion of the anterior femur is removed. **B,** The exposed bone marrow is collected with a curette.

the end of each slice to maintain the organ slices in anatomic position. We find this unnecessary, and it constrains examination and discourages photography. When using scissors, make cuts neatly. By not completely closing the blades of the scissors in a snip before advancing the scissors for the next cut, a smoother, less jagged cut is obtained. Also, use the proper scissors for the job at hand. Blades of different sizes and types (straight, curved, or enterotome) each have their ideal purpose.

Weigh organs accurately after first removing excess fat and tissue (such as long vascular segments). When cutting an organ, know and keep its proper orientation. Do not cut through a twisted or disoriented organ or organ block. Organ dissection includes removing obscuring tissues before making final cuts. For example, do not try to cut a heart covered with adherent pericardium. Take a few moments to prepare the specimen. It is then easier to dissect the specimen accurately, and you are rewarded with a fine specimen for demonstration or photography. Finally, when examining the cut surface of an organ, rinsing excess blood from the surface aids in distinguishing the more subtle findings.

# REFERENCES

1. Virchow R: *Description and explanation of the method of performing post-mortem examinations in the dead house of the Berlin Charite Hospital, with especial reference to medico-legal practice*, London, 1880, Churchill (Translated from the second German edition by TP Smith).

2. Weber DL, Fazzini EP, Reagan TJ: *Autopsy pathology procedure and protocol*, Springfield, Ill, 1973, Charles C Thomas.

3. Mallory FB: *A practical manual for workers in pathological histology including directions for the performance of autopsies and for microphotography*, Philadelphia, 1938, WB Saunders.

4. Wilson RR: *Methods in morbid anatomy*, New York, 1972, Appleton-Century-Crofts.

5. Gresham GA, Turner AF: *Post-mortem procedures*, Chicago, 1979, Year Book Medical.

6. Letulle MEJL: *La pratique des autopsies*, Paris, 1903, C Naud.

7. Saphir O: *Autopsy diagnosis and technic*, ed 4, New York, 1958, Hoeber-Harper.

8. Baker RD: *Postmortem examination: Specific methods and procedures*, Philadelphia, 1967, WB Saunders.

9. Chiari H: *Pathologisch-Anatomische Sektionstechnik*, Berlin, 1894, H Kornfeld.

10. Culora GA, Roche WR: Simple method for necropsy dissection of the abdominal organs after abdominal surgery, *J Clin Pathol* 49:776-779, 1996.

11. Shimuzu M, Sakurai T, Tadaoka Y: A simple technique for identifying the adrenal glands at necropsy, *J Clin Pathol* 50:263-264, 1997.

12. Finkbeiner WE: Morphological procedures in respiratory anatomy and pathology. In Gold W, Murray J, Nadel J, editors: *Atlas of procedures in respiratory medicine*, Philadelphia, 2002, WB Saunders, pp 1-34.

13. McCulloch TA, Rutty GN: Postmortem examination of the lungs: A preservation technique for opening the bronchi and pulmonary arteries individually without transection problems, *J Clin Pathol* 51:163-164, 1998.

14. Gresham GA: The tubule plucking test for testicular atrophy, *Arch Pathol* 64:63-66, 1957.

# 5

# Postmortem Examination of Fetuses and Infants

*"Accuracy of observation, completeness of detail, and sound conclusions can be obtained only when the post-mortem examination is made according to some definite and systematic plan so that regions and organs are successively examined without disturbing the relations and appearances yet to be investigated."*

Ludvig Hektoen[1]

The autopsy of the fetus, infant, or young child should be approached somewhat differently from that of the adult. At these developmental stages, the presence of malformations is often the major consideration, and the dissection should be made to preserve anatomic relationships in order to define the abnormal anatomy. Thus, organs are usually left together en bloc. This does not mean that there is less dissection than in the adult; on the contrary, dissections to investigate the anatomy on a small scale are usually quite detailed and tedious. The general pathologist who does occasional postmortem examinations on fetuses and infants, therefore, should have a good working knowledge of normal anatomy—enough so that he or she is able to recognize the abnormal and preserve the anatomic relationships until a consultation can be obtained if necessary.

## FACILITIES AND EQUIPMENT

The standard autopsy suite used for postmortem examinations of adults should be adequate for pediatric autopsies. Access to a photography setup and a specimen X-ray machine must be available. The entire body of the fetus or small infant can be placed on an elevated dissection table to bring the work area up to chest level. Good lighting is essential; a portable operating room spot to light the field works well. In addition to a standard kilogram scale and linear measuring device, a gram-milligram scale, a flexible ruler, and a tape measure are necessary. Instruments of appropriate scale for the size of the body include round-tip and pointed small scissors, scalpel, forceps, and probes. Regarding the latter, a woman's hairpin of small caliber that has been straightened makes a fine probe for very small structures provided one is careful with the relatively sharp end. A magnifying glass is necessary, and a dissecting microscope may be useful in some cases.

## POSTMORTEM EXAMINATION

The following section details a protocol that is useful in a postmortem examination of a fetus or infant. Although generally applicable, the protocol may have to be tailored for certain cases with unusual anomalies. The various measurements and observation are used to document either normal anatomy or various pathologic conditions (listed in Appendix A and described in standard texts), which will not be presented here. Further information regarding how to perform an autopsy of a fetus or infant can be found in standard texts[2-4] or numerous articles on the topic.

A proper postmortem examination is always documented with photographs. Photographs of the external features are routine: Frontal pictures of the entire body and closeups of the face and side of the head, as well as any other unusual aspects, should be taken before the autopsy commences. Photographs provide an accurate record, not only for future conferences but also for the occasional case in which review of the gross and histologic findings prompts a reevaluation of the external features. Similarly, photographs should be made of any major abnormality encountered in the evisceration and dissection.

Whole-body radiographs (anteroposterior and lateral) are routine in stillborn infants and in neonates who have not been examined radiographically during life; close-up views of abnormal features may also be appropriate. In many instances skeletal abnormalities identified in radiographs provide the first clue to a malformation complex or syndrome, and in some cases radiographs provide data supporting a particular diagnosis. Although the literature is replete with articles describing various radiographic abnormalities in fetuses and infants,[5] consulting colleagues in radiology can be extremely helpful in correctly identifying the lesions.

Many fetuses and neonates present a dysmorphic appearance that heralds a syndrome. In addition to pictures, the abnormal features may be documented through measurements of certain structures that can be compared with reference standards. For this reason these autopsies require additional linear measurements using a tape measure, as described later. In many cases consultation by a geneticist is useful.

Maceration (organ softening due to decomposition) is a confounding problem in fetuses that have been retained in utero following fetal demise. The degree of autolysis is variable depending upon intrauterine conditions. Nevertheless, sequential gross and microscopic changes help one estimate the time of death (Table 5-1).[6-8] Following delivery, the autolytic process can progress at room temperature but is slowed considerably by refrigeration of the body. Thus, in cases of perinatal death, the delivery room staff can assist the pathologist by putting the body in the refrigerator as soon after delivery as possible. Despite deformation due to maceration, many malformations may be discerned upon careful inspection. Linear measurements and weights may be artifacted, however, and histologic results are usually suboptimal.

## EXTERNAL EXAMINATION

Some indication of the degree of autolysis should be given to frame the context of the postmortem examination. We use a rough index that may be helpful to the clinician: mild (skin sloughing only), moderate (skin sloughing and organ softening), and marked (skin sloughing, organ softening, and joint laxity) maceration. The external examination of the fetus or infant includes measurements of head, chest, and abdominal circumferences, as well as length (crown-rump, crown-heel, and foot for fetuses) and weight of the body. Abnormal body parts should also be measured. The positions of penetrating tubes and wires are recorded. The distribution and quality of hair over the head and rest of the body are noted. The fontanelle dimensions are measured. Abnormalities of the shape of the head related to molding, trauma, soft tissue edema, hemorrhage, or autolysis are noted; the basis for these changes may be investigated later. The facial features are examined and abnormalities recorded. The distances between inner and outer canthi are measured. These and other common facial measurements are shown in Figure 5-1. If the palpebral fissures can be opened, the color of the sclera and iris and relative sizes of the pupils are recorded. The color of the conjunctiva is noted. By late intrauterine development, the crest of the external ear should be superior to the level of the lateral canthus. The configuration of the ear is examined and plasticity (indicating amount of cartilage) evaluated as an index to developmental stage (Fig. 5-2). Patency of each external auditory canal should be ascertained. The position and shape of the nose are noted; patency of the choanae should be determined by probing. The configuration of the philtrum and mouth are observed, and the philtrum length and mouth width are measured (see Fig. 5-1). Examination of the oral cavity consists of digital palpation of the palate and direct observation of the gingiva.

| Table 5-1 | Timing of death in autopsies of stillborn infants* | |
|---|---|---|
| **Elapsed time** | **Gross findings** | **Microscopic findings** |
| ≥4 hours | | Kidney: loss of cortical tubular nuclei basophilia |
| ≥6 hours | Desquamation ≥1 cm Brown or red umbilical cord discoloration* | Placenta: intravascular karyorrhexis |
| ≥12 hours | Desquamation of face, back, or abdomen | |
| ≥18 hours | Desquamation over ≥5% of body or 2 or more of 11 body zones† | Lung: bronchial mucosal epithelial detachment* |
| ≥24 hours | Skin color brown or tan* Moderate desquamation* | Liver: loss of hepatocyte nuclear basophilia Heart: loss of nuclear basophilia on inner half of myocardium |
| ≥36 hours | Cranial compression* | Pancreas: maximal loss of nuclear basophilia‡ |
| ≥48 hours | Desquamation over 10% of body* | Heart: loss of nuclear basophilia on outer half of myocardium Placenta: multifocal stem vessel luminal abnormalities |
| ≥72 hours | Desquamation over 75% of body* | Gastrointestinal tract: transmural bowel wall loss of nuclear basophilia |
| ≥96 hours | Overlapping cranial sutures | Liver: loss of nuclear basophilia in all liver cells Bronchus: loss of epithelial nuclear basophilia |
| ≥1 week | Widely open mouth* | Gastrointestinal tract: maximal loss of nuclear basophilia Adrenal: maximal loss of nuclear basophilia |
| ≥2 weeks | Mummification (any) | Placenta: extensive stem vessel luminal abnormalities; extensive villous fibrosis |
| >4 weeks | | Kidney: maximal loss of nuclear basophilia |

*Intermediate to poor predictor.
†Scalp, face, neck, chest, abdomen, back, arms, hand, leg, foot, and scrotum.
‡Intermediate predictor.
Modified from Genest DR, Williams MA, Greene MF: Estimating the time of death in stillborn fetuses: I. Histologic evaluation of fetal organs; an autopsy study of 150 stillborns, *Obstet Gynecol* 80:575-584, 1992; Genest DR: Estimating the time of death in stillborn fetuses: II. Histologic evaluation of the placenta; a study of 71 stillborns, *Obstet Gynecol* 80:585-592, 1992; and Genest DR, Singer DB: Estimating the time of death in stillborn fetuses: III. External fetal examination; a study of 86 stillborns, *Obstet Gynecol* 80:593-600, 1992.

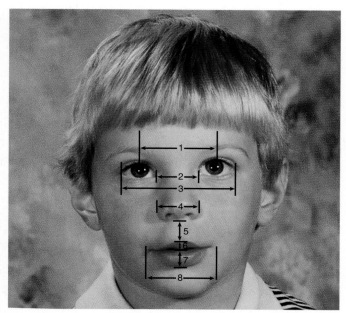

**Figure 5-1** Common facial measurements. *1,* Interpupillary distance; *2,* inner canthal distance; *3,* outer canthal distance; *4,* interalar distance; *5,* philtral length; *6,* upper lip thickness; *7,* lower lip thickness; *8,* intercommissural distance.

The position of the trachea and thyroid within the neck is palpated. Symmetry or abnormal shape of the thorax is noted. The separation of the nipples is recorded and the presence of any mammary tissue determined. The amount of subcutaneous tissue over the chest and abdomen is noted. The shape of the abdomen is noted. The liver and spleen are palpated to determine approximate size; abnormal masses are noted. Lymphadenopathy or hemorrhage at a catheter access site may be palpable in the inguinal areas. The genitalia are inspected. The contents of the bladder may be gently expressed (Credé method) to document urethral patency. In boys, the position of the meatus is determined and scrotal contents assessed. In girls, the position of the meatus and configuration and relative size of the labia and clitoris are observed. The perineal area is inspected and the anal opening probed to document patency. The back of the body is examined for midline defects or discoloration of the skin.

The extremities must be examined for muscle bulk, as well as symmetry and configuration. The mobility of the joints should be evaluated, as well as possible, and the amount and distribution of the skin and subcutaneous tissues around joints noted. The position of the hands and feet, as well as the fingers must be noted. The appearance of each digit must be considered, including the number of phalanges and their form, as well as the shape and length of the nails; the hand length and foot length should be recorded. The palmar and plantar markings should be observed.

## INTERNAL EXAMINATION AND EVISCERATION

After completion of the external examination, a standard Y-shaped incision is made, and a smaller connecting incision on the other side of the umbilicus is made to isolate this structure in the fetus and neonate. The skin and subcutaneous tissue are reflected off the thorax and abdomen. When suspected, pneumothorax may be evaluated either by immersing the body in a basin of water and observing bubbles escaping from a small intercostal incision or by aspirating the air in a water-containing syringe. The body may have to be rotated to move the air bubble to the opening in the thoracic wall. The peritoneal cavity is opened with a pair of scissors. The intestines in situ may be injected with formalin for preemptive fixation in cases in which mucosal damage is suspected. For this purpose, a tie is placed tightly around the proximal jejunum and another around the upper rectum and formalin gently injected by syringe from both ends. The abdominal contents should then remain undisturbed until the chest and neck have been dissected. The breast plate is removed by cutting through the cartilaginous portion of the ribs at the

**Figure 5-2** Anatomic landmarks of the external ear.

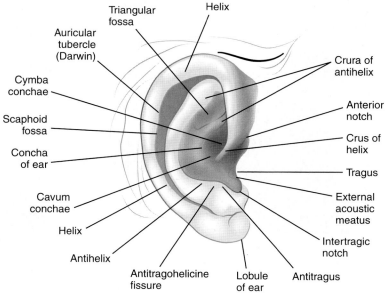

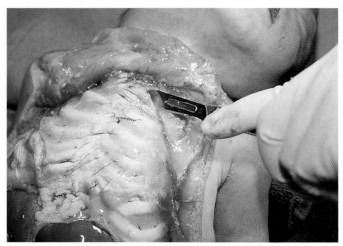

**Figure 5-3** Opening the thorax. With the neck and shoulders elevated by a towel roll and the bone landmarks exposed, incise each rib cartilage at the costochondral junction to provide a generous opening.

costochondral junction (Fig. 5-3). Fluid contents of the pleural cavities should be measured or at least estimated as accurately as possible. The thymus should be carefully dissected off the pericardium: elevating the thymus off the mediastinum, cut against the thymus and let the pericardial sac fall back into the thorax (Fig. 5-4). This approach minimizes the risk of cutting the brachiocephalic vein just behind the thymus. Before any vessels are cut, the pericardial sac should be opened; the free parietal pericardium then can be trimmed.

To facilitate the neck dissection, the shoulders should be placed on a block (or, for small bodies, a towel roll) with the neck somewhat hyperextended, and the skin incision should be carried almost to the acromial process. The relative positions of the great arteries as they arise from the heart should be noted. The large veins and arteries of the neck should then be carefully dissected and identified starting at the heart (Fig. 5-5). These vessels should not be cut until all have been identified correctly. Reflect the left lung completely out of the hemithorax, observe the shape of the lobes, and establish that the thoracic portion of the aorta courses along the left side of the vertebral column. By reflecting the apex of the heart toward the right shoulder (Fig. 5-6), check the connections of the pulmonary veins between the left lung and left atrium; with the heart back in anatomic position, the right pulmonary veins can be seen in the window between the superior vena cava and pericardium if the parietal pericardium is retracted rightward (Fig. 5-7). Reflecting the right lung out of the thorax enables complete inspection of the lobes.

The positions of the abdominal organs should be inspected in situ. In fetuses and young infants the liver is relatively large, extending well across the midline. Marked by the gallbladder, the right hepatic lobe should be in the right upper quadrant. Check that there is a solitary spleen in the left upper quadrant, lateral to the stomach. By the second trimester, the cecum and appendix should be fixed to the posterior peritoneum in the

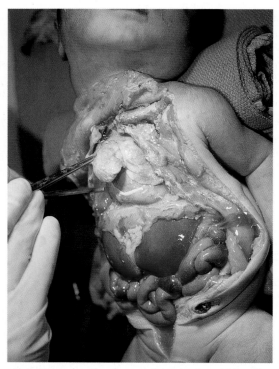

**Figure 5-4** Removing the thymus. In order to avoid cutting the brachiocephalic vein just behind the thymus, lift the thymus away from the mediastinum as you cut against the thymus. The intact brachiocephalic vein and pericardial sac will fall back into the thorax.

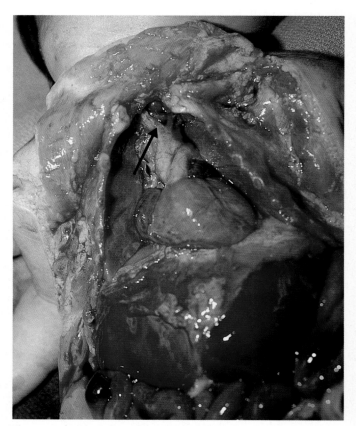

**Figure 5-5** Dissection of the aortic arch in situ. The pericardium is removed in order to dissect the great arteries. The branches *(arrow)* of the aortic arch should be dissected enough to define the anatomy and exclude anomalies.

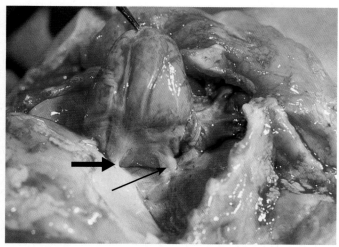

**Figure 5-6** Checking the connection between the left pulmonary veins and the heart. With the apex of the heart reflected toward the right shoulder, trace the left pulmonary veins *(thin arrow)* from the left lung to the left atrium. The inferior caval vein *(thick arrow)* is present in the middle of the inferior (diaphragmatic) surface.

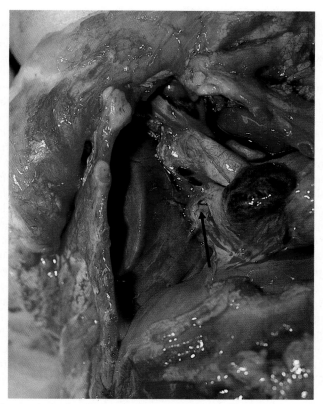

**Figure 5-7** Visualizing the right pulmonary veins. With the heart back in correct anatomic position, the right pulmonary veins *(arrow)* can be seen in the groove between the superior caval vein and the parietal pericardium that has been gently retracted. The position of the right pulmonary veins behind the heart is difficult to see until the heart-lung block is removed.

right lower quadrant. While the small intestines are reflected, identify the positions of the kidneys and adrenal glands in the retroperitoneum on each side. The gonads should be located and, in females, the shape and position of the uterus between the bladder and rectum ascertained. For premature

males, intraabdominal testes should be removed before evisceration. The umbilical arteries can be identified coursing along either side of the bladder.

When the positions of the organs have been determined, the organs can be eviscerated in anatomically related groups (Ghon method) or all together en bloc (Letulle method). The entire block from tongue to rectum can be removed, as in adults (see Chapters 4 and 6).

## SEPARATION OF THE ORGAN BLOCKS

Following evisceration by the Letulle method, the entire block can be rinsed and the table cleaned in preparation for separation of the organ blocks. One disadvantage of the approach to be described is that the weight of certain organs may be impossible to determine accurately. In developmental pathology, the importance of preserving anatomic relationships sometimes outweighs the usefulness of knowing the organ weight. For example, the heart with cardiac defects is often hypertrophied, but the heart-lung block is usually of greater educational value when left intact. In these instances, cardiac hypertrophy can be documented in other ways (e.g., wall thickness, histologic appearance of the myocardial cells). Thus, the prosector should record the weights of the organs that can be reasonably isolated; later, these data are compared with reference values for a similar developmental stage (see Appendix B).

The dorsal (posterior) aspect of the block is examined first. The inferior caval vein should be opened to identify thrombi; if either kidney appears congested, the venous dissection should be carried into the renal vein on the same side. The descending aorta can also be opened along its posterior aspect (Fig. 5-8). While viewing this aspect, reflect the diaphragm, identify the adrenal glands, and remove them. These organs should be weighed and cut in cross section before fixation.

Turn the block of organs back to view the ventral (anterior) aspect. Cut the inferior caval vein, esophagus, and aorta at the level of the diaphragm to remove the heart and lungs from the rest of the block. Different from the method of dissecting adult organs, this approach maintains the relationship of the pulmonary arteries, arterial duct (i.e., *ductus arteriosus*), and aortic arch to the heart, as well as the esophagus to the trachea. Set this block aside for consideration later.

Isolate the bowel with ligatures or clamps and remove the gut at the mesenteric attachment from the ligament of Treitz to the upper rectum, leaving a short segment of rectum with the bladder-uterus. Although the full length of the gut is examined for malformations, the intestines of fetuses need not be opened unless a pathologic condition is suspected. For liveborns, if not done already, the bowel can be injected with formalin and immersed in fixative to improve preservation in cases of putative mucosal damage. Alternatively, the fresh bowel may be opened longitudinally and placed in fixative. The lengths of the small and large intestines may be recorded. Check the patency of the biliary tree by viewing the opened duodenum over the segment where the ampulla of Vater is located and manually expressing bile from the

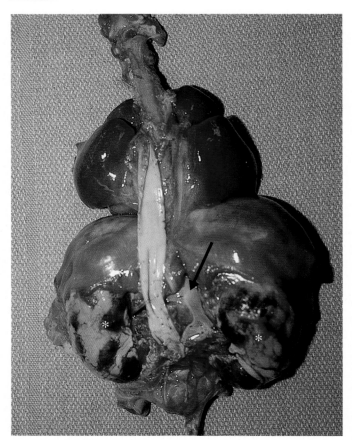

**Figure 5-8** Complete block following evisceration by the Letulle method. Viewed from behind (posterior aspect), the block shows the opened descending aorta and the kidneys *(*)* as well as the inferior caval vein *(arrow)*. If renal vein thrombosis is suspected, the inferior caval vein should be opened before the aorta and the renal vein are sectioned.

gallbladder. Dissect the extrahepatic bile ducts if indicated. The gallbladder can be dissected off the liver. Reflect the abdominal aorta away from the diaphragm, and keep it with the genitourinary block. Separate the liver from the diaphragm, and remove the liver separately. Separate the spleen from the block, paying attention to locate the tail of the pancreas. The descending abdominal aorta can be reflected to stay with the genitourinary block. Cut the remnant of distal esophagus from the diaphragm, and remove the gastrointestinal block together with the spleen. The gastrointestinal block consists of the gastroesophageal junction, stomach, duodenum, and pancreas. The diaphragm remains as a separate muscular sheet.

The kidneys, ureters, bladder, urethra, and rectum are removed en bloc together with the descending abdominal aorta. In females, this includes the internal reproductive organs. The navel is excised in a rhomboid form, including both umbilical arteries and the umbilical vein. The abdominal aorta with the iliac arteries are kept with the genitourinary block.

The testes are removed through the inguinal ring. Bone samples are taken from the costochondral junction of the ribs and from the vertebral column. A full-thickness piece of skin and subcutaneous tissue is placed in fixative. Representative

samples of femoral nerve and psoas muscle are also taken routinely. However, more extensive sampling of muscle from the proximal and distal limbs should be made in cases of suspected skeletal myopathy and neuromuscular disorders.

## DISSECTION OF ORGANS AFTER EVISCERATION

A pathologic condition in the heart is always easier to visualize when the chambers are distended to physiologic volumes. For this reason, hearts with suspected cardiovascular malformations should be perfused with formalin overnight before dissection (see Chapter 6). Because the lungs still are attached at this point, they must be perfused too. Alternatively, if there is no suspected cardiovascular malformation, or if a pathologic condition in the lung is anticipated, the fresh heart is dissected along the lines of blood flow first (see later) to confirm that there is no malformation, and then the lungs are disconnected, weighed, and fixed. Whether fixed or fresh, the neck organs are dissected while still in continuity with the heart-lung block. The esophagus is opened posteriorly and the trachea and larynx anteriorly, thus preserving any tracheoesophageal abnormality. The relationship of the great arteries is confirmed. The anterior and posterior descending coronary arteries are landmarks delimiting the interventricular septum.

While still connected to the block, the heart is opened along the lines of normal blood flow.[9] The right atrium is opened by a separate long-axis incision inferiorly (along the diaphragmatic surface), lateral to and avoiding the orifice of the inferior caval vein; the incision can be carried into the superior caval vein to open the atrium more completely. This inferior approach allows inspection of the ostium of the coronary sinus and the oval fossa and the tricuspid valve. Using the probe, check the patency of the connection between the atrium and the right-sided ventricle. The ventricle should be opened by continuing the atrial incision through the atrioventricular valve and into the ventricle along the inferior aspect, parallel to the interventricular groove (posterior descending coronary artery), to the apex. After turning the specimen back to the anterior aspect, the right ventricle is probed gently to check that the pulmonic valve is patent and the outflow tract opened by continuing the same incision from the apex into the main pulmonary artery. On this anterior surface of the heart, the anterior descending coronary artery denotes the septum and should not be cut across. The left pulmonary artery is opened into the hilum of the left lung. The arterial duct is also opened completely into the descending aorta.

Back on the inferior aspect of the heart, the left atrium should be entered through a separate Y-shaped incision showing the connection of the pulmonary veins with the left atrial cavity and exposing the mitral orifice. After the orifice is probed, the incision should be carried along the inferior surface through the valve and the left ventricle to the apex, again parallel to the ventricular septum. On the anterior aspect the left ventricular outflow tract should be opened by continuing the incision along the septum (using the anterior descending coronary artery as a landmark) toward the base, stopping at a point under the left atrial appendage. At this

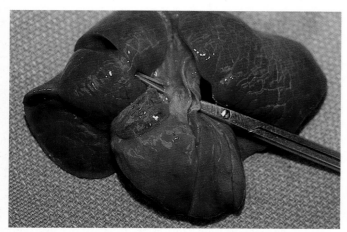

**Figure 5-9** Dissection of the left ventricular outflow tract. The relationship between the great arteries is preserved by cutting behind the main pulmonary artery, not across it. The ligamentous connections between the roots of the great arteries are bluntly dissected to create a window between the vessels (position of the scissors). When one blade of the scissors is within the left ventricular outflow tract and one blade is in the dissected channel between the great arteries, only the aortic valve and proximal ascending aorta will be cut.

juncture, the objective of preserving the relationship between the great arteries necessitates a special approach (Fig. 5-9). In order to incise the aorta *without* cutting across the pulmonary artery, the fibrous junction between aorta and pulmonary artery must be separated down to the vessel roots. When this dissection is complete, one blade of the scissors may be placed across the aortic valve into the aorta while the other blade rests in the dissected space or "tunnel" between the great arteries. Make sure that the blade between the vessels is positioned adjacent to the ascending aorta before making the single cut to the tip of the scissors. Take the scissors out and continue the incision along the anterior aspect of the ascending aorta, through the isthmus and into the descending aorta.

For histologic examination, one section from each side of the heart, including atrium, ventricle, atrioventricular valve, and coronary artery, should be taken along the inferior incisions; papillary muscle sections should also be submitted from the right and left ventricles. In cases with cardiac defects, the heart is kept together with the lungs en bloc and sections for histology taken judiciously so as to not destroy the educational value of the gross specimen.

It follows that the prosector should *not* separate lungs from heart until normal anatomy has been confirmed. Once separated and weighed, the fresh lungs (including pleural surfaces) should be inspected and gently perfused with formalin to physiologic volume. This may be accomplished manually or by a perfusion apparatus. Alternatively, each of the lobes of one fresh lung may be scored and then fixed by immersion. One section of each lung for fetuses or one section of each lobe of lung for infants and children is routinely taken for histologic examination, with additional sections as needed.

The liver and spleen should not be sliced in the short axis. Rather, both organs should be cut in half in a long-axis plane parallel to their inferior surfaces, thereby preserving the major

vessels (in the liver) and the hilum (in the spleen). The vessels on the undersurface of the liver (umbilical vein, portal sinus and venous duct [i.e., ductus venosus]) should be opened longitudinally in the fetus and neonate. For histology, submit one section from the spleen and each lobe of liver. In fetuses and neonates younger than 1 day of age, the stomach is left unopened (to retain evidence of chorioamnionitis) and the whole block fixed intact. Following fixation, the entire stomach, cut into short axis rings, is submitted for histologic examination. In infants older than 1 day of age, open the stomach and duodenum before fixing in formalin. If obscured by mucus, the mucosa may be washed gently with water or dilute acetic acid. The pancreas should be cut in half longitudinally and one half submitted for histologic examination. To preserve the generative glomeruli, the capsule of the kidney should not be stripped in the fetus or infant. Each kidney should be hemisected completely and the collecting systems opened. Sections of each kidney should include cortex, medulla, and collecting system. Each ureter should be opened or at least probed to document patency. The bladder should be opened. For histologic examination, there should be one longitudinal section through the anterior wall of the bladder and a transverse section through the prostate at the verumontanum. In female fetuses and neonates with normal anatomy, a sagittal section through the posterior wall of the bladder, uterus-cervix, and anterior wall of the rectum is often possible. One ovary should be cut longitudinally and one in cross section to include Fallopian tubes for histologic examination. The testes should be hemisected and one half submitted for histologic examination.

A portion of one rib cut longitudinally through the costochondral junction and one of vertebral column to show several vertebral bodies should be fixed, decalcified, and submitted for histologic examination. The psoas muscle is fixed well before a cross section and a longitudinal section are submitted. A section of pituitary for histologic examination should include both the anterior and posterior lobes. The umbilicus is dissected so that both umbilical arteries in cross section can be included in one section and the umbilical vein in longitudinal section in another if inflammation is suspected.

## BRAIN AND SPINAL CORD REMOVAL AND EXAMINATION

As in the adult, the goal of the removal of the brain and other cranial contents is to produce minimal distortion and artifact, enabling a careful examination and diagnosis. As described in Chapter 4, the great majority of older children's brains can be removed in a manner identical to those of adults. In fetuses and infants, once the galea has been retracted forward and backward to expose the skull, the fontanelles may be measured. In these younger age groups, although the scalp incision and dissections are the same, prior to fusion of the sutures, the bony plates of the skull can be separated by sharp dissection and retracted in a "butterfly" manner (Fig. 5-10). Further, suspected posterior fossa and cervical cord lesions may be explored by a posterior approach, as described in detail by Gilles.[10] This method is superb for demonstration of posterior fossa abnormalities, but it takes additional time.

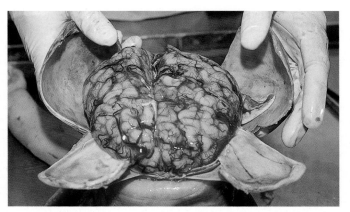

**Figure 5-10** Brain removal in infants and fetuses. Before skull ossification and suture closure is complete, the fontanelles can be separated, allowing access to the anterior and middle cranial fossae.

In newborn infants in whom sagittal sinus trauma or developmental abnormalities are suspected, the following approach preserves the critical anatomy: To preserve the superior sagittal sinus, a scalpel is used to incise the dura at the lateral angles of the anterior fontanelle. The two small incisions allow access for a pair of heavy-duty scissors to cut through bone parallel to and approximately 1 cm lateral on both sides of the midline, preserving the superior sagittal sinus between (Fig. 5-11, A). Each of these incisions is continued anteriorly and posteriorly (into frontal and occipital bones) and laterally (into the parietal bones) to create two large bone flaps, each on a "hinge" of uncut parietal bone inferiorly. After carefully inspecting the hemispheres, falx cerebri, and tentorium cerebelli through the openings, remove the midline bone and sinus (Fig. 5-11, B). Make sure that your gloves are wet before touching the brain. Fully reflect the flaps to maximize the opening, and let the occiput rest on the autopsy table. Use a

pair of scissors to release the attachments of the falx and tentorium. The cranial nerves are cut as described for the adult. As these cuts are made, the prosector must use a hand to support the brain as it slowly falls out of the cranial cavity. With the brainstem in view, transect the spinal cord as far down as possible. If the tissue is autolyzed, the soft brain may have to be eased directly into the container of formaldehyde and weighed after fixation. Alternately, with very soft fetal or infant brains, their removal from the skull can be accomplished under water, allowing flotation of the delicate brain out of the skull until separation through the low brainstem–cervical cord is achieved. The floating brain can be eased into a container for fixation. Support during fixation can be greatly enhanced by the "salting" technique described in Chapter 8.

After adequate fixation, the brain is inspected and cut, largely as described for the adult brain (see Chapter 4). Briefly, the cerebral hemispheres are separated from the brainstem and cerebellum with a scalpel. The cerebral convexities are placed down on a cutting board, and, with a long knife, serial coronal slices (approximately 1 cm thick) are made starting from the frontal tip and finishing with the occipital pole. The thickness of the cuts may need to be increased for brains that are soft and friable. Coronal cuts of the cerebellum and spinal cord complete the dissection (Fig. 5-12).

The removal of the fetal and neonatal spinal cord from either the anterior or posterior approach is essentially the same as described for the adult (see Chapter 4). However, a scalpel, heavy-duty scissors, and bone cutters substitute for the vibrating saw in these dissections. Again, the posterior approach to the brain and spinal canal is superior for the demonstration of posterior fossa and cervical cord lesions (Fig. 5-13).

Special procedures, such as removal of the temporal bone for examination and culture of the middle ear cavity, are presented in Chapter 6.

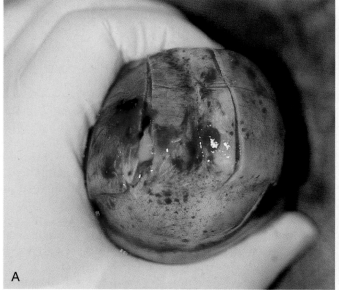

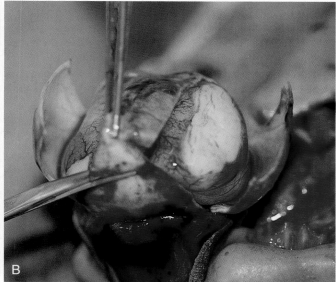

**Figure 5-11** Brain removal in infants and fetuses (examination of the sagittal sinus). **A,** The skull bone, parallel to and approximately 1 cm lateral on both sides of the midline, preserves the superior sagittal sinus between. **B,** After carefully inspecting the hemispheres, falx cerebri, and tentorium cerebelli through the openings, the midline bone and sinus are removed.

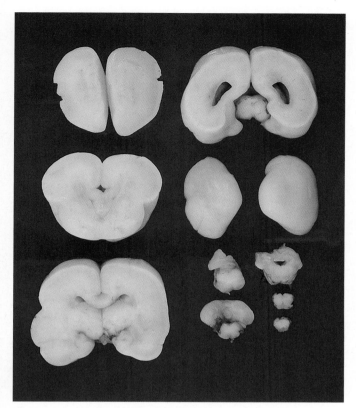

**Figure 5-12** Following fixation, fetal brain slices are displayed for examination and sampling for histology.

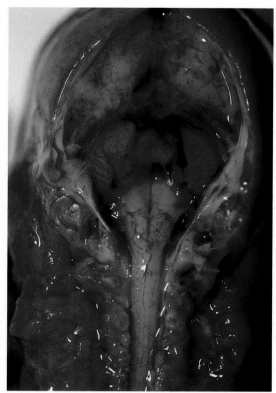

**Figure 5-13** In a fetus with Dandy-Walker malformation, the posterior cranium has been removed and the spinal canal opened from the posterior aspect to expose the contents of the posterior fossa and spinal canal. The hypoplastic cerebellum and dilated fourth ventricle, as well as the medulla and cervical and upper thoracic portions of the spinal cord, are readily visible.

## EXAMINATION OF THE PLACENTA

The examination of the placenta is an important part of the fetal and neonatal autopsy.[11] The length of the umbilical cord is measured and any unusual features of the cord (discoloration, abnormal spiraling, true knots) noted. The number of vessels is ascertained. The insertion of the cord into the placenta is examined. The membranes are carefully examined for discoloration, clumps of squamous cells, or bands. The distance of the sac opening from the placenta is noted. For multiple pregnancies, examine the membranes and vessels carefully and submit histologic sections that will allow assessment of zygosity. The membranes and cord are trimmed, and the placenta is weighed and measured. The fetal surface and its branching vessels are examined. The maternal surface is inspected for completeness of the cotyledons and excessive clot. From the maternal surface the placenta is cut serially in cross section to document infarcts, and an estimate of the amount of placenta involved by infarct should be made. A section of cord, membrane roll, and representative sections of placenta that include both decidual and fetal surfaces are submitted for histologic examination.

## EXAMINATION OF THE FRAGMENTED FETUS

Dilation and evacuation specimens consist of fragmented fetal parts and placenta. In the vast majority of these specimens anomalies are not present and a cursory surgical pathology examination is customary. However, when the procedure is performed for anomalies diagnosed prenatally, or when anomalies are unexpectedly observed in the grossing room during routine surgical pathology examination, a detailed autopsy-like examination is indicated. A systematic approach to these specimens will confirm, clarify, extend, or perhaps contradict the prenatal diagnostic studies. In fetuses or neonates with congenital anomalies that were unsuspected, the diagnoses may indicate the need for genetic counseling and specialized prenatal studies in subsequent pregnancies.

We perform these detailed fragmented fetal examinations in the autopsy suite using an approach as similar as possible to a fetal autopsy. First, the tissues and organs are laid out on a dissecting board in a manner approximating an intact fetus. Whenever possible, observations and measurements of external features are made. Complete organs are weighed or measured. Normal or abnormal anatomy, including that seen in the placenta, membranes, and umbilical cord, is described in a format similar to a regular fetal autopsy (see Appendix A). As in fetal autopsies, a dissecting microscope may be quite useful. An overview photograph and photographs of specific anomalies are taken as needed to demonstrate the gross findings. Radiographs are obtained in cases in which skeletal anomalies are in question. Microscopic examination is guided by available tissues and gross findings. If not already done, samples should be collected for any indicated supplemental laboratory studies such as chromosome analysis.

## CONCLUSION

The postmortem examination of the fetus, infant, or young child requires a sound knowledge of normal anatomy and a consistent approach for discovery of malformations, deformations, and other pathologic conditions that constitute the various sequences or syndromes seen in this age group. Specific detailed knowledge of developmental pathology is less critical; if the postmortem examination has been performed correctly, reference to a standard textbook of pediatric pathology or specialized consultant will provide the diagnosis.

## REFERENCES

1. Hektoen L: *The technique of post-mortem examination*, Chicago, 1984, W.T. Keener Co.
2. Siebert J: Perinatal, fetal and embryonic autopsy. In Gilbert-Barness E, Kapur RP, Oligny LL, Siebert JR, editors: *Potter's pathology of the fetus, infant and child*, ed 2, St. Louis, 2007, Mosby, pp 695-739.
3. Stocker JT, Macpherson TA: The pediatric autopsy. In Stocker JT, Dehner LP, editors: *Pediatric pathology*, Philadelphia, 2002, Lippincott, Williams & Wilkins, pp 5-17.
4. Gilbert-Barness E, Debich-Spicer DE: *Handbook of pediatric autopsy pathology*, Totowa, NJ, 2005, Humana Press.
5. Grønvall J, Graem N: Radiography in post-mortem examinations of fetuses and neonates. Findings on plain films and at arteriography, *APMIS* 97:274-280, 1989.
6. Genest DR, Williams MA, Greene MF: Estimating the time of death in stillborn fetuses: I. Histologic evaluation of fetal organs; an autopsy study of 150 stillborns, *Obstet Gynecol* 80:575-584, 1992.
7. Genest DR: Estimating the time of death in stillborn fetuses: II. Histologic evaluation of the placenta; a study of 71 stillborns, *Obstet Gynecol* 80:585-592, 1992.
8. Genest DR, Singer DB: Estimating the time of death in stillborn fetuses: III. External fetal examination; a study of 86 stillborns, *Obstet Gynecol* 80:593-600, 1992.
9. Virmani R, Ursell PC, Fenoglio JJ Jr: Examination of the heart. Human Pathology 18:432-440, 1987.
10. Gilles FH: Perinatal neuropathology. In Davis RL, Robertson DM, editor: *Textbook of neuropathology*, Baltimore, 1997, Williams & Wilkins, pp 331-385.
11. Benirschke K, Kauffmann P, Baergen R: *Pathology of the human placenta*, ed 5, New York, 2006, Springer.

# 6

# Special Dissection Procedures

*"The individuality of the case must often determine the plan of the examination. But we must not begin with individualising, nor make a rule of the exceptions. The expert may allow himself to make alterations, supposing they are well grounded, but he must be able to remember his motive for so doing, and also to state it."*

Rudolph Virchow[1]

The thorough standard postmortem examination provides the framework for accurately detecting and diagnosing most clinical disease. Sometimes the length of the postmortem interval or limitations placed on the extent of the autopsy hinder the pathologist in his or her efforts to investigate a disease process. However, the skillful autopsy pathologist, recognizing the limitations of the basic examination, supplements it with special studies whenever indicated and possible. This chapter describes a number of useful techniques that broaden the basic autopsy.

## SPECIAL EXAMINATIONS OF THE BRAIN AND NEUROMUSCULAR SYSTEM

### Dementia

Currently we are seeing an unprecedented increase in the proportion of the population that is older than age 65. Accompanying this is an increase in the absolute numbers of individuals with dementia. Because clinical criteria for separating the dementias are imperfect and some of the dementias have a genetic component, clinicians and families are asking pathologists to establish diagnoses of Alzheimer's and other dementias. In addition, sponsored basic and clinical research programs with the ultimate goal of developing effective treatment for these disorders require accurate diagnostic classification. Reaching an accurate diagnosis may require consultation with a neuropathologist specializing in these disorders. By properly handling postmortem brain tissue obtained from patients with dementia, the general autopsy pathologist can often make the diagnosis or tremendously aid the neuropathology specialist. Standard gross and microscopic examinations of the brain as described in Chapters 4 and 8 provide diagnostic material for accurate diagnosis in most of the diseases associated with dementia.

### Neuromuscular Disorders

In persons with suspected cases of neuromuscular disorders coming to autopsy, the pathologist must sample and preserve the critical diagnostic tissues appropriately.[2] Muscle should be sampled from both proximal and distal portions of a lower extremity (the quadriceps and gastrocnemius muscles are relatively easy to obtain) along with any other accessible muscles thought to be involved clinically. One should refrain from sampling muscles of the upper extremity (except the deltoid muscle) that require disfiguring incisions unless specific consent has been obtained. Fresh muscle tissue should be frozen separately for enzyme histochemical analysis and possible biochemical studies, the latter in multiple small pieces to avoid repetitive thawing for separate assays. One should fix and retain samples for possible electron microscopic examination (see Chapter 8).

The peripheral nervous system is not routinely sampled; some sites are too exposed to be dissected without special autopsy consent. However, the nerve roots of the spinal cord, dorsal root and sympathetic ganglia, nerve trunks, and brachial and lumbar plexuses are available during a standard autopsy. With the appropriate permission, the proximal and distal sciatic nerves and the sural nerves are also accessible. The sural nerve is a pure sensory nerve, limiting its value in the investigation of motor neuropathies. However, it is the most commonly sampled nerve during life, so the range of morphologic changes in the sural nerve is well documented.[3] To find the sural nerve, one should place the body in a lateral decubitus position or cross the legs and pronate the foot. An 8- to 10-cm incision is then made superficial to the deep fascia 1 cm proximal to the lateral malleolus parallel to the Achilles tendon.[4] The pathologist dissects into the fascial plane overlying the peroneus longus muscle to identify the nerve running adjacent to the saphenous vein. A 1-cm segment is the minimal amount needed for the various studies; however, if possible, one should sample at least 2.5 cm.

These specimens must be handled gingerly because they are susceptible to artifacts caused by crushing and stretching. To fix nerves, one should gently stretch them onto a piece of stiff paper and immerse them in buffered formalin for routine embedding of transverse and longitudinal segments in paraffin. One can routinely fix a portion of nerve in glutaraldehyde or mixed glutaraldehyde-paraformaldehyde fixative for semi-thin Epon sections and, if necessary, electron microscopy. A small (0.5 cm) segment of fresh nerve can be snap frozen for special studies.

## EXAMINATION OF THE MIDDLE AND INNER EAR

Removal of the temporal bone for examination of the middle and inner ear is necessary in cases of meningitis and otitis media and in the study of disease processes that produce deafness and vestibular disorders. If either temporal bone is acceptable for study, one should remove the left. Removing the left temporal bone reduces problems with embalming because the right side of a decedent's face is generally viewed. The standard technique for temporal bone removal[5] is outlined here. Sando and colleagues[6] described a more extensive dissection that includes the entire eustachian tube and soft and hard palates along with the inner and middle ears. The interested reader is referred to their work.

To access the middle and inner ears the brain is removed and tissue is cleaned from the base of the cranium. By using a vibrating (Stryker) saw, one can make the cuts indicated in Figure 6-1. Cut 1 is made near the apex of the petrous bone at a right angle to the superior angle of the petrous pyramid. This cut should be completely vertical and quite deep, depending on the age and size of the specimen. Cut 2 is made nearly parallel to cut 1 but through the middle mastoid region as far lateral and deep as possible without jeopardizing the face. The cut should be made vertically, or the saw can be slightly inclined away from the side of the face. Cut 3, which joins the anterior ends of cuts 1 and 2, is made vertically in the floor of the middle cranial fossa about 2.5 cm in front of the petrous ridge and laterally as close to the cranial wall as the saw will fit. Finally, cut 4 connects the posterior ends of cuts 1 and 2 starting posterolaterally and moving medially. This cut is nearly horizontal and undercuts the tissue block (Fig. 6-2). One should grasp the block with a bone forceps and rock the specimen back and forth gently to break any unsevered bone connections at the corners of the cuts. Any dense fibrous connections along cuts 3 and 4 are cut with a scalpel. A sharp bone chisel is sometimes useful in freeing the block, but if it is not used carefully it may crush the air cells or crack the specimen along the plane of the middle ear.

A temporal bone specimen may also be obtained using a vibrating saw equipped with an attached circular bone-plug blade. The cutter is centered on the arcuate eminence (see Fig. 6-1). The cut is continued, lubricating liberally with water until the loss of resistance indicates penetration of the skull base. Then the plug is grasped with a bone forceps, and the inferior attachments are cut with a scalpel or scissors.

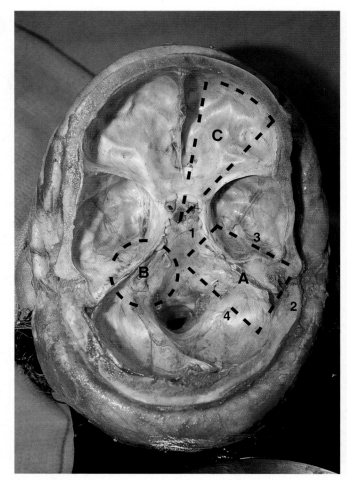

**Figure 6-1** Outline of saw cuts for removal of inner and middle ear and eye. **A,** Removal of a portion of the temporal bone containing the inner and middle ear. The cuts are performed in the numbered order. **B,** Orientation for removal of a temporal bone specimen with a circular bone-plug blade. **C,** Orientation of the saw cuts used in the posterior approach to the eye and orbital contents. (Adapted from Ludwig J: *Current methods of autopsy practice,* ed 2, Philadelphia, 1979, WB Saunders, 1979. By permission of Mayo Foundation.)

After removal of the temporal bone specimen, one ligates the carotid artery and the external auditory canal and packs the bony void with plaster gauze or clay for support and as added insurance against fluid leaks. The specimen is preserved in 10% buffered formalin, changed daily for 2 additional days, and decalcified as described in Chapter 8.

## EXAMINATION OF THE EYES

Postmortem examination of the eye is of interest in patients with a history of primary ocular disease (e.g., infection, neoplasm, macular degeneration, or optic atrophy after ophthalmologic surgery), neurologic disorders involving the eye (e.g., multiple sclerosis, neuronal storage disorders, vasculitis), and ocular complications of systemic diseases (e.g., diabetes mellitus, hypertension). Eye disease in the hospital autopsy population is significant. In a study of 277 consecutive

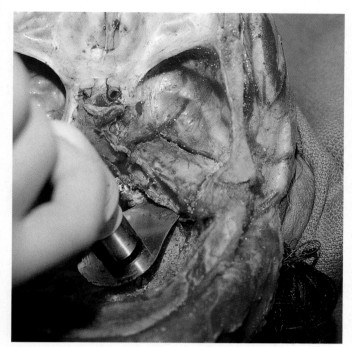

**Figure 6-2** Removal of the temporal bone. The final saw is nearly horizontal and undercuts the tissue block.

**Box 6-1** Orbital findings in infants and children following violent acceleration-deceleration forces

Ocular hemorrhage
    Subretinal hemorrhage
    Intraretinal hemorrhage
    Subhyloid hemorrhage
    Small vitreous hemorrhages
    Intraocular hemorrhages
Other ocular findings:
    Purtscher retinopathy
    Papilledema
    Retinal detachment
    Injuries simulating congenital glaucoma
    Paramacular retinal folds
    Hemorrhagic macular retinoschisis
Extraocular findings:
    Optic nerve sheath hemorrhage (subarachnoid, subdural, dural)
    Hemorrhage within sheaths of the orbital portion of cranial nerves
    Hemorrhage within extraocular muscles
    Hemorrhage in orbital fat

From Gilliland GF, et al: Guidelines for postmortem protocol for ocular investigation of sudden unexplained infant death and suspected physical child abuse, *Am J Forensic Med Pathol* 28:323-329, 2007.

autopsies in which eyes were removed and examined, Butnor and Proia[7] found that only 14% of cases disclosed no ophthalmologic diseases. If possible, both eyes are removed for examination, even if a process is considered to be unilateral. In the forensic setting, examination of the eyes is critical in the investigation of infant and early childhood deaths to help confirm and characterize or exclude traumatic injury due to repetitive violent acceleration-deceleration forces such as are seen in shaken baby syndrome (Box 6-1).[8] Prior to eye removal, a careful inspection of the eye and periorbital facial areas should take place, with appropriate photographic and diagrammatic documentation.

Some have demonstrated the feasibility of postmortem ophthalmologic examination.[9,10] Fiberoptic endoscopic imaging systems can detect retinal hemorrhages, papilledema, retinal tears, macular degeneration, diabetic retinopathy, and other ocular abnormalities.[11]

## Anterior or External Removal

Specialized instruments that aid in removing the eye by the anterior approach (Fig. 6-3) are available (Bausch & Lomb Surgical, St. Louis, Mo). To prevent inadvertent injury to the eyelids and to make eye removal easier, separate the eyelids with a Knapp or other appropriate eye speculum. Using Aebli

**Figure 6-3** Instruments useful for removing the eye for the anterior approach. *Left to right:* Adson forceps, Storz curved enucleation scissors, Knapp eye speculum, Aebli straight corneal scissors, eye muscle hook, mosquito hemostatic forceps.

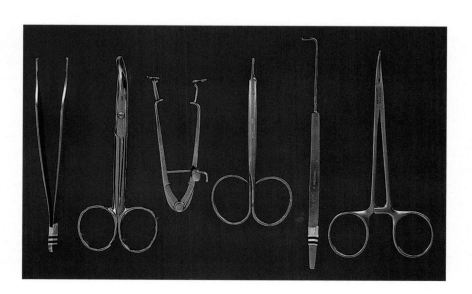

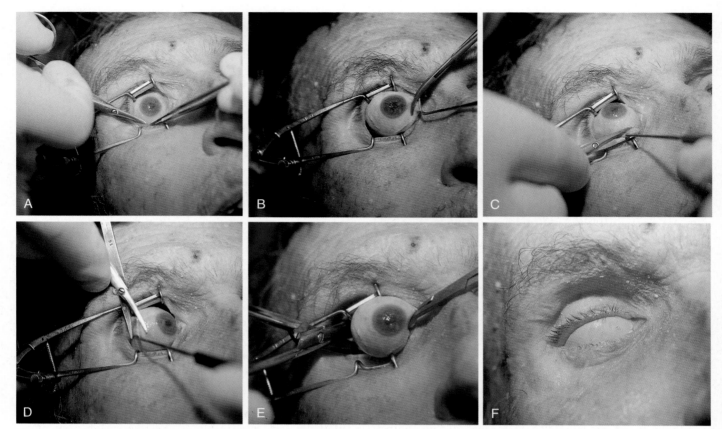

**Figure 6-4  A,** After separating the eyelids, the conjunctiva is cut from the sclera around the entire eye. **B,** The conjunctival flap is clamped, and the eye is rotated laterally to expose the medial rectus muscle. An eye muscle hook is passed behind the muscle, which is then transected. **C, D.** The muscle hook is used to rotate the eye inferiorly, superiorly, and medially; and the superior, inferior (shown in **C**), and lateral rectus muscles (shown in **D**) are transected in turn. **E,** A clamp attached to the medial rectus muscle tag allows the eye to be pulled forward. The optic nerve is transected as far posteriorly as possible and the superior and inferior oblique muscles and any remaining soft tissue attachments are severed, allowing removal of the eye. **F,** The orbit is filled with some cotton or gauze and then covered with a plastic shield.

straight corneal scissors, one should free the conjunctiva from the sclera around the entire eye (Fig. 6-4, *A*). The conjunctival flap is clamped with a small (Hartmann) mosquito hemostatic forceps, and the insertion of the medial rectus muscle is exposed. One then passes an eye muscle hook behind the medial rectus muscle and pulls the eye laterally (Fig. 6-4, *B*). The muscle is transected 1 to 1.5 cm behind the insertion. With the muscle hook, one then rotates the eye inferiorly, superiorly, and medially, transecting in turn the superior, inferior, and lateral rectus muscles (Fig. 6-4, *C*). The medial rectus muscle tag is clamped with the hemostat, and the eye is pulled forward. Using the Storz curved enucleation scissors, one should transect the optic nerve as posteriorly as possible (Fig. 6-4, *D*). Next, the superior and inferior oblique muscles are cut along with any remaining soft tissue attachments to free the eye. One then packs the orbit with some cotton or gauze and covers the area with a plastic shield (Fig. 6-4, *E*).

## Posterior or Internal Removal

The entire orbital contents (eye, optic nerve, extraocular muscles, lacrimal gland, and orbital fat) may be removed by an internal approach after removal of the brain and dura (see Fig. 6-1). In fact, this is the method of choice in the evaluation of most inflammatory or neoplastic disorders and is

particularly recommended for evaluation of suspected trauma in the pediatric age group. With a vibrating saw fitted with a narrow fan-shaped blade, one cuts through the orbital roof (see Fig. 6-3). In infants, the orbital roof can be removed with scissors or cartilage cutters. The bone overlying the optic nerve canal is included so that the entire nerve can be removed intact to the point where it was transected during brain removal. The bone flap is lifted with a forceps to expose the orbital contents (Fig. 6-5). Bluntly dissect the lateral medial and inferior orbital tissues that attach to the periosteum. With a scalpel, cut to attachments at the inferior orbital fissure, the extraocular muscles, vessels and nerves entering the orbit, and the ring of connective tissue surrounding the optic nerve. Before removing the specimen, separate the conjunctiva from the sclera as shown in Figure 6-4A, and bluntly dissect the Tenon fascia that underlies the conjunctiva. The remaining periosteal attachments are then incised and gentle digital pressure on the anterior surface of the eye delivers it into the cranial cavity, although a few inferior attachments may require cutting. Pack the orbit as described earlier.

## Fixation and Dissection of the Eye

The globe or orbital specimen is fixed in 10% buffered formalin for 24 to 48 hours. After an overnight wash in running

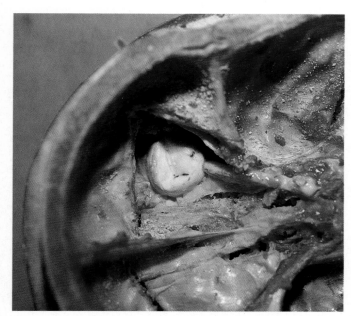

**Figure 6-5** The dura has been stripped, and cuts have been made through the roof of the orbit. The orbital soft tissues have been dissected away, exposing the eye and its optic nerve, which are now ready for removal.

water, the eye is stored in 70% alcohol until cutting. If the eye collapses, as it tends to do, inject some alcohol into the vitreous to restore the shape of the globe before dissection.

Although eye specimens are generally labeled right or left, this should be confirmed by observation. To orient the eye, identify the tendinous insertion of the superior oblique muscle and the muscular insertion of the inferior oblique muscle, both of which pass medially in the orbit. The eye is described, giving the anterior-posterior, horizontal, and vertical diameters. The vertical and horizontal diameters of the cornea are measured, noting in turn the translucency of the cornea, color of the iris, and shape of the pupil. Then transilluminate the globe and outline any opacities with a marking pencil. If the eye shows signs of trauma, obtain a radiograph to exclude a metallic foreign body. Obtain a sample of the optic nerve with a cross section just behind the globe. The eye is cut parallel to the long ciliary arteries, starting adjacent to the optic nerve and ending just inside the corneal limbus. Note the character of the vitreous, filtration angle, position of the iris, presence or absence of the lens, and position of the retina. A second cut is made parallel to the first, yielding a central section approximately 8 mm thick for light microscopic embedding. This section includes the cornea, lens, optic nerve, and macula.

## EXAMINATION OF THE NASAL SINUSES AND NASOPHARYNX

Examination of the frontal, ethmoidal, sphenoidal, and maxillary sinuses is complex, and there is great potential for damaging the face of the decedent. One approach is to use a chisel to remove the bone plates that separate the base of the skull from the nasal sinuses. Gresham and Turner[12] described a more

aggressive approach in which the base of the skull is split down the midline and pried apart, and then the sinuses are opened from their medial sides with a chisel.

Szanto[13] reviewed and described various methods for examination and removal of the nasopharynx and throat, and the reader is referred to this work. The prosector should not perform these dissections without the appropriate consent or legal authority, and then only after consulting the mortician for aid in proper reconstruction. Langlois and Little[14] developed a method for examination of the intraosseous portion of the carotid arteries that also exposes the maxillary and ethmoid facial air sinuses. The approach preserves the anterior portion of the maxilla, aiding reconstruction.

## EXAMINATION OF MANDIBLE, MAXILLA, AND TEETH

Extensive examination of the structures of the oral cavity requiring their removal is usually confined to situations in which extensive decomposition has occurred. The purpose of examination is identification of the body, and the resulting disfigurement is not typically a concern. In these cases, the mandible is disarticulated or cut posterior to the third molar area with a saw, and the maxilla is removed by cutting into the maxillary sinuses above the root apices of the teeth.[15] The mandible may also be removed using the standard postmortem neck incision and additional access through the oral cavity. Reconstruction is possible using a prefabricated jaw replica.[16]

## EXAMINATION OF THE NECK AND CERVICAL SPINE

Complete examination of the neck is not usually performed during the routine autopsy. However, in special circumstances, particularly those encountered by the pathologist evaluating trauma to the cervical region, upper respiratory tract obstruction, or tumors of, at, or near the base of the tongue, a systematic approach to the structures of the neck is desirable. In two detailed monographs, Adams[17,18] presented dissection approaches to the anterior and posterior compartments of the neck. Vanezis[19] recommends and describes a systematic approach to evaluation of neck trauma involving infrared photography, step-by-step dissection, and radiography.

Forensic cases are guided by taking into account two concepts. First, the initial incision and superficial dissection must provide generous exposure of the neck. Though some suggest a single primary midline incision from symphysis mentis to symphysis pubis, a Y-shaped incision that begins behind each ear is more versatile (Fig. 6-6). The left and right branches of the Y extend down to the lateral third of their respective clavicles and then gradually meet in the middle of the sternum to be carried along the midline as usual to the pubis. The advantages of this incision are that it can be continued up over the chin and through the buccal sulcus, allowing examination of the mouth or, if necessary, the whole face, because the tissues can be detached from the skull by continued reflection of the lateral incisions.[20] The second consideration is preventing artifacts resembling premortem trauma. Removing the brain,

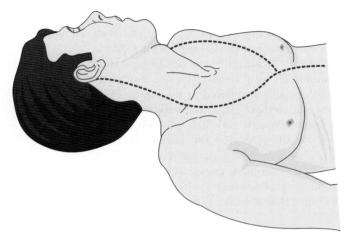

**Figure 6-6** Recommended incision for exposue and dissection of the neck.

and perhaps the heart as well, before commencing with the neck dissection prevents postmortem extravasation of blood into the neck tissues that could be mistaken for premortem hemorrhage.[21] Second, dissecting the neck in situ by reflecting individual cervical muscles from their attachments in a layer-by-layer dissection also minimizes postmortem seepage of blood and prevents inadvertent injury (e.g., postmortem fractures of the laryngeal cartilage or hyoid bone) that might result from the force required to remove the tongue and neck structures en bloc.

Berzlanovich and coworkers[22] described a method for dissection of the cervical vertebral column. The method of Yang and Steffan[23] describes removing the entire cervical spine along with the atlantooccipital joint via a posterior approach. A wooden strut and plaster are used to reconstruct the spine and stabilize the head. Angiography has been applied to evaluate both traumatic and atherosclerotic damage to the important vascular structures of the neck.[19,24,25] For the rare case requiring direct examination of the vertebral arteries, a relatively simple method has been described.[26]

## EXAMINATION OF THE THORACIC DUCT AND CISTERNA CHYLI

The cisterna chyli receives the lymphatic drainage in the abdomen, just posterior to the aorta. It passes through the aortic hiatus of the diaphragm, where it continues as the thoracic duct. The thoracic duct is identified to best advantage before evisceration. Inferiorly, it may be viewed from either side. To view it in the right side of the chest, one should lift the right lung up and to the left, displacing the mediastinal structures to the left.[27] The duct is located anterior to the thoracic vertebrae, to the left of the azygos vein and to the right of the thoracic aorta. At the level of the third or fourth thoracic vertebra, it courses to the left to enter the left subclavian or innominate vein. To view it in the left side of the chest, one should expose the left posterior mediastinum by retracting the left lung out of the chest.[28] The intercostal arteries are transected close to the aorta, clamping their stumps. One then

pulls the aorta to the right, exposing the retroaortic fat, in which the thoracic duct can be isolated and dissected.

## SPECIAL EXAMINATIONS OF THE HEART

### Dissection of Hearts with Developmental Malformations

The malformed heart presents challenges that often require a customized approach to dissection. A solid knowledge of normal cardiac anatomy is essential. Even then, if the prosector encounters a puzzling abnormality, he or she should cease dissection and wait for additional input. This may entail consulting the local pediatric cardiologist or sending the fixed, nondissected specimen to a recognized cardiac anatomist. A delay of a few hours, days, or weeks is preferable to an incorrectly dissected, and possibly useless, specimen.

The purpose of the autopsy in a patient with congenital heart disease is to (1) correlate the defects with clinical data and (2) provide a properly dissected specimen for education and research. There are still many instances in which the anatomy cannot be defined from the echocardiogram with certainty. This is particularly true for fetal echocardiograms, for which the fetus may not be positioned to present the anatomy to best advantage. Beyond medical education, the structural data obtained at autopsy are useful in family counseling—for example, to support a decision to terminate the pregnancy voluntarily.

The first step in the evaluation of the malformed heart at autopsy is to understand the clinical diagnosis. In this age of echocardiography and other sophisticated noninvasive methods, as well as cardiac catheterization and angiography, the anatomy has often been defined accurately during life. It is essential to have a modern concept of the expected cardiac anatomy, including surgical intervention, before dissection. This can be obtained from any of a number of standard textbooks of pediatric cardiology, all of which include sections describing cardiac anatomy and pathophysiology associated with the malformations.[29-33]

Regardless of prior clinical documentation of malformations, each case should be approached in a consistent manner. The possibility of unexpected malformations is the reason why the pediatric autopsy must be detailed and systematic (see Chapter 5). As in routine autopsies, the heart and lungs are inspected in situ, and the relative size of the heart within the thorax is assessed. Similarly, in every pediatric autopsy, it is important to dissect the great arteries and their major branches before evisceration; the prosector should document the relation of the great vessels and any anomalous course of branch vessels so that accommodations in the dissection may be made if necessary. In addition, the position of the descending thoracic aorta relative to the spine, course of the pulmonary veins, and location of the anterior and posterior descending coronary arteries should be noted. The position of the abdominal organs and presence of polysplenia or asplenia may be the first indication of a heart malformation; in general, these syndromes warrant stopping the autopsy and consulting a specialist.

When the anatomy has been defined in situ, the organs are removed en bloc. From the posterior aspect, the course of the inferior vena cava should be noted. If the pulmonary veins course in the usual fashion—that is, do not connect with a vessel below the diaphragm—the thoracic organs can be separated from the rest of the block. In a case of suspected cardiovascular malformation (including subdiaphragmatic connection of the pulmonary veins), these organs remain together. In our institutions, we perfuse and fix the nondissected heart overnight through a cannula usually placed in the orifice of one of the venae cavae; it is not absolutely necessary to occlude the aorta or its major branches during perfusion. Although this enhances the final appearance of the specimen, the risk of artifactual injury may not be worth the improvement. Following fixation, the heart is generally opened along the lines of blood flow, taking care to probe valve orifices before cutting. Hearts with malformations often contain shunts, and the prosector must use caution in opening the heart.

Although it is beyond the scope of this chapter to describe the approaches to dissection of the various cardiac malformations, suffice it to say that advance knowledge of the expected anatomy, as well as a common-sense approach, is adequate for all but the most complex lesions. One should never cut through a defect (or the septum). Anatomic relationships should be maintained to the best extent possible. In pediatric pathology, too little dissection is often preferable to too much. Besides the lines-of-blood-flow method of dissection, there is the "windows method," in which the chambers are opened by incisions that are not carried through the valves.[34] The windows method is superior to the standard method for keeping the specimen in proper anatomic appearance but not as good for inspecting the cardiac valves. For certain defects, it may be advisable to use an adaptation of both methods. Finally, it is important to show the autopsy specimen to the treatment group; the clinicians are usually best positioned to place the anatomic findings in proper perspective.

### Dissection of Hearts with Valve Implants

Valve implants and other prostheses usually require modification of the dissection of the heart. In most cases, it is unnecessary to sever the device or remove it. The objective is to gain an adequate view by making cuts up to but excluding the manufactured material. The type of valve implant, its position, and its diameter should be recorded; there are several good references that can be useful for identification of the valve type.[35-38] Paravalvular channels as evidence of leaks or frank dehiscence should be noted. Any other pathologic changes—such as fractures, degenerative change in the leaflets, infective material, or thrombus—should also be described and sampled for histologic examination. The mobility of the leaflets must be ascertained. Again, the valve disorder and cardiac anatomy must be considered in the appropriate pathophysiologic context.[39,40]

### Electronic Medical Devices, Including Pacemakers and Defibrillators

Electronic medical devices have become a regular part of modern therapeutics, and the autopsy pathologist should expect to encounter them at autopsy with increasing regularity. These include older instruments such as implantable cardiac pacemakers but also newer implanted devices such as defibrillators; Holter monitors; cerebellar stimulators; spinal cord, peripheral nerve, and diaphragmatic/phrenic nerve stimulators; drug infusion pumps; insulin pumps; and glucose monitors. Little has been written on how the pathologist should handle these devices at autopsy, although the excellent article by Weitzman[41] stands out. Table 6-1 describes some of the more common electronic medical devices, and Box 6-2 summarizes Weitzman's recommendations for their examination. Upon encountering an electronic medical device or, for that matter, any medical device, prosthesis, or graft, the pathologist should determine whether the device is subject to tracking by the U.S. Food and Drug Administration (FDA) and notify the appropriate health care provider and/or manufacturer. Information regarding tracking of medical devices is available at the FDA website (http://www.fda.gov/cdrh/devadvice/353.html).

In most cases, the presence of an implantable device in a decedent will not significantly alter the autopsy procedure. Defibrillators, however, present a potential risk to autopsy personnel and should be turned off by the cardiologist or cardiology technician before autopsy. (Safety recommendations are presented in Chapter 3.) Virtually all hearts in patients with defibrillators or pacing wires will have a significant pathologic lesion, and the method of dissection must be the one best suited for the underlying disease process. For the lines-of-blood-flow method, an endocardial wire can be left in place; the short-axis method requires removal of wires before slicing the ventricles. The course of the wire within the heart and the position of its point of contact with the cardiac muscle should be described; wires that have been in place for months are tethered by reactive fibrosis at the points of contact. The generator and the full length of the wire should be inspected for evidence of infection, thrombus, insulation cracks, or other abnormality. In cases of sudden unexplained death, the generator should be sent to the manufacturer for evaluation.

## EXAMINATION OF BONES AND JOINTS

The joints most readily accessible through the incision made in a routine autopsy include the intervertebral joints, the sternoclavicular joints, and the shoulder joints. Pathologic study of tissue obtained from these joints often suffices in evaluation of systemic joint disease.[42]

The technique of Hutchins[43] provides access to the femoral head through the standard abdominal incision. The peritoneal aspect of the abdominal flap is incised parallel and anterior to the ilium and pubis (Fig. 6-7). Then the joint capsule is incised, the knee flexed, and the leg rotated laterally and pushed cranially. A hook secured around the femoral neck aids in dislocation of the femoral head anteriorly. The upper femur is exposed and cut with a saw. Commercially available adjustable plastic rods or simple wood dowels facilitate reconstruction (Fig. 6-8).

The knee joint is exposed by a curved incision above or below the patella.[44] The knee is then flexed, and an incision

**Table 6-1** Electronic medical devices, indications for their use, and potential complications

| Device | Clinical indications or diagnostic utility | Medical complications |
|---|---|---|
| Cardiac pacemaker | Sinus nodal dysfunction; acquired AV block; congenital AV block; bifascicular or trifascicular block; hypersensitive carotid sinus; and neurocardiac syndromes | Early—pneumothorax, large hematoma, cardiac perforation, delayed tamponade, atrial dislodgement, ventricular dislodgement, venous thrombosis, subclavian stick complications (pneumothorax, hemothorax, air embolism, subclavian artery puncture) Later or long-term—wound dehiscence, infection, pain, high thresholds, loose set screw, lead failure, abandoned leads, pacemaker failure, diaphragmatic stimulation, skin erosion, pacemaker syndrome (adverse reaction to VVI pacing), twiddler's syndrome (patients who intentionally or unintentionally manipulate pulse generator, which can lead to dislodgement or fracture) |
| Implanted Holter monitor | Arrhythmias; distinguishing seizures of cardiac origin from epilepsy; diagnosis of bradycardia ictal syndrome | Not applicable |
| Implanted cardiac defibrillator | Life-threatening ventricular tachyarrhythmia | Early—inappropriate therapy delivery; inability to defibrillate; worsening systolic function; electromechanical dissociation on testing; subclavian stick complications (pneumothorax, hemothorax, air embolism, subclavian artery puncture); venous thromboembolism; phrenic nerve stimulation; right ventricular perforation; pericardial effusion or tamponade; hematoma in pulse generator pocket; hypotension; myocardial infarction; cerebrovascular accident; provocation of new arrhythmia; aggregation of preexisting arrhythmia Later or long-term—infection; lead erosion and migration; venous thromboembolism; endocarditis; shoulder-related problems; twiddler's syndrome; lead conductor fracture; lead insulation defect; lead perforation; loose set screw; exit block (high pacing threshold); inappropriate shock delivery; premature battery depletion; device recall; psychosocial issues |
| Spinal cord and peripheral nerve stimulators | Chronic intractable pain | Hematoma; epidural hemorrhage; paralysis; seroma; cerebrospinal fluid leakage; infection; erosion; allergic response; hardware malfunction or migration; pain at implant site; loss of pain relief; chest wall stimulation; surgical risks |
| Drug pumps | Long-term intrathecal infusion of morphine sulfate for treatment of chronic intractable pain; intrathecal injection for severe spasticity; long-term epidural infusion of morphine sulfate for treatment of chronic intractable pain; long-term intravascular infusion of chemotherapeutic agents for primary or metastatic cancer; long-term intravenous infusion of antibiotics for treatment of osteomyelitis | Component failure; pocket seroma; hematoma; erosion or infection; complete or partial catheter occlusion, kinking, breakage, or disconnection; catheter dislodgement or migration; bleeding; arachnoiditis; meningitis; spinal headache; drug toxicity |
| Insulin pump | Diabetes mellitus | Hypoglycemic or hyperglycemic events |
| Ambulatory glucose monitor | Diabetes mellitus (takes and records glucose measurements every 5 minutes for up to 3 days) | Not applicable |

is made through the quadriceps tendon to gain access to the joint for sampling of articular surfaces, joint capsule, bursae, and tendons. The entire knee can be removed through an anteromedial incision, but this requires reconstruction to restore normal contours.

## SPECIAL CIRCUMSTANCES

### Detection of Air Emboli

In cases of sudden death after pneumothorax, pneumoperitoneum, intravenous infusions, childbirth, operations, or sharp instrument injuries to the neck and thorax, it is important to check for air embolism to the heart. A postmortem chest radiograph should be taken and inspected for larger quantities of air in the heart and great vessels. Baker[44] described a simple technique for detection of air emboli during a modified postmortem dissection. In suspected cases, the initial superior portion of the body incision should be limited to just below the sternal notch to reduce the possibility of air reaching the heart from a severed superficial neck vein. One should reflect the skin and muscles but cut only the rib cartilages from the second rib inferiorly. The sternum and anterior ribs are removed, exposing the pericardium. One then ligates the aorta securely and makes a small incision in the anterior pericardial sac. The cut edges of the pericardium are grasped with clamps and the pericardial contents are inspected, noting in particular any bulging of the right ventricle, indicating possible

distention by entrapped air. The pericardial cavity is filled with water, submerging the heart entirely. The left circumflex and anterior descending arteries are transected in turn, and their contents are milked toward the incisions. The prosector must look carefully for intravascular air bubbles that escape. The same test is performed with the right coronary artery. Keeping the heart submerged, one incises in turn the right atrium, the right ventricle, and the pulmonary artery, pressing slightly to release any pockets of trapped air. The same maneuver is performed on the left atrium, the left ventricle, the superior vena cava, the inferior vena cava, and the pulmonary veins.

Another method involves using a large (30 mL), airtight syringe fitted with a needle and filled halfway with water.[45] After introduction of the needle into the right ventricle, the appearance of bubbles within the syringe indicates entrapped air. Alternatively, the needle can be hooked in series through tubing to a stopper-topped bottle and separatory funnel. The system is filled with oil, allowing collection of any air. Van Ieperen[46] also described a simple apparatus for collection and measurement of heart gas that does not require a needle, eliminating the possibility of the needle clogging with fibrin clots. Bajanowski and colleagues[47] have reviewed other more complicated methods that include analysis of collected gas.

## Detection of Pneumothorax

Detection of a pneumothorax is easily done by holding the dissected skin and subcutaneous tissues of the chest to form a pocket adjacent to the ribcage.[48] The pocket is filled with water, and a scalpel is used to incise the thoracic cavity. The presence of air bubbles indicates a pneumothorax. For neonates and small infants, the thorax may be submerged in a basin of water. The apparatuses described previously for detection of air emboli work equally well for detecting pneumothoraces. Chest radiographs provide the most reliable method for determining the extent of pneumothoraces and whether or not a pneumothorax has resulted in mediastinal shift.[49]

## The Maternal Autopsy

Autopsy technique in cases of maternal death does not require significant deviation from a standard postmortem examination. Of course, special attention must be given to known causes of maternal death (Table 6-2).[50-52] As seen from the data summarized in Table 6-2, in developing countries the cause of death associated with pregnancy is much more likely to be associated with infection. In any case, the pathologist must use appropriate autopsy techniques and ancillary studies in the investigation of any maternal death.[53]

Before starting the autopsy, one must obtain a detailed medical history. Consulting directly with obstetricians, midwives, anesthesiologists, or other physicians who provided the decedent's care is always good practice and may indicate the need for special studies or dissections. The pathologist should plan on which samples and laboratory tests are necessary. Consider the need for toxicological studies on peripheral blood, vitreous humor, urine, and stomach contents. If in doubt, discuss the case with a toxicologist to ensure that any

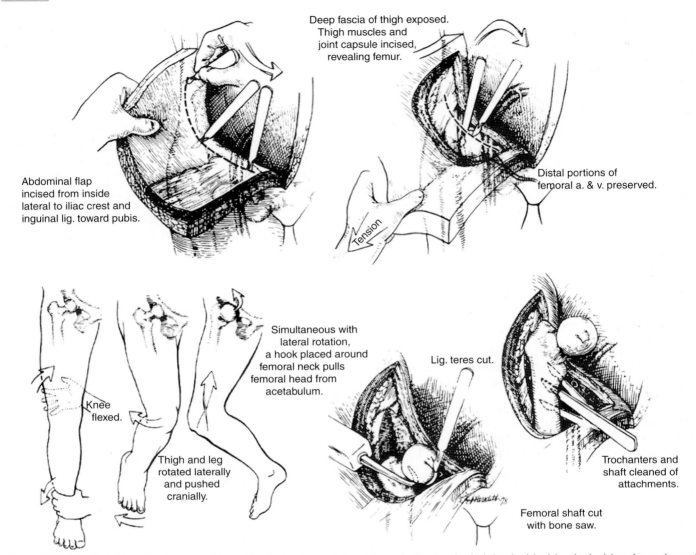

**Figure 6-7** The Hutchins technique provides access to the femoral head through the standard abdominal incision by incising the peritoneal aspect of the abdominal flap parallel and anterior to the ilium and pubis. Dissection of the soft tissues and fascia exposes the thigh muscles and joint capsule, which are incised to expose the femur. Care is taken to preserve the femoral vessels located at the medial aspect of the incision. After the joint capsule has been excised, the leg is flexed at the knee, rotated laterally, and simultaneously pushed cranially. A hook placed around the femoral neck allows the operator to pull the femoral head from the acetabulum. The upper portion of the femur is freed from any muscle attachments, and a vibrating saw is used to cut the shaft of the femur. (From Hutchins GM: Removal of the femoral head at autopsy, *Am J Clin Pathol* 85:598-601, 1986. © 1986 American Society of Clinical Pathologists; reprinted with permission.)

toxicology samples are properly obtained and preserved. Procure blood, genital tract swabs, and appropriate tissue samples for microbiological studies.

The external examination may reveal purpura or petechial hemorrhages indicative of disseminated intravascular coagulation due to sepsis. Careful examination of the external genitalia may demonstrate signs of infection (e.g., discharge), unusual amounts of hemorrhage, or evidence of trauma. The initial prosection should include appropriate tests to determine if there are any signs of pneumothorax or air embolism (see earlier). Next, open the main pulmonary artery and check for thromboemboli. Rarely, lanugo hairs, vernix, or meconium may indicate amniotic fluid emboli. From this point, the standard autopsy should suffice. Though some recommend routine en bloc removal of the perineum with the internal genitalia, specific abnormal findings should determine if this is truly warranted. Table 6-3 summarizes some findings associated with maternal mortality.

## CONCLUSION

The autopsy, as routinely performed, provides an excellent evaluation of most organ systems and identifies pathologic processes responsible for the majority of diseases leading to death. However, unless supplemented by special procedures, the postmortem examination fails to correlate pathologic changes of

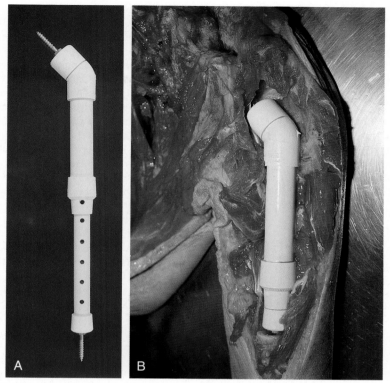

**Figure 6-8** Commercially available adjustable plastic rods or simple wood dowels facilitate reconstruction after removal of long bones. **A,** Adjustable plastic rod with screw ends. **B,** Postmortem reconstruction of the proximal left humerus after its removal.

| **Table 6-2** | Causes of maternal death and their proportion in three countries | | |
|---|---|---|---|
| **Cause of death** | **United States %** (20 states 2000-2006) | **United Kingdom %** (2000-2002) | **Mozambique %** (10/2002-12/2004) |
| Complications of preeclampsia | 16 | 5.4 | 8.7 |
| Amniotic fluid embolism | 14 | 1.9 | 0.7 |
| Obstetric hemorrhage | 12 | 6.5 | 16.6 |
| Cardiac disease | 11 | 16.9 | 0 |
| Pulmonary thromboembolism | 9 | 11.5 | 0 |
| Nonobstetric infection | 7 | Not given | 46 |
| Obstetric infection | 7 | 4.2 | 10.1 |
| Accident/suicide | 6 | 6.1 | 0 |
| Medication error/reaction or anesthesia related | 5 | 2.3 | None listed |
| Ectopic pregnancy | 1 | 4.2 | 1.4 |
| Other | 12 | 39.9 | 10 |
| Acute fatty liver of pregnancy | Not given | 1.1 | 0.7 |
| Unknown | None listed | None listed | 5.8 |
| Total | 100 | 100 | 100 |

Data from Clark SL, Belfort MA, Dildy GA, et al: Maternal death in the 21st century: Causes, prevention and relationship to cesarean delivery, *Am J Obstet Gynecol* 199:36.el-5, 2008; Lewis G: Introduction and key findings, 2000-2002. From *Why mothers die 2000-2002 report,*http://www.cemach.org.uk/Publications/Saving-Mothers-Lives-Report-2000-2002.aspx (accessed October 1, 2008); and Menéndez C, Romagosa C, Ismail MR, et al: An autopsy study of maternal mortality in Moazmbique: The contribution of infectious diseases. PLOS Med:5:e44, 2008, http://medicine.plosjournals.org/perlserv/?request=getdocument&doi=10.1371/journal.pmed.0050044 (accessed October 1, 2008).

**Table 6-3**    Some possible findings in cases of maternal death

| Organ system or site | Pathology |
|---|---|
| Body cavities | Pneumothorax<br>Intraabdominal hemorrhage |
| Cardiovascular system | Saddle thromboembolus<br>Cardiomyopathy<br>Coronary artery dissections<br>Aortic dissections<br>Ruptured aneurysms (mesenteric splenic, hepatic, uterine, or ovarian arteries) |
| Respiratory system | Amniotic fluid emboli<br>Pulmonary thromboemboli<br>Diffuse alveolar damage<br>Aspiration of gastric contents<br>Problems with intubation<br>Pulmonary hypertension |
| Gastrointestinal system | Trauma |
| Hepatobiliary system | Necrosis, hemorrhage<br>Acute fatty change in pregnancy |
| Urinary system | Ureteral, bladder, or urethral trauma following caesarean section or forceps delivery<br>Acute pyelonephritis<br>Hypertensive changes due to eclampsia<br>Renal cortical necrosis |
| Reproductive system | Trauma<br>Hemorrhage<br>Retained placenta<br>Tubal pregnancy<br>Abnormalities of placental attachment |
| Central nervous system | Venous sinus thrombosis<br>Cerebral hemorrhage due to choriocarcinoma<br>Pituitary necrosis |

many degenerative diseases with the patient's clinical findings. In some cases, relatively simple special postmortem dissections can complete or tremendously enhance clinicopathologic correlations. The modern autopsy pathologist should have these techniques in his or her repertoire.

## REFERENCES

1. Virchow R: *Description and explanation of the method of performing post-mortem examinations in the dead house of the Berlin Charite Hospital, with especial reference to medico-legal practice*, London, 1880, Churchill (Translated from the second German edition by TP Smith).
2. Powers JM: Practice guidelines for autopsy pathology: Autopsy procedures for brain, spinal cord, and neuromuscular system. Autopsy Committee of the College of American Pathologists, *Arch Pathol Lab Med* 119:777-783, 1995.
3. Hilton DA, Weller RO: Autopsy investigation of disorders of skeletal muscle and peripheral nerves. In Love S, editor: *Current topics in pathology*, Berlin, 2001, Springer-Verlag, pp 207-237.
4. de la Monte SM: Postmortem evaluation of neuromuscular diseases. In Hutchins GM, editor: *Autopsy performance and reporting*, Northfield, Ill, 1990. College of American Pathologists, pp 99-105.
5. Schuknecht H: Temporal bone removal at autopsy: Preparation and uses, *Arch Otolaryngol* 87:129-137, 1968.
6. Sando I, Doyle WJ, Okuno H, et al: A method for the histopathological analysis of the temporal bone and the eustachian tube and its accessory structures, *Ann Otol Rhinol Laryngol* 95:267-274, 1986.
7. Butnor KJ, Proia AD: Unexpected autopsy findings arising from postmortem ocular examination, *Arch Pathol Lab Med* 125:1193-1196, 2001.
8. Gilliland MG, Levin AV, Enzenauer RW, et al: Guidelines for postmortem protocol for ocular investigation of sudden unexpected infant death and suspected physical child abuse, *Am J Forensic Med Pathol* 28:323-329, 2007.
9. Gilliland MGF, Folberg R: Retinal hemorrhages: Replicating the clinician's view of the eye, *Forensic Sci Int* 56:77-80, 1992.
10. Amber R, Pollak S: Postmortem endoscopy of the ocular fundus: A valuable tool in forensic postmortem practice, *Forensic Sci Int* 124:157-162, 2001.
11. Tsujinaka M, Bunai Y: Postmortem ophthalmologic examination by endoscopy, *Am J Forensic Med Pathol* 27:287-291, 2006.
12. Gresham GA, Turner AF: *Post-mortem procedures*, Chicago, 1979, Year Book Medical.
13. Szanto PB: A modified technic for the removal of the nasopharynx and accompanying organs of the throat, *Arch Pathol* 38:313-320, 1944.
14. Langlois NEI, Little D: A method for exposing the intraosseous portion of the carotid arteries and its application to forensic case work, *Am J Forensic Med Pathol* 24:35-40, 2003.
15. Stimson PG: Oral autopsy protocol, *Dent Clin North Am* 21:177-179, 1977.
16. de Jonge HK, van Merkesteyn JP, Bras J: Reconstruction of the lower half of the facial skeleton after removal at autopsy, *Int J Oral Maxillofac Surg* 19:155-157, 1990.
17. Adams VI: Autopsy technique for neck examination. I. Anterior and lateral compartments and tongue, *Pathol Annu* 25:331-349, 1990.
18. Adams VI: Autopsy technique for neck examination. II. Vertebral column and posterior compartment, *Pathol Annu* 26:211-226, 1991.
19. Vanezis P: Post mortem techniques in the evaluation of neck injury, *J Clin Pathol* 46:500-506, 1993.
20. Camps FE: *Gradwohl's legal medicine*, ed 2, Bristol, UK, 1968, J. Wright.
21. Prinsloo I, Gordon I: Post-mortem dissection artefacts of the neck: Their differentiation from ante-mortem bruises, *South African Med J* 25:358-361, 1951.
22. Berzlanovich AM, Sim E, Muhm MA: Technique for dissecting the cervical vertebral column, *J Forensic Sci* 43:190-193, 1998.
23. Yang K, Steffen T: Harvesting the intact cadaveric cervical spine (C0-Th1), *Spine* 25:1447-1449, 2000.
24. Hutchinson EC, Yates PO: The cervical portion of the vertebral artery: A clinico-pathological study, *Brain* 79:319-331, 1956.
25. Choi SS, Crampton A: Atherosclerosis of arteries of neck, *Arch Pathol* 72:379-385, 1961.
26. Bromilow A, Burns J: Technique for removal of the vertebral arteries, *J Clin Pathol* 38:1400-1402, 1985.
27. Weber DL, Fazzini EP, Reagan TJ: *Autopsy pathology procedure and protocol*, Springfield, Ill, 1973, Charles C Thomas.

28. Ludwig J: *Current methods of autopsy practice*, Philadelphia, 1979, WB Saunders.

29. Becker AE, Anderson RH: *Pathology of congenital heart disease*, London, 1981, Butterworths.

30. Anderson RH, Macartney FJ, Shinebourne EA, Tynan M: *Paediatric cardiology*, Edinburgh, 1987, Churchill Livingstone.

31. Emmanouilides G, editor: *Heart disease in infants, children and adolescents*, Baltimore, 1995, Williams & Wilkins.

32. Bharati S, Lev M: *The pathology of congenital heart disease*, Armonk, NY, 1996, Futura.

33. Moller JH, Hoffman JIE: *Pediatric cardiovascular medicine*, New York, 2000, Churchill Livingstone.

34. Valdés-Dapena M, Huff D: *Perinatal autopsy manual*, Washington, DC, 1983, Armed Forces Institute of Pathology.

35. Schoen FJ, Hobson CE: Anatomic analysis of removed prosthetic heart valves: Causes of failure of 33 mechanical valves and 58 bioprostheses, 1980-1983, *Hum Pathol* 16:549-559, 1985.

36. Mehlman DJ: A pictorial and radiographic guide for identification of prosthetic heart valve devices, *Prog Cardiovasc Dis* 30:441-464, 1988.

37. Schoen FJ: Approach to the analysis of cardiac valve prostheses as surgical pathology or autopsy specimens, *Cardiovasc Pathol* 4:241-255, 1995.

38. Vongpatanasin W, Hillis LD, Lange RA: Prosthetic heart valves, *N Engl J Med* 335:407-416, 1996.

39. Walley VM, Masters RG: Complications of cardiac valve surgery and their autopsy investigation. Cardiovasc Pathol 4:269-286, 1995.

40. Schoen FJ, Levy RJ: Tissue heart valves: Current challenges and future research perspectives, *J Biomed Mater Res* 47:439-465, 1999.

41. Weitzman JB: Electronic medical devices: A primer for pathologists, *Arch Pathol Lab Med* 127:814-825, 2003.

42. Sokoloff L, Gleason IO: The sternoclavicular articulation in rheumatic diseases, *Am J Clin Pathol* 24:406-414, 1954.

43. Hutchins GM: Removal of the femoral head at autopsy, *Am J Clin Pathol* 85:598-601, 1986.

44. Baker RD: *Postmortem examination: Specific methods and procedures*, Philadelphia, 1967, WB Saunders.

45. Kulka W: A practical device for demonstrating air embolism, *Arch Pathol* 48:366-369, 1949.

46. Van Ieperen L: Venous air embolism as a cause of death—a method of investigation, *S Afr Med J* 63:442-443, 1983.

47. Bajanowski T, West W, Brinkmann B: Proof of fatal air embolism, *Int J Legal Med* 111:208-211, 1998.

48. Box CR: *Post-mortem manual: A handbook of morbid anatomy and post-mortem technique*, ed 1, London, 1910, J & A Churchill.

49. Ludwig J, Miller WE, Sessler AD: Clinically unsuspected pneumothorax: A postmortem roentgenographic study, *Arch Pathol* 90:274-277, 1970.

50. Clark SL, Belfort MA, Dildy GA, et al: Maternal death in the 21st century: Causes, prevention and relationship to cesarean delivery, *Am J Obstet Gynecol* 199:36.el-5, 2008.

51. Lewis G: Introduction and key findings 2000-2002. From *Why mothers die 2000-2002 report*, http://www.cemach.org.uk/Publications/Saving-Mothers-Lives-Report-2000-2002.aspx (accessed October 1, 2008).

52. Menéndez C, Romagosa C, Ismail MR, et al: An autopsy study of maternal mortality in Moazmbique: The contribution of infectious diseases. PLOS Med:5:e44,2008, http://medicine.plosjournals.org/perlserv/?request=getdocument&doi=10.1371/journal.pmed.0050044 (accessed October 1, 2008).

53. Rushton DI, Dawson IMP: The maternal autopsy, *J Clin Pathol* 35:909-921, 1982.

# 7
# Autopsy Photography and Radiology

*"Verbal descriptions, by themselves, may become boring and soporific."*

John P. Vetter[1]

## AUTOPSY PHOTOGRAPHY

The purposes of autopsy photography are twofold: documentation of findings and preparation of educational or research aids. Pathologists generally use photographic records to demonstrate morbid anatomy, but it may be equally important to document normal anatomy. In either case, to be successful, autopsy photography must demonstrate the subject accurately, enhance written or verbal descriptions, and be performed easily and economically.[2]

Some pathology departments have a full-time medical photographer. Most do not, however, and the duties of photography fall on the prosector. Although this may be perceived as a disadvantage by some, we feel that responsibility for photography can enhance the pathology training program. Thinking about how a specimen is to be presented assists pathology residents in developing their own expertise. However, without adequate training in the art of specimen photography, pathology house staff produce pictures of low quality or neglect specimen photography entirely, failing to document important findings. The photographic product also reflects departmental quality in general. A dramatic, resplendent photograph, presented at hospital conferences, goes a long way toward enhancing the pathology department's image in the medical center. It is our hope that the material presented briefly herein will help the pathologist-in-training become a more capable medical photographer. For those desiring a more detailed discussion of photographic principles and specialized techniques, we recommend a number of excellent textbooks.[3-5]

## Photographic Equipment and Supplies

### Camera

The most versatile camera choice for specimen photography is a 35-mm single-lens reflex (SLR) camera. These cameras are light and small but still allow critical focusing of the specimen. With the maturation of digital photography, this medium has become the choice of many if not most individuals documenting autopsy findings. With digital photography, the quality of an image can be immediately reviewed by the photographer, and if it is found to

be wanting, a new photograph can be taken. The low cost, in the long term, of digital media, and their readiness for storage on CDs or DVDs, with their long lives, are very attractive. We urge that cameras with at least 5 megapixels on the recording "chip" be utilized. The cost of digital SLR cameras has now dramatically decreased, allowing pathology departments to consider switching to digital specimen photography while maintaining the versatility of the SLR format. Some institutions have used a dual system with 35-mm and digital cameras mounted side by side,[6] and combined units are available commercially. Whether one uses film-based or digital methods to document gross autopsy findings, the considerations and recommendations that follow are generally relevant.

Many SLR cameras on the market today are fully automatic. However, high-end technology is not required. In fact, exposure determinations by automatic equipment may not adequately account for the influences of a light specimen on a dark background.[4] A black camera is desirable because it reduces the possibility of reflection in the background. Waist-level viewfinders permit one to look horizontally into the camera and, when equipped with a magnifier, facilitate focusing.[7] With our equipment, we use an eye-level viewfinder and a step stool that allows the photographer to see through the viewfinder at higher camera elevations. A cable shutter release is mandatory because it reduces camera motion and eliminates reflections on the background from the operator's hand.

Commercially available automated systems that include foot pedal control of video cameras linked to a computer allowing zoom control, auto focus, image capture, automatic downloading, and recognition of specimen accession numbers are available.[8] Alternatively, homemade systems utilizing either video or digital systems have been described.[9,10]

### Lens

A wide range of lenses are available for SLR cameras. Lenses for specimen photography should have high resolution at short focal length. The 50-mm lens is probably the most versatile choice for photography of small and large specimens.

Lenses of longer focal lengths, 80 to 105 mm, increase the working distance, avoiding the possibility of obstruction of the illumination and increasing the safety margin when photographing infectious specimens.[4,11] However, these lenses are not ideal for photography of small specimens such as coronary arteries or for extreme close-ups of lesions. An alternative is a macrozoom lens, which allows one to vary the size of the image at a fixed working distance. Compared with fixed-length lenses, macrozoom lenses have a number of disadvantages, including bulkiness, smaller maximum aperture, lower reproduction ratios, less sharpness in the corners, and greater cost.[12]

### Film

As noted earlier, digital media are, in the long run, less expensive and easier to store than film, as well as slides and prints made from film. Important factors in the consideration of film for specimen photography include color balance, film speed, reciprocity characteristics, format, processing, resolving power, granularity value, and long-term stability of dyes.[4,13] The most versatile type of film for routine specimen photography is the color transparency (slide) film designed for projection. Films with low International Standards Organization (ISO) speed provide fine grain and high resolution and are generally the films preferred by most pathologists. However, the choice of specific film is somewhat subjective and should probably be made after testing several brands and types.

### Photographic Stand and Specimen Box

Photographic stands from a number of manufacturers are available through suppliers of professional photographic equipment. For specimen photography, one requires a stand with a vertical column. These may be freestanding (copy stands) or mounted on a wall. In either case, they should be sturdy and placed in areas free from vibrations. In addition to vertical movement, a good photographic stand allows camera movement toward and away from the front of the column and rotation on this axis. A stand that permits camera movement to the left and right of the column is desirable but not necessary for most work, particularly with a free-moving specimen or light box. Specimen boxes can be purchased or hand made according to the specifications supplied by Vetter.[14] For autopsy photography, specimen boxes should provide even background illumination and have a surface area that accepts large specimens. The ideal specimen box has a removable top plate that is easily changed and cleaned.

### Copy Stand and Lighting

Specimen illumination should be bright, even, and with minimal specular highlights. Photoflood lamps (500 watt, 3200 K or 3400 K rating) that match tungsten films are inexpensive but do not last long and shift colors as they age.[15] Although adequate for black-and-white photography, fluorescent lamps may distort colors. Tungsten-halogen lamps or electronic flash units with modeling lights are best. Compared with tungsten-halogen lamps, flash units develop less heat during operation and produce less spectral reflection.[14] For photography of very small specimens, LeBeau[16] advocated the use of supplemental fiber-optic lighting or specialized macrophotography lighting systems. For illuminating cavities, axial lighting systems offer considerable advantages and are easy to incorporate into a basic illumination setup.[17] Note that when using a digital camera the white balance needs to be adjusted for "flash" or comparable setting for optimal color balance.

### Background

The ideal background isolates the subject, avoids distraction, and is free of clutter.[18] Backgrounds in use for specimen photography include white, black, gray, and colored. There is considerable disagreement among specimen photographers about the ideal background choice. Each has its advantages and disadvantages, and ultimately one's choice is based on personal preference. However, regardless of which color background is chosen, make sure that it is easily cleaned. This condition is most easily achieved when the top plate or surface in contact with the specimen is easily removable and washable. Glass or Plexiglas plates fulfill this requirement.

White backgrounds do not compete with the color of the specimen, although specimens may appear lighter. They are effective in isolating the specimen but achieve a better definition of contour and outline for dark specimens than they do for light specimens. One of the advantages of white backgrounds is that they convert well to black-and-white publication prints. The major disadvantages include distracting shadows and glare that may be difficult to eliminate. Typically, white backgrounds are obtained through the use of a transilluminated light box, a relatively easy system to assemble and maintain.

Black backgrounds provide a dramatic impact. When projected in a dark room, specimens photographed against a dark background have the appearance of floating, providing a three-dimensional effect. Like white backgrounds, black backgrounds do not compete with the color of the specimen. However, they provide better isolation of lighter specimens than dark specimens. Black backgrounds may place too much emphasis on the outline of the subject, particularly if it is light colored. This has the effect of distracting the viewer from important internal details. Some find it difficult to obtain consistent black backgrounds except with deep-nap velvet, which has the disadvantage of requiring frequent washing.[8] Vetter[14] relies on a glass-topped black box made by placing clear glass over a wooden box with its insides painted flat black and its bottom lined with black velvet. The distance separating top plate and background adds to the three-dimensional effect. Others spray the back of the glass with flat black paint and then place the specimen on the other side.[19]

Most who use colored backgrounds for specimen photography prefer blue or bluish green because these colors complement the pink to red colors of most tissues. Colored backgrounds provide vividness and clarity to the subject. They also increase the visibility of important white, black, or gray areas present in the specimens that tend to be lost against white, black, or gray backgrounds. When projected on a screen, the reflected light from the background adds brightness and helps maintain viewers' interest.[4] However, colored backgrounds cause viewer color adaptation, which influences true color perception. For this reason, many deem colored backgrounds undesirable. Colored backgrounds are easily obtained with transillumination and colored glass or Plexiglas sheets or with colored mat board placed in a specimen box.

Gray backgrounds avoid many of the pitfalls mentioned for black and colored backgrounds in that they do not concentrate undue attention on the specimen border or produce false color perception. However, like white backgrounds, gray backgrounds produce visible shadows that are difficult to eliminate. Furthermore, uniform gray backgrounds are difficult to repeat from photograph to photograph because of color cast and reflectivity of specimens.[4]

## Photographic Technique

In general, by using a photographic setup, one can establish a standardized set of photographic conditions that can yield excellent results, even for the novice photographer. However, those with little previous experience should be familiar with some basic concepts. The film is like the retina; it receives an image that has been focused by a lens. The photographer focuses the lens of the camera while viewing the image through the viewfinder, rotating the lens, and observing the image come into sharp focus. The camera lens has a lens aperture (*f*) controlling how much light reaches the film. Thus, it functions like the iris, controlling the size of the pupil and the light reaching the retina. In low light, the lens aperture must be opened widely, and in very bright light it must be opened only narrowly. The photographer opens and closes the lens aperture by twisting a ring located on the lens. The lens aperture ring clicks into various numbered positions that are referred to as *f*-stops. The highest numbered *f*-stop indicates the minimum or narrowest aperture and the lowest the greatest or widest aperture. The camera has a shutter (eyelid) that covers the film at all times except when a picture is being taken (i.e., during an exposure). The length of this exposure is controlled on the camera by adjustment of the shutter speed. Shutter speed dials are marked in fractions of a second. However, the numerator is always 1 and is not shown. Thus, typical shutter speed markings of 1, 2, 4, 8, 16, 30, 60, 125, 250, and 500 refer to times ranging from 1 to 1/500 second. Properly exposing the film requires one to determine the appropriate lens aperture and shutter speed settings.

Focusing is easy with most 35-mm SLR cameras because the lens aperture automatically opens to its widest setting and provides a bright image. However, the inexperienced specimen photographer should know that only one plane of the specimen is in perfect focus. There is a distance both above and below this plane of perfect focus where the specimen is in acceptable focus. This distance is referred to as the depth of field. Depth of field is not a problem with a flat specimen such as a cut section of liver. It may be a major problem in close-ups of specimens with multiple focal planes, such as the heart opened to expose chambers and valves. In simple terms, the camera setting that provides the greatest depth of field is one where the *f*-stop is set maximally. However, this must be done while still allowing a reasonable exposure time. In some instances, flattening the specimen so that focal planes are closer to one another may also help.

## Specimen Preparation

Proper preparation of the specimen is the first step in obtaining a high-quality gross photograph. No matter how perfectly a photograph is composed, if the specimen is poorly dissected, the photograph serves mainly to demonstrate the poor preparation. One should strive to maintain the appearance of the specimen as it existed in situ, demonstrating any lesions to advantage. Remove any unnecessary adipose and connective tissues. Carefully rinse, wipe, or blot away blood, mucus, and other secretions unless they constitute an integral part of the pathologic findings. A sharp knife and proper cutting technique eliminate marks that may mar otherwise excellent photographs of cut surfaces.

Photographs of fresh specimens demonstrate natural colors and are more dramatic than photographs of fixed specimens, which often appear artificial and bland. However, the problem of oozing fluids may make photography of unfixed organs difficult or impractical. Color-preserving fixatives such as modified Jore's solution partially solve this problem (Table 7-1).[14] The color of tissues placed in modified Jore's solution is stable for several weeks, allowing temporary storage of specimens prior to photography. Because color-preserving solutions provide poor fixation for histology, one must obtain and fix samples for histology separately. For specimens previously fixed in formalin, immersion in 80% ethanol for 30 minutes partially restores natural colors.[11] Other color-preserving fixatives and color rejuvenation solutions are discussed by Ludwig.[20]

## Composition
### Orientation

As nearly as possible, the photograph should depict the organ in its anatomic position.[21] Typically organs are situated as if the viewer were facing the patient.[1] But in fact there is great disparity in how pathologists orient organs in photographs. For example, many (including us) photograph brain slices so that their caudal sections are viewed and the left side of the brain is to the viewer's left. In any case, the photographer should line up the long axis of an organ with the longitudinal axis of the camera to minimize the amount of background. Later, one can rotate the transparency or print 90 degrees and display the specimen with its long axis either horizontal or vertical as dictated by anatomic considerations.

### Cropping

All the important details of the specimen should be present in the photograph. For photographs that provide an overview of

| Table 7-1 | Modified Jore's solution |
| --- | --- |
| Water | 20 L |
| Sodium chloride | 90 g |
| Sodium bicarbonate | 162 g |
| Sodium sulfate (desiccated) | 200 g |
| Chloral hydrate | 360 g |
| 40% formaldehyde | 400 ml |

the specimen, a good rule to follow is to get as close to the specimen as possible, limiting unwanted background but isolating the subject. The subject should not touch the border of the frame because this leads the eye out of the picture. Usually it is best to position the area of interest in the center of the frame, although some advocate the "thirds rule," which states that the point of interest belongs at the junction of thirds.[22] Often both an overview and a close-up view photograph are necessary. Close-up views must include enough of the surrounding anatomy to permit orientation. One should pay particular attention to depth of focus and increased illumination requirements of close-up photographs.

### Distracters

Eliminate distracting objects from the photographic field. Generally this means pointers, probes, labels, rulers, surgical clamps, or fingers that lead the eye away from the subject. Good dissections coupled with good photographs usually obviate the need for pointers or probes by directing the viewer to the important features. Pointers have two unwanted consequences. First, they are difficult to attach in proper orientation.[21] Second, they hide a portion of the specimen. Small communicating defects are exceptions that often require a probe for identification. McGavin and Thompson[4] use urinary catheters as probes because they are unobtrusive, flexible, easily cut to the appropriate length, and available in a variety of diameters. A number of methods using overlays allow one to add pointers or other identifying symbols to publication prints or transparencies.

Some circumstances (e.g., legal) may necessitate inclusion of identifying labels. Many photographers take photographs with and without labels. In either case, labels should be as small and unobtrusive as possible. Rulers elicit significant controversy among professional biomedical photographers. Haber[2] includes a ruler at the lower edge of the frame when it is necessary to provide a size relationship but otherwise excludes them. Others use them routinely.[4,14] Like labels, rulers should be unobtrusive. This is best achieved by using rulers with graduations and no numbers so that the size of the ruler in the photograph can be controlled by moving it up or down to reveal an appropriate and nondistracting length of the graduations.[4] Some photographers combine labels and rulers but risk creating a distraction by adding too much written information. Photographic labels and rulers require elevation to the same focal plane as the specimen. A number of systems, including corks, copper tubing, wooden blocks, specially constructed stands, and modeling clay, have been recommended.[4]

Organs with cavities or lumens may require retraction to demonstrate the pertinent anatomy. Obtaining aesthetic photographs of these specimens presents a challenge to the photographer. Surgical instruments such as clamps or forceps should be avoided. The viewer's attention is unnecessarily attracted to the instruments, which often contain imperfections or produce unwanted highlights. Gloved fingers in the photographic field are acceptable to some; however, the gloves must be opaque, well fitting, and clean.[4] Kennedy[23] has designed a traction apparatus that is relatively easily assembled. Black silk sutures

(00 or 000) with an attached curved needle are placed on tissue that needs retracting, and tension is applied to the suture by securing it under cleats. Coupled with a black background, the sutures are essentially invisible and the small needles relatively unobtrusive. We use a simpler system in which the free ends of the sutures are stayed by being tied to suction cup hooks (Adams Manufacturing, Portersville, Penn., or Jersey Wood & Metal Specialties, Paterson, N.J.) that are readily available at hardware or houseware stores. These movable suction cup hooks facilitate traction in any direction. We keep a set of five hooks handy, enough for even the most difficult hearts (Fig. 7-1).

### Specular Highlights

Specular highlights, the reflections of light sources from surfaces of subjects, provide special problems for the specimen photographer. A number of techniques reduce or eliminate specular highlights. Drying the specimen surface, eliminating surface contours, changing the angle of illumination, illuminating through diffusing screens, and using small reflectors may reduce highlights. The use of polarizing filters on the light source and on the camera lens also reduces reflections (Fig. 7-2). Some feel that complete elimination of highlights renders specimens unnaturally flat; they add some nonpolarized lights to produce some controlled reflections that add relief and structural effect.[11]

Photography of specimens placed under fluid reduces undesirable highlights. Although numerous liquids have been tried, water, saline, and 95% alcohol are the most practical for specimen photography. In addition to reduction of specular highlights, immersion photography accentuates lesion borders and the three-dimensional structure of villous or papillary lesions.[24,25] Adhering small specimens to glass plates through surface tension, inverting the plate, and photographing through the plate eliminate highlights.[26] Technical obstacles include cutting a flat slice and adhering the specimen to the glass without trapping air bubbles between tissue and glass.

### Photography at the Autopsy Table

Often there are pathologic findings at autopsy that cannot be photographed at a copy stand. External signs of disease; processes involving large, contiguous regions of the viscera; the body cavities; the effects of surgery or other therapeutic interventions; and any findings altered during organ removal or evisceration might require documentation. Thus, the pathologist should be prepared to photograph at the autopsy table. A 35-mm SLR camera coupled with a battery-powered electronic flash provides an easily operated system for performing in situ photography. However, the newer digital cameras are perhaps a better choice for in situ photography because they provide excellent images in low-light conditions. A ladder or step stool is necessary for some overhead views. A macro-zoom lens may afford some flexibility but is not absolutely required.

The same principles that characterize good specimen photography distinguish in situ autopsy photography. One should dissect with care and expose the photographic field. Excess blood is removed. Distracting backgrounds that are often

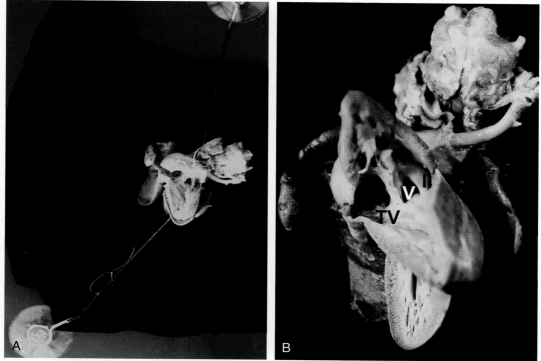

**Figure 7-1** A simple method of positioning a specimen for photography. **A,** A photograph of the top of the copy stand shows suction cup hooks outside the photographic field and a black velvet background. A suture with a curved needle bent to function as a hook is used to retract the heart with cardiac defects. **B,** In this classic view of tetralogy of Fallot, the free wall of the right ventricle has been reflected to reveal the ventricular septum. The anteriorly malpositioned outlet septum narrows the infundibulum *(I)* and creates a perimembranous ventricular septal defect *(V)*. *TV,* Tricuspid valve and inlet portion of the right ventricle.

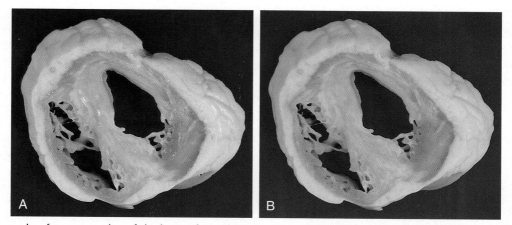

**Figure 7-2** Photographs of a cross section of the heart of a patient with myocardial scars. **A,** In this photograph taken without polarization, the specular highlights are distracting and partially obscure the areas of fibrosis. **B,** In this photograph, polarization has reduced the specular highlights, and the areas of fibrosis are clearly and distinctly seen.

necessarily contained in photographs of large areas may be cropped out of the transparency or photographic print after processing and printing. Unfortunately, unwanted highlights are more difficult to remedy. This problem may be compounded by the need to retract tissues with stainless steel surgical instruments, which often create disturbing reflections. Altering the position of the retractors can often reduce the amount of reflected light. Illumination of cavities for in situ photography presents another problem. A spotlight or a ring flash may provide sufficient supplemental light.

## Storing and Preserving Photographic Images

Color transparencies are sensitive to temperature and fluctuations in humidity. Long-term storage at a relative humidity of 35% at a temperature as low as possible prolongs color stability.[27] Systems for creating a manageable collection of photographic images are discussed by Morton and Dorrington.[28] New developments for electronic capture and storage of images have revolutionized biomedical photography during the late twentieth and early twenty-first centuries. Most assuredly, digital imaging will continue to alter the way pathologists document postmortem findings. The lifespan of a burnable CD or DVD is dependent on the type of disk (CD-R and DVD-R last longer than CD-RW, DVD-RW, DVD+RW, and DVD-RAM), the quality of the disk material, and the manufacturing process. Some manufacturers estimate a lifespan of 100 years for their highest quality products but only 30 years for others. Because the technology advances rapidly, it is advisable to consult information technology experts to determine the most cost effective and stable methods of storing and backing up digital image files.

### Manipulation of Digital Photographic Images

Because images can be used as evidence in court, it is important that the original, unaltered image is saved. For medical examiners and coroners, the usual identifiable chain of custody for evidence must be preserved. Of course, medical images, whether they are digital, film, or prints, are covered under the Health Information Portability and Accountability Act (HIPAA) and must be treated as confidential.[29]

## AUTOPSY RADIOLOGY

Autopsy radiology is an effective supplement to gross and microscopic examination. Postmortem radiographs are of particular importance in autopsies of fetuses and neonates who may have a syndrome with characteristic or complex skeletal malformations.[30,31] Imaging studies are also useful for evaluation of acquired diseases of the bones and joints and for medicolegal death investigations.

### Postmortem Radiographs

A low-voltage cabinet X-ray machine (Faxitron, X-Ray LLC, Wheeling, Ill.) is an indispensable piece of equipment for a modern autopsy service (Fig. 7-3). We routinely obtain anteroposterior radiographs of all fetuses and stillborn infants to aid

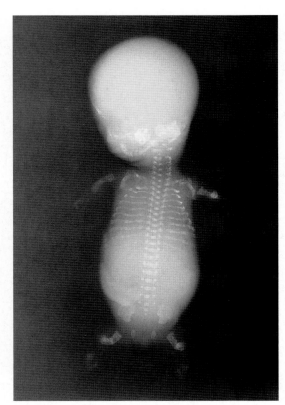

**Figure 7-4** This radiograph of a fetus with osteogenesis imperfecta congenita discloses osteopenic bones and multiple healing or healed fractures. Cranial bones are largely inconspicuous.

in the diagnosis of skeletal abnormalities (Fig. 7-4). Radiographs of dissected specimens also provide useful information for evaluation of skeletal lesions in the older child and adult. Lytic, inflammatory, degenerative, and developmental lesions of bones and joints are particularly well demonstrated by radiographs (Fig. 7-5). If a cabinet X-ray machine is not available, the autopsy pathologist should approach the radiology department for assistance with postmortem radiographic studies. The cooperation of the radiology department is also helpful when the size of the specimen (e.g., a full-term stillborn infant) precludes examination in a cabinet X-ray machine.

### Forensic Radiology

Postmortem radiology is such an important part of a thorough forensic examination that all well-equipped medical examiners' offices should have access to a radiology table or a portable X-ray machine. In the medicolegal setting, postmortem radiographs are useful for localizing bullets or other metallic foreign objects; confirming suspected air embolism; documenting pneumothorax, pneumomediastinum, and pneumoperitoneum; and examining bones for signs of recent and old trauma.[32,33] Data obtained from radiographs may aid in determining the cause of death or help verify the identity of the deceased. Without radiographs, the prosector may easily miss subtle fractures of the facial bones, skull, spine, and pelvis.[34] The forensic pathologist should also employ radiographs in cases of mutilated, decomposed, or burned bodies and in cases in which one suspects the presence of human remains but verification is difficult by visual inspection only.[35]

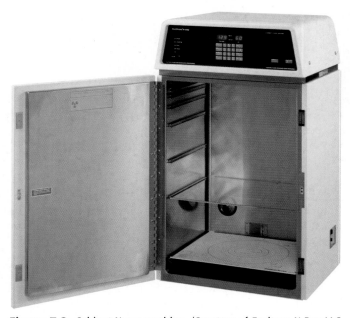

**Figure 7-3** Cabinet X-ray machine. (Courtesy of Faxitron X-Ray LLC, Wheeling, Ill.)

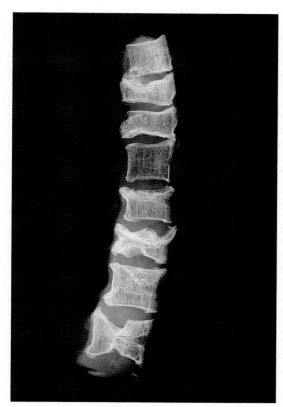

**Figure 7-5** Cabinet radiograph of a portion of the vertebral column removed at autopsy from an elderly man who had received recent radiation to the spine for treatment of metastatic prostate cancer. Marked osteopenia, several collapsed vertebral bodies, and a few scattered osteolytic lesions are present. Tumor masses are not seen. Microscopic study of the vertebral bone showed widespread necrosis, hemorrhage, and reactive change along with residual foci of poorly differentiated adenocarcinoma.

## Specialized Imaging Techniques

Although they are prohibitively expensive for routine work, pathologists and radiologists have used specialized procedures such as postmortem computed tomography (CT) and magnetic resonance imaging (MRI) for research and specialized forensic applications. Ros and colleagues[36] found postmortem MRI to be superior to autopsy in detecting air and fluid in body cavities or potential body spaces. Similarly, postmortem CT demonstrated the distribution of gas within the brain in a diving fatality.[37] However, the most useful application of these techniques appears to be in the investigation of traumatic deaths.[38] Postmortem cranial MRI,[39] whole-body MRI,[40] and whole-body CT scanning[41] can be effective adjuncts to autopsy examination, helping to direct the postmortem examination or adding valuable information not detected by postmortem dissection and examination.

## Angiography

Angiography is underused in the autopsy suite. It extends the autopsy pathologist's ability to evaluate vascular disease and is extremely useful for determining the degree of narrowing in coronary and other small arteries[42-45] and locating the origin

of bleeding, as in cases of gastrointestinal hemorrhage related to angiodysplasia.[46-48] In cases of suspected vascular injury, angiography may help localize the site of perforation or dissection.[49,50] In cases of complex congenital vascular malformations, angiography may help define the abnormalities or locate sites of obstruction.[51] The lungs,[52-55] liver,[56] kidneys,[57,58] and brain[59] all lend themselves to postmortem angiography (Fig. 7-6). The vastness and complexity of the collateral circulation of the celiac and mesenteric arteries[60] complicate postmortem angiography of the upper and lower gastrointestinal organs. However, the partitioning technique of Reiner and colleagues,[61,62] although still challenging, helps in overcoming these impediments (Fig. 7-7).

Ludwig[63] outlined various techniques for in situ and ex vivo arteriography, venography, and lymphangiography. However, many of these methods are too complicated for routine use. For most purposes, we find that a handheld syringe is adequate for injecting contrast material into vessels. Rissanen[64] described a simple instrument made out of a Foley catheter, large-bore needle, and rubber stopper that is useful for injections into the aorta or other large vessels. For smaller vessels, we use discarded catheters obtained from the cardiology or radiology department. Barium-gelatin solution (Box 7-1) is an ideal contrast agent for postmortem angiography. It solidifies after injection but does not interfere with subsequent processing of the tissue for microscopic examination. Others

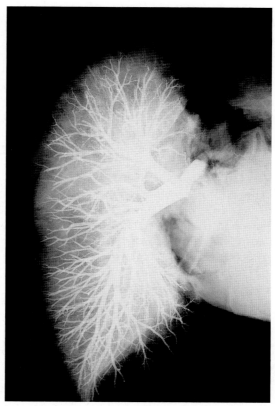

**Figure 7-6** Postmortem pulmonary arteriography. The lung was inflated with air before the pulmonary artery was injected with a mixture of barium sulfate and gelatin.

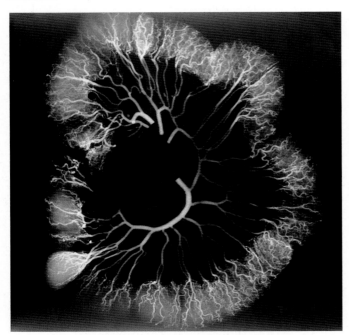

**Figure 7-7** Postmortem superior mesenteric artery angiogram showing arborizing arterial branches.

---

**Box 7-1**   Barium sulfate-gelatin contrast material

1. Dissolve 50 g of gelatin in hot water and bring up to a volume of 200 mL.
2. Add 800 mL of 100% (w/v) barium sulfate suspension.
3. Divide into appropriate-volume aliquots and store frozen.
4. Heat to 45°C before use.

---

**Box 7-2**   A method for postmortem coronary subtraction angiography

1. Separate the unfixed heart and proximal aorta from the lungs and adjacent tissues.
2. Using either water or saline solution, flush the heart chambers along the direction of blood flow to remove blood.
3. Open the proximal aorta longitudinally from its free end until the coronary artery ostia are accessible. Test the patency of the proximal 0.5 cm of each coronary arterial ostium.
4. Place string ligatures under the proximal right and left coronary arteries within 0.5 to 1.0 cm of the ostia.
5. Prepare two syringes with contrast material, attach to catheters, and completely fill the catheters with contrast material, making sure that they do not contain air bubbles.
6. Pass the catheter tips into the coronary artery ostia and tie them in securely. Retract the catheters until their tips abut the ligatures.
7. Place the specimen on a raised polyurethane (Plexiglas) platform and secure the catheters and syringes with tape.
8. Place unexposed X-ray film under the platform and take a preinjection radiograph. Remove the exposed film and replace it with unexposed film.
9. Inject 1.5 to 3 mL of contrast material into each coronary artery (4 to 6 mL for coronary arterial bypass grafts), and take a postinjection radiograph. Injections may also be documented sequentially.

From Prahlow JA, Scharling ES, Lantz PE: Postmortem coronary subtraction angiography, *Am J Forensic Med Pathol* 17:225-230, 1996.

---

have used liquid vulcanizable silicone rubber made radiopaque to prepare vascular casts.[65,66] In many situations, solidification of the contrast material is unnecessary. In such cases, we use contrast solutions (Omnipaque, Winthrop Pharmaceuticals, New York, or Gastrografin, Mallinckrodt, St. Louis, Mo.). Again, clinical angiographers and radiologists can often provide materials left over from studies of patients.

Box 7-2 describes and Figure 7-8 demonstrates a technique of Prahlow and coworkers[50] for coronary angiography that can be easily adapted to other arteries. We use this technique routinely before dissection of hearts with significant coronary artery disease. It is also an ideal method for evaluating coronary artery bypass grafts, being particularly useful for determining patency or occlusion at the graft-artery anastomosis. By simply taking a preangiogram film, one also obtains sufficient imaging data to perform subtraction angiography. This technique is effective in locating subtle lesions that might be missed by visual inspection alone or obscured by preexisting vascular disease detected on routine angiograms. Most hospital radiology departments or cardiac catheterization facilities have the computer hardware and software needed for the subtraction analysis. The addition of different colored dyes (Stat Lab Medical Products, Lewisville, Tex.) to right and left coronary artery injections allows the pathologist to determine the coronary artery distribution within the myocardium at both gross and microscopic levels.[67]

### Other Radiographic Contrast Studies

The methods for angiography apply equally well for techniques such as bronchography,[68] cholangiography,[69] pancreatography,[70,71] and urography (Fig. 7-9).[63]

### Virtopsy

The field of postmortem imaging is growing and finding some practical usefulness in forensic cases.[72-74] The term *virtopsy* (a combination of "virtual" and "autopsy") has been coined to describe body volume documentation and analysis using CT, MRI, and microradiology and three-dimensional body surface documentation using forensic photogammetry and three-dimensional optical scanning.[75] Sophisticated postmortem angiography using a modified heart-lung machine has yielded detailed images of the vascular system.[76] A number of investigators have used postmortem MRI and suggested that its use as a supplement to regular autopsy or even as a minimally invasive substitute for autopsy when autopsy consent cannot be obtained.[77-79]

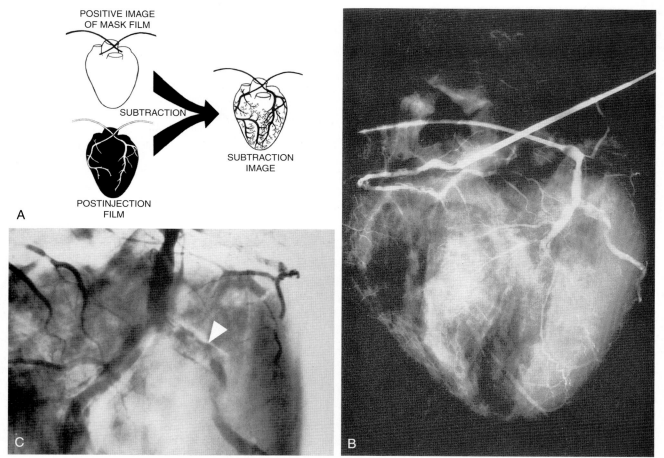

**Figure 7-8 A,** Diagrammatic representation of subtraction angiography. Structures seen in the positive image of the preinjection film are digitally subtracted from the postinjection film to create the subtraction angiogram. **B,** Routine postinjection film. **C,** Subtraction coronary angiogram demonstrating contrast material within the wall of an atherosclerotic coronary artery diagnostic of a dissection. (From Prahlow JA, Scharling ES, Lantz PE: Postmortem coronary subtraction angiography, *Am J Forensic Med Pathol* 17:225-230, 1996.)

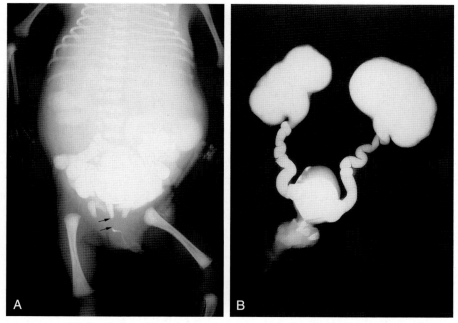

**Figure 7-9** Postmortem urograms performed on a 28-week gestational age male fetus with obstructive uropathy due to posterior urethral valves. **A,** Whole fetal urogram obtained after suprapubic injection of radiopaque dye into the urinary bladder and retrograde injection of radiopaque dye into the urethra through the urinary meatus. The lower urinary tract is well visualized, including the area of severe urethral narrowing in the region of the verumontanum *(arrows)*. Gross dissection demonstrated posterior urethral valves with a central aperture (type III Young valves). **B,** Radiograph of the urinary specimen removed en bloc shows dilated ureters and kidneys to better advantage.

## REFERENCES

1. Vetter JP: An integrated method of preserving and photographing gross specimens, *J Biol Photogr Assoc* 28:21-27, 1960.
2. Haber MH: Five mistakes to avoid in macrophotography, *Pathologist* 38:172-197, 1984.
3. Hansell P: *A guide to medical photography*, Baltimore, 1979, University Park Press.
4. McGavin MD, Thompson SW: *Specimen dissection and photography for the pathologist, anatomist and biologist*, Springfield, Ill, 1988, Charles C Thomas.
5. Vetter JP: *Biomedical photography*, Boston, 1992, Butterworth-Heinemann.
6. Belanger AJ, Lopes AE, Sinard JH: Implementation of a practical digital imaging system for routine gross photography in an autopsy environment, *Arch Pathol Lab Med* 124:160-165, 2000.
7. Haber SL: Choosing a camera body, *Pathologist* 37:339-341, 1983.
8. Leong FJW-M, Leong AS-Y: Digital imaging in pathology: Theoretical and practical considerations, and applications, *Pathology* 36:234-241, 2004.
9. Leong AS-Y Visinoni F, Visinoni C, Milios J: An advanced digital image-capture computer system for gross specimens: A substitute for gross description, *Pathology* 32:131-135, 2000.
10. Park R, Eom J, Park P, Lee K, Joo H: Automation of gross photography using a remote-controlled digital camera system, *Arch Pathol Lab Med* 127:726-731, 2003.
11. Häberlin C: Specimen photography. In Hansell P, editor: *A guide to medical photography*, Baltimore, 1979, University Park Press, pp 77-97.
12. Haber SL: Choosing a lens for your camera, *Pathologist* 37:570-579, 1983.
13. Haber SL: Choosing film for your camera, *Pathologist* 38:186-188, 1984.
14. Vetter JP: Gross specimen photography. In Vetter JP, editor: *Biomedical photography*, Boston, 1992, Butterworth-Heinemann, pp 359-368.
15. deVeer WH: Photographic copying. In Vetter JP, editor: *Biomedical photography*, Boston, 1992, Butterworth-Heinemann, pp 77-90.
16. LeBeau LJ: Photography of very small biomedical objects, *J Biol Photogr Assoc* 59:77-87, 1991.
17. Frederickson RM: Axial lighting for in situ photography of heart valves, *J Biol Photogr Assoc* 57:69-73, 1989.
18. Blaker AA: *Handbook for scientific photography*, San Francisco, 1977, WH Freeman.
19. LeBeau LJ, Eimmrt AD: Photography of tiny reflective biomedical objects, *J Biol Photogr* 50:101-120, 1982.
20. Ludwig J: *Handbook of autopsy practice*, Totowa, NJ, 2002, Humana Press.
21. Martin D: Gross pathological specimens. In Linssen EF, editor: *Medical photography in practice*, London, 1961, Fountain Press, pp 247-276.
22. Kodak: *Composition*, Rochester, NY, 1971, Eastman Kodak.
23. Kennedy LA: A traction apparatus for specimen photography, *J Biol Photogr Assoc* 54:85-87, 1986.
24. Ellis J: Under-fluid gross specimen photography—recent observations, *J Biol Photogr Assoc* 45:98-99, 1977.
25. Kennedy LA: Techniques for photography of immersed specimens, *J Biol Photogr Assoc* 52:67-71, 1984.
26. Burry AF, Stewart B: A simple method of eliminating highlights in photography of fresh specimens, *Med Biol Illus* 23:55, 1973.
27. Irvine RF: Conserving and storing photographic images. In Vetter JP, editor: *Biomedical photography*, Boston, 1992, Butterworth-Heinemann, pp 475-486.
28. Morton R, Dorrington JA: The management of collections of photographic images. In Vetter JP, editor: *Biomedical photography*, Boston, 1992, Butterworth-Heinemann, pp 487-498.
29. Scheinfeld N: Photographic images, digital imaging, dermatology, and the law, *Arch Dermatol* 140:473-476, 2004.
30. Kjaier I, Graem N: Simple autopsy method for analysis of complex fetal cranial malformations, *Pediatr Pathol* 10:717-727, 1990.
31. Dugoff L, Thieme G, Hobbins JC: Skeletal anomalies, *Clin Perinatol* 27:979-1005, 2000.
32. Sanes S, Eschner EG: Roentgen-ray examination in medicolegal autopsies, *N Y State J Med* 55:628-633, 1955.
33. Saliba NA, Maya G: Air embolism during pneumoperitoneum refill, *Am Rev Respir Dis* 92:810-812, 1965.
34. Rose EF: The medicolegal autopsy. In Race GJ, editor: *Laboratory medicine*, Hagerstown, Md, 1980, Harper & Row, pp 3-19.
35. Morgan TA, Harris MC: The use of X-rays as an aid to medicolegal investigation, *J Forensic Med* 1:28-38, 1953.
36. Ros P, Li KC, Vo P, et al: Preautopsy magnetic resonance imaging: Initial experience, *Magn Reson Imaging* 8:303-308, 1990.
37. Krantz P, Hotås S: Postmortem computed tomography in a diving fatality, *J Comput Assist Tomogr* 7:132-134, 1983.
38. Stäbler A, Eck J, Penning R, et al: Cervical spine: Post-mortem assessment of accident injuries—comparison of radiographic, MR imaging, anatomic, and pathological findings, *Radiology* 221:340-346, 2001.
39. Hart BL, Dudley MH, Zumwalt RE: Postmortem cranial MRI and autopsy correlation in suspected child abuse, *Am J Forensic Med Pathol* 17:217-224, 1996.
40. Patriquin L, Kassarjian A, Barish M, et al: Postmortem whole-body magnetic resonance imaging as an adjunct to autopsy: Preliminary clinical experience, *J Magn Reson Imaging* 13:277-287, 2001.
41. Donchin Y, Rivkind AI, Bar-Ziv J, et al: Utility of post-mortem computed tomography in trauma victims, *J Trauma* 37:552-556, 1994.
42. Schlesinger MJ: An injection plus dissection study of coronary artery occlusions and anastomoses, *Am Heart J* 15:528-568, 1938.
43. Robbins SL, Fish SJ: A new angiographic technic providing a simultaneous permanent cast of the coronary arterial lumen, *Am J Clin Pathol* 42:156-163, 1964.
44. Thomas AC, Pazios S: The postmortem detection of coronary artery lesions using coronary arteriography, *Pathology* 24:5-11, 1992.
45. Katsuragawa M, Fujiwara H, Miyamae M, Sasayama S: Histologic studies in percutaneous transluminal coronary angioplasty for chronic total occlusion: Comparison of tapering and abrupt types of occlusion and short and long occluded segments, *J Am Coll Cardiol* 21:604-611, 1993.
46. Boley SJ, Sammartano R, Adams A, et al: On the nature and etiology of vascular ectasias of the colon: Degenerative lesions of aging, *Gastroenterology* 72:650-660, 1977.
47. Mitsudo SM, Boley SJ, Brandt LJ, et al: Vascular ectasias of the right colon in the elderly: A distinct pathologic entity, *Hum Pathol* 10:585-600, 1979.
48. Pounder DJ, Rowland R, Pieterse AS, et al: Angiodysplasias of the colon, *J Clin Pathol* 35:824-829, 1982.
49. Resnick JM, Engeler CE, Derauf BJ: Postmortem angiography of catheter-induced pulmonary perforation, *J Forensic Sci* 37:1346-1351, 1991.

50. Prahlow JA, Scharling ES, Lantz PE: Postmortem coronary subtraction angiography, *Am J Forensic Med Pathol* 17:225-230, 1996.

51. James CL, Keeling JW, Smith NM, Byard RW: Total anomalous pulmonary venous drainage associated with fatal outcome in infancy and early childhood: An autopsy study of 52 cases, *Pediatr Pathol* 14:665-678, 1994.

52. Liebow AA, Hales MR, Lindskog GE, Bloomer WE: Plastic demonstrations of pulmonary pathology, *Bull Int Assoc Med Mus* 27:116-129, 1947.

53. Milne ENC: Circulation of primary and metastatic pulmonary neoplasms, *Am J Roentgenol Radium Ther Nucl Med* 100:603-619, 1967.

54. Hendin AS, Greenspan RH: Ventilatory pumping of human pulmonary lymphatic vessels, *Radiology* 108:553-557, 1973.

55. Reeves JT, Noonan JA: Microarteriographic studies of primary pulmonary hypertension, *Arch Pathol* 95:50-55, 1973.

56. Mann JD, Wakim KG, Baggenstoss AH: Alterations in the vasculature of the diseased liver, *Gastroenterology* 25:540-546, 1953.

57. Holley KE, Hunt JC, Brown AL Jr, et al: Renal artery stenosis, *Am J Med* 37:14-22, 1964.

58. Bauer FW, Robbins SL: A postmortem study comparing renal angiograms and renal artery casts in 58 patients, *Arch Pathol* 83:307-314, 1967.

59. Wollschlaeger G, Wollschlaeger PB, Lucas FV, Lopez VF: Experience and result with postmortem cerebral angiography performed as routine procedure of the autopsy, *Am J Roentgenol Radium Ther Nucl Med* 101:68-87, 1967.

60. Michels NA, Siddharth P, Kornblith PL, Parke WW: Routes of collateral circulation of the gastrointestinal tract as ascertained in dissection of 500 bodies, *Int Surg* 49: 8-28, 1968.

61. Reiner L, Rodriguez FL, Platt R, Schlesinger MJ: Injection studies on the mesenteric arterial circulation. I. Technique and observations on collaterals, *Surgery* 45:820-833, 1959.

62. Reiner L: Mesenteric vascular occlusion studied by post-mortem injection of the mesenteric arterial circulation, *Pathol Annu* 1:193-220, 1966.

63. Ludwig J: *Current methods of autopsy practice*, Philadelphia, 1979, WB Saunders.

64. Rissanen VT: Double contrast technique for postmortem coronary angiography, *Lab Invest* 23:517-520, 1970.

65. Weman SM, Salminen U-S, Pentitilä A, et al: Post-mortem cast angiography in the diagnostics of graft complications in patients with fatal outcome following coronary artery bypass grafting (CABG), *Int J Legal Med* 112:107-114, 1999.

66. Saimanen E, Järvinen A, Pentitilä A: Cerebral cast angiography as an aid to medicolegal autopsies in cases of death after adult cardiac surgery, *Int J Legal Med* 114:163-168, 2001.

67. Smith M, Trummel DE, Dolz M, Cina SJ: A simplified method for postmortem coronary angiography using Gastrografin, *Arch Pathol Lab Med* 123:885-888, 1999.

68. Leopold JG, Gough J: Post-mortem bronchography in the study of bronchitis and emphysema, *Thorax* 18:172-177, 1963.

69. Legge DA, Carlson HC, Ludwig J: Cholangiographic findings in diseases of the liver: A postmortem study, *Am J Roentgenol Radium Ther Nucl Med* 113:34-40, 1971.

70. Stimec B, Bulajic M, Korneti V, et al: Ductal morphometry of ventral pancreas in pancreas divisum. Comparison between clinical and anatomical results, *Ital J Gastroenterol* 28:76-80, 1996.

71. Stimec B, Bulajic M, Tatic S, Markovic M: Unusual variants of the tributaries of the main pancreatic duct revealed by postmortem and endoscopic pancreatography, *Anat Anz* 178:169-171, 1996.

72. Yen K, Lövblad K-O, Scheurer E, et al: Post-mortem forensic neuroimaging: correlation of MSCT and MRI findings with autopsy results, *Forensic Sci Int* 173:21-35, 2007.

73. Levy AD, Virtual autopsy: Two- and three-dimensional multidetector CT findings in drowning with autopsy comparison, *Radiology* 243:862-868, 2007.

74. Harcke HT, Levy AD, Abbott RM, et al: Autopsy radiography: Digital radiographs (DR) vs multidetector computed tomography (MDCT) in high-velocity gunshot-wound victims, *Am J Forensic Med Pathol* 28:13-19, 2007.

75. Dirnhofer R, Jackowski C, Vock P, Potter K, Thali MJ: VIRTOPSY: Minimally invasive, imaging-guided virtual autopsy, *RadioGraphics* 26:1305-1333, 2006.

76. Grabherr S, Gygax E, Sollberger B et al: Two-step postmortem angiography with a modified heart-lung machine: Preliminary results, *AJR Am J Roentgenol* 190:345-351, 2008.

77. Brookes JS, Hagmann C: MRI in fetal necropsy, *J Magn Reson Imaging* 24:1221-1228, 2006.

78. Sebire NJ: Towards the minimally invasive autopsy? *Ultrasound Obstet Gynecol* 28:865-867, 2006.

79. Cohen MC, Paley MN, Griffiths PD, Whitby EH: Less invasive autopsy: Benefits and limitations of the use of magnetic resonance imaging in the perinatal postmortem, *Pediatr Dev Pathol* 11:1-9, 2008.

# 8

# Microscopic Examination

*"Pathologic Histology deals with departures from the normal in the various tissues of the body, which, occurring as the sequelae of disease processes, or standing in the closest causal relationship to the clinical symptoms and physical signs, constitute the foundation of all diagnostic conclusions, and of all rational therapeutic treatment."*

Alfred S. Warthin[1]

## BRIGHTFIELD MICROSCOPY

Brightfield or light microscopic analysis of organs and tissues supplements the gross autopsy examination and is an integral part of a complete postmortem examination. Although the focus and extent of the microscopic examination vary from case to case, microscopy of diseased tissues often aids the pathologist in correlating pathologic abnormalities with clinical findings. For the pathologist in training, microscopic examination of tissues obtained at autopsy helps build a broad foundation in normal and abnormal microanatomy. A general discussion of tissue preparation and staining is included in this chapter; however, the pathologist in training may want to consult specialized works for in-depth discussions of these topics.

## Tissue Fixation

Unlike tissues obtained from surgery, autopsy material has generally undergone considerable postmortem autolysis, the degree influenced by the time interval since death, body size, conditions in which the body has been stored, and to a certain extent the underlying disease processes. In view of this, careful handling and fixation of tissues obtained at autopsy are important to avoid further tissue degradation. First, one should avoid excessive handling or forceful rinsing of tissues, particularly those with delicate mucosal membranes. It should be noted, however, that gentle rinsing of tissues with water probably does little damage to histologic preparations of autopsy specimens.[2] Second, the tissues should not be allowed to dry out. Third, the tissues should be fixed in an adequate amount of fixative. Save small (i.e., 3 × 3 × 0.5 cm) pieces of representative tissues and specific lesions for microscopic examination in an adequate amount of fixative, typically at least 20 volumes of fixative to 1 volume of tissue. For gross pathology demonstrations, whole or large portions of organs may be fixed and then stored in less than the optimal amount of fixative. Finally, large collections of blood should be gently removed from the external surfaces of tissue (e.g., circle of Willis in case of vessel rupture) before fixation. Not only does this improve visualization of the anatomy, but it also facilitates fixation. Bloody fixatives fix poorly. If the fixative becomes heavily contaminated with blood from congested postmortem tissues, it should be replaced after 12 to 24 hours.

The aims of chemical fixation include arresting autolysis so that gross organs retain their shape and microanatomy is preserved and preventing postmortem bacterial overgrowth in preparation for tissue processing and subsequent staining reactions. Typically, 10% neutral buffered formalin (about 4% formaldehyde) has been the most commonly used fixative in autopsy practice. The advantages of formaldehyde-based fixatives include relatively rapid tissue penetration and thus good preservation of cell organelles, limited tissue shrinkage, and minimal tissue hardening. Formalin-fixed tissues are also still suitable for many immunohistochemical and molecular studies. However, biosafety concerns, environmental protection, and cost of disposal has heightened interest in the development of formalin-free fixatives. Most of these are alcohol-based. Compared with formaldehyde, alcohol has the advantage of lower toxicity but the disadvantages of causing increased tissue shrinkage and brittleness. A number of commercially available alcohol-based fixatives contain additives to counter these disadvantages.[3] Environmental and biosafety concerns limit the usefulness of aqueous fixatives based on mercuric chloride (Zenker, Helly), picric acid (Bouin), or chloroform (Carnoy).

Microwave energy speeds fixation and has been used successfully for diagnostic work. Optimal microwave fixation occurs at temperatures between 45°C and 55°C, but the ideal conditions for the tissue of interest must be worked out for each model. Underheating renders soft, poorly fixed tissue, making sectioning difficult. Overheating produces tissue vacuoles, pyknotic nuclei, and overstained cytoplasm.[4] To cool the tissue after microwaving, the heated fixative should be replaced with fixative at room temperature as soon as possible.

It has generally been recommended that whole brains remain in fixative for 2 to 4 weeks before cutting.[5,6] This practice lengthens the time needed to complete the examination and final report, however. To shorten the time needed to fix brains before optimal sectioning for gross and microscopic examination, Boon and colleagues[7] used microwave energy in combination with formalin- or alcohol-fixation. Garzón-de la Mora and colleagues[8] have explored electrochemical methods for rapidly fixing human brains. Others[9-13] have fixed the brain by vascular perfusion either by positive pressure through a syringe or electric pump or by an apparatus employing gravity. Compared with fixation by immersion, perfusion fixation shortens the interval required for fixation of the deep-seated regions of the brain. This not only allows the brain to be cut sooner but also improves immunohistochemical staining.[10] However, in a few brains fixed by perfusion, we have noted an artifact—irregular white matter pallor seen by hematoxylin and eosin stain. Although this appearance simulated white matter disease, there was no attendant gliosis to signify antemortem injury. Finally, vascular diseases such as atherosclerosis or injuries such as inadvertent laceration of the circle of Willis during brain removal make perfusion difficult or even impossible. Thus, in cases of suspected cerebral emboli or thrombi, perfusion fixation of the brain is contraindicated.

An easier alternative to perfusion fixation, immersion fixation in a large reservoir of formalin also reduces the time needed to preserve whole brains. A string is slipped under the basilar artery to suspend the brain in a $2 \times 2 \times 1$ foot acrylic plastic (Plexiglas) tank filled with 10% formalin and covered with an acrylic sheet. The tank is located within a fume hood, and the formalin is continually recirculated. Recirculation promotes faster fixation than immersion alone, and this technique is free of the technical difficulties of perfusion or microwave fixation. Brains are fixed for a minimum of 4 days, rinsed overnight, and then cut. Trimmed tissues are fixed for an additional 24 hours before processing.

Immersion fixation of the fetal or neonatal brain can be facilitated by adding kosher salt to the fixative. This "floats" the brain, minimizing artifacts produced by compression of the soft unmyelinated brain tissue against the walls of the vessel. Some pathologists fix the fetal or neonatal brain and spinal cord in situ by percutaneously injecting fixative into the lateral ventricles. The advantage of this technique is that it preserves delicate pathologic anatomy in cases of hydrocephalus or porencephalic cysts.[14] Because the injection can be done shortly after death and without any disfigurement, in situ fixation of the central nervous system may also be useful in cases in which autopsy permission has been obtained but postmortem dissection is delayed.[15] However, this is of practical significance only in situations in which special diagnostic studies such as electron microscopy or in situ hybridization are required.

## Decalcification

Bone and other mineralized tissue contain insoluble calcium salts that make them too hard to cut with an ordinary microtome; they must be softened or decalcified. This is accomplished by chemical removal of the calcium salts in solutions of acid, chelating agents, or ion exchange resins. The decalcification step is performed only after adequate fixation; otherwise, the decalcifying solutions denature the tissue proteins, adversely affecting the histology. To ensure proper fixation and subsequent ease in decalcification, small tissue samples approximately 4 mm thick should be prepared using a bone knife or saw. After fixation and before decalcification, the fixed tissue should be washed in running tap water to completely remove fixative that would otherwise react unfavorably with the decalcifying agent. Next, the tissue should be placed in the decalcifying solution (100 parts solution to 1 part tissue, or as otherwise directed by the manufacturer). The solution should be changed at least twice a day until the tissue has been sufficiently softened. Suspending the tissue (e.g., by wrapping it in gauze) ensures adequate decalcification of all surfaces of the sample.

Testing the softness of an additional small piece of similar tissue placed in the decalcifying solution is a convenient way to check the progress and yet preserve the integrity of the specimen. Samples that are cut easily with a scalpel will be cut readily on a microtome. Alternatively, one can insert a narrow-caliber needle into several representative regions of the specimen itself. If any grittiness is detected, decalcification is incomplete. The extent of decalcification can also be detected radiographically or chemically.[16] These methods are rarely required, and then only for samples that are difficult to decalcify, such as temporal bones. For chemical assessment of decalcification, aspirate 5 ml of decalcification fluid from the bottom of the container in which a sample has been suspended for at least 6 hours and in only five times the volume of the specimen to ensure that any calcium is in high concentration. Then add 5 ml each of 5% ammonium hydroxide and 5% ammonium oxalate and mix well. Formation of a cloudy precipitate indicates incomplete decalcification. If the solution is clear, decalcification is complete. After determining that decalcification is adequate, the tissue is placed in a labeled cassette and rinsed well under running tap water. The rinsing removes the decalcifying solution and allows adequate infiltration of paraffin during the later stages of processing. After rinsing, samples are stored in fixative until final tissue processing.

In cases of metabolic bone disease, alternative methods may be preferable to standard processing. For example, embedding in plastics (methyl methacrylate, glycol methacrylate, or a combination of the two) and preparation of sections with glass knives allow examination of nondecalcified bone.[17] Specialized grinding techniques allow the cutting of large sections.[18]

## General Guidelines for Microscopic Sampling of Tissues

In preparation for sampling for histology, trim the fixed tissues carefully. Use a sharp scalpel, and do not crush the tissue when cutting. Cut tissue to a thickness of approximately 3 mm, or less if the tissue is particularly dense or fatty. Do not overload the tissue cassettes because compressed tissues cannot be adequately dehydrated, infiltrated with paraffin, or properly embedded for optimal sectioning. Putting tissues of similar density together in cassettes makes for easier sectioning. If labeling cassettes by hand, pay particular attention to numbers such as 4 and 9 and letters *C* and *G*; *D*, *O*, and *Q*; and *U* and *V*, which are often unclear. Box 8-1 lists standard sections (excluding the central nervous system) that are submitted from pediatric and adult autopsies in our university hospital; additional sections from areas of pathology may be warranted. Box 8-2 and Figure 8-1 provide guidelines for microscopic sampling of the brain and spinal cord.

Except as indicated in Boxes 8-1 and 8-2, there are no set rules for determining where tissue from normal-appearing organs should be selected for microscopy. Whenever possible, however, organ capsules are sampled along with the underlying parenchyma and serosal or adventitial surfaces along with

mucosa or endothelium. In other words, full-thickness sections should be taken from hollow viscera, if possible. Microscopic sections of the kidney include cortex, medulla, and calyx. Use a hammer and bone knife to take samples of bone for decalcification rather than a vibrating or bone saw, which leaves bone dust as an artifact. Careful dissection, visual examination, and knowledge of pathologic processes guide the autopsy pathologist in the selection of sites and extent of sampling for microscopy. For example, sample primary malignancies in such a way that tumor progression and stage can be assessed. For discrete lesions, sample the edge of the lesion along with the adjacent transition into "normal" tissue, because this demonstrates the host response to the injury, often useful in dating the onset of the disease process. A number of manuals of surgical pathology offer guidelines for tissue sampling of individual organs and provide useful suggestions for microscopic sampling of organs containing primary neoplasms.[19-21]

---

**Box 8-1** Suggested method of trimming tissues, excluding brain and spinal cord, for standard microscopic sections using 2.5 × 3 cm plastic tissue processing cassettes

### Older child or adult (17 cassettes)*

Heart (1 section including left atrium, left circumflex coronary artery, mitral valve, and left ventricle)
Heart (1 section including right atrium, right coronary artery, tricuspid valve, and right ventricle)
Lung, left, hilus and periphery
Lung, right, hilus and periphery
Gastroesophageal junction/stomach
Small intestine/large intestine/appendix
Liver/head of pancreas
Thyroid gland/tail of pancreas
Parathyroid glands/pituitary gland
Adrenal gland/kidney, left
Adrenal gland/kidney, right
Breast/gonad, left/urinary bladder
Breast/gonad, right
Uterus (cervix, corpus) or prostate/seminal vesicles
Muscle (cross and longitudinal sections)/skin/nerve
Spleen/lymph nodes
Vertebra including bone marrow (decalcified)

### Fetus or infant (10 cassettes)*

Lung, left/heart, left including papillary muscle
Lung, right/heart, right including papillary muscle
Esophagus/stomach†/small intestines/large intestines
Liver/pancreas/thyroid gland/pituitary gland
Adrenal gland/kidney (including cortex, medulla, and papilla)/gonad, left
Adrenal gland/kidney (including cortex, medulla, and papilla)/gonad, right
Uterus or prostate/urinary bladder
Thymus/spleen/lymph nodes
Vertebra including bone marrow (decalcified)/rib including costochondral junction
Placenta/membranes/umbilical cord

*Additonal sections to demonstrate abnormalities that cannot be included in the preceding sections or for additional studies.
†Stillborn fetus/neonate younger than 1 day old—entire unopened stomach submitted in short-axis cross sections. Neonate older than 1 day—gastroesophageal junction, body, pyloris.

---

**Box 8-2** Suggested method of trimming central nervous system tissues

### Central nervous system (8 or more cassettes depending on brain size and lesions present)*

1. Parasagittal frontal lobe from anterior horn of lateral ventricle to midline apex (samples corpus callosum, lateral ventricular wall, cingulate gyrus, indusium griseum, parasagittal neocortex, and centrum semiovale)†
2. Temporal lobe including hippocampus at level of lateral geniculate body (samples hippocampus, transitional allocortex, temporal neocortex, lateral geniculate body, temporal horn wall, choroid plexus, and often tail of caudate nucleus)†
3. Midline mamillary bodies through insular cortex (samples hypothalamus, anterior thalamus, third ventricular wall, internal capsule, optic tract, globus pallidus, putamen, claustrum, insular cortex, and both external and extreme capsules)†
4. Midbrain (samples crus cerebri, substantia nigra, aqueduct of Sylvius, red nucleus or decussation of brachium conjunctivum)†
5. Pons at level of fifth nerve exit (samples pontine tegmentum, floor of fourth ventricle, trapezoid body [ascending sensory pathways], pyramidal tracts, and cerebellar afferent nuclei and tracts)
6. Medulla oblongata (samples pyramidal tracts, inferior olivary nuclei, medial lemniscus, various cranial nerve nuclei, medial longitudinal fasciculus, choroid plexus, floor of fourth ventricle, and inferior cerebellar peduncle)
7. Cerebellum (samples vermal and newer cerebellar cortex, white matter, and dentate nucleus)†
8. Spinal cord, cervical, thoracic, lumbar (samples several levels of spinal cord)
9. Additional sections to demonstrate abnormalities that cannot be included in the preceding sections or for additional studies

*It is most desirable to have identifying anatomic features visible on each section if at all possible.
†Cut in half for two cassettes; for midbrain, only half need be used for routine case.
Note: The sections as originally devised were for the "old" style paraffin Els used in most neuropathology laboratories in past eras; they can be modified as described to fit in the "new" almost universally used plastic cassettes.

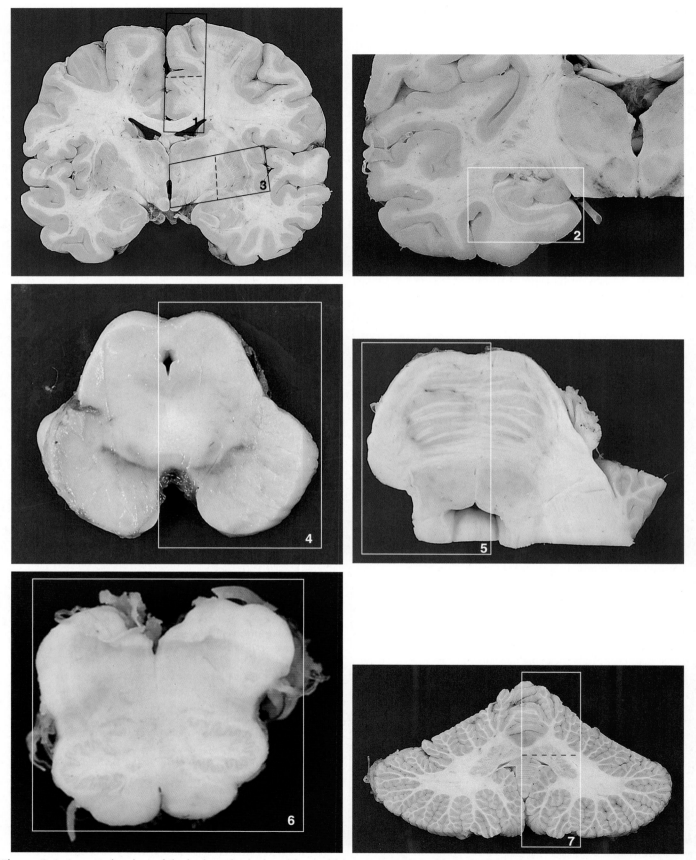

**Figure 8-1** Suggested regions of the brain and spinal cord from which to prepare tissue blocks for light microscopy. *1*, Parasaggital cortex and corpus callosum; *2*, temporal lobe including hippocampus; *3*, hypothalamus/basal ganglia/insular cortex; *4*, midbrain; *5*, pons; *6*, medulla oblongata; *7*, cerebellum. Two tissue blocks (as indicated by *dashed lines*) may be required for regions 1, 3, and 7. See also Box 8-2 for detailed descriptions of sections.

## Specialized Microscopic Examination of the Heart

Often, microscopic examination of the heart requires more detailed study than outlined in Box 8-1; the actual areas for evaluation depend on the type or location, or both, of the disease processes. Various methods for microscopic examination of the heart are described next.

### Examination of Cardiac Valves

Cardiac valves may contain vegetations, rupture sites, fused commissures, or degenerative changes such as fibrosis or calcification. The gross description is key. For valve lesions, decalcify as needed, and submit full-thickness cross sections through the valve and the adjacent heart muscle. Include chordae tendineae, and the superior portion of papillary muscles, with atrioventricular valves, if possible. In cases of valvular stenosis, consider preserving the valve and its malformed, fused, or calcified leaflets because this displays the extent of narrowing to best advantage. The friable nature of many valve vegetations necessitates care during trimming and subsequent handling. Gross and coworkers[22] recommended standard sections for evaluation of the heart with valvular disease, especially as a consequence of rheumatic fever. This extensive sampling is seldom necessary today because of the decreasing incidence of rheumatic heart disease.

### Examination of the Myocardium

Coronary artery disease is seen by the pathologist more commonly than valvular heart disease. Generally, the gross findings should guide sampling for microscopy. If an infarct is identified, sections from its central and peripheral zones are useful in dating the onset of ischemic damage and determining any recent extension. When a coronary artery is significantly narrowed (luminal stenosis greater than 50%) but there is no gross evidence of a myocardial infarct, sample the myocardium adjacent and distal to the arterial lesion. In the presence of generalized coronary artery atherosclerosis of significant degree but without obvious ischemic damage, it is best to sample myocardium supplied by each of the coronary arteries. Reiner[23] and Lie and Titus[24] have proposed standard methods for sampling the heart muscle on the basis of its blood supply. The procedure of the latter is demonstrated in Figure 8-2.

### Examination of Coronary Arteries and Coronary Artery Bypass Grafts

Pathologists vary in their methods of examining the native coronary arteries that usually have some degree of atherosclerosis.[25-28] The easiest is to perpendicularly transect the epicardial coronary arteries on the heart at regular (approximately 5 mm) intervals and describe the extent of plaque along the vessel and the severity of narrowing (the percentage of luminal stenosis); the narrowest segments and any areas containing thrombi should be selected for microscopic examination. Extensively calcified arteries, however, cannot be transected easily and may be damaged by the dissection. In this situation, the large coronary arteries of the fixed heart should be dissected free of the epicardium and removed intact before decalcification and subsequent transection of the arteries. The major disadvantage of this technique is that it dissociates the arteries from the myocardium; the specimens may have to be marked if the orientation is not clear. In this regard

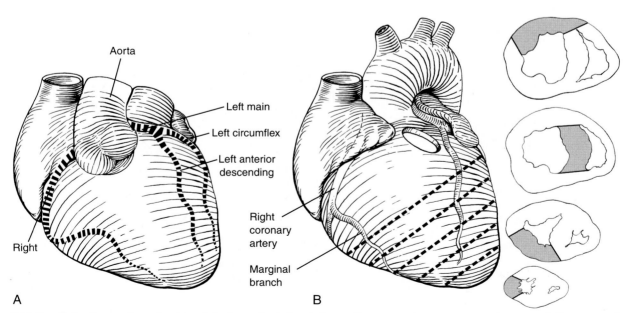

**Figure 8-2** Detailed microscopic evaluation of the heart for ischemic heart disease. **A,** The coronary arteries are serially cross-sectioned at 2- to 3-mm intervals and sampled for microscopic examination at points of severe stenosis or occlusion. **B,** After transverse sectioning of the heart at 1-cm intervals, the myocardium is sampled for histologic examination. The crosshatched areas in successive heart slices shown in the ventricular maps indicate areas of spiral-step histologic sampling of the anterior, septal, posterior, and lateral walls of the left ventricle. Gross evidence of recent infarcts necessitates directed sampling of the lesion and its borders.
(Modified from Lie JT, Titus JL: Pathology of the myocardium and the conduction system in sudden coronary death, *Circulation* 52[Suppl III]:41-52, 1975.)

postmortem angiography for evaluation of the extent and severity of atherosclerotic plaques in coronary arteries (or bypass grafts) can be useful as a guide for selecting areas for microscopic study.

In most hearts with bypass grafts, the grafts (being more superficial) should be examined before the native coronary arteries. In cases for postmortem angiography, bypass grafts should be injected before the proximal native coronary arteries to allow more detailed study of the native coronary arteries distal to the grafts.[29] Regarding dissection, grafts that are recent or appear to be free of significant atherosclerosis may be opened longitudinally with small scissors, taking care not to dislodge any thrombus. Grafts with suspected atherosclerosis are perpendicularly transected at 5-mm intervals, and the extent of plaque and degree of vessel narrowing are documented. Sampling of anastomotic sites is performed in different ways depending on the type of surgical connection (Fig. 8-3).

### Dissection and Examination of the Cardiac Conduction System

Because the cardiac conduction system is not easily identifiable grossly, blocks of tissue from anatomic locations known to contain the specialized muscle must be dissected and presented in proper orientation for embedding. The classic transverse plane of section through areas containing the sinoatrial and atrioventricular nodes, as well as the atrioventricular bundle and bundle branches, includes histologic landmarks for easy recognition of the specialized muscle.[30,31] This method may be performed in either the fresh heart or the fixed specimen.

### Sinoatrial Node

The sinoatrial node is located along the lateral aspect of the junction between the superior caval vein and the right atrium. The terminal sulcus (an epicardial groove often filled with fat in the adult) may be identified at this junction, and the specialized muscle is located on the epicardial surface within the groove. A block of tissue centered about the groove (i.e., including 1 cm of vena cava and 1 cm of right atrial tissue) is cut from the heart (Fig. 8-4). Viewed from the endocardial aspect, this block of tissue contains the crista terminalis, a relatively thick band of muscle separating the smooth caval vein surface from the ridgelike pectinates of the right atrium. The block is subdivided into strips of tissue across this band, each piece containing both cava and atrium. Each strip must be embedded on edge so that a full-thickness cross section is present in the glass slide.

Located on the caval side of the crista terminalis, the specialized muscle of the sinoatrial node is characterized by a basket-weave configuration of smaller-diameter muscle fibers admixed with collagen and surrounding the artery to the sinoatrial node (Fig. 8-5). Whereas the working atrial muscle appears fascicular, the specialized muscle fibers are arranged in a seemingly haphazard array. A trichrome stain may be necessary to distinguish the muscle from the interstitial collagen of the node.

No anatomically recognizable tracts of specialized muscle are present between the sinoatrial and atrioventricular nodes.

### Atrioventricular Node

The atrioventricular node is located between the atria and the ventricular septum adjacent to the point where the tricuspid, aortic, and mitral valve annuli meet.

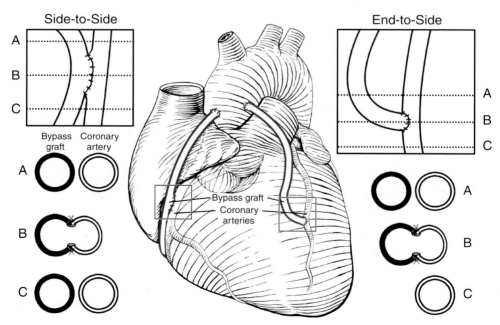

**Figure 8-3** Diagram illustrating coronary bypass grafts that have end-to-side and side-to-side anastomosis in two separate grafts *(boxes)* to the left anterior descending and right coronary arteries, respectively. The figure demonstrates the sampling method used for end-to-side and side-to-side anastomosis for detection of any of the three mechanisms for anastomotic site obstruction (i.e., compression or loss of arterial lumen if the majority of the arterial wall has been used for anastomosis; thrombosis of the site of anastomosis; dissection of the native coronary artery at the site of anastomosis) and if the coronary artery has severe narrowing at the site of anastomosis secondary to severe atherosclerosis. (Modified from Bulkley BH, Hutchins GM: Pathology of coronary artery bypass surgery, *Arch Pathol* 102:273-280, 1978.)

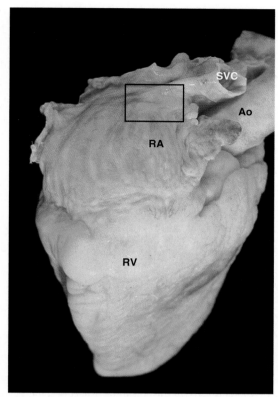

**Figure 8-4** The position of the sinoatrial node is identified by the terminal groove at the junction between superior vena cava *(SVC)* and right atrium *(RA)*. Although in many adults the groove is obscured by adipose tissue, the specialized muscle is contained in a 2-cm-wide block of tissue *(box)* dissected from the lateral aspect of this junction, including approximately 0.5 cm of vessel and 0.5 cm of atrium. Laid flat on the table, this block is cut into strips (each oriented to include both SVC and atrium) before processing. *Ao,* Ascending aorta; *RV,* right ventricle.

Access to this region of the heart necessitates opening the chambers in the usual fashion so that the septal structures remain intact. Again, because the tiny structures making up the conduction axis cannot be visualized grossly, a block of tissue containing the atrioventricular node and bundle must be removed and sectioned for histologic identification of the specialized muscle. This critical area in the center of the heart may be approached from either the right atrioventricular septum or the left ventricular outflow tract. Key to successful dissection of the conduction axis is making sure that the atrioventricular septum is flat against the cutting surface. Viewed from the endocardial aspect medially, the right atrioventricular septal region demonstrates several landmarks useful as boundaries for dissection. If tension is placed on the inferior caval vein orifice by gently pulling the atrial wall posteriorly, the endocardial surface is lifted up by a subendocardial tendon (tendon of Todaro), creating a ridge from the inferior caval vein to the annulus of the tricuspid valve. The angle formed by the tendon and the annulus is the apex of the triangle of Koch and corresponds to the point at which the atrioventricular bundle penetrates the septum of the heart.

For an adult heart, the prosector uses a sharp scalpel to remove a block of tissue including approximately 1 cm of atrial tissue and 1 cm of ventricular tissue on either side of the annular attachment of the septal leaflet of the tricuspid valve; it should extend from the orifice of the coronary sinus to the papillary muscle of the conus (just anterior to the apex of the triangle of Koch) (Figs. 8-6 and 8-7). Alternatively, the dissection may be done while viewing the left ventricular outflow tract. From this side, holding the right atrioventricular septum against the cutting surface and cutting perpendicular to the aortic valve annulus, the prosector removes a block of tissue containing the membranous portion of the ventricular septum from the commissure between the left and noncoronary leaflets of the aortic valve through the noncoronary leaflet to include one half of the right coronary leaflet. No matter which side the tissue is dissected from, the prosector then subdivides the block into strips by cutting perpendicular to the endocardial surface running from atrium to ventricle (see Fig. 8-7). Each piece should be marked so that it can be embedded and cut in the same direction as all the other pieces. Multiple step sections are made from each piece, and the slides are viewed in order.

The atrioventricular node appears as a somewhat discrete semicircular collection of cardiac muscle cells adjacent to the central fibrous body, the area of dense collagen at the intersection of the tricuspid, mitral, and aortic valve annuli (Fig. 8-8, *A*). Smaller in diameter than the working atrial and ventricular muscle fibers, the specialized muscle is arranged in basket-weave array with abundant interstitial collagen (Fig. 8-8, *B*). The specialized muscle of the atrioventricular node is continuous with that of the atrioventricular bundle anteriorly, which appears encased in the dense collagen as it courses from the atrial to the ventricular side of the central fibrous body (Fig. 8-9, *A*). Where adjacent to the crest of the ventricular septum, the specialized muscle of the bundle appears triangular in cross section. Several millimeters farther on, the left bundle branches course in the subendocardial tissue along the left ventricular aspect of the septum (Fig. 8-9, *B*). Still more anteriorly, the right bundle branches do the same on the right.

### Specialized Examination of the Autonomic Nervous System in Perinatal Deaths and Sudden Infant Death Syndrome

Some unexpected fetal deaths, including stillbirths and intrauterine fetal deaths after 22 gestational weeks, early neonatal death, and deaths categorized as due to the sudden infant death syndrome (SIDS), may be related to underlying abnormalities in the cardiac conduction system or the central autonomic nervous system.[32,33] In particular, a high incidence of hypoplasia in the arcuate nucleus is seen in these patients. Thus, in addition to cardiac conduction system examination, Matturri and colleagues[34] recommend and provide a detailed protocol for specialized microscopic examinations of the brainstem, cerebellum, and spinal cord. Although it may not be practical for the nonneuropathologist to perform the detailed morphometric analysis of the central autonomic nervous system as outlined by these investigators, a basic knowledge of how to appropriately sample the tissues is a useful starting point. Tissue sampling

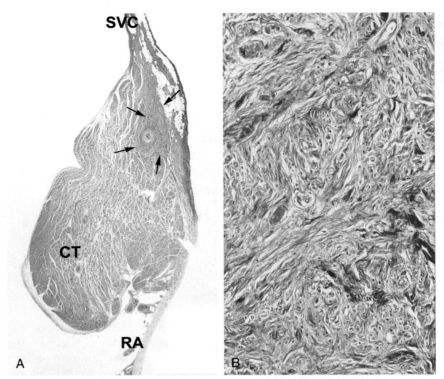

**Figure 8-5** Histology of the sinus node. **A,** At low magnification, a cross section of the junction between the superior vena cava *(SVC)* and the right atrium *(RA)* includes the distinctive bundle of muscle known as the crista terminalis *(CT)*. On the epicardial aspect of the junction, the sinus node *(arrows)* surrounds the sinus node artery. **B,** At high magnification, the specialized muscle consists of narrow myofibers coursing in many directions with abundant interstitial collagen. Masson's trichrome.

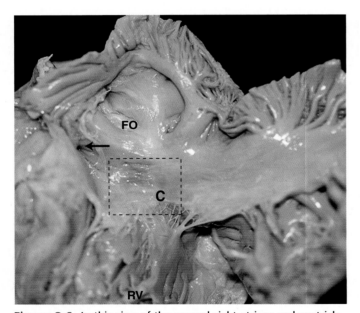

**Figure 8-6** In this view of the opened right atrium and ventricle, the atrioventricular node is contained within the triangle of Koch (bounded by the tendon of Todaro superiorly, the annulus of the septal leaflet of the tricuspid valve apically, and the ostium of the coronary sinus inferiorly). For this dissection the heart should be held with the opened aorta against the table. As shown by the box, the block removed includes 1 cm each of atrium and ventricle and extends from the coronary sinus ostium *(arrow)* to a point just beyond the commissure *(C)* between the septal and anterosuperior leaflets of the tricuspid valve. *FO,* fossa ovale; *RV,* right ventricle.

methods of the brainstem are described in Figure 8-10. The various brainstem nuclei and other structures present in the sections are depicted in Figure 8-11. The cerebellum, including both cortex and nuclei, is obtained in a sample that includes cerebellar hemisphere extending all along its major diameter. The spinal cord samples should include the entire cervical and the first five thoracic levels. Sectioning and staining protocols are included; the interested reader is referred to the original article.

## Tissue Processing, Sectioning, and Staining

After fixation and trimming, tissues destined for routine microscopic examination are dehydrated (stepwise in graded alcohols), cleared (usually in xylene), infiltrated with paraffin wax, and finally embedded in the wax. Sections, typically 5 μm thick but occasionally as thin as 3 μm, are cut and floated on warm water to remove wrinkles. The sections are picked up on glass microscopic slides and allowed to dry. Because histochemical reagents are prepared as aqueous solutions, the paraffin-embedded tissues on slides are rehydrated by reversing the process—that is, equilibrating them first in the clearing agent and then passing them through the graded alcohols into water before staining.

Histochemical staining techniques have evolved over the past 175 years and are described in detail in a number of reference works.[4,35-38] The stains rely on one of four types of chemical reactions: (1) simple ionic interactions, (2) reactions of aldehydes with Schiff's reagent or silver compounds,

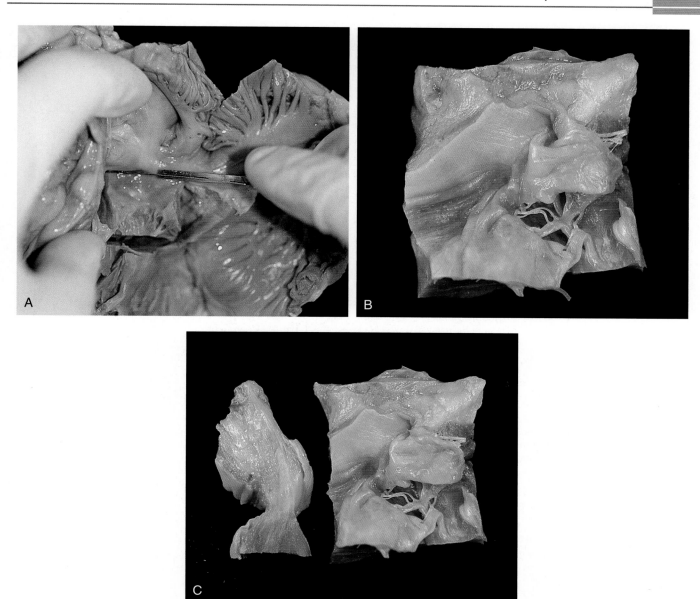

**Figure 8-7** Dissection of the atrioventricular node. **A,** The partially cut block containing the atrioventricular conduction axis is shown. **B,** The excised tissue block. **C,** When the block has been completely cut and removed from the heart, it is cut into strips (each oriented to include both atrium and ventricle); one strip is shown as separate from the rest of the block. The same side of each strip is embedded down. Depending on the size of the heart, step sections may need to be prepared.

(3) coupling of aromatic diazonium salts with aromatic residues on proteins, or (4) conversion of the primary reaction product of an enzyme acting on a substrate to form a colored precipitate.[37] The mainstay of light microscopic diagnostic autopsy pathology is the hematoxylin-eosin stain. It is quick, easy, and inexpensive. It demonstrates cell nuclei, cytoplasm, and connective tissues adequately. Histochemical stains for specific applications are listed in Table 8-1.

## Polarized Light Microscopy

Brightfield microscopy with polarized light is useful for identification of exogenous dusts or endogenous crystals within tissues or fluids (Tables 8-2 and 8-3).[39,40] The optics of polarized light and the characteristics of polarizing microscopes are reviewed in detail elsewhere.[40-42] Briefly, polarized light is ordinary light that is oriented into parallel panels. The polarizing system has a polarizing filter (the polarizer) below the stage and one above the microscopic stage (the analyzer), both in the path of illumination. One of these polarizers can be easily rotated. When the analyzer is orientated 90 degrees to the polarizer, light transmission is blocked. Thus, in the presence of two crossed polarizers in the light path of a microscope, the viewer does not see light through the eyepiece (Fig. 8-12, A and B). As shown in Figure 8-12, C, some types of crystals split and rotate the light wave into two rays; the ray with the greater angle of deviation (slow ray) passes through the crystal more slowly than the ray with the lesser angle of deviation (fast ray). This effect is referred to as birefringence.

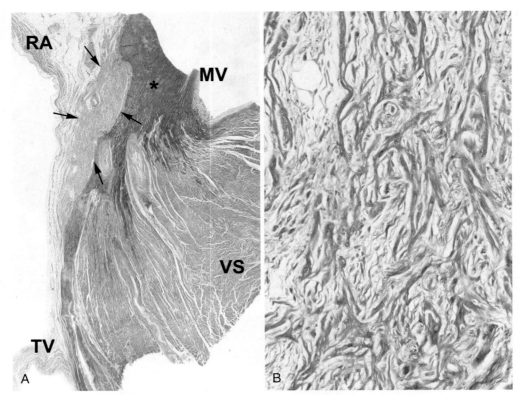

**Figure 8-8** Histology of the atrioventricular node. **A,** In a transverse section through the atrioventricular septum, the atrioventricular node *(arrows)* abuts the central fibrous body *(*)* between the right atrium *(RA)* and the crest of the ventricular septum *(VS)*. **B,** High magnification of the specialized muscle discloses a multidirectional array of myofibers with interstitial collagen. Masson's trichrome. *MV,* Mitral valve hinge-point; *TV,* tricuspid valve hinge-point.

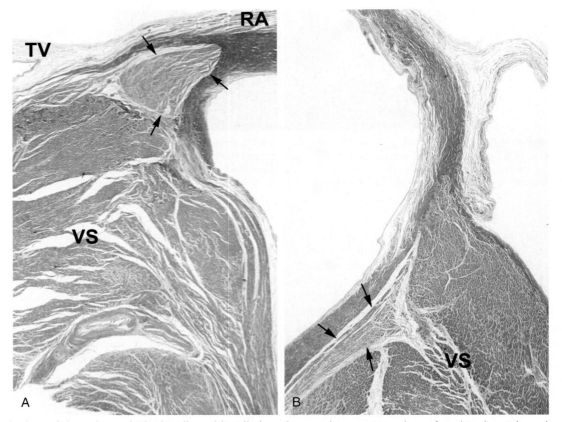

**Figure 8-9** Histology of the atrioventricular bundle and bundle branches. **A,** The transverse plane of section shows the atrioventicular bundle *(arrows)* astride the crest of the ventricular septum *(VS)*. **B,** In a section farther anterior, a bundle branch *(arrows)* consists of specialized muscle with collagen in a tract just beneath the endocardial surface. Masson's trichrome. *RA,* right atrium; *TV,* Tricuspid valve hinge-point.

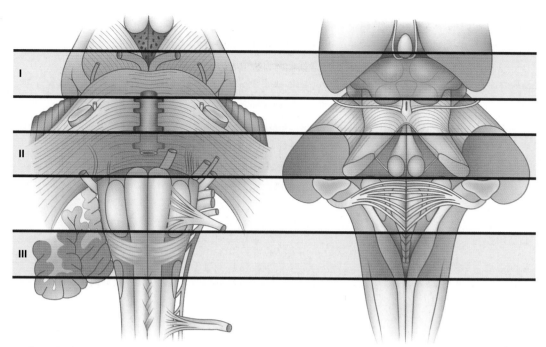

**Figure 8-10**  Sampling of the brainstem: ventral (left) and dorsal (right) surfaces of the brainstem. *I,* The first block, pontomesencephalic, includes the upper third of the pons and the adjacent portion of midbrain. *II,* The second block contains the upper third of the medulla oblongata to the portion adjacent to the pons. *III,* The third block includes the tissue 2 to 3 mm above and below the obex. (Modified from Testut L: *Anatomia umana, unione tipografico-editrice torinese,* Torino, 1923.)

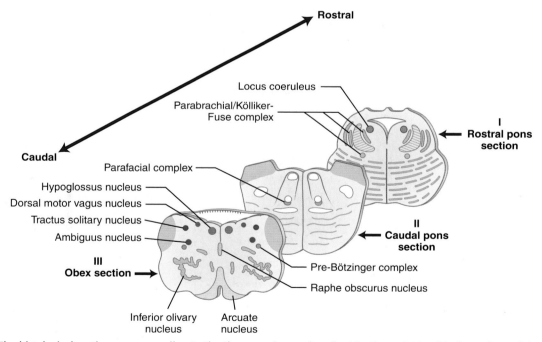

**Figure 8-11**  The histological sections corresponding to the three specimens described in Figure 8-10, with the main nuclei and structures to be examined indicated.
(Modified from Matturri L, Ottaviani G, Lavezzi AM: Guidelines for neuropathologic diagnostics of perinatal unexpected loss and sudden infant death syndrom (SIDS)—a technical protocol, *Virchows Archiv* 452:19-25, 2008. Used with permission from Springer Science and Business Media.)

Birefringent material appears white against the black background of crossed polarizers.

For compensated polarized microscopy, a compensator oriented 45 degrees to the axes of the polarizer and analyzer is added to the system. Compensators are efficient birefringent materials, typically quartz, mica, or gypsum, that retard one of the colors of the spectrum of white light a full wavelength, erasing it from the background illumination. Compensators also produce interference colors through addition to the incident slow ray and subtraction from the incident fast ray when

**Table 8-1**   Application of histochemical stains in evaluation of tissues obtained at autopsy

| Application | Histochemical stain |
|---|---|
| *Specific tissues and tissue components* | |
| Basement membrane | Periodic acid–Schiff (PAS); PAS-Jones |
| Collagen | Masson trichrome |
| Elastin | Weigert elastic van Gieson |
| Fat | Sudan black B; oil red O (frozen tissue) |
| Glial elements | Mallory phosphotungstic acid hematoxylin (PTAH)* |
| Muscle | Masson trichrome |
| Myelin | Luxol fast blue |
| Nerve fibers | Bielschowsky; Bodian |
| Nissl substance | Cresyl violet |
| Reticulin | Wilder reticulin |
| *Minerals (endogenous)* | |
| Calcium | Von Kossa |
| Copper | Rubeanic acid |
| Iron (hemosiderin) | Perls Prussian blue |
| *Carbohydrates* | |
| Glycogen | PAS with diastase |
| Glycosaminoglycans | Alcian blue pH 2.5 |
| Hyaluronic acid | Alcian blue pH 2.5 with and without hyaluronidase |
| Mucins | Mayer mucicarmine; Alcian blue pH 2.5–PAS |
| Neutral mucins | PAS |
| Acid mucins | Alcian blue pH 2.5 |
| *Pigments, other metabolic products* | |
| Amyloid | Congo red |
| Bile | Gmelin |
| Ceroid | Sudan black B |
| Cholesterol | Perchloric acid–naphthoquinone; digitonin reaction |
| Fibrin | Mallory PTAH; Lendrum Martius yellow–brilliant crystal scarlet–soluble blue (MSB) |
| Lipofuscin | Long Ziehl-Neelsen |
| Melanin | Masson-Fontana |
| *Microorganisms* | |
| Gram-positive and gram-negative bacteria | Brown-Brenn-Gram |
| *Mycobacterium* species | Fite |
| *Legionella* species | Dieterle |
| Spirochetes and *Rochalimaea* species | Warthin-Starry |
| Fungi | Grocott methenamine silver; PAS with diastase |
| Protozoa | Giemsa[†] |

*Replaced by immunodetection of glial fibrillary acidic protein (GFAP).
[†]Replaced by immunodetection with specific antisera if available.

**Table 8-2** Identification of common minerals or dusts in histologic sections

| Mineral/dust | Color, shape | Birefringence |
|---|---|---|
| Asbestos | Colorless fibers | Positive or weak |
| Barium sulfate | Yellow-white plates | Strong |
| Carbon/smoke/lignite/anthracite coal | Black | Negative |
| Bituminous coal | Yellow/brown | Negative |
| Crystalline silica (e.g., quartz, cristobalite) | Colorless needles and plates | Weak |
| Graphite | Black | Positive |
| Gypsum ($CaSO_4$) | Red-brown to black, granular | Negative |
| Iron | Red-brown to black, granular | Negative |
| Coal fly ash | Usually black, spheres or lacy forms | Negative |
| Nonfibrous silicates such as talc, mica, feldspars | Colorless or very pale yellow plates or needles | Strongly positive |
| Starch | Colorless or white, round | Strongly positive (Maltese cross) |
| Microcrystalline cellulose | Colorless (periodic acid–Schiff and Congo red positive) | Positive |

Data from Churg A, Green FHY: Analytic methods for identifying and quantifying mineral particles in lung tissue. In Churg A, Green FHY, editors: *Pathology of occupational lung disease,* Baltimore, 1998, Williams & Wilkins, pp. 45-55.

**Table 8-3** Characteristics of crystals sometimes found in body fluids or tissues

| Crystal | Elongation | Brightness | Morphology | Extinction | Size |
|---|---|---|---|---|---|
| MSUM | Negative | Strong | Needle, rod, spherule | On axis sharply | Submicroscopic—40 μm |
| CPPD | Positive | Weak | Rod and rhomboid | Gradual | Submicroscopic—40 μm |
| HA individual crystal clusters | | | Rod Shiny coins | | Submicroscopic 1.9-15.6 μm |
| Brushite* | Positive | Strong | Rod | | |
| Calcium oxalate | Positive | Variable | Tetrahedron, rod | | 1.0-2.0 μm |
| Cholesterol | Negative or positive | Weak or strong | Plates (notched corners) | | 5-40 μm |
| Lipid liquid | Maltese cross positive | Variable | Round extracellular or intracellular | | 0.5-30 μm |
| Lithium heparin | Positive | Weak | Polymorphic | | 2-5 μm |
| Talc or starch | Maltese cross positive | Strong | Ovoid | | |
| Corticosteroid | Variable | Usually strong | Polymorphic | | 1-40 μm |

*CPPD,* Calcium pyrophosphate dehydrate; *HA,* hydroxyapatite; *MSUM,* monosodium urate monohydrate.
*Calcium hydrogen phosphate dihydrate.
Data from Gatter RA, Schumacher HR: *A practical handbook of joint fluid analysis,* Philadelphia, 1991, Lea & Febiger, p 118.

each in turn is positioned parallel to the slow-ray orientation of the compensator. In practical terms, this is achieved by rotating the stage containing the specimen (crystal). This rotation produces color shifts that are dependent on the color of the compensator and the character of the crystal.

Microscopes for clinical applications are typically fitted with red compensators of the first order. Under these conditions, the microscopic field becomes rose colored and crystals turn either blue or yellow, depending on their identity and orientation relative to the compensator (Fig. 8-13). The direction of vibration of the slower component of the compensator is usually denoted by an arrow, and the stage is rotated so that the long axis of the crystal is parallel to the axis of slow vibration of the compensator. If, in this position, the crystal is blue, it is said to have a positive elongation; if the crystal is yellow, it is said to have negative elongation. Conversely, if the long axis of the crystal is lined up perpendicular to the slow vibration orientation of the compensator, crystals with positive elongation are yellow and those with negative elongation are blue. Midway between the sites of elongation on the axes of the polarizer and analyzer, neither blue nor yellow color is seen. This effect is called extinction.

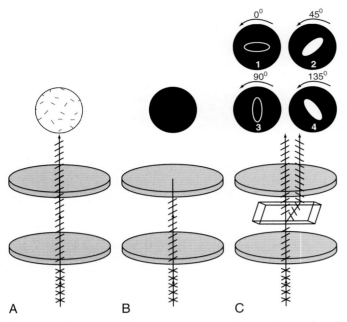

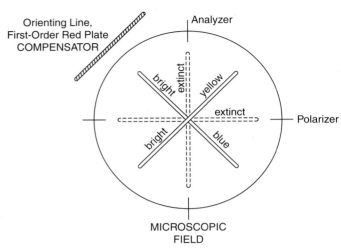

**Figure 8-13** A crystal with negative elongation rotated through 360 degrees under compensated polarized light showing positions of maximum brilliance and extinction.
(© 1972-1999 American College of Rheumatology Clinical Slide Collection. Used with permission.)

**Figure 8-12** Polarized light microscopy. **A,** The polarizer and analyzer are parallel, and light rays vibrating in the parallel plane pass through. **B,** The polarizer and analyzer are crossed, and light rays passing through the polarizer are blocked by analyzer. **C,** A birefringent crystal splits a ray of light into two light paths (slow and fast rays) vibrating at right angles to each other and in different planes than the analyzer, allowing the image of the crystal to reach the observer. A birefringent crystal is visible when its planes of rotation are halfway (45 degrees) between the vibration planes of the polarizers. Extinction occurs when one of its planes of vibration is parallel to either polarizer. Both conditions occur four times in a complete revolution of 360 degrees.
(Modified from Bancroft JD: Light microscopy. In Bancroft JD, Gamble M: *Theory and practice of histological techniques,* ed 5, London, 2002, Churchill Livingstone, p 56.)

## Immunohistochemistry

The adaptation of immunologic methods to histochemical techniques has revolutionized diagnostic pathology. Immunohistochemical stains rely on the specificity of an antibody for a specific epitope in the tissue and a secondary reaction that allows detection of the antibody-antigen reaction with a microscope.[43] Both direct and indirect detection methods are available (Fig. 8-14). In the direct method, antibodies are conjugated with an indicator such as fluorescein. Fluorescence is observed using a microscope equipped with an ultraviolet light source and specialized filters. The more sensitive indirect method uses a secondary heterologous antiserum for recognition of the primary antibody. Again, one can use a fluorescein-conjugated antibody. However, enzymes such as peroxidase are favored for diagnostic pathology, because they involve a durable reaction product that is visible by standard light microscopy. After incubation of the tissue section in the appropriate substrate, enzyme reactions evident as a precipitated color change are observed with a light microscope. Recognition of specific antibody binding with the peroxidase-antiperoxidase or alkaline phosphatase method or the avidin-biotin complex method in paraffin-embedded or fresh frozen tissues has found great usefulness. These methods increase sensitivity of the indirect method about tenfold. The immunogold technique uses antibodies labeled with colloidal gold particles. The immunogold reagent may be difficult to see in light microscopic sections; however, antigen localization can be enhanced using silver intensification. Immunogold reagents are readily detected by electron microscopy, and this technique is most often used at the ultrastructural level. Enhanced polymer one-step staining provides sensitivity similar to that of the avidin-biotin technology but requires fewer procedural steps.

Improved immunohistochemical technology employing antigen retrieval and peroxidase-antiperoxidase or avidin-biotin complex methods together with an increasingly diverse array of commercially available antibodies that react with formalin-fixed, paraffin-embedded antigens has greatly expanded the role of immunohistochemistry in diagnostic pathology.[44] For example, immunohistochemistry is particularly useful in tumor diagnosis. It is also finding additional uses in predicting tumor behavior (e.g., markers of cell proliferation) and response to therapy (e.g., hormone receptors). This makes it an important adjunct to the routine hematoxylin- and eosin-stained microscopic section. Immunohistochemical markers are useful when the autopsy pathologist is faced with the task of classifying primary neoplasms and identifying site of origin in cases of cancer widely disseminated from an unknown primary site. Another major diagnostic application of immunohistochemistry, namely detection of infective agents, continues to see more and more use in anatomic pathology. Antibodies directed against a number of microorganisms are available commercially (Table 8-4).[45] Less well-established uses of immunocytochemistry at autopsy include detection of early ischemic myocardial necrosis[46,47] and estimation of the age of skin wounds.[48]

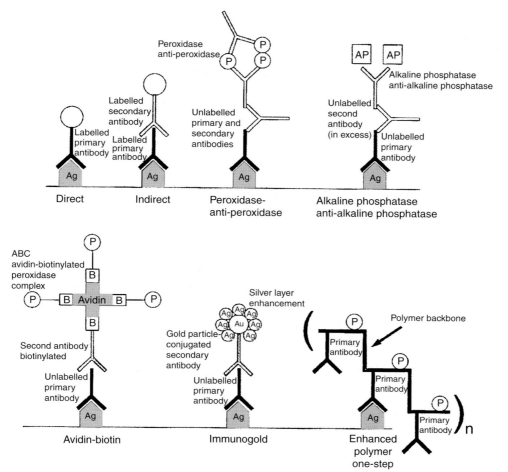

**Figure 8-14** Immunocyto(histo)chemical staining of cells and tissues. See text for explanation.
(From Finkbeiner WE: Morphological procedures in respiratory anatomy and pathology. In Gold WM, Murray JF, Nadel JA, editors: *Atlas of procedures in respiratory medicine,* Philadelphia, 2002, WB Saunders, pp 1-34.)

**Table 8-4     Some antibodies useful in immunohistochemical detection of infectious organisms**

| Antibody target | Source | Localization |
|---|---|---|
| Adenovirus | Chemicon | Nuclear |
| Aspergillus | Dako | Septate hyphae |
| *Bartonella henselae* | Biocare Medical | Intact bacteria |
| BK virus | Lee Biomolecular Research | Nuclear (tubular cells) |
| *Candida albicans* | Chemicon | Yeast forms |
| Cytomegalovirus | Novocastra | Nuclear and cytoplasmic |
| Hepatitis B core Antigen | Dako | Nuclear and cytoplasmic |
| Hepatitis B surface Antigen | Dako | Cytoplasmic |
| Herpes simplex 1 and 2 | Dako | Nuclear and cytoplasmic |
| *Helicobacter pylori* | Dako | Intact bacteria |
| Human herpesvirus 8 | Novocastra | Nuclear (spindle and endothelial cells) |
| JC virus | Lee Biomolecular Research | Nuclear (oligodentocytes) |
| *Listeria monocytogenes* | Difco | Intact bacteria |
| *Mycobacterium tuberculosis* | Biocare Medical | Intact bacteria |

*table continues*

| Antibody target | Source | Localization |
|---|---|---|
| Parvovirus B19 | Novocastra | Nuclear (normoblasts and pronormoblasts) |
| *Pneumocystis jiroveci* | Novocastra | Cysts and trophozoites |
| Respiratory syncytial virus | Novocastra | Cytoplasm (syncytial giant cells) |
| *Toxoplasma gondii* | BioGenex | Pseudocysts and tachyzoites |
| *Treponema pallidum* | Biocare Medical | Intact bacteria |
| Varicella-zoster | Chemicon | Cytoplasmic |
| West Nile virus | Bioreliance | Neuronal cytoplasm and processes |

**Table 8-4**  *(continued)*

Data from Eyzaguirre E, Haque AK: Application of immunohistochemistry to infections, *Arch Pathol Lab Med* 132:424-431, 2008.

## In Situ Hybridization

In situ hybridization is becoming more feasible as a supplement to routine histochemistry and immunohistochemistry as simpler techniques are developed for paraffin-embedded tissue sections. It allows cellular localization of nucleic acid sequences and is useful for studies of gene expression in disease or identification of microorganisms. DNA is generally more stable than messenger RNA, but the sensitivity of in situ hybridization techniques allows detection of as few as 10 DNA or RNA copies per cell.[49] Numerous factors contribute to the degeneration of the nucleic acids within tissue samples. The best results are obtained with optimally prepared tissues. Either snap-freezing of fresh tissue or fixation should be performed as soon as possible. Nonetheless, successful hybridizations have been achieved with autopsy material.[50,51] One may also need to vary published in situ hybridization protocols when using different fixatives. Fortunately, standard 10% buffered formalin is an excellent fixative for purposes of in situ hybridization. At this time, the role of in situ hybridization for diagnostic autopsy pathology is limited; its value is primarily for detection of viruses in cases of infection of unclear etiology and interphase cytogenetics in the evaluation of fetal abnormalities.[52,53]

The TUNEL method (in situ end-labeling of fragmented DNA with biotinylated nucleotides and subsequent staining with 3,3'-diaminobenzidine through peroxidase-conjugated avidin) may be utilized to detect cells that have undergone programmed cell death or apoptosis.[54,55] In an experimental animal model, Kajstura and coworkers[56] have used this in situ apoptosis assay to detect myocardial cell death within 2 hours of coronary artery occlusion. Others[57-59] have applied this technique after death to detect myocardial cell death that occurred 2 hours before death. Because detection of myocardial necrosis by routine hematoxylin-eosin light microscopy is typically reliable only when patients survive for at least 4 to 6 hours, the in situ apoptosis assay may offer significant improvement in cases of early death.

## Frozen Sections, Needle Biopsies, Cytology, and Smears

Frozen sections prepared from autopsy tissue are useful as an adjunct to gross examination for establishing diagnoses for the preliminary or provisional report. They are also used in detection of immune complexes and immunoglobulin deposits by immunofluorescence microscopy (see below) or fat by oil red O histochemistry in tissues.

A percutaneous needle biopsy autopsy provides a very limited postmortem examination but usually is better than no autopsy at all. When physicians are unsuccessful in obtaining consent for a conventional autopsy, they may be able to obtain permission for organ sampling via needle biopsy. This method not only presents technical difficulties for the inexperienced but also is subject to sampling error.[60-62] The guidance or help of clinicians who specialize in percutaneous biopsy procedures should be sought until the pathologist gains confidence in his or her ability to obtain adequate tissue samples using the specialized equipment. Despite the limitations of needle biopsy autopsies, Huston and colleagues[63] were able to confirm the cause of death and identify a number of diseases, particularly when the diseases were either neoplastic or infective. Cina and Smialek[64] obtained diagnostic information from percutaneous core biopsies of the liver in a substantial number of cases.

Cytologic examination has little use in standard autopsy practice, with the exception of cases in which families agree to tissue sampling by needle aspiration only. To facilitate accurate preliminary diagnoses, some pathologists[65-67] have used cytologic methods as a supplement to gross examination. Imprints or scrapings of tumors or certain other lesions may be helpful in rapid diagnosis.[68] Imprints of bone marrow retain good cytologic detail, and a simple technique is described by Kao.[69] Briefly, a 0.5- to 1-cm$^3$ sample of marrow is squeezed out of a rib and is placed on a piece of cardboard. A clean glass microscopic slide is lightly applied to the bone marrow, allowing a small amount of marrow to adhere to the slide. Next, this slide is applied directly to another glass slide, and the marrow is allowed to spread under light pressure. The slides are lifted apart, air dried, and stained.

## IMMUNOFLUORESCENCE MICROSCOPY

Immunofluorescence microscopy in autopsy pathology is primarily of use in the evaluation of renal or other diseases in which there is abnormal deposition of immunoglobulins (Fig. 8-15). The prosector must anticipate the need for

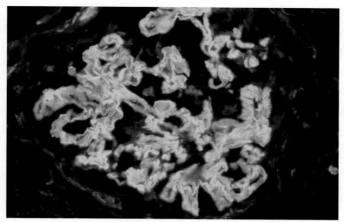

**Figure 8-15** Immunofluorescence microscopy in anti-glomerular basement membrane nephritis (Goodpasture syndrome) in a postmortem kidney specimen. There is linear deposition of immunoglobulin G (IgG) along the glomerular capillary endothelial basement membranes (fluorescein-labeled anti-IgG).

immunofluorescence studies, because at autopsy fresh (unfixed) tissue should be embedded in a suitable freezing medium and then quickly frozen. Alternatively, tissue can be temporarily stored (up to 5 days but preferably less) in l transport fixative (Zeus Scientific, Raritan, N.J.) but must be adequately rinsed before freezing.[70] For routine studies, staining of thin frozen sections for immunoglobulins (IgG, IgA, IgM), complement (C1q, C3), and fibrinogen is demonstrated using fluorescein isothiocyanate–labeled antisera. Antibodies

against κ and λ light chains are useful in the diagnosis of light chain disease and amyloid light-chain (AL) amyloidosis. Antibodies against albumin provide a useful control for evaluation of nonspecific entrapment of plasma proteins.

## ELECTRON MICROSCOPY

### Transmission Electron Microscopy

In the current age, electron microscopy has largely been superseded by immunohistochemistry and in situ hybridization as a diagnostic tool. Occasionally, ultrastructural examination can be a useful adjunct to light microscopy, particularly when its use is anticipated and tissue samples are acquired and properly fixed expeditiously. Even in cases with extensive postmortem autolysis, electron microscopy may play an important role in the diagnosis of diseases encountered by the autopsy pathologist, particularly those in which there are accumulations of normal and abnormal metabolites. The use of electron microscopy to detect viral inclusions has been largely supplanted by immunocytochemical or molecular biologic techniques. Table 8-5 lists ultrastructural findings for a number of diseases in which electron microscopy may be useful.

Buffered glutaraldehyde at a concentration of 2.5% provides excellent fixation of cellular organelles for ultrastructural examination, although tissue penetration of the fixative is quite slow. Thus, tissue samples should be carefully minced into pieces that are $1 \times 1 \times 1$ mm or smaller. Formaldehyde penetrates tissue more rapidly, but organelle preservation is not as good as that provided by glutaraldehyde. Nonetheless, formalin-fixed tissues

| **Table 8-5** | Electron microscopic findings in some nonneoplastic and noninfectious diseases |
|---|---|
| **Disease** | **Ultrastructural findings** |
| *Lysosomal storage diseases* | |
| *Diseases with specific electron microscopic findings* | |
| Cystinosis | Polygonal and rectilinear electron-lucent crystals |
| Fabry's disease | Complex, pleomorphic, rectilinear lamellae, spherules and tubular structures or prismatic inclusions |
| Fucosidosis | Clear and dense, heterogeneous inclusions |
| GM$_2$ gangliosidosis | Membranous cytoplasmic bodies (regular parallel lamellae associated with granular structures) |
| Gaucher's disease | Enlarged, elongated, fusiform lysosomes containing tubular inclusions |
| Krabbe's disease | Distended endoplasmic reticulum; geometric or needlelike inclusions |
| Metachromatic leukodystrophy | Geometric or herringbone inclusions |
| Mucolipidosis IV | Lamellar whorls within scant fibrillogranular material |
| Neuronal ceroid-lipofuscinosis | Curvilinear or fingerprint inclusions |
| Niemann-Pick disease types A and B | Vacuolated and whorled irregular electron-dense material alternating with electron-lucent inclusions |
| Niemann-Pick disease type C | Multivesicular and plurilobulated inclusions |
| Pompe's disease (infantile type II glycogenosis) | Small glycogen granules in lysosomes |

*table continues*

**Table 8-5** *(continued)*

| Disease | Ultrastructural findings |
|---|---|
| *Diseases with nonspecific electron microscopic findings* | |
| GM$_1$ gangliosidosis | Clear or lamellar lysosomal inclusions |
| Mannosidosis | Clear or fibrillogranular inclusions |
| Mucolipidoses II and III | Fibrillogranular and lamellar inclusions |
| Mucopolysaccharidoses | Fibrillogranular inclusions |
| *Primarily nervous system diseases* | |
| Infantile neuroaxonal dystrophy | Spheroids (terminal axonal dilatations) |
| Adrenoleukodystrophy | Membrane-bound curvilinear lamellar inclusions |
| Myoclonic epilepsy (Lafora's disease) | Lafora's bodies (concentric rounded inclusions) |
| *Primarily liver diseases* | |
| Cholesterol ester storage disease | Membrane-bound lipid deposits in hepatocytes |
| $\alpha_1$-Antitrypsin deficiency | Storage material within endoplasmic reticulum |
| Reye syndrome | Enlarged, irregular hepatocyte mitochondria lacking matrix granules |
| Wilson's disease | Enlarged, pleomorphic hepatocyte mitochondria with dilated and separated inner and outer membranes, containing flocculent material and large matrix granules |
| *Primarily skeletal muscle diseases* | |
| Nemaline myopathy | Nemaline rods (electron-dense rectangular or cylindrical proliferations of Z-band material) |
| Mitochondrial myopathies | Variable mitochondrial abnormalities including increased numbers, increased size, aberrant orientation of cristae, crystalline mitochondrial inclusions |
| *Primarily renal diseases* | |
| Cryoglobulinemia | Mesangial, subendothelial, intramembranous, and sometimes subepithelial cylindrical deposits (mixed cryoglobulinemia) or fibrillar bundles (monoclonal cryoglobulinemia) |
| Immunoglobulin A nephropathy/Henoch-Schönlein purpura | Subendothelial and mesangial dense deposits |
| Membranous glomerulopathy | Dense and irregular subepithelial deposits |
| Postinfectious glomerulopathy | Discrete subepithelial deposits |
| Lupus nephritis | Subendothelial, subepithelial, and mesangial deposits, tubulovesicular bodies |
| Immunotactoid (fibrillary) glomerulonephritis | Fibrils or microtubules (16-50 nm) |
| *Respiratory disease* | |
| Ciliary dyskinesia | Absence of central microtubules, dynein arms, or radial spokes |
| *Miscellaneous diseases* | |
| Amyloid | Nonbranching fibrils 7-10 nm in diameter |
| Carnitine deficiency | Abnormal lipid accumulations with minimal or no increase in mitochondrial number |
| Carnitine palmitoyltransferase deficiency | Normal, swollen, or pleomorphic mitochondria containing dense deposits in matrix and abnormal cristae |
| Fatty acid beta-oxidation defects | Abnormal lipid accumulations |
| Peroxisomal disorders | Absent or abnormal peroxisomes |

and even formalin-fixed, paraffin-embedded material may be adequate for electron microscopic examination. In these situations, we try to select tissue from the edge of the sample, presumably the site of initial fixation. The formalin-fixed sample is then fixed secondarily in a glutaraldehyde. In the case of paraffin-embedded material, however, the wax must be removed and the tissue rehydrated first.[71]

## Specialized Electron Microscopic Techniques

At this time, immunoelectron microscopy is not of any practical use in autopsy diagnosis. Scanning electron microscopy offers a unique view of the surfaces of cells and other structures. Although this is of little importance in routine autopsy diagnosis, it has potential research applications for evaluation of biomaterials and prosthetic devices collected as part of a postmortem examination. Among the many uses of analytic scanning electron microscopy in forensic pathology are the identification of gunshot residues,[72] firearm identification from examination of bullet fragments,[73] and identification and characterization of human hair.[74,75] Analytic transmission and scanning electron microscopes allow identification of a wide range of inorganic fibers and particulate materials and therefore are of great value in the analysis of mineral dusts (e.g., within lung tissue in suspected cases of pneumoconiosis).[39,76] A detailed discussion of analytic electron microscopy, however, is beyond the scope of this book.

## REFERENCES

1. Warthin AS: *Practical pathology: A manual of autopsy and laboratory technique for students and physicians*, Ann Arbor, Mich, 1911, George Wahr.
2. Cotton DWK, Stephenson TJ: Impairment of autopsy histology by organ washing—a myth, *Med Sci Law* 28:319-323, 1988.
3. Bostwick DG, al Annouf NA, Choi C: Establishment of the formalin-free surgical pathology laboratory. Utility of an alcohol-based fixative, *Arch Pathol Lab Med* 118:298-302, 1994.
4. Bancroft JD: *Theory and practice of histological techniques*, ed 5, London, 2002, Churchill Livingstone.
5. Hedreen JC: Examination of brain and spinal cord. In Hutchins GM, editor: *Autopsy: Performance and reporting*, Northfield, Ill, 1990, College of American Pathologists, pp 85-92.
6. Smith C: Examination of the nervous system. In Cotton DWK, Cross SS, editors: *The hospital autopsy*, Oxford, 1993, Butterworth Heinemann, pp 88-98.
7. Boon ME, Kok LP, Marani E: Three strategies for microwave irradiation of human brains producing paraffin slides within one day. In Bullock GR, Leathem AG, van Velzen D, editors: *Techniques in diagnostic pathology*, London, 1989, Academic Press, pp 201-210.
8. Garzón-de la Mora P, Garcia-Estrada J, Ballesteros-Guadarrama A, et al: Electrochemical fixation techniques. I. Electrochemical fixation of human brain, *Arch Med Res* 27:37-42, 1996.
9. Okazki H, Campbell RJ: Nervous system. In Ludwig J, editor: *Current methods of autopsy practice*, Philadelphia, 1979, WB Saunders, pp 95-129.
10. Beach TG, Tago H, Nagai T, et al: Perfusion-fixation of the human brain for immunohistochemistry: Comparison with immersion-fixation, *J Neurosci Methods* 19:183-192, 1987.
11. McKenzie JC, Berman NEJ, Thomas CR, et al: Atrial natriuretic peptide-like (ANP-LIR) and ANP prohormone immunoreactive astrocytes and neurons of human cerebral cortex, *Glia* 12:228-243, 1994.
12. Adickes ED, Folkerth RD, Sims KL: Use of perfusion fixation for improved neuropathologic examination, *Arch Pathol Lab Med* 121:1199-1206, 1998.
13. Sharma M, Grieve JHK: Rapid fixation of brains: A viable alternative? *J Clin Pathol* 59:393-395, 2006.
14. Whitehouse SR, Kissoon N, Singh N, Warren D: The utility of autopsies in a pediatric emergency department. *Pediatr Emerg Care* 10:72-75, 1994.
15. Bass T, Bergevin MA, Werner AL, et al: In situ fixation of the neonatal brain and spinal cord, *Pediatr Pathol* 13: 699-705, 1993.
16. Kiernan JA: *Histological and histochemical methods. Theory and practice*. Oxford, UK, 1981, Pergamon Press.
17. Gruber HE, Mekikian P: Application of stains—all for demarcation of cement lines in methacrylate embedded bone, *Biotech Histochem* 66:181-184, 1991.
18. Hahn M, Vogel M, Delling G: Undecalcified preparation of bone tissue: Report of technical experience and development of new methods, *Virchows Arch A Pathol Anat Histopathol* 418:1-7, 1991.
19. Leong AS-Y, James CL, Thomas AC: *Handbook of surgical pathology*, New York, 1996, Churchill Livingstone.
20. Rosai J: Guidelines for handling of most common and important surgical specimens. In Rosai J, editor: *Ackerman's surgical pathology*, St. Louis, 1996, Mosby, pp 2629-2725.
21. Hruban RH, Westra WH, Phelps TH, Isacson C: *Surgical pathology dissection: an illustrated guide*, New York, 1996, Springer.
22. Gross L, Antopol W, Sacks B: A standardized procedure suggested for microscopic studies of the heart: With observations on rheumatic hearts, *Arch Pathol* 10:840-852, 1930.
23. Reiner L: Selection of blocks from heart for microscopic study, *Bull Pathol* 9:198-200, 1968.
24. Lie JT, Titus JL: Pathology of the myocardium and the conduction system in sudden coronary death, *Circulation* 52(Suppl III):41-52, 1975.
25. Roberts WC, Buja LM: The frequency and significance of coronary arterial thrombi and other observations in fatal acute myocardial infarction. The study of 107 necropsy patients, *Am J Med* 52:425-443, 1972.
26. Vlodaver Z, Frech R, Van Tassel RA, Edwards JE: Correlation of the antemortem coronary arteriogram and the postmortem specimen, *Circulation* 47:162-169, 1973.
27. Thomas AC, Davies MJ: Post-mortem investigation and quantification of coronary artery disease, *Histopathology* 9:959-976, 1985.
28. Giraldo AA, Higgins MJ, Humes JJ: Anatomical methods in the study of cardiovascular pathology: A refined technique, *Ann Clin Lab Sci* 16:13-25, 1986.
29. Virmani R, Ursell PC, Fenoglio JJ: Examination of the heart, *Hum Pathol* 18:432-440, 1987.
30. Lev M, Widran J, Erickson EE: A method for the histopathologic study of the atrioventricular node, bundle, and branches, *Arch Pathol* 52:73-83, 1951.
31. Hudson REB: The human conducting system and its examination, *J Clin Pathol* 16:492-498, 1963.
32. Ottaviani G, Matturri L: Histopathology of the cardiac conduction system in sudden intrauterine unexplained death (SIUD), *Cardiovasc Pathol* 17(3):146-155, 2008.
33. Matturri L, Ottaviani G, Lavezzi AM: Techniques and criteria in pathologic and forensic-medical diagnostics in sudden unexplained infant and perinatal death, *Am J Clin Pathol* 124:259-268, 2005.
34. Matturri L, Ottaviani G, Lavezzi AM: Guidelines for neuropathologic diagnostics of perinatal unexpected loss and sudden infant

death syndrome (SIDS)—a technical protocol, *Virchows Arch* 452:49-25, 2008.

35. Pearse AGE: *Histochemistry, theoretical and applied*, ed 4, Edinburgh, 1980, Churchill Livingstone.

36. Filipe MI, Lake BD: *Histochemistry in pathology*, Edinburgh, 1983, Churchill Livingstone.

37. Spicer SS, editor: *Histochemistry in pathologic diagnosis. Clinical and biochemical analysis*, New York, 1987, Marcel Dekker.

38. Beckstead JH: Histochemistry. In Damjanov I, Linder J, editors: *Anderson's pathology*, St. Louis, 1996, Mosby, pp 176-189.

39. Churg A, Green FHY: Analytic methods for identifying and quantifying mineral particles in lung tissue. In Churg A, Green FHY, editors: *Pathology of occupational lung disease*, Baltimore, 1998, Williams & Wilkins, pp 45-55.

40. Gatter RA, Schumacher HR: *A practical handbook of joint fluid analysis*, ed 2, Philadelphia, 1991, Lea & Febiger.

41. Phelps P, Steele AD, McCarty DJ Jr: Compensated polarized light microscopy, *JAMA* 203:166-170, 1968.

42. Nunn RE, Bancroft JD: Light microscopy. In Bancroft JD, Stevens A, editors: *Theory and practice of histological techniques*, New York, 1996, Churchill Livingstone, pp 1-21.

43. Finkbeiner WE: Morphological procedures in respiratory anatomy and pathology. In Gold W, Murray J, Nadel JA, editors: *Atlas of procedures in respiratory medicine*, Philadelphia, 2002, WB Saunders, pp 1-34.

44. Dabbs D: *Diagnostic immunohistochemistry*, Philadelphia, 2006, Churchill Livingstone, 2006.

45. Eyzaguirre E, Haque AK: Application of immunohistochemistry to infections, *Arch Pathol Lab Med* 132:424-431, 2008.

46. Hansen SH, Rossen K: Evaluation of cardiac troponin I immunoreaction in autopsy hearts: A possible marker of early myocardial infarction, *Forensic Sci Int* 99:189-196, 1999.

47. Ribeiro-Silva A, Martin CCS, Rossi MA: Is immunohistochemistry a useful tool in the postmortem recognition of myocardial hypoxia in human tissue with no morphological evidence of necrosis? *Am J Forensic Med Pathol* 23:72-77, 2002.

48. Betz P: Immunohistochemical parameters for the age estimation of human skin wounds. A review. *Am J Forensic Med Pathol* 16:203-209, 1995.

49. Nuovo GJ: *PCR In Situ Hybridization: Protocols and Applications*, ed 3, Philadelphia, 1997, Lippincott-Raven.

50. Ternghi G, Polak JM: In situ hybridization. In Rapley R, Walker MR, editors: *Molecular diagnostics*, Oxford, UK, 1993, Blackwell Scientific, pp 41-49.

51. Nuovo G: The utility of immunohistochemistry and in situ hybridization in placental pathology, *Arch Pathol Lab Med* 130:979-983, 2006.

52. McNicol AM, Farquharson MA: In situ hybridization and its diagnostic applications in pathology, *J Pathol* 182:250-261, 1997.

53. Guovo GJ: The utility of in situ-based methodologies including in situ polymerase chain reaction for the diagnosis and study of viral infections, *Hum Pathol* 38:1123-1136, 2007.

54. Gavrieli Y, Sherman Y, Ben-Sasson SA: Identification of programmed cell death in situ via specific labeling of nuclear DNA fragmentation, *J Cell Biol* 3:493-501, 1992.

55. Wijsman JH, Jonker RR, Keijzer R, et al: A new method to detect apoptosis in paraffin sections: In situ end-labeling of fragmented DNA, *J Histochem Cytochem* 41: 7-12, 1993.

56. Kajstura J, Cheng W, Reiss K, et al: Apoptotic and necrotic myocyte cell deaths are independent contributing variables of infarct size in rats, *Lab Invest* 74:86-107, 1996.

57. Bardales RH, Hailey LS, Xie SS, et al: In situ apoptosis assay for the detection of early acute myocardial infarction, *Am J Pathol* 149:821-829, 1996.

58. Rodríguez-Calvo MS, Tourret MN, Concheiro L, et al: Detection of apoptosis in ischemic heart: Usefulness in the diagnosis of early myocardial injury, *Am J Forensic Med Pathol* 22:278-284, 2001.

59. Edston E, Gröntoft L, Johnsson J: TUNEL: A useful screening method in sudden cardiac death, *Int J Legal Med* 116:22-26, 2002.

60. Terry R: Needle necropsy, *J Clin Pathol* 8:38-41, 1955.

61. Wellmann KF: The needle autopsy. A retrospective evaluation of 394 cases, *Am J Clin Pathol* 52:441-444, 1969.

62. Foroudi F, Cheung K, Duflou J: A comparison of the needle biopsy post mortem with the conventional autopsy, *Pathology* 27:79-82, 1995.

63. Huston BM, Malouf NN, Azar HA: Percutaneous needle autopsy sampling, *Mod Pathol* 9:1101-1107, 1996.

64. Cina SJ, Smialek JE: Postmortem percutaneous core biopsy of the liver, *Mil Med* 164:419-422, 1999.

65. Walker E, Going JJ: Cytopathology in the post mortem room, *J Clin Pathol* 47:714-717, 1994.

66. Suvarna SK, Start RD: Cytodiagnosis and the necropsy, *J Clin Pathol* 48:443-446, 1995.

67. Schnadig VJ, Molina CP, Aronson JF: Cytodiagnosis in the autopsy suite: A tool for improving autopsy quality and resident education, *Arch Pathol Lab Med* 131:1056-1062, 2007.

68. Suen KC, Yermakov V, Raudales O: The use of imprint technic for rapid diagnosis in postmortem examinations. A diagnostically rewarding procedure, *Am J Clin Pathol* 65:291-300, 1976.

69. Kao YS: A technic for bone marrow imprints from post-mortem specimens, *Am J Clin Pathol* 63:832-835, 1975.

70. Michel B, Milner Y, David K: Preservation of tissue-fixed immunoglobulins in skin biopsies of patients with lupus erythematosus and bullous diseases—preliminary report, *J Invest Dermatol* 59:449-452, 1972.

71. Wang N-S, Minassian H: The formaldehyde-fixed and paraffin-embedded tissues for diagnostic transmission electron microscopy, *Hum Pathol* 18:715-727, 1987.

72. Germani MS: Evaluation of instrumental parameters for automated scanning electron microscopy/gunshot residue particle analysis, *J Forensic Sci* 36:331-342, 1991.

73. Taylor RL, Taylor MS, Noguchi TT: Firearm identification by examination of bullet fragments and SEM/EDS study, *Scanning Electron Microsc* 2:167-174, 1979.

74. Seta S, Sato H, Yoshino H: Quantitative investigation of sulfur and chlorine in human head hairs by energy dispersive X-ray microanalysis, *Scanning Electron Microsc* 2:193-201, 1979.

75. Seta S, Sato H, Yoshino M, Miyasaka S: SEM/EDX analysis of inorganic elements in human scalp hairs with special reference to the variation with different location on the head, *Scanning Electron Microsc* 1:127-140, 1982.

76. Howell DN, Payne CM, Miller SE, Shelburne JD: Special techniques in diagnostic electron microscopy, *Hum Pathol* 29: 1339-1346, 1998.

# 9

# Supplemental Laboratory Studies

*"For the field of pathology includes not merely pathologic anatomy but pathologic physiology and pathologic chemistry as well. And it is the autopsy which furnishes the problems for all three. It should be emphasized that the autopsy has not been completed when the organs have been inspected, removed, and dissected: rather the investigation has just begun. Methods may now be borrowed from any source to assist in the solution of questions raised on gross examination."*

Sidney Farber[1]

## COLLECTION OF SAMPLES

The hospital autopsy pathologist should take full advantage of modern chemical, microbiologic, cytogenetic, and molecular analysis of body fluids, tissues, and cells as a supplement to anatomic dissection and microscopic examination if necessary. Careful review of the case records usually indicates to the prosector whether special studies are called for. In most instances, the collection and proper storage of samples for such studies requires little in the way of additional work for the pathologist and offers the possibility of valuable diagnostic information. However, proper acquisition of diagnostic material and appropriate analytic methods are keys to obtaining reliable results.

### Blood

Postmortem analysis of blood samples has shown that there are significant differences between specimens taken from various body sites. In particular, analysis of postmortem glucose, enzymes, and drugs shows significant differences between specimens taken from the right side of the heart, the left side of the heart, and the peripheral blood vessels.[2] Peripheral venous or arterial specimens best approximate the antemortem values. The best samples for toxicologic analysis are obtained from the femoral artery or vein. The subclavian vessels serve as secondary collection sites. Samples are collected percutaneously with a large-bore needle and syringe. Gentle, rather than vigorous, aspiration helps keep the thin vascular walls from collapsing. If large volumes of blood are necessary, samples can also be collected from the heart after the chest cavity is opened. However, it is important to label each container with the anatomic site and time of collection and not mix samples.

The amount of blood collected depends on the particular biochemical analysis needed. For toxicology studies performed as part of the forensic autopsy, collection of 40 to 50 mL is usually more than adequate. Some of the sample should be placed in fluoride preservative and some placed in anticoagulant. It may also be of value to spot blood routinely (300 µL) on specialized filter papers (Whatman, Ann Arbor, Mich., or Schleicher & Schuell, Keene, N.H.). Several samples can be collected, dried overnight, wrapped in plastic wrap, and stored at -20°C. Such samples are useful for genotype and protein analyses available through academic and commercial laboratories. In a study of infants who died unexpectedly, Chace and colleagues[3] used tandem mass spectrometry to analyze postmortem blood spotted on filter paper and successfully identified specific enzyme defects, allowing diagnosis of disorders of fatty acid oxidation. Filter blots of liver tissue, bile, and vitreous humor may also be used.[3,4]

### Vitreous Humor

Vitreous humor provides one of the best samples for postmortem chemical analysis because it comes from a closed space and postmortem values often approximate the antemortem levels. Despite controversy, there does not appear to be any between-eye differences, at least between electrolytes and calcium.[5] Vitreous humor may not become contaminated after embalming, so it may still provide material for analysis in these cases. However, a sample of the embalming fluid should also be submitted to the laboratory as a control.[6]

Collection is with a small syringe attached to an 18-gauge needle. The tip of the needle is inserted into the approximate center of the globe, and gentle suction is applied until all the vitreous (generally 2 to 5 mL in an adult; approximately 1 mL in newborns) is removed. All the fluid from each eye should be removed because there is regional variation in vitreous solute concentration.[2] To restore the contour of the eyes, simply remove the syringe without removing the needle and introduce a roughly equivalent amount of saline solution into the globes with a second syringe. Then, using a fresh syringe and needle, fluid is withdrawn from the other eye, and the right and left eye samples are stored in individual tubes rather than pooled.

## Synovial Fluid

Rarely used for postmortem studies, synovial fluid can be acquired as a substitute when vitreous humor is unavailable.[7] Approximately 1 mL can be aspirated from each knee joint.

## Urine

Urine should be collected with a large-bore needle attached to a syringe after the bladder is exposed at autopsy. Alternatively, it may be collected by urethral catherization prior to autopsy. In cases in which the bladder contains only a small amount of urine, it may be necessary to open the bladder to collect the residual urine. If the bladder must be opened to obtain the urine, care must be taken to prevent contamination of the urine sample with blood or other fluids present in the peritoneal cavity.

## Cerebrospinal Fluid

Using a needle of appropriate length, one can aspirate cerebrospinal fluid (CSF) from the cisterna magnum. The decedent is placed in a prone position with a block under the chest. The neck is flexed, and the skin at the junction of the back of the head and posterior neck is punctured. The needle is directed at an angle toward the bridge of the nose, and entry into the cisterna is appreciated as a loss of resistance.[8] CSF can also be withdrawn by (1) standard percutaneous posterior lumbar puncture, (2) aspiration through the spinal foramina between the first and second lumbar vertebrae after organ evisceration, or (3) inserting a needle connected to a sterile syringe into a lateral ventricle after removing the skull cap, reflecting the dura, and parting the cerebral hemispheres.

## Bile

Collection of bile may be useful for some toxicology studies but is not generally relevant for the standard hospital autopsy. It can be aspirated from the gallbladder or, in decedents who have undergone cholecystectomy, directly from the common bile duct.

## Gastric Contents

Stomach contents are easily collected by clamping the distal esophagus and the pylorus before the stomach is removed. Once removed, the stomach is rinsed with water and then held inside a sturdy plastic bag or container. A hole is made in the stomach wall, and the contents are collected.

## Hair and Fingernails

Hair samples should not be obtained by cutting but rather by pulling so as to include the hair roots. An adequate sample (0.5 g for DNA analysis, up to 10 g for analysis of heavy metals) should be tied together to maintain orientation and aid the laboratory in the identification of the hair roots. Fingernails can be collected by clipping or, if necessary, removing the entire nail.

## Fibroblasts for Tissue Culture

Karyotyping, metabolic assays, enzyme assays, and diagnostic ultrastructural studies can be performed on cultured fibroblasts. Skin, fascia, lung, diaphragm, muscle, and cartilage all provide sources for initiating fibroblast cell cultures as long as care is taken to prevent contamination by careful cleaning of the skin surface with an appropriate antimicrobial solution before dissection. If skin is collected, one should clean it only with sterile saline because alcohol or other antimicrobial solutions are toxic and may impede growth of the fibroblasts. Small tissue samples suffice, and these should be placed in a sterile tube containing a culture medium such as Roswell Park Memorial Institute (RPMI) medium or minimal essential medium (MEM). Samples can be stored briefly in a refrigerator (4°C) until they can be transported to the laboratory. Unfortunately, in about one quarter of cases, fibroblasts will fail to grow from postmortem fetal tissue.[9] Chorionic placental villous sampling performed as soon as intrauterine fetal demise is confirmed provides a greater likelihood of generating successful cultures, so clinicians should be advised to consider this approach.[10-12]

## Tissues for Metabolic Studies and Nucleic Acid Analysis

Tissue (liver, brain, kidney, cardiac muscle, skeletal muscle, peripheral nerve) obtained at autopsy may be used for biochemical studies in the diagnosis of inborn errors of metabolism. Generally, two or more 1-cm$^3$ pieces or two or more 1-cm segments of nerve provide adequate material for analysis. Increasingly, molecular analysis provides important diagnostic information. Tissues should be obtained soon after death, particularly for studies of messenger RNA (mRNA). The tissue should be frozen rapidly in liquid nitrogen or dry ice and stored at −70°C. When in doubt about whether or not to obtain tissue for freezing, one should collect and freeze it; it can always be discarded later if it is not deemed useful.

## POSTMORTEM CHEMISTRY

Chemical analysis of blood and other body fluids is primarily a component of the forensic autopsy. The typical hospital autopsy is performed on decedents who have had sufficient laboratory tests before death, and postmortem chemical analysis of blood or other fluids is usually superfluous. Nevertheless, the hospital autopsy pathologist should be aware of the value and limitations of postmortem biochemistry because he or she will inevitably encounter a number of cases that require investigation into the decedent's metabolic state. Before beginning postmortem chemical analysis, the pathologist should determine the appropriate fluid or tissue for analysis. Comparisons of premortem and postmortem fluids have shown which components remain relatively constant, which undergo predictable change, and which are too altered to be of diagnostic use. Coe,[2,13,14] in a number of reviews and chapters, has provided useful discussions of the subject.

## Carbohydrates and Related Metabolites

### Glucose

Postmortem serum glucose decreases rapidly because of glycolysis, preventing detection of antemortem hypoglycemia. Even elevated levels of postmortem blood glucose require careful interpretation. Death from asphyxia, cerebral hemorrhage, congestive heart failure, electrocution, or terminal cardiopulmonary resuscitation may increase postmortem peripheral vascular glucose and falsely indicate hyperglycemia. Of course, glycosuria, ketonuria, or elevated serum acetone level helps confirm diabetic ketoacidosis. Coe[2] recommended determinations of glycosylated hemoglobin and glycosylated fructosamine when blood is the only fluid available for analysis. Blood samples taken from the right atrium or inferior vena cava may have a high glucose content because of glycogenolysis in the liver and subsequent diffusion of glucose into adjacent vessels. Thus, a low glucose level in blood from the right atrium and a positive test for ketones may support starvation in the setting of abuse or neglect.[2]

Vitreous humor provides more reliable data for determination of antemortem hyperglycemia. Glycolysis reduces the postmortem concentration of vitreous humor glucose; however, values greater than 200 mg/dL usually indicate that the decedent had uncontrolled diabetes.[14]

### Ketones and Lactic Acid

In the autopsy suite, dipstick tests of urine allow a quick determination of possible ketoacidosis. Total ketone bodies (acetone, acetoacetate, and b-hydroxybutyrate) can be measured in postmortem blood, vitreous, pericardial fluid, and urine.[15] Serum lactic acid increases rapidly after death, and antemortem levels are increased 20 times and 50 to 70 times at 1 and 24 hours, respectively. Vitreous humor lactic acid increases from its initial values of 80 to 160 mg/dL to 210 to 260 mg/dL 20 hours after death. Brinkmann and coworkers[16] noted that lactic acidosis and ketoacidosis may be the cause of sudden unexpected death in chronic alcoholics.

## Electrolytes and Trace Elements

### Sodium, Chloride, and Potassium

The concentrations of sodium, chloride, and potassium in postmortem blood do not accurately reflect antemortem levels because of variable instability after death. The blood potassium level rises extremely rapidly after death as cell membranes lose integrity. Sodium and chloride blood concentrations decrease slowly but variably after death. In vitreous humor, potassium levels rise gradually after death, allowing estimation of agonal concentration and time since death. However, because of numerous factors, as outlined by Coe,[14] the margin of error in these calculations is high and vitreous potassium levels should not be used to estimate time of death. Vitreous sodium and chloride concentrations remain relatively constant during the early postmortem period.

The postmortem vitreous humor concentrations of sodium, chloride, potassium, and nitrogenous compounds fall into four general patterns (Table 9-1), allowing some assessment of the terminal metabolic condition of the decedent.[14]

| Table 9-1 | Terminal metabolic condition of decedent as assessed by postmortem analysis of vitreous sodium, potassium, chloride, urea nitrogen, and creatinine |
|---|---|
| Dehydration pattern | Increased sodium and chloride concentrations  Moderate elevation of urea nitrogen levels |
| Uremic pattern | No substantial increase in sodium and chloride values  Urea nitrogen and creatinine levels increased |
| Low-salt pattern | Low sodium and chloride concentrations  Relatively low potassium level (<15 mEq/L or 15 mmol/L) |
| Decomposition pattern | Low sodium and chloride concentrations  High potassium level (>20 mEq/L or 20 mmol/L) |

### Carbon Dioxide Content

Postmortem vitreous carbon dioxide content averages 15 mEq/L (range 4 to 27 mEq/L) and remains relatively stable for at least 15 hours after death.[17]

### Calcium, Magnesium, Phosphorus, and Sulfur

Measurements of these electrolytes are of little use. After death, the serum calcium concentration remains briefly stable and then rises slowly.[18] Initial vitreous calcium levels range from 6 to 8 mg/dL (1.5 to 2 mmol/L), and the values rise very slowly until decomposition ensues.[19] Magnesium levels in vitreous humor rise slowly but erratically after death.[19] Inorganic and organic phosphorus levels increase quickly after death; sulfate levels are stable during the initial postmortem period.[2]

### Trace Elements

Coe[2] has tabulated concentrations of trace elements measured in postmortem blood and vitreous humor. A number of authors[20-23] have measured essential and toxic elements in autopsy tissues.

## Nitrogenous Compounds

### Urea Nitrogen and Creatinine

Urea nitrogen is perhaps the most stable blood constituent following death as it approximates premortem levels, even after moderate decomposition.[2] Urea nitrogen also remains stable in CSF, vitreous humor (even after embalming), and synovial fluid.[24-26] In addition to their use in assessing renal function, urea nitrogen concentrations aid in the interpretation of hypernatremia (see later). Similarly, creatinine levels in the blood remain stable after death, as they do in CSF and vitreous humor, making creatinine a valid postmortem marker of nitrogen retention and renal function.[2]

### Other Nitrogenous Compounds

Serum concentrations of ammonia, amino acids, glutamine, creatine, and oxypurines (uric acid, xanthine, and hypoxanthine) increase after death. However, during the first 24 hours after death, ammonia levels in vitreous humor increase linearly.[27] Although relatively stable after death, uric acid levels are higher in blood samples from the right side of the heart than in samples taken from the left side of the heart or periphery.[28] Postmortem hyperuricemia may also be elevated after death caused by asphyxiation or drowning, but further studies of this finding are required.

## Cholesterol and Other Lipids

Postmortem measurements of serum total cholesterol, although somewhat unpredictable, have been used to identify familial hypercholesterolemia.[29] Correlation of postmortem serum lipid levels with the antemortem state is difficult because the decedents may not have been in a fasting state at the time of death. Thus, unless the stomach and small intestine are empty at the time of autopsy, elevated postmortem serum lipid levels must be interpreted with caution. Nevertheless, familial hyperlipoproteinemias have been identified from postmortem studies, and, as one would expect, elevated levels of postmortem lipids in serum and other fluids have been associated with the presence of coronary heart disease and sudden cardiac death.[30-32]

## Proteins

### Serum Proteins

Postmortem measurement of total serum protein, serum protein electrophoresis, and immunoglobulin electrophoresis provides valid data that can be interpreted in the clinical context. Postmortem studies show that the values for total proteins and the albumin/globulin ratio are similar to those of antemortem specimens.[13,33] If hemolysis is minimal, postmortem electrophoresis patterns remain similar to antemortem patterns, showing only a 4% fall in albumin and a 5% increase in β-globulin, with other fractions remaining the same.[34,35] Thus, serum electrophoresis has been useful in the postmortem diagnosis of agammaglobulinemia,[2] monoclonal gammopathy,[2] and hemoglobinopathies.[36] Total immunoglobulin E (IgE) is elevated in some cases of fatal asthma.[37] Measurement of specific IgE antibodies in postmortem serum may help corroborate the diagnosis of anaphylaxis following insect stings or ingestion of allergenic food (see also mast cell tryptase paragraph).[38-40] Postmortem measurement of C-reactive protein in the blood or liver may indicate a natural mode of death in decedents with evident traumatic injury; in those with obvious trauma, it suggests a vital reaction.[41,42]

### Enzymes

Few enzymes lend themselves to postmortem assay because their levels change rapidly and unpredictably. Levels of cholinesterase remain constant for weeks after death and provide tests for organic phosphorus or carbofuran poisoning.[2] Piette and Schrijver[43] suggested that γ-glutamyltransferase is useful as a postmortem marker of chronic alcoholism; however, Sadler and colleagues[44] found carbohydrate-deficient transferrin a more useful marker. Elevated levels of creatine kinase, lactic dehydrogenase, and their isozymes in pericardial fluid and serum have been correlated with myocardial injury related to trauma or the early stages of myocardial infarcts.[45,46] However, Osuna and coauthors[47] found that the pericardial fluid/serum ratio of myosin concentration was a better indicator of widespread cardiac muscle damage. In one study, postmortem pericardial levels of cardiac troponin I correlated closely with pericardial concentrations of myoglobin, with elevated troponin levels supporting a diagnosis of cardiac injury.[48] The highest levels

of cardiac troponin I in pericardial fluid followed myocardial infarcts that were confirmed histologically. Other investigators found postmortem pericardial fluid levels of cardiac troponin I to be an inaccurate indicator of cardiac-related deaths.[49] However, postmortem serum concentrations of cardiac troponin I greater than 40 ng/mL and a positive rapid assay for cardiac troponin T were helpful in detecting cardiac-related deaths.[50,51]

Mast cell tryptase (combined assay for α- and β-tryptase) has been used to detect anaphylactic reactions.[38,52-54] However, postmortem serum mast cell tryptase levels may be elevated in other conditions, including coronary artery thrombosis,[55] heroin injection,[56] sudden infant death syndrome,[57] amniotic fluid embolism,[58] and asphyxia,[59] as well as nonspecifically.[60] In cases of suspected anaphylaxis, serum tryptase concentrations should be correlated with available history (particularly atopic disposition of the decedent and temporal relationship of possible allergen exposure and death), findings at autopsy, total IgE levels, and, if possible, analysis of relevant IgE antibodies.[38,61] Analysis of peripheral (femoral) blood is optimal because heart blood is elevated in a greater number of control subjects and typtase concentrations in femoral blood are not altered by resuscitation efforts.[59,62] Even better than blood collected at autopsy is blood that may have been collected and sent to the clinical laboratory during the terminal event.[63]

### Other Proteins

Biochemical analyses for specific metabolites in postmortem liver, bile, vitreous humor, and blood have established disorders of fatty acid oxidation.[3,4,64,65] Serum and urine myoglobins are both markedly elevated after death. Myoglobinuria greater than that related to autolysis alone is seen in deaths caused by heat stroke, electrocution, massive trauma, or thermal injury and in deaths associated with possible exertional muscle hyperactivity or convulsions such as drowning or cerebral hemorrhage.[66] Elevated glycosylation levels of the short-lived serum proteins α$_1$-antitrypsin and haptoglobin in postmortem samples are a reliable indicator of antemortem hyperglycemia.[67] Enzyme-linked immunosorbent assays (ELISAs), Western blot analysis, and various radioimmunoassays designed for antemortem laboratory diagnosis have been applied successfully to autopsy cases as aids in diagnosis. These include tests to identify infections caused by viruses (e.g., hepatitis B virus,[68] hepatitis C virus,[69] human immunodeficiency virus[70]) and bacteria (e.g., meningococcemia,[71] syphilis[72]). Immunoassays have also been used to identify antibodies associated with disease (e.g., acute myasthenia gravis by detection of antibodies against striated muscle and acetylcholine receptor units[73]). Acute-phase proteins and mediators of inflammation can be detected in postmortem serum and provide evidence supporting the diagnosis of sepsis or other inflammatory conditions.[74,75]

## Bile Pigments and Other Indicators of Hepatic Function

Levels of serum bilirubin increase slowly after death but allow determination of the extent of antemortem jaundice; however, minimal elevations of postmortem bilirubin are difficult to interpret.[14] Urobilinogen remains stable in the urine but diffuses from blood to CSF whenever the blood level is high. Mild liver dysfunction cannot be readily assessed using postmortem chemical analysis because the enzymes used to assess liver function become elevated after death. However, total cholesterol, low serum protein levels with inversion of the albumin/globulin ratio, high serum bilirubin level, and the presence of abnormal levels of bile and urobilinogen in the urine confirm severe liver damage. Elevation of glutamine level in the postmortem CSF samples correlates with hepatic coma.[14]

## Hormones

Coe[2] has reviewed the status of various hormones after death. Serum cortisol, parathormone, chorionic gonadotropin, thyroid-stimulating hormone, and luteinizing hormone concentrations remain stable in the early postmortem period. Serum growth hormone levels decrease after death. Catecholamines and 17-hydroxycorticosteroid levels in serum generally rise in the postmortem period. Urine catecholamines are also elevated after death.[76] The free thyroxine ($T_4$) and free triiodothyronine ($T_3$) levels in postmortem blood are comparable to premortem levels, but the upper limits of normal, especially for $T_4$, must be adjusted upward.[77] Vitreous levels of the thyroid hormones cannot be used because values do not correlate with blood hormone levels. Serum insulin is extremely difficult to measure accurately because it degrades rapidly at room temperature.[78] Peripheral blood samples should be collected in tubes containing sodium fluoride or ethylenediaminetetraacetic acid (EDTA), and serum should be separated from red blood cells as soon as possible. Samples should be refrigerated or, preferably, frozen. The measurement of C peptide has been used to support a diagnosis of exogenous insulin overdose.[79,80] In postmortem blood, C peptide is more stable than insulin, although collections still require special handling: collection in heparinized tubes, separation of plasma, and, without delay, storage of the serum sample in a freezer.

## POSTMORTEM TOXICOLOGY

Exceedingly important in forensic pathology, postmortem toxicology is a well-developed science beyond the scope of this book. The reader is referred to several excellent textbooks[81-83] and comprehensive reviews[84-86] of forensic toxicology for additional information. In all forensic cases, even when drug overdose or exposure to poisons is not suspected, collection of blood should be supplemented with collections of vitreous humor, urine, bile, gastric contents, and, in some instances, CSF. As mentioned earlier, femoral blood is generally the sample of choice. Because considerable redistribution of drugs occurs after death, collected samples must be site labeled, and the site of origin must be considered when interpreting the results.[87,88]

Solid tissue should be saved for possible toxicologic analysis. It is advisable to obtain and freeze a portion of liver from the right lobe routinely and other tissues as indicated. Muscle tissue can be analyzed as a last resort when internal organs are badly decomposed. Brain tissue is sometimes saved for toxicology testing because many of the drugs act on the central nervous system. However, concentrations in the blood are probably more meaningful for interpreting the extent of toxicity. Analysis of adipose tissue is useful and sometimes warranted when the presence of fat-soluble drugs (e.g., thiopental) or chlorinated hydrocarbons and other pesticides is suspected. Kidney tissue should be saved for analysis of heavy metals. If blood is not available, muscle, brain, lung, and kidney are the most useful tissues for diagnosising death from carbon monoxide exposure and may also be used to determine deaths due to carbon monoxide inhalation before thermal injury.[89] Lung tissue (50 g) stored in a nylon but not a plastic bag may aid in evaluation of volatile substance abuse or exposure.[6]

For suspected injections of poisonous substances, an elliptical resection of the needle puncture mark and surrounding skin should be performed along with a similar resection at a distant or contralateral site as a control.

## POSTMORTEM MICROBIOLOGY

There is disagreement regarding the accuracy and, thus, usefulness of postmortem cultures. Factors affecting the validity of microbiologic studies performed on postmortem fluids and tissues include the postmortem interval (though less than might be expected), degree of organ manipulation before sampling, technique of obtaining the sample, and therapy with antibiotics prior to death.[90,91] Interpretation of the results obtained from a positive microbiologic culture must be correlated with the patient's history and gross and microscopic pathology findings. Geller[90] emphasized the importance of preparing smears for Gram staining to aid in the interpretation.

Obviously, the best postmortem culture results are obtained from grossly infected tissues and body cavity fluids rather than from routine cultures of fluids or tissues. If possible, tissue specimens should be obtained in situ.[92] Abscesses and granulomata should be cultured from both their center and periphery and instruments should be changed or flame sterilized before sampling different sites.[93] Fluid in a body cavity can be collected using a sterile syringe and needle. Purulent material in a body cavity or from an abscess can be swabbed with a sterile, cotton-tipped applicator. To culture tissue from an organ, one should first clean and dry the surface. We have discontinued the standard practice of searing the organ surface with a hot spatula to prevent potential aerosols containing infectious organisms. Rather, we wipe the surface of the organ with an iodine-containing disinfectant and, after cutting the surface or capsule of the organ, obtain a piece of tissue with a sterile scalpel and forceps, taking care not to include any tissue exposed to disinfectant. The tissue (1 $cm^3$) is placed in a sterile plastic cup and submitted for viral, bacterial, or fungal culture. If meningitis is suspected, CSF should be obtained as described previously. Swabs should also be taken from the subarachnoid space. The subarachnoid space is reached by lifting the leptomeninges and making a small cut into the meninges.

Blood cultures often yield mixed growth of organisms that are nondiagnostic. However, if the body is refrigerated at 4°C to 10°C shortly after death, postmortem invasion by endogenous microorganisms is delayed.[94] In fact, postmortem interval has only a minimal effect on the isolation rate of blood cultures.[95] Postmortem blood cultures are generally obtained from the inferior vena cava after the pericardium is opened and the heart is reflected upward. Using aseptic technique, the pathologist introduces a needle into the right atrium and aspirates blood into a sterile syringe. However, data from Hove and Pencil[96] demonstrated that during the early postmortem period, percutaneous, aseptic sampling of subclavian blood provides more reliable samples. Roberts[97] found good correlation of postmortem cultures of spleen with clinically documented bacteremia.

Despite the difficulties associated with postmortem microbiology studies, their use should not be uniformly discouraged. The autopsy pathologist who takes the time to submit appropriate specimens to the microbiology laboratory is sometimes rewarded with information that not only improves the final autopsy report but also provides vital information to hospital infection control personnel and local public health authorities.

## POSTMORTEM CYTOGENETIC AND MOLECULAR STUDIES

In cases of dysmorphic fetuses or infants, careful anatomic dissections may be aided by chromosomal analysis.[98] The tissue sample should be placed in RPMI or other appropriate tissue culture medium for transport to a cytogenetics laboratory. Short-interval storage should be in a refrigerator at 4°C. Because initiating successful fibroblast cultures is time sensitive, the pathologist should work with his or her colleagues in obstetrics to ensure prompt collection of appropriate samples.

Advances in molecular biology research have quickly transformed medicine and provided many useful diagnostic tests. Molecular techniques such as the polymerase chain reaction (PCR) allow identification of abnormal genes, infectious microorganisms, and contaminating DNA from samples or evidence collected from the body of the deceased. Newer techniques allow analysis of archived paraffin tissue blocks.[99] With adequate preservation and handling, even mRNA species can be isolated from autopsy tissues and profiled.[100] Kapur[101] strongly advocated routinely freezing a sample of liver and placenta from every fetal and perinatal autopsy case and selected tissues as dictated by the gross autopsy findings. Samples should be collected carefully and as soon after death as possible. Tissue samples for nucleic acid analysis can be snap frozen and stored at −70°C.

## GENETIC/METABOLIC DISEASE AUTOPSY

Genetic metabolic disorders or inborn errors of metabolism are a large (greater than 400) group of diverse diseases that may cause death in the fetal or perinatal period (Table 9-2).[102]

| Table 9-2    Presenting features and examples of some important genetic metabolic disorders presenting in fetuses and infants | |
|---|---|
| **Predominant clinical or biochemical presentation** | **Examples** |
| *Acute encephalopathy* | |
| Hypoglycemia | Fatty acid oxidation defects; organic acidopathies; gluconeogenic disorders; glycogen storage disorders; hereditary fructose intolerance (also consider hyperinsulinism, pituitary insufficiency) |
| Hyperammonemia | Urea cycle disorders; transient hyperammonemia of the newborn; lysinuric protein intolerance |
| Ketosis | Maple syrup urine disease |
| Disorders of acid-base status | Mitochondrial respiratory chain disorders, defects of pyruvate metabolism; organic acidoses |
| Seizures (as early predominant feature) | Nonketotic hyperglycinemia; pyridoxine-dependent epilepsy; peroxisomal disorders; sulphite oxidase deficiency; molybdenum cofactor defect; folinic acid responsive seizures; glucose transporter defect |
| *Acute hepatocellular disease* | |
| | Galactosemia; fatty acid oxidation defects; tyrosinemia type I; hereditary fructose intolerance; peroxisomal disorders; $\alpha_1$-antitrypsin deficiency; mitochondrial respiratory chain disorders; Niemann-Pick disease type C; neonatal hemochromatosis; defects of bile acid metabolism; congenital defects of glycosylation |
| *Sudden death, including cardiomyopathy* | |
| | Fatty acid oxidation defects; mitochondrial respiratory chain disorders; glycogen storage disorder type IV; lysosomal storage disorders; Barth syndrome; heart-specific phosphorylase kinase deficiency |
| *Severe hypotonia* | |
| | Peroxisomal disorders; nonketotic hyperglycinemia; sulphite oxidase deficiency; molybdenum cofactor defect; congenital defects of glycosylation; congenital lactic acidosis; glycogen storage disease type II |
| *Nonimmune hydrops fetalis* | |
| | Lysosomal storage disorders; hemoglobinopathies, red blood cell glycolytic defects; neonatal hemochromatosis; glycogen storage disorder type IV; mitochondrial respiratory chain disorders |
| *Facial dysmorphism, with or without congenital malformations* | |
| | Lysosomal storage disorders; peroxisomal disorders; congenital defects of glycosylation; maternal phenylketonuria; pyruvate dehydrogenase deficiency; mevalonic aciduria; Smith-Lemli-Opitz syndrome |

From Christodoulou J, Wilcken B: Perimortem laboratory investigation of genetic metabolic disorders, *Semin Neonatol* 9:275-280, 2004.

In other instances, genetic metabolic disorders may lead to sudden unexpected death in infants and children and become the jurisdiction of the medical examiner and coroner systems.[103] In either case, autopsy diagnosis becomes critical not only for elucidating the cause of death but also for providing critical information needed in subsequent genetic counseling of the parents. Ideally, the genetic metabolic autopsy (or at least the specialized fluid and tissue collections) should be performed within 2 hours of death. In the hospital setting, this requires cooperation among the clinical, pathology, and decedent affair services and readiness to perform the initial specimen collection and processing. Table 9-3 lists the major components of a genetic metabolic autopsy.[104,105]

| Table 9-3 | Components of the genetic metabolic autopsy | |
|---|---|---|
| **Component** | **Specific instructions** | **Uses** |
| ***Clinical and imaging data*** | | |
| Family history with three-generation pedigree | | Determine mode of inheritance |
| Photographs | Multiple anterior, lateral, and posterior external views including whole body, face, hands, feet, ears, genitalia; internal in situ views of any anomalies; external and cut surfaces of organs | Evaluation and documentation |
| Radiographs | Complete skeletal survey | Skeletal dysplasia syndromes |
| Clinical geneticist consultation | | Evaluate for dysmorphic syndromes, initiate parental investigations (hemoglobinopathies, thrombophilic disorders) |
| ***Fluid samples*** | | |
| Dried blood spots on filter paper (newborn screening cards) | Store at room temperature but *not* in a plastic bag | Fatty acid oxidation disorders, organic acid disorders, galactosemia, others |
| Whole blood (5 mL) in lithium heparin tube | Separate within 20 minutes of collection and store at -70°C | Carnitine, quantitative aminoacids, very long chain fatty acids |
| Whole blood (5 mL) in EDTA tube | Can be stored at 4°C for 48 hours | DNA extraction |
| Whole blood (5 mL) in lithium heparin | Test must be started within 4 hours of sample collection | Chromosome analysis |
| Urine (5 mL or more) | Freeze and store at -70°C | Amino acid and organic acid profiles, acylglycines, orotic acid |
| Vitreous fluid | Freeze and store at -70°C | Organic acid disorders |
| Cerebrospinal fluid (1 mL) | Freeze and store at -70°C | Amino acid profile |
| Bile | Freeze and store at -70°C | Fatty acid disorders |
| ***Tissue samples*** | | |
| Skin (full thickness), fascia, lung, diaphragm, muscle or cartilage, blood, bone marrow | Send to cytogenetics laboratory for generation of fibroblast cultures and archiving in liquid nitrogen | Cell (fibroblast)–based assays, DNA source, chromosome analysis |
| Brain, spinal cord, peripheral nerve (sural or sciatic), skeletal muscle, heart, bone, cartilage, liver, kidney, others as indicated | 5-mm cubes placed in plastic vials or wrapped in aluminum foil and snap-frozen in isopentane and stored at -70°C; consider freezing larger quantities of tissue, e.g., one frontal lobe of brain depending on type of suspected metabolic disease | Molecular and DNA analysis, enzymatic studies (tricarboxylic acid cycle and electron transport chain complexes analyzed by spectrophotometry) |
| Muscle | Snap freeze in cryoembedding medium. Store at -70°C | Enzyme histochemistry in skeletal muscle disease |

*table continues*

**Table 9-3**   *(continued)*

| Component | Specific instructions | Uses |
|---|---|---|
| Brain (gray and white matter), skeletal muscle, heart, bone, cartilage, liver, kidney, placenta, others as indicated | 1-mm cubes fixed in 2.5% glutaraldehyde for electron microscopy | |
| Tissues for routine autopsy microscopy | Routine formalin-fixation, paraffin embedding | Routine histochemistry and immunohistochemistry |
| Tissues for specific histochemistry (alert histology laboratory of need for special tissue processing) | Alcohol fixation for glycogen storage diseases and cystinosis; cetyltrimethylammonium bromide (CTAB) for mucopolysaccharidosis | Histochemistry |

Data from Christodoulou J, Wilcken B: Perimortem laboratory investigation of genetic metabolic disorders, *Semin Neonatol* 9:275-280, 2004; Ernst LM, Sondheimer N, Deardorff MA, et al: The value of the metabolic autopsy in the pediatric hospital setting, *J Pediatr* 148 (6):779-83, 2006; Gilbert-Barness E, Debich-Spicer DE: *Handbook of pediatric autopsy pathology,* Totowa, NJ, 2005, Humana Press.

## REFERENCES

1. Farber SB: *The postmortem examination,* Springfield, Ill, 1937, Charles C Thomas.
2. Coe JI: Postmortem chemistry update, *Am J Forensic Med Pathol* 14:91-117, 1993.
3. Chace DH, DiPerna JC, Mitchell BL, et al: Electrospray tandem mass spectrometry for analysis of acylcarnitines in dried postmortem blood specimens collected at autopsy from infants with unexplained cause of death, *Clin Chem* 47:1166-1182, 2001.
4. Bennett MJ, Rinaldo P: The metabolic autopsy comes of age, *Clin Chem* 47:1145-1146, 2001.
5. Mulla A, Massey KL, Kalra J: Vitreous humor biochemical constituents: Evaluation of between-eye differences, *Am J Forensic Med Pathol* 26:146-149, 2005.
6. Forrest ARW: Toxicological and biochemical analysis. In Burton J, Rutty G, editors: *The hospital autopsy,* ed 2, London, 2001, Arnold, pp 126-133.
7. Madea B, Kreuser C, Banaschak S: Postmortem biochemical examination of synovial fluid—a preliminary study, *Forensic Sci Int* 118:29-35, 2001.
8. Forrest ARW: Obtaining samples at post mortem for toxicological and biochemical analyses, *J Clin Pathol* 46:292-296, 1993.
9. Kyle PM, Sepulveda W, Blunt S, et al: High failure rate of postmortem karyotyping after termination for fetal abnormality, *Obstet Gynecol* 88:859-897, 1998.
10. Johnson MP, Drugan A, Koppitch FC 3d, Uhlmann WR, Evans MI: Postmortem chorionic villus sampling is a better method for cytogenetic evaluation of early fetal loss than culture of abortus material, *Am J Obstet Gynecol* 163:1505-1510, 1990.
11. Brady K, Duff P, Harlass FE, Reid S: Role of amniotic fluid cytogenetic analysis in the evaluation of recent fetal death, *Am J Perinatol* 8:68-70, 1991.
12. Greenwold N, Jauniaux E: Collection of villous tissue under ultrasound guidance to improve the cytogenetic study of early pregnancy failure, *Hum Reprod* 17:452-456, 2002.
13. Coe JI: Postmortem chemistry of blood, cerebrospinal fluid, and vitreous humor. In Tedeschi CG, Eckert WG, Tedeschi LGP, editors: *Forensic medicine,* Philadelphia, 1977, WB Saunders, pp 1033-1060.
14. Coe JI: Time of death and changes after death: Part 2: Chemical considerations. In Spitz WU, editor: *Spitz and Fisher's medicolegal investigation of death.* Springfield, Ill, 1993, Charles C Thomas, pp 50-64.
15. Pounder DJ, Stevenson RJ, Taylor KK: Alcoholic ketoacidosis at autopsy, *J Forensic Sci* 43:812-816, 1998.
16. Brinkmann B, Fechner G, Karger B, DuChesne A: Ketoacidosis and lactic acidosis—Frequent causes of death in chronic alcoholics? *Int J Legal Med* 111:115-119, 1998.
17. Coe JI: Postmortem chemistries on human vitreous humor, *Am J Clin Pathol* 51:741-750, 1969.
18. Hodgkinson A, Hambleton J: Elevation of serum calcium concentration and changes in other blood parameters after death, *J Surg Res* 9:567-574, 1969.
19. Farmer JG, Benomran F, Watson AA, Harland WA: Magnesium, potassium, sodium and calcium in postmortem vitreous humor from humans, *Forensic Sci Int* 27:1-13, 1985.
20. Ingrao G, Belloni P, Di Pietro S, Santaroni GP: Levels of some trace elements in selected autopsy organs, and in hair and blood samples from adult subjects of the Italian population, *Biol Trace Elem Res* 26:699-708, 1990.
21. Bush VJ, Moyer TP, Batts KP, Parisi JE: Essential and toxic element concentrations in fresh and formalin-fixed human autopsy tissues, *Clin Chem* 41:284-294, 1995.
22. Benes B, Jakubec K, Smid J, Spevackova V: Determination of thirty-two elements in human autopsy tissue, *Biol Trace Elem Res* 75:195-203, 2000.
23. Garcia F, Ortega A, Domingo JL: Accumulation of metals in autopsy tissues of subjects living in Tarragona County, Spain, *J Environ Sci Health Part A Tox Hazard Subst Environ Eng* 36:1767-1786, 2001.
24. Naumann HN: Studies on postmortem chemistry, *Am J Clin Pathol* 20:314-324, 1950.
25. Coe JI: Use of chemical determinations on vitreous humor in forensic pathology, *J Forensic Sci* 17:541-546, 1972.
26. More DS, Arroyo MC: Biochemical changes of the synovial liquid in corpses with regard to the cause of death. 1: Calcium, inorganic phosphorus, glucose, cholesterol, urea nitrogen, uric acid, proteins and albumin, *J Forensic Sci* 30:541-546, 1985.
27. van den Oever R: Postmortem vitreous ammonium concentrations in estimating time of death, *Z Rechtsmed* 80:259-263, 1978.
28. Zhu B-L, Ishida K, Quan L, et al: Postmortem serum uric acid and creatinine levels in relation to causes of death, *Forensic Sci Int* 125:59-66, 2002.
29. Leadbeatter S, Williams DW, Stansbie D: Incidence of familial hypercholesterolaemia in premature deaths due to coronary heart disease, *Am J Forensic Med Pathol* 8:280-282, 1987.

30. Valenzuela A, Hougen HP, Villanueva E: Lipoproteins and apolipoproteins in pericardial fluid: New postmortem markers for coronary atherosclerosis. *Forensic Sci Int* 66:81-88, 1994.

31. Takeichi S, Nakajima Y, Osawa M, et al: The possible role of remnant-like particles as a risk factor for sudden cardiac death, *Int J Legal Med* 110:213-219, 1997.

32. Tsuji A, Ikeda N, Nakamura T: Plasma lipids, lipoproteins and apolipoproteins and sudden cardiac death, *Int J Legal Med* 112:151-154, 1999.

33. Naumann HN: Postmortem liver function tests, *Am J Clin Pathol* 26:495-505, 1956.

34. Robinson DM, Kellenberger RE: Comparison of electrophoretic analysis of antemortem and postmortem serum proteins, *Am J Med Sci* 38:371-377, 1962.

35. Coe JI: Comparison of antemortem and postmortem serum proteins, *Bull Bell Mus Pathobiol* 2:40-42, 1973.

36. Perry GW, Vargas-Cuba R, Vertes RP: Fetal hemoglobin levels in sudden infant death syndrome, *Arch Pathol Lab Med* 121:1048-1054, 1997.

37. Salkie ML, Mitchell I, Revers CW, et al: Postmortem serum levels of tryptase and total and specific IgE in fatal asthma, *Allergy Asthma Proc* 19:131-133, 1998.

38. Yunginger JW, Nelson DR, Squillace DL, et al: Laboratory investigation of deaths due to anaphylaxis, *J Forensic Sci* 36:857-865, 1991.

39. Yunginger JW, Sweeney KG, Sturner WQ, et al: Fatal food-induced anaphylaxis, *JAMA* 260:1450-1452, 1988.

40. Prahlow JA, Barnard JJ: Fatal anaphylaxis due to fire ant stings, *Am J Forensic Med Pathol* 19:137-142, 1998.

41. Fujita MQ, Zhu B-L, Ishida K, et al: Serum C-reactive protein levels in postmortem blood—an analysis with special reference to the cause of death and survival time, *Forensic Sci Int* 130:160-166, 2002.

42. Astrup BS, Thomsen JL: The routine use of C-reactive protein in forensic investigations, *Forensic Sci Int* 172:49-55, 2007.

43. Piette M, Schrijver G: Gamma-glutamyl transferase: Applications in forensic pathology: I. Study of blood serum recovered from human bodies, *Med Sci Law* 27:152-160, 1987.

44. Sadler DW, Girela E, Pounder DJ: Postmortem markers of chronic alcoholism, *Forensic Sci Int* 82:153-163, 1996.

45. Luna A, Villanueva E, Castellano M, Jimenez G: The postmortem determination of CK, LDH and its isoenzymes in pericardial fluid and its application to postmortem diagnosis of myocardial infarction, *Forensic Sci Int* 19:85-91, 1982.

46. Stewart RV, Zumwalt RE, Hirsch CS, Kaplan L: Postmortem diagnosis of myocardial disease by enzyme analysis of pericardial fluid, *Am J Clin Pathol* 82:411-417, 1984.

47. Osuna E, Pérez-Cárceles MD, Vieira DN, Luna A: Distribution of biochemical markers in biologic fluids: Application to the postmortem diagnosis of myocardial infarction, *Am J Forensic Med Pathol* 19:123-128, 1998.

48. Osuna E, Pérez-Cárceles MD, Alvarez MV, et al: Cardiac troponin I (cTN I) and the postmortem diagnosis of myocardial infarction, *Int J Legal Med* 111:173-176, 1998.

49. Cina SJ, Thompson WC, Fischer JR Jr, et al: A study of various morphologic variables and troponin I in pericardial fluid as possible discriminators of sudden cardiac death, *Am J Forensic Med Pathol* 20:333-337, 1999.

50. Cina SJ, Chan DW, Boitnott JK, et al: Serum concentrations of cardiac troponin I in sudden death: A pilot study, *Am J Forensic Med Pathol* 19:324-328, 1998.

51. Cina SJ, Brown DK, Smialek JE, Collins KA: A rapid postmortem cardiac troponin T assay: Laboratory evidence of sudden cardiac death, *Am J Forensic Med Pathol* 22:173-176, 2001.

52. Ansari MQ, Zamora JL, Lipscomb MF: Postmortem diagnosis of acute anaphylaxis by serum tryptase analysis: a case report, *Am J Clin Pathol* 99:101-103, 1993.

53. Schwartz HJ: Elevated serum tryptase in exercise-induced anaphylaxis, *J Allergy Clin Immunol* 95:917-919, 1995.

54. Schwartz HJ, Yunginger JW, Schwartz LB: Is unrecognized anaphylaxis a cause of sudden unexpected death? *Clin Exp Allergy* 25:866-870, 1995.

55. Edston E, van Hage-Hamsten M: Immunoglobulin E, mast cell-specific tryptase and the complement system in sudden death from coronary artery thrombosis, *Int J Cardiol* 52:77-81, 1995.

56. Edston E, van Hage-Hamsten M: Anaphylactoid shock—a common cause of death in heroin addicts? *Allergy* 52:950-954, 1997.

57. Edston E, Gidlund E, Wickman M, et al: Increased mast cell tryptase in sudden infant death—anaphylaxis, hypoxia or artefact? *Clin Exp Allergy* 29:1648-1654, 1999.

58. Nishio H, Matsui K, Miyazaki T, et al: A fatal case of amniotic fluid embolism with elevation of serum mast cell tryptase, *Forensic Sci Int* 126:53-56, 2002.

59. Edston E, Eriksson O, van Hage M: Mast cell tryptase in postmortem serum—reference values and confounders, *Int J Legal Med* 121:275-280, 2007.

60. Randall B, Butts J, Halsey JF: Elevated postmortem tryptase in the absence of anaphylaxis, *J Forensic Sci* 40:208-211, 1995.

61. Pumphrey RS, Roberts IS: Postmortem findings after fatal anaphylactic reactions, *J Clin Pathol* 53:273-276, 2000.

62. Edston E, van Hage-Hamsten M: beta-Tryptase measurements post-mortem in anaphylactic deaths and in controls, *Forensic Sci Int* 93:135-142, 1998.

63. Pumphrey RSH, Roberts ISD: Investigating possible anaphylactic deaths. In Burton J, Rutty G, editors: *The hospital autopsy*, ed 2, London, 2001, Arnold, pp 147-158.

64. Boles RG, Martin SK, Blitzer MG, Rinaldo P: Biochemical diagnosis of fatty acid oxidation disorders by metabolite analysis of postmortem liver, *Hum Pathol* 25:735-741, 1994.

65. Rashed MS, Ozand PT, Bennett MJ, et al: Inborn errors of metabolism diagnosed in sudden death cases by acylcarnitine analysis of postmortem bile, *Clin Chem* 41:1109-1114, 1995.

66. Zhu B-L, Ishida K, Quan L, et al: Post-mortem urinary myoglobin levels with reference to the causes of death, *Forensic Sci Int* 115:183-188, 2001.

67. Ritz S, Mehlan G, Martz W: Postmortem diagnosis of diabetic metabolic derangement: Elevated alpha 1-antitrypsin and haptoglobin glycosylation levels as an index of antemortem hyperglycemia, *J Forensic Sci* 41:94-100, 1996.

68. Watkins BP, Haushalter RE, Bolender DL, et al: Postmortem blood tests for HIV, HBV, and HCV in a body donation program, *Clin Anat* 11:250-252, 1998.

69. Takamatsu J, Tsuda F, Okudaira M: Infection with GB virus C, hepatitis C and B viruses in 1,044 cases autopsied at the medical examiner's office in Tokyo, *J Med Virol* 55:123-128, 1998.

70. Scheer S, McQuitty M, Denning P, et al: Undiagnosed and unreported AIDS deaths: Results from the San Francisco Medical Examiner, *J Acquir Immune Defic Syndr* 27:467-471, 2001.

71. Challener RC, Morrissey AM, Jacobs MR: Postmortem diagnosis of meningococcemia by detection of capsular polysaccharides, *J Forensic Sci* 33:336-346, 1988.

72. Gormsen H: Postmortem diagnosis of syphilitic aortitis, including serological verification on postmortem blood, *Forensic Sci Int* 24:51-56, 1984.

73. Torry JM: Acute myasthenia gravis: A postmortem diagnosis in a case of sudden death, *Med Sci Law* 23:111-113, 1983.

74. Tsokos M, Reichelt U, Jung R, et al: Interleukin-6 and C-reactive protein serum levels in sepsis-related fatalities during the early postmortem period, *Forensic Sci Int* 119:47-56, 2001.

75. Uhlin-Hansen L: C-reactive protein (CRP), a comparison of pre- and post-mortem blood levels, *Forensic Sci Int* 124:32-35, 2001.

76. Tormey WP, Carney M, FitzGerald RJ: Catecholamines in urine after death, *Forensic Sci Int* 103:67-71, 1999.

77. Edston E, Druid H, Holmgren P, Öström M: Postmortem measurements of thyroid hormones in blood and vitreous humor combined with histology, *Am J Forensic Med Pathol* 22:78-83, 2001.

78. Winston DC: Suicide via insulin overdose in nondiabetics, *Am J Forensic Med Pathol* 21:237-240, 2000.

79. Haibach H, Dix JD, Shah JH: Homicide by insulin administration, *J Forensic Sci* 32:208-216, 1987.

80. Iwase H, Kobayashi M, Nakajima M, Takatori T: The ratio of insulin to C-peptide can be used to make a forensic diagnosis of exogenous insulin overdosage, *Forensic Sci Int* 115:123-127, 2001.

81. Karch SB: *Drug abuse handbook*, ed 2, Boca Raton, Fla, 2006, CRC Press.

82. Baselt RC: *Disposition of toxic drugs and chemicals in man*, ed 7, Foster City, Calif, 2004, Biomedical Publications.

83. Karch SB: *Karch's pathology of drug abuse*, ed 3, Boca Raton, Fla, 2002, CRC Press.

84. Leikin JB, Watson WA: Post-mortem toxicology: What the dead can and cannot tell us, *J Toxicol* 41:47-56, 2003.

85. Drummer OH: Postmortem toxicology of drugs of abuse, *Forensic Sci Int* 142:101-113, 2004.

86. Drummer OH: Requirements for bioanalytical procedures in postmortem toxicology, *Anal Bioanal Chem* 388:1495-1503, 2007.

87. Cook DS, Braithwaite RA, Hale KA: Estimating ante-mortem drug concentrations from postmortem blood samples: The influence of postmortem redistribution, *J Clin Pathol* 53:282-285, 2000.

88. Karch SB: Alternate strategies for postmortem drug testing, *J Anal Toxicol* 25:393-395, 2001.

89. Vreman HJ, Wong RJ, Stevenson DK, et al: Concentration of carbon monoxide (CO) in postmortem human tissues: Effect of environmental CO exposure, *J Forensic Sci* 51:1182-1190, 2006.

90. Geller SA: Sampling for microorganisms during the autopsy. In Hutchins GM, editor: *Autopsy performance and reporting*, Northfield, Ill, 1990, College of American Pathologists, pp 127-128.

91. Wilson SJ, Wilson ML, Reller LB: Diagnostic utility of postmortem blood cultures, *Arch Pathol Lab Med* 117: 986-988, 1993.

92. Sogaard P, Larsen KE, Buhl L, et al: Bacteriological autopsy. I. A methodological study, *APMIS* 99:541-544, 1991.

93. Mazuchowski EL II, Meir PA: The modern autopsy: What to do if infection is suspected, *Arch Med Res* 36:713-723, 2005.

94. Spencer RC: The microbiology of the autopsy. In Cotton DWK, Cross SS, editors: *The hospital autopsy*, Oxford, UK, 1993, Butterworth-Heinemann, pp 144-157.

95. Morris JA, Harrison LM, Partridge SM: Postmortem bacteriology: A re-evaluation, *J Clin Pathol* 59:1-9, 2006.

96. Hove M, Pencil SD: Effect of postmortem sampling technique on the clinical significance of autopsy blood cultures, *Hum Pathol* 29:137-139, 1998.

97. Roberts FJ: The association of antimicrobial therapy with postmortem spleen culture in bacteremic patients, *Am J Clin Pathol* 87:770-772, 1987.

98. Valdés-Dapena M, Kalousek DK, Huff DS: Perinatal, fetal and embryonic autopsy. In Gilbert-Barness EG, editor: *Pathology of the fetus and infant*, St. Louis, 1997, Mosby, pp 482-524.

99. Bonin S, Petrera F, Niccolini B, Stanta G: PCR analysis in archival postmortem tissues, *Mol Pathol* 56:184-186, 2003.

100. Haller AC, Kanakapalli D, Walter R, et al: Transcriptional profiling of degraded RNA in cryopreserved and fixed tissue samples obtained at autopsy, *BMC Clin Path* 6:9, 2006, http://www.biomedcentral.com/1472-6890/6/9 (accessed October 1, 2008).

101. Kapur RP: Practicing pediatric pathology without a microscope, *Mod Pathol* 14:229-235, 2001.

102. Christodoulou J, Wilcken B: Perimortem laboratory investigation of genetic metabolic disorders, *Semin Neonatol* 9:275-280, 2004.

103. Norman MG, Taylor GP, Clarke LA: Sudden, unexpected, natural death in childhood, *Pediatr Pathol* 10:769-784, 1990.

104. Ernst LM, Sondheimer N, Deardorff MA, et al: The value of the metabolic autopsy in the pediatric hospital setting, *J Pediatr* 148 (6):779-83, 2006.

105. Gilbert-Barness E, Debich-Spicer DE: *Handbook of pediatric autopsy pathology*, Totowa, NJ, 2005, Humana Press.

# 10

# The Autopsy Report

*"The postmortem records of hospitals and other institutions constitute, when properly kept, available sources of scientific information of importance and value."*

L. Hektoen[1]

The autopsy report is a description and interpretation of the findings at necropsy and provides a record of the completed case as seen from the perspective of the anatomic pathologist. The document is part of the patient's medical record or, in the case of fetuses, the mother's medical record. As such, it is confidential; the information is shared with the patient's clinicians, appropriate hospital committees (quality of care, infection control), next of kin, immediate family members acknowledged by the next of kin, or legal appointee. Government agencies may request autopsy reports. Beyond these individuals and institutions, however, the pathologist or medical records representative should release the autopsy only under the authority of the proper writ or court order. The data contained within the report may be processed for general use if kept anonymous.

The main purpose of generating an autopsy report is to record and communicate the postmortem findings in an organized fashion. The expectation is that the report will provide definitive answers to medical issues. Thus, the autopsy pathologist must become proficient in diverse fields. Accurate information must be conveyed with clarity, insight, and authority. The autopsy report is the product of intense labor, thoughtful assessment, and purposeful reporting of clinicopathologic information.

There is considerable variation in the format and length of autopsy reports, depending on the needs of the institution and its personnel. For example, a teaching hospital that uses the autopsy for educational purposes and research may require a more detailed report that covers all systems, even normal ones. In contrast, other institutions (community hospitals, medical examiner's offices, military hospitals) may use an abbreviated report focused on the major clinical problem just before death. Thus, each institution must establish a standard for autopsy reports to fit its own needs, as well as to meet the requirements of the accrediting agencies. The Autopsy Committee of the College of American Pathologists has suggested a format including a list of headings for the autopsy report.[2]

The final report should be versatile enough to accommodate the different interests of the individuals expected to use it. For example, the health care delivery team is likely to expect an analysis of the impact of disease and effect of treatment, as well as a cause of death. The patient's physician and social worker may use the autopsy report as a vehicle for communication with family members; interpretation of the anatomic data within the clinical context by the doctor is helpful to the family in understanding the disease course. The autopsy report is often perceived as the final word, providing answers to questions that family or friends may have regarding the disease process or the care rendered. In fact, the report can be useful in reassuring a family upset over the patient's management. The autopsy report may facilitate an end to the grieving process. The institution can use the report for quality improvement. Furthermore, in academic centers, autopsy reports can be used in teaching exercises. The various data contained within the autopsy report can be used for future study by scientists, the institution, or the public health authority. Such diverse uses of the autopsy report demand a consistent approach.

## OVERVIEW OF THE AUTOPSY REPORT

In complete form, the standard autopsy report includes six parts:

1. Final Anatomic Diagnosis
2. Clinical Summary
3. Gross Findings
4. Microscopic Findings
5. Additional Findings
6. Clinicopathologic Correlation or Case Discussion

The first section of the report, Final Anatomic Diagnosis (FAD), is a list of anatomic diagnoses—the findings from the postmortem examination in telegraphic form. Although this list refers to what follows, the FAD is often placed first in the autopsy report, immediately after demographic data or incorporated with demographic data as the *autopsy face sheet.* This front page position provides an accessible digest of the entire case. Clinical Summary, the second section, consists of a summary of the patient's medical record. It provides an overview of historical aspects, physical signs, and laboratory data relevant to the clinical issues including pathologic diagnoses from surgical specimens. Gross Findings provides a description of the anatomic findings at postmortem examination, including radiographs and other imaging studies. It is the only permanent record of the pathologist's observations and measurements of the body cavity and organs. Microscopic Findings relates the histologic data primarily; immunohistochemical and electron microscopic findings would also be included in this section. Additional Findings provides an optional section for communication of ancillary studies such as microbiologic, toxicologic, molecular, chromosomal, or other laboratory studies performed on material obtained from the postmortem examination. The last section of the report, Clinicopathologic Correlation, is an interpretation of the significant anatomic findings within the clinical setting. Some reports include a discussion of the case within a wider context based on individual or departmental experience or a literature review.

Considering its various uses and the variety of institutions that perform autopsies, the autopsy report has evolved in many different ways. The College of American Pathologists, through its Autopsy Committee, provides a template for the Autopsy Face Sheet with recommended and desirable information (Fig. 10-1). The FAD must be included because it is the barest list of results. One concept of an autopsy report is that of a list of diagnoses with no description; the raw data (including description) are retained by the pathology department for dissemination on request. Another is a checklist or outline with extended description only for abnormal organs. These formats have the advantage of a short completion time. Alternatively, there is the complete report in prose, including clinical history, all anatomic data, and the final anatomic diagnoses. The conclusion or wrap-up is another source of considerable variation among

---

Institution Name and Address
(Provisional) Autopsy Diagnosis

| Patient's Name | Hosp/Med Records No. | Social Security No.* | Autopsy No. |

| Age (as appropriate) | Gestational Age | Birth Date |
| ___Yrs ___Mos ___Days ___Hrs | Weeks | Mo/Day/Year |

Race/Ethnicity_____  Hispanic?_____  Gender_____

| Final Admission | Death Date & Time | Place of Death/Ward/Service | Autopsy Date & Time |
| Mo/Day/Year | Mo/Day/Year/Military | | Mo/Day/Year    Military |

| Forensic Case | Extent of Autopsy Permit:_____ | Prosector(s) |
| Yes___ No___ | Embalmed: Yes___ No_____ | |

Patient's Usual Occupation(s)*                    Patient's Zip Code*

Patient's Physicians** Pending Studies          In Attendance at the Autopsy

| Conference Presentation** | Report Distribution** | Autopsy Completed |
| | | /    / |
| | | Mo/Day/Year _____ |
| | | Pathologist |

CLINICAL HISTORY (H/O):

AUTOPSY DIAGNOSES AND FINDINGS (A/D):

CAUSE-OF-DEATH STATEMENT:

SUMMARY STATEMENT

*Asterisks indicate optional but desirable information. Inclusion on the face sheet of items marked with a double asterisk may be useful but should be decided by individual institution.*

**Figure 10-1** The Autopsy Face Sheet format suggested by the College of American Pathologists. (Modified from Collins KA, Hutchins GM: *Autopsy performance & reporting,* ed 2, Northfield, Ill, 2003, College of American Pathologists, p 266.)

different types of autopsy reports. It may not include a discussion of the anatomic findings at all. Other reports contain a final note—a terse summary of the major pathologic findings and clinicopathologic correlation. Still others include a final note in the first paragraph and continue with a more extensive discussion of the interesting aspects of the case, including a literature review.

Pictorial representations used alone or in combination with a narrative have been suggested but have not found favor.[3] In the future, widespread use of digital images as supplements may enhance the presentation of the data and even facilitate shortening of the report. Protocols designed as extensions to the Problem-Oriented Medical Record System[4-6] have not been widely accepted. The classic autopsy report is narrative in form, although only experienced pathologists are able to dictate a report without cues. Most pathologists rely on a template or synoptic report. The generalized use of computerized pathology information systems makes generation of the autopsy narrative from a template relatively easy.[7]

In practice, few individuals read the entire autopsy report. Some sections must seem rather irrelevant, even dry, to the nonpathologist. Yet the data must be presented in such a way that they will be accessible in the future to individuals with special interests (e.g., subspecialty consultants, research scientists). The FAD and final note are probably the most commonly read sections. These high-profile sections should be intelligible to a general audience with a medical, but not necessarily pathology, background.

The following provides the basis for the autopsy report that we use in the university hospital. The finished product has the hallmarks of the "academic" style—fairly detailed description, analysis, and clinicopathologic discussion—all of which make the report somewhat lengthy. One of the objectives of the autopsy service in the teaching hospital is pathology resident and fellow training; our approach is to teach the complete autopsy so that trainees will be able to handle varied cases in future practice. Preparation of the autopsy report is instructional in several ways. Formulation organizes the pathologist's view of the case and directs the focus. It also prompts the pathologist to update his or her knowledge of the relevant area of medicine.

## FINAL ANATOMIC DIAGNOSIS

This first section of the autopsy report provides an overview of the case. In addition to the patient's demographic data, the first page of the report includes a short list of significant clinical diagnoses and procedures—a summary of the clinical issues. Starting immediately after the clinical diagnoses, the FAD is a union of the gross anatomic diagnoses made at the time of postmortem examination (essentially the provisional anatomic diagnoses) and the histologic diagnoses.

There are a number of different ways of organizing the individual diagnoses, but each should present the diagnoses in a hierarchy starting with the major pathology that explains the patient's terminal course and ending with incidental findings of lesser consequence in the patient's life. The first

approach is to list anatomic diagnoses related by pathogenetic themes, as shown in the following example:

- Example 1
  - I. Consequences of hypovolemic shock following rupture of abdominal aortic aneurysm
    - A. Diffuse alveolar damage, lungs
    - B. Acute subendocardial myocardial infarct, left ventricle, anteroseptal
    - C. Acute tubular necrosis, kidneys
  - II. Hypertensive atherosclerotic cardiovascular disease
    - A. Severe atherosclerosis, aorta
    - B. Hypertrophy, heart, left ventricle
    - C. Benign nephrosclerosis, kidneys

The objective is to provide the basis for a logical overview of each disease process, enabling the pathologist to show a connection between diagnoses or relate them to a procedure. This formulation clearly organizes consequences of disease process; however, some overlap may occur among categories, requiring repetition of diagnoses under different themes. For example, left ventricular cardiac hypertrophy may reflect both systemic hypertension and ischemic heart disease.

A second approach to organizing the FAD is to list anatomic diagnoses by organ systems, a scheme that does not emphasize pathogenetic relationships. Adding a phrase such as "in association with," "following," or "secondary to," however, can link consequences with pertinent disease processes that may not be obvious, as in the following example:

- Example 2
  - I. Diffuse alveolar damage following hypovolemic shock in association with ruptured abdominal aortic aneurysm
    Centriacinar emphysema, lungs

In this approach, there are three notable exceptions to organ system listings. The first exception encompasses diagnoses that apply to the body as a whole, such as edema, jaundice, sepsis, maceration, nutritional status, malformation complexes, or systemic diseases. The second includes combining diagnoses of the body cavities as a single group. Finally, the third involves neoplastic disease, for which sites of local extension or metastasis, or both, are grouped under the organ system of the primary tumor as in the following:

- Example 3
  - I. Prostatic adenocarcinoma, Gleason grade 7, with extension to right seminal vesicle and bladder wall, as well as metastasis to:
    - A. Pelvic and paraaortic lymph nodes
    - B. Thoracic and lumbar spine, diffuse
    - C. Lungs, diffuse
  - II. Acute bronchopneumonia, right lower lobe
  - III. Fibrinous adhesions, right pleural cavity
    Serosanguineous effusions, pleural cavities
    Fibrous adhesions, pericardial cavity
    Serous ascites
  - IV. Cachexia

A third approach to organizing the FAD is to list findings under the headings of immediate and intervening causes of death, followed by contributing conditions and then miscellaneous incidental findings.

- Example 4
  *Immediate Cause of Death*
  Cardiac tamponade (clinical)
  *Intervening and Underlying Cause(s) of Death*
  Rupture of anterior wall of left ventricle with hemopericardium due to:
  Acute myocardial infarct, anteroseptal wall, left ventricle due to:
  Severe atherosclerosis (>90% stenosis), left anterior descending coronary artery
  *Other Significant Conditions Contributing to Death*
  Hyperlipidemia (clinical)
  Chronic tobacco use (clinical)
  *Miscellaneous Findings*
  Moderate atherosclerosis, aorta
  Acute congestion, lungs
  Nodular thyroid gland

The specific format for listing each finding in the FAD is a function of departmental preference. A standard format such as

- Modifier(s), Diagnosis, Anatomic Site, Modifier(s)

imposes a rigid structure on the sequence for listing diagnoses and anatomic sites but allows easy categorization and specific diagnostic coding, such as with *SNOMED International*[8,9] or the *International Classification of Diseases*.[10,11] An example is illustrated as follows:

- Example 5
  I. Atherosclerotic cardiovascular disease
     A. Severe atherosclerosis, heart, left anterior descending coronary artery
        1. Acute infarct, heart, left ventricle, anteroseptal wall.
     B. Moderate atherosclerosis, aorta, abdominal

Some pathologists find this format stilted and argue that it can be difficult for the general reader, creating a barrier between pathologist and others. In the current age of automated diagnosis coding and natural language searching by computer, it may be preferable to use standard medical language and straightforward syntax to create a format that is easier to read. The following illustrates this approach as applied to the preceding example:

- Example 6
  I. Atherosclerosis involving aorta (grade 4) and anterior descending coronary artery (95% narrowed).
     A. Acute myocardial infarct involving anteroseptal region of left ventricle.

Pediatric cases should be presented in a manner that highlights the developmental context. In our institution, the first line of the pediatric FAD includes the developmental stage at birth, gender, birth weight, and whether the newborn was average, large, or small for gestational age. The second line of the pediatric FAD includes the stage at death, age, and weight and length measurements at death, as well as corresponding percentiles, as illustrated in the following:

- Example 7
  I. Premature female, 32 weeks gestation, 1600 grams, average for gestational age.
     Neonatal death, 6 days, 2100 grams (75th percentile), 44 cm (50th percentile).

This format is followed for infants and young children because the status at delivery is often relevant to the subsequent clinical course.

Whatever the age group of the patient, the remainder of the FAD is organized in a hierarchy by pathogenetic theme or organ system, starting with the one that dominates in terms of clinical issues and pathology and listing each diagnosis under that heading (see preceding example 5). The order of diagnoses conveys the pathologist's bias concerning the relative importance of each disease process. In this regard, inconsequential diagnoses should be omitted from the list; they are contained in the gross description and list of histologic diagnoses. These minor diagnoses tend to clutter the list and obfuscate the FAD. The addition of objective data such as degree of vascular narrowing, weight of a hypertrophied organ, or volume of intracavitary fluids is a matter of personal preference. As a general rule, however, avoid including too much detail, which makes the FAD look like a gross description. Although many pathologists incorporate names of procedures in the FAD, our practice is that procedures are never given as diagnoses in themselves; in some instances, the prosector cannot be absolutely certain of the history of a lesion—for example, cannot distinguish remote surgical intervention from malformation. Procedures, including the proper name if known with certainty, may be included in a qualifying phrase at the end of the line, highlighting the association for the reader, as in the following:

- Example 8
  I. Anastomosis, side-to-side, between ascending aorta and main pulmonary artery, intact, consistent with Norwood procedure.
     Atrial septal defect, following atrial septectomy.

It is important to emphasize, however, that it is safest to report only observations made at postmortem examination. Misinterpretation is a basis for error. Thus, in the preceding example, had the pathologist not known of the atrial septectomy, the diagnosis would have been written:

- Atrial septal defect.

In other instances, a fairly high degree of certainty can be reflected in the phrase "consistent with":

- Atrial septal defect, consistent with atrial septectomy.

An *interpretation* may follow the FAD. This short comment on the face sheet summarizes the essence of the case and minimally includes a cause-of-death statement.

- Example 9

This 46-year-old man with a lung allograft and respiratory insufficiency due to diffuse alveolar damage following preservation injury died of hypovolemic shock resulting from a massive upper gastrointestinal hemorrhage secondary to a duodenal ulcer.

## CLINICAL SUMMARY

The clinical summary is the second section of our autopsy report. It is abstracted from the patient's medical record; interviews with the health care delivery team and, in cases of death outside the hospital, the family or friends of the deceased; and the report of the individual who found the body. It should be brief (perhaps no longer than one-half page) but include details pertinent to the clinical issues, as well as the pathologic findings. By definition it is a synopsis, not a substitute for the medical record, which contains all the clinical information. Jargon and abbreviations should be avoided.

For adults, the first line of the clinical summary should include the age, gender, significant underlying condition, and chief complaint of the patient on the final admission to the hospital. The history of patient's present illness is next, followed by the systems review (pertinent positives only) and occupation at work. Other significant aspects of the medical history (surgical procedure dates, if known) and family and social history should be included if they provide information that correlates with the pathologic disorder. The admission physical examination lists the vital signs and a summary of the findings with more detail in the area related to the clinical issues. Pertinent admission laboratory data and radiographic findings are listed. The differential diagnosis, as well as the working diagnosis, is next. The hospital course is briefly summarized, including pertinent lab values, the principal therapies, and response to treatment. For patients with lengthy medical histories, a summary of problems is most efficient and should be tailored to fit the main clinical issues and pathologic findings from the FAD. Near the end of the clinical summary, the overwhelming clinical problem and the presumed cause of death should be indicated. The last line of the clinical summary should list the time of death.

For fetuses and young infants, the first line of the clinical summary should include the birth weight, developmental stage, maternal gravidity and parity, maternal age, and significant underlying conditions of the mother or patient. The perinatal history includes type of delivery, Apgar score, and condition of the neonate in the delivery room. This information may be relevant to the autopsies of older infants and children as well. Growth and development should be commented on, if pertinent.

## GROSS FINDINGS

Together with photographs and radiographs, this part of the report serves as the sole permanent record of the gross anatomic data, and it must be inclusive and accurate. At our hospitals, templates are employed as dictation guides for the anatomic findings (see Appendix A). This method leads the pathologist through the report step by step, ensuring that important details are included; as a result, the structure of final reports is fairly uniform. This is helpful not only to the pathologist but also to the regular reader of reports (e.g., pathologist, clinician, researcher). The disadvantage is that templates tend to stifle original thinking about the findings.

Several general rules, if followed, make for better reports. Organ pathology is described systematically, starting from the external surface. Any departure from normal should be clearly indicated. All lesions should be described; if numerous similar lesions are present, the first reported should be described in the greatest detail. Also, pertinent negative findings may be reported. Descriptions of gross pathology should be concise, as well as accurate. Because the gross description reports the anatomic data, it should contain sufficient, but not excessive, detail so that the reader can draw an independent conclusion regarding the diagnosis. Thus, neither diagnosis nor interpretation should be stated in this section. The weight of an organ is a good indicator of size and often alludes to pathologic findings; other measurements (linear in three dimensions or volume) may be useful as well. Finally, postmortem radiographic data can be included at an appropriate position in the text (e.g., coronary artery angiograms following description of the course of these vessels) or after the gross description in a separate section.

The report is organized to parallel the progression of the dissection at autopsy. Thus, it should start with a description of the external features and the findings on physical examination. Measurements can be given either at the appropriate points in the text or in a table at the end. For pediatric cases, the corresponding normal mean is also given. Following a report of the external examination, the position of the thoracic organs, as well as pathologic findings of the thorax, is given; pleural and pericardial effusions are quantified and their character described. For the peritoneal cavity, organ positions are noted and the amount and character of excess fluid recorded. Cardiac pathologic findings are approached from the pericardium; pathologic findings of the coronary arteries are described. Despite the various dissection methods, the description of the heart progresses sequentially chamber by chamber in the order of blood flow—cavities, valves, and myocardium. The condition of the large vessels of the body is noted; configuration of vessels and vascular connections is important in pediatric cases. Next, the appearance of the lungs and lung weights are reported: pleural lesions, bronchial and vessel abnormalities, and parenchymal pathologic findings as seen or palpated on cut slices. The other organ systems—alimentary, liver-biliary, urinary, reproductive, endocrine, and musculoskeletal—and pancreas, spleen, and lymph nodes are described in turn. The amount and character of the cerebrospinal fluid are recorded together before a description of pathologic findings in the dura and leptomeninges. The external features of the brain and spinal cord are described, followed by the pathologic findings in the coronal slices.

It stands to reason that the description of abnormal organs is much more extensive than that of normal ones. Nevertheless, clinical issues may relate to organ systems that are deemed relatively normal at postmortem examination. Thus, the report must convey the impression that the examination was complete. The pathologist learns that a certain amount of detail is needed to describe even normal organs—weight, dimension, shape, color, texture, consistency, and surface appearance. Examples of the Gross Findings section of our reports are in Appendix A.

## MICROSCOPIC FINDINGS

In contrast to the gross organs, glass slides are retained indefinitely. The histopathologic findings are reported in abbreviated form as diagnoses, and the normal histologic findings may be summarized by the phrase "no pathologic diagnosis." These data are recorded in tabular form, simplifying this section of the autopsy report for the nonpathologist. The diagnoses are indexed by slide number for future reference. One example is a three-column list, as shown in Table 10-1. If warranted, additional description of the histopathologic findings may be reported in a note at the end. The results of special studies—immunohistochemistry or electron microscopy—should also be at the end of this section.

## ADDITIONAL FINDINGS

As mentioned earlier, this optional section provides a place to report ancillary studies, such as microbiologic, toxicologic, molecular, chromosomal, or other laboratory studies performed on autopsy material. Although these data may come from various outside laboratories, they are pertinent to the interpretation of the anatomic findings. The autopsy report is a logical repository for this information because it should be a comprehensive summary of all aspects of the case. In those instances in which the results of ancillary studies are not available at the time that the autopsy report is finalized, it is helpful to state that a particular study is pending so that the clinician and family can temper their interpretation of the anatomic findings. The final result is then communicated as an addendum to the autopsy report.

| Table 10-1 | Example of a tabular listing of autopsy microscopic findings |  |
|---|---|---|
| Slide | Organ and site | Diagnosis |
| A | Heart, right atrium and ventricle | No pathologic diagnosis |
| B | Heart, left atrium and ventricle | Myxoid change in mitral valve |
| C | Lung, right lower lobe, periphery | Diffuse alveolar damage, centriacinar emphysema |
| D | Lung, left lower lobe, hilar and periphery | Acute bronchopneumonia with gram-negative rods |
| E | Stomach | Acute gastritis |
|  | Duodenum | Acute ulcer |

## CASE DISCUSSION

The case discussion is the section used for clinicopathologic correlation. It begins with a "final note." This is a succinct paragraph summarizing the entire case: one sentence relating the clinical setting and major issues, another listing the principal findings at postmortem examination, and one or two sentences relating the anatomic findings to the clinical course. Complex cases may require more extensive correlation. Often, the final sentence of this first paragraph is a statement of the cause of death.

The final note should clearly indicate the pathologist's interpretation of the data. An unambiguous conclusion resolves the intellectual tension that exists before the postmortem examination. Sensitive issues uncovered by the anatomic findings should be discussed with a gentle yet forthright approach. The autopsy report should never leave an impression of a cover-up. On the other hand, overinterpretation of anatomic data may lead to error, which can carry a high price. In this regard, it is often advisable for the pathologist to discuss the anatomic findings with the clinician before the final note is formulated. The consensus attained by reconciling two perspectives reinforces the result.

On occasion, the postmortem examination fails to resolve a clinical issue definitively. Certain entities can be ruled out on the basis of the anatomic data but not all the possibilities. In this circumstance, the final note may provide a short differential diagnosis and evidence for and against each item in the list. Although the possibilities are stated, a conclusion is never established. Frustrating for the pathologist, this type of report with an unanswered question may nevertheless satisfy the clinician, who uses the information to rule out key clinical issues.

In our reports, the rest of the discussion consists of a brief overview of an interesting topic relevant to the case. The purpose is primarily education; the pathologist learns by reviewing the experience of others, and the reader gains insight into the case within a particular context. Because pathology's strength is structure, this part of the discussion should focus on an interesting aspect of the anatomic findings. This part of the autopsy report requires a review of the literature, and a few pertinent up-to-date references should be cited at the end of the discussion. In most instances, discourses related to clinical aspects (e.g., epidemiology or treatment, which the clinicians know well) are avoided. Nevertheless, to make a good report, the pathologist must be familiar with all clinical areas, and these topics constitute background necessary for the pathologic analysis.

## CONCLUSION

As noted, the autopsy report described in this chapter is a comprehensive exposition of the diagnoses, clinical history, anatomic findings, and clinicopathologic correlation that serves the purpose of our particular academic institutions. Autopsy pathologists in other settings may prefer a different model. Whatever its form, the autopsy report serves as the permanent record of the anatomic data that is the basis for clinicopathologic correlation used by the health care delivery team, scientists, medicolegal professionals, and others. To be useful, its information must be accurate and presented clearly. The autopsy report should convey an intelligent approach to a problem. Its quality reflects not only that of the autopsy service but also that of the department of pathology and the institution. An outstanding autopsy report casts the institution in a very favorable light.

## REFERENCES

1. Hektoen L: *The technique of post-mortem examination*, Chicago, 1894, Chicago Medical Book.
2. Hanzlick RL: The autopsy lexicon: Suggested headings for the autopsy report, *Arch Pathol Lab Med* 124:594-603, 2000.
3. Ludwig J: *Handbook of autopsy practice*, Totowa, NJ, 2002, Humana Press.
4. Gravanis MB, Rietz CW: The problem-oriented postmortem examination and record: An educational challenge, *Am J Clin Pathol* 60:522-535, 1973.
5. Christie RW: The problem-oriented autopsy audit, *Am J Clin Pathol* 60:536-542, 1973.
6. Saladino AJ, Dailey ML: The problem oriented postmortem examination, *Am J Pathol* 69(Suppl 2):253-257, 1978.
7. Brown AG, Berry CL: Production of necropsy reports by medical staff using a computer system, *J Clin Pathol* 38:1394-1396, 1985.
8. College of American Pathologists. *SNOMED terminology solutions*, http://www.cap.org/apps/cap.portal?_nfpb=true&_pageLabel=snomed_page (accessed October 2, 2008).
9. Coté RA, Rothwell DJ, Polotay JL, Beckett RS, editors: *SNOMED International (Systematized Nomenclature of Human and Veterinary Medicine)*, ed 3, vols 1 and 2, Numeric indices, vols 3 and 4, Alphabetic indices, Northfield, Ill, 1993, College of American Pathologists.
10. *International classification of diseases*, rev 9, Clinical modification: Physician ICD-9 CM, vols 1 and 2, Chicago, 2001, AMA Press.
11. World Health Organization: *International statistical classification of diseases and related health problems*, rev 10, Geneva, 1992-1994, World Health Organization.

# 11

# Postmortem Examination in Cases of Sudden Death Due to Natural Causes

*"It is very much to be regretted that the knowledge of morbid structure does not lead with certainty to the knowledge of morbid actions, although the one is the effect of the other; yet surely it lays the most solid foundation for prosecuting such enquiries with success."*

Matthew Baillie[1]

The occurrence of sudden death presents a challenge to the general autopsy pathologist, who usually examines hospitalized patients with detailed medical records. In this chapter we discuss the approach to the patient who dies within 1 hour of the onset of symptoms, an arbitrary definition of "sudden."[2] This group may be subdivided into the patients for whom death can be considered an expected outcome of a known illness and those for whom death is unexpected. This distinction is important because unexpected death due to unnatural causes, unintentional and intentional, usually falls within the purview of forensic pathology.

## PREPARING FOR THE AUTOPSY

Whether expected or unexpected, natural sudden death is due to a catastrophic complication of a disease process or congenital malformation. As with any autopsy, the pertinent medical history of the patient should give the prosector some indication of the differential diagnosis of the lethal complication. In fact, the autopsy provides anatomic data that must be considered not only together with medical information but also in light of other social history and circumstances of the terminal event.[3] Thus, if the available history is incomplete, the pathologist should ask a relative or other person who knew the patient well. The possibility of recent signs and symptoms that might indicate a prodrome should be explored. Moreover, family history of sudden death is characteristic in certain syndromes.

Even after uncovering information regarding the patient's underlying condition, the pathologist should initiate the postmortem examination as if any cause of death is possible. There should be no restrictions on the extent of the examination. The prosector should be experienced in autopsy pathology, and it is important that objectivity be maintained.

Treating the case as a mystery puts the prosector on guard for unexpected pathologic findings. As is true in general autopsy practice, the initial dissection provides the best and sometimes only opportunity to examine organs, tissues, or body fluids properly. Thus, it is imperative to have a systematic approach to this detailed examination. Such an approach has been presented elsewhere in this book (see Chapters 4 and 5), but adaptation of the general procedure to the specific instance of sudden death and the possibility of subtle pathologic findings remains to be discussed.

Before starting, the prosector should make certain special preparations. Pictures of the exterior body surface can serve as documentation for future reference, and in infants and young children radiographs are useful for not only hidden trauma but also syndromes affecting the skeleton. Sterile syringes for cultures and vials for collection and storage of body fluids should be part of the setup in case they are needed. The pathologist should collect and store fluid and tissue samples as outlined in Chapter 9.

## THE APPROACH TO AUTOPSY IN CASES OF SUDDEN DEATH DUE TO NATURAL CAUSES

A list of natural causes of sudden death is given in Box 11-1. This chapter is not intended to be a complete discourse on pathologic findings in these entities; rather it describes an approach to the problem of determining the cause of sudden death. In fact, the great majority of sudden death occurs by a limited number of mechanisms: hemorrhage, sepsis, and ischemia or arrhythmia (Table 11-1).[4] Some of these are readily apparent at autopsy, but some have to be inferred (as a diagnosis of exclusion) from the gross and microscopic pathologic findings. The following discussion assumes a certain sequence of discovery and should serve as an algorithm useful in consideration of sudden death at autopsy.

**Box 11-1** Natural causes of sudden death

**Cardiovascular**
Ischemic heart disease
   Myocardial infarct—acute, chronic
Inflammatory heart disease
   Myocarditis
   Arteritis
   Endocarditis
Tumor
Hypertrophied heart
   Cardiomyopathy—hypertrophic, dilated, infiltrative
   Systemic hypertension
   Valvular heart disease—aortic stenosis
   Obesity
Right ventricular dysplasia
Anatomic anomalies
   Malformations of coronary arteries
   Anomalous atrioventricular muscle bundles
   Mitral valve prolapse syndrome
Conduction tissue abnormalities
   Age-related changes—sclerosis, calcification of mitral annulus
   Systemic disease—collagen-vascular disorders
   Hemorrhage
   Sick sinus syndrome
Functional disorders: anatomic basis may not be recognized
   Low-output state due to sepsis
   Surgically repaired congenital heart defects
   Coronary artery spasm, including drug-related
   Excess sympathetic discharge, including catecholaminergic
      polymorphic ventricular tachycardia
   Vagal inhibition
   Spontaneous ventricular fibrillation, including Pokkuri disease
   Hereditary or acquired predisposition to arrhythmia (long QT
      interval; Brugada, Wolff-Parkinson-White, Timothy syndromes)
Vascular
   Dissection, rupture
   Thromboembolism

**Pulmonary**
Asthma
Pulmonary hypertension, including Eisenmenger's syndrome
Pneumonia
Pneumothorax
Tumor

Epiglottitis
Functional disorder: anatomic basis may not be recognized
   Respiratory arrest, including drug-related
   Anaphylaxis
   Asphyxiation (including positional asphyxia)

**Gastrointestinal**
Peptic ulcer
Acute pancreatitis
Strangulated hernia, intussusception, volvulus
Tumor
Vascular malformation

**Hepatobiliary**
Tumor
Cirrhosis, including ruptured varices

**Reticuloendothelial, hematopoietic**
Splenic rupture
Sickle cell disease (and rarely sickle cell trait)

**Genitourinary**
Pyelonephritis
Ruptured ectopic pregnancy
Amniotic embolism

**Endocrine**
Functional disorder: anatomic basis may not be recognized
   Hyper- and hypothyroidism
   Pituitary insufficiency
   Diabetic ketoacidosis

**Central Nervous System**
Cerebrovascular accident
Encephalomyelitis, meningitis, brain abscess
Tumor
Functional disorder: anatomic basis may not be recognized
   Seizure disorder, including drug-related

**Miscellaneous**
Drug overdose
Drowning
Diabetic ketoacidosis
Electrocution (especially low voltage)
Inhalational toxicity (volatiles)
Sudden infant death syndrome

## Pathologic Findings on External Body Surface

Before cutting, the prosector should perform a careful examination of the external body surface. Signs of trauma to the body or head (e.g., localized ecchymosis, fracture, or dislocation) raise the possibility of foul play, and on discovery of suspicious lesions the autopsy must be stopped for notification of the medical examiner. Similarly, needle puncture wounds or other evidence of recreational drug use necessitates a toxicology analysis, although many of the individuals who abuse drugs die of natural causes from diseases to which they are susceptible. Skin rash or purpura should alert the prosector to the possibility of overwhelming infection or disseminated intravascular coagulopathy.

## Pathologic Findings in the Body Cavity

Before opening the thorax, the prosector should consider the possibility of *tension pneumothorax* and document air within the thorax (see Chapter 4); for infants, a radiograph taken before autopsy is helpful in this regard. The postmortem examination should proceed with a thorough inspection of the body cavities, including the organs in situ. *Hemorrhage* may be evident within the body cavities at first view (e.g., hemoperitoneum, hemopericardium). Because dissection may disrupt the anatomy and thereby obscure the source of the blood, the site of initial hemorrhage should be investigated in situ. For example, hemoperitoneum necessitates inspection of the organ surfaces to detect signs of trauma (e.g.,

| Table 11-1 | Relative incidence of natural causes of sudden death | |
|---|---|
| **Disease** | **Relative Incidence (%)** |
| Cardiovascular | 56 |
| Respiratory | 16 |
| Central nervous system | 8 |
| Malignancy | 8 |
| Gastrointestinal | 4 |
| Renal | 1.5 |
| Sudden infant death syndrome | 0.5 |
| Miscellaneous | 6 |

Data from Craig-Hunter C: Deaths due to sudden or unexpected natural causes. In Mart AK, editor: *Taylor's principles and practice of medical jurisprudence,* Edinburgh, 1984, Churchill Livingstone, pp 111-127.

laceration). In some cases, selective postmortem angiography (see Chapter 7), which should be performed before much dissection has been done, may be helpful in localizing vessel lesions.

Alternatively, the origin of hemorrhage may not be apparent until dissection of the organs (e.g., hepatic tumor). In some cases hemorrhage may become apparent within the viscera after dissection, and the source should be determined while the organ is fresh. Manual removal of loose blood and gentle washing may reveal a small lesion suspicious as the origin of hemorrhage. Fixation usually obscures the pertinent anatomy in an area of hematoma. For example, a cerebral aneurysm should be investigated for rupture in the area of hematoma while the vessels are fresh and the blood clot is easier to remove. On the other hand, dissection may make the underlying pathologic disorder less obvious (e.g., esophageal varices); special techniques to preserve the gross pathologic findings may be helpful. It is surprising how little additional information is provided by histologic analysis; when the gross pathologic findings are unrevealing, histologic examination is usually not very helpful. Only in a minority of cases does judicious sectioning of the area in question disclose pathologic findings that can account for hemorrhage. Thus, in cases of massive hemorrhage leading to sudden death, the gross pathologic findings usually provide the most important clue to pathogenesis; in a few cases microscopy may be required to ascertain the underlying condition.

## Overwhelming Infection

Less obvious than massive hemorrhage as a cause of sudden death is *sepsis* complicating overwhelming infection. Although cases may demonstrate only minimal pathologic changes, in a surprising number of instances, established organ pathology provides a clue to infection as a cause of sudden death. As noted previously, skin rash or purpura may be the initial evidence. Associated with meningococcemia, adrenal hemorrhage often complicates disseminated intravascular coagulopathy of diverse causes and thus is nonspecific. *Lobar pneumonia* or other major infection (including *abscess* or *meningitis*) may

be recognized for the first time at autopsy. The setting is often one in which the patient's health has been neglected; the mechanism of sudden death is probably sepsis or, sometimes, hemorrhage.

In cases in which the cause of death is not readily apparent on inspection of the body cavities, it is wise to obtain a blood culture before removing any organ (see Chapter 9). The culture tube may be discarded if significant pathologic findings that explain the patient's sudden death are encountered later in the autopsy. Occasionally, a positive blood culture is the only significant finding at autopsy, and sepsis (such as that known to complicate urologic infection) is the cause of sudden death. Although overwhelming viral infection can also lead to sudden death, the low yield of meaningful results makes routine viral cultures of little diagnostic usefulness in most cases.

## Respiratory Disease

*Asthma, pulmonary thromboemboli,* and *pulmonary hypertension* may cause sudden death. However, most established diseases of the lung parenchyma are not causes of sudden death as defined here, unless massive hemorrhage is a complication. Before slicing the lungs of a victim of sudden death, one should inspect the pleural surfaces carefully for subtle pathologic findings such as petechiae, which may be the only evidence of terminal hypoxia. Increased lung weight may be the first indication of intrinsic pulmonary disease. *Pulmonary edema,* such as that complicating anaphylactic shock or massive aortic or mitral valve insufficiency, is suggested by the gross appearance and is confirmed by histologic examination. Measurement of postmortem serum tryptase level has been useful in establishing a diagnosis of anaphylaxis when used in conjunction with supporting clinical or historical data.[5,6]

Hyperinflated lungs that billow out from the opened thorax and contain interspersed areas of atelectasis are indicative of air trapping, such as that associated with *asthma.* According to Sur and colleagues,[7] sudden-onset fatal asthma (death occurring within 1 hour of an attack) is distinguished by the presence of a neutrophil-rich submucosal infiltrate on a background of the classic histopathologic changes of the asthmatic airways (mucosal edema, mucus plugging, mucous gland enlargement, smooth muscle hyperplasia, and thickening of the subepithelial collagen layer). Others[8] attribute the increased neutrophils to intubation and cardiopulmonary resuscitation, however, and suggest that the true distinguishing features of sudden-onset fatal asthma are inflammatory infiltrates of large numbers of $CD8^+$ T lymphocytes. In slow-onset fatal asthma (longer than 2½ hours), eosinophils predominate in the submucosa.

*Pulmonary artery thromboembolism* remains a difficult disease to prevent and continues to be a significant cause of death.[9] Emboli are readily apparent on dissection of the pulmonary arteries, and the main issues at autopsy become determination of the site of origin and predisposing condition. Whereas most patients with *pulmonary hypertension* have recognizable clinical symptoms before death, some may die suddenly and unexpectedly without exhibiting any recognized signs of the disease.[10] During or shortly after induction of general anesthesia or during imaging procedures such as cardiac catheterization, angiography, or radioisotopic lung scanning, patients with pulmonary hypertension may experience sudden cardiovascular collapse and sudden death.[11,12] Presumably, these interventions stimulate additional constriction of the already compromised pulmonary vascular bed, exacerbating right heart failure or eliciting lethal arrhythmias, or both. At autopsy pulmonary hypertension can be suspected from right ventricular hypertrophy or atherosclerotic plaques in the pulmonary arterial tree, or both; in this instance, the cause is disclosed by dissection of the heart (e.g., congenital heart defect) or histopathologic examination (e.g., chronic thromboembolism, plexogenic arteriopathy, venoocclusive disease).

Patients with *obstructive sleep apnea syndrome* often have cardiac dysrhythmias during cyclic nocturnal hypoxemia but do not have an increased risk of dying during sleep.[13] However, these individuals are prone to motor vehicle accidents while asleep at the wheel.[14]

## Cardiovascular Disease

As a cause of sudden death, cardiovascular disease is the most important in terms of incidence (see Table 11-1). Many of these deaths result from lethal arrhythmias, most commonly ventricular tachycardia or fibrillation. Again, gross pathologic findings may provide important clues to underlying disease. If the lungs appear unremarkable, increased heart weight should focus the prosector's attention on this organ, and hypertrophy almost always indicates underlying heart disease. (Conditioned athletes may have hearts weighing somewhat more than the normal, but this physiologic hypertrophy does not seem to be associated with sudden death.[15]) Several authors have provided guidelines for investigating and examining cases of sudden cardiac death.[16-18]

### Ischemic Heart Disease

The most common cause of sudden death in the United States is ischemic heart disease.[19,20] Coronary artery *atherosclerosis* is commonly identified at autopsy in victims of sudden death.[21] It is important to point out, however, that because of the high prevalence of atherosclerosis in our society, the pathologist should not be blind to the possibility of a coexisting lethal process.[22] Because atherosclerosis provides an important clue to cardiac ischemia, close inspection of the coronary arteries is imperative; if calcified, the arteries should be removed intact and decalcified before sectioning. Whether the arteries are examined on the heart or in isolation after decalcification, the interval between cuts depends on the diameter of the vessels; the prosector should be able to see through the lumen of each segment. How much atherosclerosis is significant? At least 50% narrowing of the artery's luminal radius (i.e., 75% reduction in luminal area) should raise the prosector's suspicion because this is the degree of compromise known to be associated with complications of ischemia.[22-24] Histopathologic findings, such as thrombosis, plaque instability (erosions, fissures, rupture),[25-27] and cholesterol emboli in the coronary arteries, establish the significance of the vessel disease.

In the setting of significant coronary artery atherosclerosis and no pathologic disorders in any other organ, arrhythmia related to acute ischemia is the likely cause of sudden death. After examination of the coronary arteries, the ventricles must be cut in short axis (cross section) up to the tips of the papillary muscles. The base should be cut through the valves along the lines of blood flow. Hearts from patients with chronic ischemic heart disease are usually hypertrophied, and most contain a healed or healing myocardial infarct. If the duration of infarction before sudden death is truly 1 hour, the classic histopathologic changes associated with acute myocardial infarction, including wavy fibers and contraction bands, will not have evolved. Other methods—apoptosis detection,[28] histochemical reactions,[29] and immunohistochemistry[30]—may provide evidence of acute ischemia. Analysis of postmortem serum and pericardial fluid for biochemical markers of myocardial injury have not proven useful in differentiating acute myocardial necrosis from other types of intramyocardial injury though they do have a high negative predictive value.[31,32] Under certain circumstances, however, myocardial infarction of longer duration may go unrecognized during life, and the pathologist can date the onset from the gross and microscopic findings.

The rate of coronary thrombosis associated with sudden coronary death varies from 20% to 70% depending on the interval between onset of symptoms and death, the type of prodromal symptoms, and the presence or absence of acute myocardial infarct.[33] Approximately 70% of patients who die suddenly with acute myocardial infarction demonstrate acute coronary artery thrombosis, whereas those with healed infarcts tend not to have thrombi.[34] Rarely, acute myocardial infarction is associated with myocardial rupture or massive cardiac failure as a cause of sudden death; more often, patients with these complications are symptomatic for longer than 1 hour. Also, in patients with healed infarcts, there is evidence that new ischemia is the major cause of ventricular arrhythmia leading to sudden death.[35]

Death from cardiac ischemia may also result from nonatherosclerotic abnormalities of the coronary arteries (e.g., vasculitis, emboli); however, usually these conditions are associated with a prodrome. Again, the coronary arteries should be thoroughly examined. Myocardial bridging, in which heart muscle surrounds a coronary artery (most often the left anterior descending)[36,37] is a relatively common incidental finding at autopsy—not the cause of sudden death in the vast majority of cases.[38] Occasionally, the intramural or small coronary arteries may become critically narrowed by fibromuscular dysplasia.[39]

### Hypertrophy of the Heart

Virtually every chronic heart condition is associated with hypertrophy, and whatever the cause, cardiac hypertrophy is a substrate for ventricular arrhythmias and sudden cardiac death.[22,40] An important cause of cardiac hypertrophy is *systemic hypertension*; however, in most cases, its relationship to sudden death derives from its being a risk factor for coronary atherosclerosis.[41] Thus, at autopsy extramural coronary artery atherosclerosis often is present in addition to left ventricular hypertrophy and nephrosclerosis indicative of hypertension. Often silent and afflicting virtually any age group, hypertension may occasionally be associated with sudden death without coronary atherosclerosis.[42] Hearts with hypertrophy related to hypertension should be distinguished from those with cardiomyopathy (see later). In this regard, review of the patient's medical record is very important; in some cases, hypertension may be documented even if it was not treated successfully.

Chronic diseases of valves may also cause hypertrophy. Of these, noninflammatory lesions causing aortic stenosis and insufficiency are most prevalent. Fibrosis of the valve leaflets is the hallmark. *Mitral valve prolapse*, another cause of sudden death, is distinguished by myxomatous thickening of the posterior leaflet, hooding of its interchordal portions, and attenuation of the chordae tendineae, which may rupture.[43] *Chronic rheumatic heart disease* is also associated with hypertrophy, which can be the basis for arrhythmia.

Finally, *idiopathic left ventricular hypertrophy* is associated with sudden death. In these unusual cases it is important to exclude hypertension following a thorough review of the medical record. Idiopathic left ventricular hypertrophy likely reflects cardiomyopathy (see later).

### Inflammatory Heart Disease

Inflammatory heart disease is also a substrate for sudden death in three distinct settings. The first is *active myocarditis*, including granulomatous myocarditis, which may be complicated by lethal ventricular arrhythmia. Because myocarditis can be a rapidly progressive disease, the cardiac muscle may not be hypertrophied. Thus, the heart often appears relatively normal on gross inspection, and histopathologic examination establishes the diagnosis.[44] Second, coronary *arteritis* may lead to either thromboembolism or vessel narrowing with catastrophic consequences. Arteritis, however, is part of systemic illness that usually arises over a longer term. Third, *infective endocarditis* has a longer natural history but may rarely lead to sudden death either by thromboembolism to the coronary arteries or intracranial circulation or massive valvular insufficiency associated with a necrotizing process. In cases of thromboembolism, close inspection of the valve surfaces provides evidence of the underlying disease process, even though only the base of the vegetation remains; careful dissection of the coronary and intracranial arteries may disclose the thrombus. In cases of acute valvular insufficiency, both perforation of the valve leaflet and pulmonary edema are characteristic.

### Malformations of the Heart

Most heart malformations do not lead to sudden death because they are associated with a long-standing clinical syndrome. Infrequently, a case of pulmonary hypertension in association with an undiagnosed cardiac defect may present with sudden death. Much more rare than valvular malformations or septal defects, congenital malformations of the coronary arteries are associated with a relatively high incidence of sudden death. Inspection of the aortic root to confirm the origin of each coronary artery from the correct aortic sinus of Valsalva is critical. The significant malformations

are readily identified in patients who die suddenly, usually after vigorous exercise. *Anomalous origin of the left coronary artery from the pulmonary artery* is the classic defect, a serious problem with manifestations in infancy in the great majority of cases; left ventricular dilation, hypertrophy, or an established myocardial infarct may be present. *Anomalous origin of the left coronary artery from the right (or anterior) sinus of the aortic valve* often involves a slitlike orifice and angulated extended course through the aortic wall before traversing the epicardial surface between the aorta and pulmonary artery.[45] Although also involving a course between the great arteries, *anomalous origin of the right coronary artery from the left sinus* is associated with sudden death less commonly. *Hypoplastic coronary arteries* are also associated with sudden cardiac death, often related to exercise.[33]

### Cardiomyopathy

Another basis for sudden death, *cardiomyopathy* refers to heart muscle disease in the absence of significant ischemic heart disease, history of systemic hypertension, valvular heart conditions, congenital heart disease, and pericardial disease.[46] Usually the substrate for sudden death is ventricular hypertrophy. Among conditioned athletes younger than 35 years who die suddenly, *hypertrophic cardiomyopathy* is the most common underlying problem.[47] Almost always increased in weight, these hearts show either concentric hypertrophy of the left ventricle or hypertrophy involving the septum disproportionately. The anatomic criterion for significant septal thickening is a septal–to–free wall ratio greater than 1.3. The cavity may be small. A plaquelike area of sclerosis on the endocardial surface in the left ventricular outflow tract just below the aortic valve signifies dynamic left ventricular outflow tract obstruction even when anatomic obstruction is not apparent; the lesion arises where there has been repeated trauma between the abnormally moving mitral valve septal leaflet and the bulging septum. The distinctive histologic feature of hypertrophic cardiomyopathy is myofiber disarray, which occurs extensively throughout the septum in this condition.[46] Sections of upper septum should be taken in the horizontal plane, away from septal–free wall junctions where disarray occurs normally. The mechanism of sudden death is arrhythmia, which occurs in a relatively high percentage of affected but asymptomatic individuals. The basis for arrhythmia likely is ischemic damage.[48] Because there is a high proportion of heredofamilial disease among patients with hypertrophic cardiomyopathy, the fact that even asymptomatic patients may develop lethal arrhythmia underscores the importance of obtaining a complete family history and making the appropriate referral in cases of hypertrophic cardiomyopathy (see later). Some patients with gene mutations associated with hypertrophic cardiomyopathy have normal-appearing hearts.

In contrast, patients with *dilated cardiomyopathy* or *infiltrative heart disease* (cardiomyopathy with restrictive hemodynamics) usually develop congestive failure and thus come to medical attention before death. Among these patients, arrhythmia is a common cause of sudden death.[35] As with other types of cardiac disease discussed previously, the hypertrophy that results from these forms of heart muscle disease is a risk factor for ventricular arrhythmias. Occasionally, in stoic individuals or those with inadequate medical care, dilated cardiomyopathy presents with sudden death, and the diagnosis is established at autopsy. Again, the exclusion of ischemic, valvular, pericardial, congenital, and hypertensive heart disease, as well as primary pulmonary disease, is key; there is virtually no active myocardial inflammation. Rarely, thromboembolism as a complication of dilated cardiomyopathy may account for acute ischemia of either heart or brain with resulting sudden death.

An unusual cardiomyopathy *right ventricular dysplasia* is associated with sudden death (especially in young people), probably through ventricular arrhythmia, to which these patients are susceptible.[49-51] In this sometimes subtle condition, the gross pathologic findings provide the first clue to the diagnosis. Fatty or fibrofatty infiltration of the right ventricular myocardium of the diaphragmatic aspect, infundibulum, or apex is characteristic. Although the left ventricle may be involved by a similar process, what really identifies these hearts is the disproportionate degree of pathologic changes in the right ventricle.

## Normal-Appearing Hearts

The heart of normal size may not attract the attention of the prosector, but careful inspection and appropriate sampling for histopathologic examination may disclose a cause of sudden cardiac death in certain settings. As discussed earlier, *active myocarditis without fibrosis* (acute myocarditis) and *right ventricular dysplasia* are diseases that can be manifest in grossly normal-appearing hearts.

The heart with no identifiable pathologic changes presents a challenge. Before discounting this organ as the cause of sudden death, the conduction tissues should be examined (see Chapter 8). Although the chance of discerning a structural basis for arrhythmia (e.g., *atrioventricular bypass tract*) in the heart at autopsy is small, focal diseases such as *sarcoidosis*, which can affect the conduction system preferentially, may be missed in the routine examination of the heart that does not include conduction system analysis.[52,53] Even common processes (e.g., aging) affect the conduction system and may, in some instances, account for sudden death. Whatever the cause, discontinuity of the atrioventricular conduction axis interrupts transmission of the electrical impulses from the atria to the ventricles, thereby facilitating idioventricular rhythms that may be lethal.

The heart that is normal even after complete postmortem examination may still harbor the cause of sudden death; the current standard of general autopsy practice is not sufficient to detect certain abnormalities. Ventricular arrhythmia is the mechanism, occurring either spontaneously or in the setting of long QT interval, Brugada syndrome, preexcitation, or other electrophysiologic syndrome that can be documented during life. Many of these arrhythmias are inherited, and diagnosis is of paramount importance to the family. Knowledge regarding these cardiomyopathies due to gene mutations that affect ion channel function is rapidly expanding. For example,

phenotypes associated with mutation in SCN5A encoding the voltage-gated Na$^+$ channel include Brugada syndrome, conduction system disease, long QT syndrome, certain atrial arrhythmias, and sudden infant death syndrome.[54] Clearly, there is overlap among these syndromes, and the mechanism by which a gene mutation leads to electrocardiogram abnormality and/or arrhythmia remains unknown. Nonetheless, molecular studies performed on fresh or paraffin-embedded tissue facilitate classification of cases related to inherited gene defects.[55-58] In these situations, a piece of fresh heart muscle should be stored frozen until analysis can be performed by a laboratory with appropriate expertise. Regrettably, the cost of doing these tests on a fee-for-service basis is high.[58] Finally, the importance of obtaining a complete medical history, including laboratory data, cannot be overemphasized.

## Central Nervous System

In cases in which there are no other significant pathologic findings, the normal-appearing brain (without hemorrhage, infarct, or other cause of increased intracranial pressure) may account for the cause of sudden death. In this group, seizure is the most frequent mechanism. In fact, sudden death accounts for 7% to 17% of deaths among patients with epilepsy.[59] Unfortunately, anatomic correlates of *epilepsy* in the brain are exceedingly difficult to document,[60,61] particularly when the brain is examined unfixed.[62] Occasionally, associated pathologic changes (pulmonary edema, bitten tongue) may suggest the possibility of seizure, but only a compatible clinical history or eyewitness account of the fatal event really lends credence. Absent or nontherapeutic serum levels of anticonvulsant medications at the time of death often lend further support.[63] Again, the importance of considering the patient's medical record, using proper technique (i.e., cutting the brain after fixation), and consulting a neuropathologist cannot be overemphasized.

Other central nervous system causes of sudden natural death are much more rare. *Primary intracranial neoplasms* are an infrequent cause of sudden, unexpected death.[64] In retrospect, most patients exhibit symptoms attributable to the tumor. The venous sinuses should be inspected because thrombosis of these vascular channels may lead to sudden death even before infarction occurs; marked venous engorgement in both hemispheres is the first indication. As mentioned previously, occult meningitis and encephalitis typically have a longer clinical course but rarely lead to sudden death; if suddent death occurs, it is usually in individuals who neglect their health.[65]

## Sudden Infant Death Syndrome

*Sudden infant death syndrome (SIDS)* refers to the sudden death of an infant under 1 year of age, which remains unexplained after a thorough case investigation, including performance of a complete autopsy, examination of the death scene, and review of the clinical history.[66] The diverse themes that run through myriad studies (e.g., hypoxia, cardiovascular or central nervous system abnormalities, risk factors, genetic background, and so on) make SIDS appear to be a heterogenous group of conditions that end in a final common pathway. In the United States each case of possible SIDS must be referred to the coroner or medical examiner who performs an extensive investigation, including a death scene examination and interviews of relatives and friends. Virtually every infant undergoes detailed postmortem examination, which should be done according to a standardized protocol.[67] Common autopsy findings include petechial hemorrhages of the thymus, visceral pleura, and epicardium (68% to 95% of cases) and pulmonary congestion (89%), but there is no pathology pathognomonic for SIDS. Research studies have documented a high percentage of patients with abnormalities in the serotonin or 5-hydroxytryptamine system that affects autonomic regulation, relative neuronal immaturity, increased neuronal apoptosis, and evidence of neuronal pathophysiology that, in sum, suggest SIDS may reflect autonomic dysfunction, immune system abnormalities, and/or malfunctioning arousal pathways.[68] These abnormalities will not be detected even on standardized protocol postmortem examination, however, and SIDS remains a diagnosis of exclusion. Matturri and colleagues[69] have recently described a protocol for microscopic sampling of critical areas of the brainstem that can be done in three blocks and report its use in the investigation of SIDS deaths (see Chapter 8).

The death of an infant is always devastating, and the lack of diagnostic criteria and established etiology in SIDS is frustrating. Investigations of SIDS should be carried out with great thoroughness, objectivity, and sensitivity.

## CONCLUSION

At autopsy in the great majority of cases of sudden death, the experienced prosector discovers significant pathologic changes. Because these changes may be subtle, the pathologic analysis requires a methodical approach so that no possibility is left unexplored. Furthermore, the initial dissection provides the best opportunity for success; second looks are usually problematic. Thus, the prosector must be prepared and maintain objectivity. As with autopsies in general, the postmortem examination in cases of sudden death provides anatomic data that must be considered together with the available clinical information, including circumstances at the time of death. Enlightenment often comes on discovery of the major pathologic changes at the autopsy table; at that point, the pieces fit together to form a coherent picture. Occasionally, the autopsy pathologist encounters cases in which there is no obvious cause of death. Molecular analysis plays an increasing role in some of these unusual cases.

## REFERENCES

1. Baillie M: *The morbid anatomy of some of the most important parts of the human body*, Albany, NY, 1795, Barbeer & Southwick (First American edition based on the London edition of 1793).
2. Goldstein S: The necessity of a uniform definition of sudden coronary death: Witnessed death within one hour of the onset of acute symptoms, *Am Heart J* 103:156-159, 1982.
3. Davis JH, Wright RK: The very sudden cardiac death syndrome—a conceptual model for pathologists, *Hum Pathol* 11:117-121, 1980.
4. Craig-Hunter C: Deaths due to sudden or unexpected natural causes. In Mart AK, editor: *Taylor's principles and practice of medical jurisprudence*, Edinburgh, 1984, Churchill Livingstone, pp 111-127.
5. Yunginger JW, Nelson DR, Squillace DL, et al: Laboratory investigation of deaths due to anaphylaxis, *J Forensic Sci* 36:857-865, 1991.
6. Schwartz HJ, Yunginger JW, Schwartz LB: Is unrecognized anaphylaxis a cause of sudden unexpected death? *Clin Exp Allergy* 25:866-870, 1995.
7. Sur S, Crotty TB, Kephart GM, et al: Sudden-onset fatal asthma: A distinct entity with few eosinophils and relatively more neutrophils in airway submucosa, *Am Rev Respir Dis* 148:713-719, 1993.
8. Faul JL, Tormey VJ, Leonard C, et al: Lung immunopathology in cases of sudden asthma death, *Eur Respir J* 10:301-307, 1997.
9. Sperry KL, Key CR, Anderson RE: Toward a population-based assessment of death due to pulmonary embolism in New Mexico, *Hum Pathol* 21:159-165, 1990.
10. Brown DL, Wetli CV, Davis JH: Sudden unexpected death from primary pulmonary hypertension, *J Forensic Sci* 26:381-386, 1981.
11. Child JS, Wolfe JD, Tashkin D, Nakano F: Fatal lung scan in a case of pulmonary hypertension due to obliterative pulmonary vascular disease, *Chest* 67:308-310, 1975.
12. Grossman W, Braunwald E: Pulmonary hypertension. In Braunwald E, editor: *Heart disease: A textbook of cardiovascular medicine*, Philadelphia, 1992, WB Saunders, pp 790-816.
13. Gonzalez-Rothi RJ, Foresman GE, Block AJ: Do patients with sleep apnea die in their sleep? *Chest* 94:531-538, 1988.
14. Wu H, Yan-Go F: Self-reported automobile accidents involving patients with obstructive sleep apnea, *Neurology* 46:1254-1257, 1996.
15. Maron BJ: Structural features of the athlete heart as defined by echocardiography, *J Am Coll Cardiol* 7:190-203, 1986.
16. Puranik R, Chow CK, Duflou J, et al: Sudden death in the young, *Heart Rhythm* 2:1277-1282, 2005.
17. Saffitz JE: The pathology of sudden cardiac death in patients with ischemic heart disease—arrhythmology for anatomic pathologists, *Cardiovasc Pathol* 14:195-203, 2005.
18. Basso C, Burke M, Fornes P, et al: Guidelines for autopsy investigation of sudden cardiac death, *Virchows Arch* 452:11-18, 2008.
19. Myerburg RJ, Kessler K, Basset AL, Castellanos A: A biological approach to sudden cardiac death: structure, function and cause, *Am J Cardiol* 63:1512-1516, 1989.
20. Myerburg RJ, Castellanos A: Cardiac arrest and sudden cardiac death. In Braunwald E, editor: *Heart disease: A textbook of cardiovascular medicine*, Philadelphia, 1992, WB Saunders, pp 756-789.
21. Liberthson RR, Nagel EL, Hirschman JC, et al: Pathophysiologic observations in prehospital ventricular fibrillation and sudden cardiac death, *Circulation* 49:790-798, 1974.
22. Davies MJ: Anatomic features in victims of sudden coronary death: Coronary artery pathology, *Circulation* 85 (Suppl 1):I19-24, 1992.
23. Solberg LA, Strong JP, Holme I, et al: Stenoses in the coronary arteries. Relation to atherosclerotic lesions, coronary heart disease and risk factors. The Oslo study, *Lab Invest* 53:648-655, 1985.
24. Warnes CA, Roberts WC: Morphologic findings in sudden cardiac death: A comparison of those with and those without previous symptoms of myocardial ischemia, *Cardiol Clin* 4:607-615, 1984.

25. Davies MJ, Thomas A: Plaque fissuring: the cause of acute myocardial infarction, sudden cardiac death and crescendo angina, *Br Heart J* 53:363-373, 1985.

26. Farb A, Burke AP, Tang AL, et al: Coronary plaque erosion without rupture into a lipid core. A frequent cause of coronary thrombosis in sudden coronary death, *Circulation* 93:1354-1363, 1996.

27. Burke AP, Farb A, Malcom GT, et al: Coronary risk factors and plaque morphology in patients with coronary disease dying suddenly, *N Engl J Med* 336:1276-1282, 1997.

28. Bardales RH, Hailey LS, Xie SS, et al: In situ apoptosis assay for the detection of early acute myocardial infarction, *Am J Pathol* 149:821-829, 1996.

29. Kubat K, Smedts F: The usefulness of the lactate dehydrogenase macroreaction in autopsy practice, *Mod Pathol* 6:743-747, 1993.

30. Hansen SH, Rossen K: Evaluation of cardiac troponin I immunoreaction in autopsy hearts: A possible marker of early myocardial infarction, *Forensic Sci Int* 99:189-196, 1999.

31. Vargas SO, Grudzien C, Tanasijevic MJ: Postmortem cardiac troponin-I levels predict intramyocardial damage at autopsy, *J Thromb Thrombolysis*, http://www.springer.com/content/u541 pg448414xn02/ (accessed October 2, 2008).

32. Pérez-Cárceles MD, Noguera J, Jiméniz JL, Martínez P: Diagnostic efficacy of biochemical markers in diagnosis post-mortem of ischaemic heart disease, *Forensic Sci Int* 142:1-7, 2004.

33. Virmani R, Burke AP, Farb A: Sudden cardiac death, *Cardiovasc Pathol* 10:275-282, 2001.

34. Davies MJ, Bland JM, Hangartner JRW, et al: Factors influencing the presence or absence of acute coronary artery thrombi in sudden ischaemic death, *Eur Heart J* 10:203-208, 1989.

35. Davies MJ: Anatomic features in victims of sudden coronary death. Coronary artery pathology, *Circulation* 85(Suppl I):I-19-I-24, 1992.

36. Morales AR, Romanelli R, Boucek R: The mural left anterior descending coronary artery, strenuous exercise and sudden death, *Circulation* 62:230-237, 1980.

37. Tauth J, Sullebarger T: Myocardial infarction associated with myocardial bridging: Case history and review of the literature, *Cathet Cardiovasc Diagn* 40:364-367, 1997.

38. Cohle SD, Graham MA, Pounder D: Nonatherosclerotic sudden coronary death, *Pathol Annu* 23(Pt 2):217-249, 1986.

39. Michaud K, Romain N, Brandt-Casadevall C, Mangin P: Sudden death related to small coronary artery disease, *Am J Forensic Med Pathol* 22:225-227, 1980.

40. Myerburg RJ: Sudden cardiac death: Epidemiology, causes and mechanisms, *Cardiology* 74(Suppl 2):2-9, 1987.

41. Kannel WB, McGee DL: Epidemiology of sudden death: Insights from the Framingham study, *Cardiovasc Clin* 15:93-105, 1985.

42. Kragel AH, Roberts WC: Sudden death and cardiomegaly unassociated with coronary, valvular congenital or specific heart muscle disease, *Am J Cardiol* 61:659-660, 1988.

43. Scheurman EH: Myxoid heart disease: A review with special emphasis on sudden cardiac death, *Forensic Sci Int* 40:203-210, 1989.

44. Aretz HT, Billingham ME, Edwards WD, et al: Myocarditis: A histopathologic definition and classification, *Am J Cardiovasc Pathol* 1:3-14, 1986.

45. Cheitlin MD, De Castro CM, McAllister HA: Sudden death as a complication of anomalous left coronary origin from the anterior sinus of Valsalva. A not-so-minor congenital anomaly, *Circulation* 50:780-787, 1974.

46. Isner JM, Maron BJ, Roberts WC: Comparison of amount of myocardial cell disorganization in operatively excised septectomy specimens with amount observed at necropsy in 18 patients with hypertrophic cardiomyopathy, *Am J Cardiol* 46:42-47, 1980.

47. Maron BJ, Epstein SE, Roberts WC: Causes of sudden death in competitive athletes, *J Am Coll Cardiol* 7:204-214, 1986.

48. Basso C, Thiene G, Corrado D, et al. Hypertrophic cardiomyopathy and sudden death in the young: Pathologic evidence of myocardial ischemia, *Hum Path* 31:988-998, 2000.

49. Thiene G, Nava A, Corrado D, et al: Right ventricular cardiomyopathy and sudden death in young people, *N Engl J Med* 318:129-133, 1988.

50. Goodin JC, Farb A, Smialek JE, et al: Right ventricular dysplasia associated with sudden death in young adults, *Mod Pathol* 4:702-706, 1991.

51. Pawel BR, de Chadarévian J-P, Wolk JH, et al: Sudden death in childhood due to right ventricular dysplasia: Report of two cases, *Pediatr Pathol* 14:987-995, 1994.

52. Roberts WC, McAllister HAJ, Ferrans VJ: Sarcoidosis of the heart: A clinicopathologic study of 35 necropsy patients (group I) and review of 78 previously described necropsy patients (group II), *Am J Med* 63:86-108, 1977.

53. Cohle SD, Sampson BA: The negative autopsy: Sudden cardiac death or other? *Cardiovasc Pathol* 10:219-222, 2001.

54. Lehnart SE, Ackerman MJ, Benson DW Jr, et al: Inherited arrhythmias. A National Heart, Lung, and Blood Institute and Office of Rare Diseases workshop consensus report about the diagnosis, phenotyping, molecular mechanisms, and therapeutic approaches for primary cardiomyopathies of gene mutations affecting ion channel function, *Circulation* 116:2325-2345, 2007.

55. Ackerman MJ, Tester DJ, Driscoll DJ: Molecular autopsy of sudden unexplained death in the young, *Am J Forensic Med Pathol* 22:105-111, 2001.

56. Basso C, Calabrese F, Corrado D, Thiene G: Postmortem diagnosis in sudden cardiac death victims: Macroscopic, microscopic and molecular findings, *Cardiovasc Res* 50:290-300, 2001.

57. Towbin JA: Molecular genetic basis of sudden cardiac death, *Cardiovasc Pathol* 10:283-295, 2001.

58. Tester DJ, Ackerman MJ. The role of molecular autopsy in unexplained sudden cardiac death, *Curr Opin Cardiol* 21:166-172, 2006.

59. Tomson T: Mortality in epilepsy, *J Neurol* 247:15-21, 2000.

60. Hirsch CS, Martin DL: Unexpected death in young epileptics, *Neurology* 21:682-690, 1971.

61. Leestma JE, Annegers JF, Brodie MJ, et al: Sudden unexplained death in epilepsy: Observations from a large clinical development program, *Epilepsia* 38:47-55, 1997.

62. Terrence CF, Rao GR, Perper JA: Neurogenic pulmonary edema in unexpected, unexplained death of epileptic patients, *Ann Neurol* 9:458-464, 1981.

63. Black M, Graham DI: Sudden unexplained death in adults. In Love S, editor: *Current topics in pathology*, Berlin, 2001, Springer-Verlag, pp 125-148.

64. DiMaio SM, DiMaio VJM, Kirkpatrick JB: Sudden, unexpected deaths due to primary intracranial neoplasms, *Am J Forensic Med Pathol* 1:29-45, 1980.

65. Luke JL, Helpern M: Sudden unexpected death from natural causes in young adults. A review of 275 consecutive autopsied cases, *Arch Pathol* 85:10-17, 1968.

66. Willinger M, James LS, Catz C: Defining the sudden infant death syndrome (SIDS): Deliberations of an expert panel convened by the National Institute of Child Health and Human Development, *Ped Pathol* 11:677-684, 1991.

67. Bajanowski T, Vege Å, Byard RW, et al: Sudden infant death syndrome (SIDS)—standardised investigations and classification: Recommendations, *For Sci Int* 165:129-143, 2007.

68. Moon RY, Horne RSC, Hauck FR: Sudden infant death syndrome, *Lancet* 370:1578-1587, 2007.

69. Matturri L, Ottaviani G, Lavezzi AM: Guidelines for neuoro-pathologic diagnostics of perinatal unexpected loss and sudden infant death syndrome (SIDS)—a technical protocol, *Virchow Arch* 452:19-25, 2008.

# 12

# Postmortem Examination in Cases of Sepsis or Multiple Organ Dysfunction

*Andrew Connolly, MD, PhD*

*"Some [microorganisms] will get into our deepest tissues and set forth in the blood, but it is our response to their presence that makes the disease. Our arsenals for fighting off bacteria are so powerful, and involve so many different defense mechanisms, that we are in more danger from them than from the invaders."*

Lewis Thomas[1]

Multiple organ dysfunction, either from infectious or noninfectious causes, has been increasing in incidence in hospitals in developed countries[2] and is present in an increasing proportion of hospital-based autopsies. It is the most common cause of death in noncoronary critical care units in Europe and the United States.[3] This is largely because of increased use of critical care supportive measures, particularly in high-risk populations. In this chapter we will discuss sepsis and multiple organ dysfunction, including their definitions, their pathophysiology, and considerations important for postmortem examination in such cases.

## SEPSIS

The term *sepsis* has been used loosely over the years, but since 1992 a consensus has been established about proper terminology.[4] First, the systemic inflammatory response syndrome (SIRS) is defined as having two or more of the following clinical criteria: (1) temperature greater than 38°C or less than 36°C; (2) heart rate greater than 90 beats/min; (3) respiratory rate greater than 20 breaths/min or $Pa_{CO_2}$ less than 32 torr; (4) white blood cell count greater than 12,000 or less than 4000 cells/mm$^3$ or more than 10% immature (band) forms. SIRS is a pathophysiologic response that arises due to release of overwhelming amounts of circulating proinflammatory cytokines, such as tumor necrosis factor-$\alpha$ and various interleukins. This leads to widespread vasodilation and hypotension.

These cytokines also affect function of microvascular endothelial cells with inappropriate activation of their inflammatory and procoagulant functions. This leads to accumulation of inflammatory cells within organs, microvascular leakage, and microvascular obstruction, with worsening hypoperfusion of organs. In addition, parenchymal cells within organs are directly affected by the circulating factors, causing further dysfunction. Activation of coagulation factors in the microvasculature has a positive feedback increasing systemic inflammation; hence the efficacy of recombinant activated protein C in sepsis. SIRS may be caused by noninfectious processes, including acute pancreatitis, major trauma, and burns, but it is usually found in the setting of infection.

Sepsis is then defined as SIRS in response to infection. Severe sepsis is defined as sepsis associated with organ dysfunction, hypotension (blood pressure less than 90 mm Hg or reduction greater than 40 mm Hg from baseline), *or* hypoperfusion abnormalities (including lactic acidosis, oliguria, or altered mental status). Septic shock is defined as sepsis with hypotension refractory to fluid resuscitation *and* hypoperfusion abnormalities. One exception is that children can be in frank septic shock without hypotension but with severe hypoperfusion abnormalities.[5] Importantly, the diagnosis of sepsis requires an infectious etiology but does not require bacteremia. Sepsis can be from infectious agents other than bacteria or can be from a local bacterial infection without seeding of the blood. In fact, even in conscientious studies, bacteremia was documented in only 17%, 25%, and 69% of patients with sepsis, severe sepsis, and septic shock, respectively.[6] This is one reason autopsy pathologists are asked to look for the possible "source of sepsis" in patients with negative blood cultures. In septic hospitalized patients with positive blood cultures, the causative organisms are gram-positive (47%), gram-negative (41%), mixed bacteria (5%), anaerobic bacteria (2%), and fungus (5%).[7]

## MULTIPLE ORGAN DYSFUNCTION

Multiple organ dysfunction syndrome (MODS) was also defined in the 1992 consensus meeting[4] as the presence of altered organ function in an acutely ill patient such that homeostasis cannot be maintained without intervention. As critical care supportive measures progress, increasing numbers of deaths are largely attributed to the progressive failure of several interdependent organ systems rather than a dominant effect of a single underlying illness. MODS has many acceptable names, such as *multiorgan failure* and *multiple systems organ failure,* that refer to the same syndrome defined by clinical criteria. In MODS, dysfunction is present in two or more of the following organ systems: (1) respiratory, (2) cardiovascular, (3) renal, (4) hepatic, (5) hematologic, and (6) neurologic. In many clinical settings, scores have been developed to gauge the severity of MODS, such as the popular Sequential Organ Failure Assessment (SOFA) that combines scores from 0 to 4 in the six organ systems just listed, assessing: (1) lowered $Pa_{O_2}/Fi_{O_2}$, (2) hypotension or vasopressor requirement, (3) elevated serum creatinine, (4) elevated serum bilirubin, (5) thrombocytopenia, and (6) Glasgow Coma Scale score.[8]

Rarely, MODS may be primary, in which an insult injures multiple organs directly, such as with large-scale physical or chemical injuries or widely disseminated disease. Usually MODS is secondary to a combination of SIRS, accumulated effects of various injurious agents (such as drug or oxygen toxicity), episodes of cardiogenic or hypovolemic hypotension, and the effects of failing organ systems on each other. Mechanical ventilation, vasopressors, intravenous fluids, hemodialysis, nutritional supplementation, and a variety of supportive medications sustain high-risk patients into phases of complex interdependent organ dysfunction with compounded insults.

In an increasing percentage of hospital autopsies, autopsy pathologists are asked to account for multiple organ dysfunctions, including whether there is an infection causing sepsis. In the future, serologic or biochemical markers of SIRS and infection may clarify this, but currently clinical presentation is unclear enough that we are often on a hunt for the possible "septic source," concurrent organ pathologies, and complex interactions.[9] In these cases the pathologist needs to consider much of the available clinical information in addition to the morphologic findings.

### Preparing for the Autopsy

A complete review of the medical record is critical in these cases. Particular attention should be paid to chronic diseases, preexisting pathologic conditions of major organs,

immunosuppressive influences, recent indicators of organ dysfunction, therapeutics applied, and the possibilities for infectious causes. Results from microbiology, chemistry, radiology, and anatomic pathology should be reviewed. After review of the medical record, it is important to confer with the responsible clinicians. Many times the clinicians have a specific interest in findings in particular organs, rather than a broad interest in the anatomic consequences of MODS. Some of the most popular clinical reasons for autopsy of late read: "reason for pulmonary infiltrates" or "cause of renal failure."

In the autopsy room, prepare for cultures suggested by your clinical review. Remember that some cultures (e.g., anaerobic bacteria, virus) require special handling. Chapter 9 describes proper methods for postmortem microbiology, and this has been reviewed elsewhere.[10] To interpret positive cultures the pathologist must consider whether the sampling was adequate, the clinical course and site are compatible with the organism, the organism is present on tissue sections, and there is a tissue response consistent with the organism. If the organism is a common contaminant, such as *Staphylococcus* or *Enterococcus,* this is particularly important. Polymicrobial growth should also raise suspicion, except when infection resulted from inoculation by an invasive procedure or from the mouth, genitals, anus, or biliary tree. Before the case starts, discuss plans with any pathology assistants or trainees, including special dissections, needs for culture, and any personal protective measures needed beyond typical universal precautions.

The general categories of infectious sources of sepsis, and their incidences, are outlined in Table 12-1.[11] A more specific anatomic guide to potential sources of sepsis is shown in Box 12-1. Note that many other infections may be found that are less likely to have severe systemic consequences, such as superficial skin infections, conjunctivitis, rhinitis, some pharyngitis, some bronchitis, otitis media, some sinusitis, uncomplicated wound infections, vaginitis, some cystitis, and urethritis. However, some typically minor infections can have huge systemic consequences in special circumstances: in immunocompromised hosts; through superantigen mechanisms for some bacteria; by direct actions of elaborated toxins on tissues; or if the infection leads to extensive seeding of the blood, such as with intravascular devices.

### Pathologic Findings on the External Body Surface

The entire external body surface should be examined for possible sources of infection, such as cellulitis (see Fig. 15-10), skin ulcers, open wounds, surgical drains, and percutaneous lines. For this reason, do not allow others to remove lines and tubing before autopsy. All clothing, patches, and bandages should be removed to allow examination of the underlying structures for signs of infection. Good photographs that include a plain white ruler are helpful. Materials for culture or histologic sampling from superficial sites should be taken at this time, although for many catheter tips, it is better to gain sterile access to them during the evisceration to prevent accidental dislodgement of infected material. Decubitus ulcers may be severe enough to cause sepsis and those of a severe

| Table 12-1 | Sources of infection underlying severe sepsis in U.S. hospitals | | |
|---|---|---|---|
| **Site of infection** | **Adult (%)** | **Children 1-9 years old (%)** | **Infant (%)** |
| Respiratory | 44 | 51 | 27 |
| Primary bacteremia | 17 | 18 | 34 |
| Genitourinary | 9 | 2 | 4 |
| Abdominal | 9 | 6 | 3 |
| Wound/soft tissue | 7 | 4 | 6 |
| Device related | 2 | 5 | 4 |
| Central nervous system | 0.8 | 3 | 5 |
| Endocarditis | 0.6 | 0.2 | 0.6 |
| Other/unspecified | 11 | 11 | 17 |

Based on 1995 hospital discharges from seven U.S. states. Data from Angus DC, Linde-Zwirble WT, Lidicker J, et al: Epidemiology of severe sepsis in the United States: analysis of incidence, outcome, and associated costs of care, *Crit Care Med* 29:1303-1310, 2001; and Watson RS, Carcillo JA, Linde-Zwirble WT, et al: The epidemiology of severe sepsis in children in the United States, *Am J Resp Crit Care Med* 167:695-701. 2003.

| Box 12-1 | Specific common sources of severe sepsis |
|---|---|
| Respiratory<br>  Pneumonia<br>  Lung abscess<br>  Empyema<br>Primary bacteremia<br>Genitourinary<br>  Pyelonephritis<br>  Cystitis<br>  Acute prostatitis<br>  Female pelvic abscess<br>  Postpartum endometritis<br>Abdominal<br>  Diverticulitis<br>  Cholangitis and cholecystitis<br>  Peritonitis or perforated viscus<br>  Enterocolitis or bowel infarct<br>  Appendicitis<br>  Hepatitis and hepatic abscess<br>Wound/soft tissue<br>  Cellulitis<br>  Wound infection<br>  Infective arthritis<br>  Osteomyelitis<br>  Oropharyngeal abscess<br>  Perirectal abscess<br>Device related<br>  Intravenous line sepsis<br>  Intravascular devices<br>  Peritoneal dialysis<br>  Infected prosthetics<br>Central nervous system<br>  Meningitis<br>  Brain abscess<br>Endocarditis | |

stage should have their deeper tissues sampled for histologic examination. The eyes, ears, nose, mouth, anus, and genitalia should be examined for signs of infection, including discharge or swelling. Nasal intubation is a risk factor for sinusitis, and the nasal cavity should be examined carefully in such cases. The extremities should be examined for deformities and asymmetries prompting exploration, including possibly infected joints and prosthetic parts. If prosthetic orthopedic parts are loose in their bony attachments, the underlying bone should be examined for infection.

The skin and mucous membranes may also demonstrate signs of systemic disease: rashes, petechiae, and certain hemorrhages can be indicative of particular infections, such as in meningococcemia (see Fig. 15-13). Petechiae are a common finding correlating with thrombocytopenia and disseminated intravascular coagulation (DIC) in MODS and sepsis. Jaundice is a good indicator of hepatic dysfunction, and peripheral edema (see Fig. 15-6) is commonly found in MODS.

## Pathologic Findings in the Body Cavities

After opening the body cavities, but before evisceration, the peritoneal, pleural, and pericardial cavities should be explored for signs of infection. Peritonitis (see Fig. 15-27), pericarditis (see Fig. 15-18), and empyema (see Fig. 15-21) are quite striking, but loculation can make them focal. The pelvis requires particularly careful examination for abscesses, and all viscera should be examined for perforations or fistulas. Record the amount and characteristics of effusions and include them in the report. Take cultures from organs in situ as early in the case as possible because evisceration and handling of organs is likely to increase contamination. Lung cultures should be taken from focal consolidation identified by recent prior radiographs or postmortem palpation with clean gloves. Blood is best sampled either from the right atrium or spleen, and grossly obvious foci of infection should be sampled and cultured for types of organisms common for each area.

During evisceration, fascial planes and spaces between organs should be carefully examined for foci of infection that will not be obvious when the organs are separated. After evisceration, the body cavity should be reexamined, with visual examination and palpation of the perirectal fascia, the iliopsoas muscle, and the retropharyngeal space. Bimanual examination, with a hand outside and one inside the neck or mouth, can make sure the neck does not harbor major lesions.

## Pathologic Findings in the Respiratory Tract

In hospitalized patients, lungs are the most common source of sepsis.[3] In addition, the lungs are commonly affected in MODS and often have multiple significant pathologies in the critically ill. Given this, gross examination of the respiratory tract benefits from a thorough systematic approach. Therefore, the favored approach is to remove the lungs as in Figure 4-15, weigh them, and inflate both lungs with formalin before cutting so that subtle or focal areas of pathology will not be missed. Meanwhile, the upper airway should be examined fresh from hypopharynx to bronchi. Laryngitis and tracheitis (see Figs. 15-75 and 15-76) are easily appreciated fresh, but beware of overinterpretation of clinically insignificant posterior vocal fold ulcerations seen with prolonged endotracheal intubation. Mucus plugs in the airways should be noted along with any aspirated materials. In the cut lungs, be sure to account for dependent postmortem congestion and then inspect all slices carefully, both visually and by gentle palpation. Pulmonary emboli and associated pulmonary infarcts may be found. Pneumonia comes in many gross morphologies (see Figs. 15-89 through 15-95) depending on the infectious agent and host response, but histologic sections should be taken from areas suspicious for pneumonia. Histologic sections with inflammatory foci should be carefully scanned at high power for viral cytopathic changes, and Gram stain for bacteria and GMS stain for fungus should be ordered. Immunohistochemistry is particularly useful for detecting or confirming viral infections.

Diffuse alveolar damage (DAD) due to SIRS will involve all five lobes, although some lobules may be less involved. Lungs with DAD are diffusely firm and often slippery from mucopolysaccharide production. Microscopically, DAD will be dominated by exudates and inflammatory infiltrates in the first days and by fibroblastic foci and organization after 1 week. It is often difficult to distinguish a healing widespread pneumonia, such as viral pneumonia, from DAD caused by SIRS. In general, hyaline membranes and organization centered in alveoli are more suggestive of DAD, whereas interstitial organization and airway squamous metaplasia are more consistent with viral causes. Many pneumonias, however, also cause DAD, making this distinction difficult. Concurrent pathologic conditions that also affect respiratory function should be noted, such as congestion, pleural effusions, atelectasis, mucus plugging, emphysema, bronchitis, and pulmonary fibrosis.

## Pathologic Findings in the Urinary Tract

The urinary tract is another common source of sepsis and is also heavily affected in MODS. Routine dissection (see Figs. 4-18 through 4-20) will show whether there is hydronephrosis, hydroureter, or bladder dilation leading to susceptibility to ascending infections. Chronic pyelonephritis may be evident by scarring and papillary blunting (see Fig. 15-173). The capsular and cut surfaces should be examined for signs of hematogenous or ascending acute pyelonephritis (see Fig. 15-170). Cystitis associated with sepsis may be quite striking grossly (see Fig. 15-179), but clinically insignificant mild cystitis is found in many autopsies. Prosectors should be careful with gross interpretation of the bladder: transitional epithelium is routinely shed postmortem and combines with urine to look like purulent fluid, and indwelling catheters often irritate the posterior wall of bladder without causing significant inflammation (see Fig. 15-180).

The usual kidney finding in MODS is ischemic acute tubular necrosis (ATN). This may be evident sometimes on gross examination as a pale swollen cortex with congested medulla,

but this is nonspecific. The microscopic findings in ischemic ATN are often masked by postmortem autolysis, but some reliable features can be found in many cases, including dilated tubules containing proteinaceous debris, regenerative changes, or even mitoses within tubular epithelium and margination of mononuclear cells within the vasa recta of the outer medulla (Fig. 12-1).[12] It is important to assess concurrent pathologic conditions that also have an effect on kidney function, including interstitial nephritis from drug therapies and chronic diseases such as diabetes and hypertension.

## Pathologic Findings in the Gastrointestinal Tract

The adventitial and serosal (outside) surfaces of the entire gastrointestinal tract should be examined carefully for transmural pathologic conditions. Postmortem changes make the mucosal surfaces quite variable, with sloughed epithelium, autolysis, staining by luminal contents, and effects of bacterial overgrowth, but the outer surfaces usually have much less artifact. Focal peritonitis is evident by a roughened or erythematous serosal surface. Ischemic bowel segments are sometimes hard to demonstrate histologically but are usually evident grossly as segmental portions of the bowel, with thickening and dark discoloration (see Fig. 15-123). In general, mucosal areas that are raised, depressed, or discolored should be examined closely and histologic sections taken as needed. Pseudomembranous colitis from antibiotic therapy is still a common finding and has distinct gross pathologic characteristics with patches of mucoid mucosal material. Esophagitis (see Figs. 15-102 and 15-103), gastritis, enterocolitis (see Fig. 15-119), diverticulitis, and appendicitis should all be considered. Cultures are usually not applied in gastrointestinal tissues, but rather histologic sections with special stains are used. Viral and fungal causes should be considered, particularly in esophagitis.

Although not a defining clinical feature of MODS, gastrointestinal pathologic conditions play an important role in these patients. SIRS and bowel hypoperfusion lead to intestinal mucosal dysfunction that allows seeding of the bloodstream with enteric organisms, providing further stimulus for SIRS. In addition, bowel infarction in the critically ill is usually inoperable and fatal, with no effective supportive measures.

## Pathologic Findings in the Cardiovascular System

Endocarditis comprises less than 1% of sepsis cases in hospitalized patients. By checking both sides of all valves it can be found grossly with great sensitivity (see Figs. 15-59 through 15-64), but histologic examination is prudent to confirm inflammation and infection and distinguish it from nonbacterial thrombotic (marantic) endocarditis. All intravascular catheters and devices should be examined for adherent infected material and sampled as needed for culture and histologic examination.

The cardiovascular system is heavily involved in MODS. Much of the pathogenesis of organ dysfunction in SIRS is due to microvascular defects, with endothelial activation and dysfunction, which is not evident on light microscopy of most autopsy tissues. As SIRS progresses, thrombi become obvious in small vessels as part of DIC. In cases with coagulopathy,

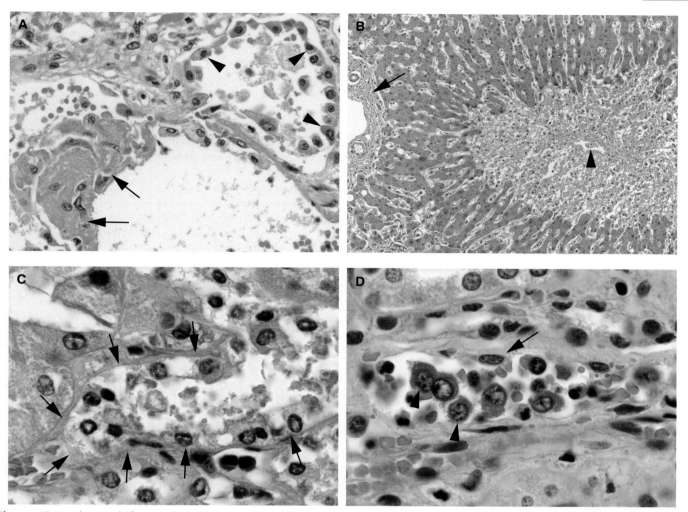

**Figure 12-1** Microscopic features in multiorgan failure (MOF). The features depend on the duration of organ dysfunction. Shown are microphotographs from a patient after 7 days of MOF in an intensive care unit. **A,** Lung with diffuse alveolar damage, early proliferative phase, with organizing hyaline membranes *(arrows)* and type II pneumocyte hyperplasia *(arrowheads).* **B,** Liver with centrilobular necrosis around central vein *(arrowhead)* with normal portal tract *(arrow).* **C,** Kidney with acute tubular necrosis most evident in the distal tubule *(arrows)* by dilation, proteinaceous debris, epithelial necrosis, and regenerative changes. **D,** Vasa recta *(arrow on endothelial cell)* containing marginated leukocytes and hematopoietic cells *(arrowheads).*

spontaneous hemorrhage may be found in many organs. With episodes of hypotension, particularly requiring vasopressor support, small myocardial infarcts can be seen. They may be scattered but are usually subendocardial and frequent in the papillary muscles of the left ventricle. It should be remembered that hypotension is a key finding in SIRS, due to decreased peripheral vascular resistance, but other contributors to hypotension should be investigated, such as hypovolemia, cardiac conditions, or even anaphylactic episodes.

## Pathologic Findings in the Hepatobiliary System

Although cholecystitis and cholangitis continue to be common sources for sepsis, hepatic abscesses (see Fig. 15-140) are becoming rare in developed countries. The biliary tree should be explored from liver hilum to gallbladder to ampulla for evidence of stones, strictures, dilations, compressions, or inflammation (see Fig. 15-151). The liver often suffers terribly in MODS, with extensive centrilobular hemorrhage and

necrosis (see Fig. 15-142) seen in many autopsies of patients from the intensive care unit. This pathologic condition, resulting largely from hypoperfusion, often overlaps with acute and chronic congestive changes. In a large autopsy study, atrophy of centrilobular hepatocytes, distension of sinusoids, and fibrosis were features of passive congestion and were associated with right-sided heart failure, whereas centrilobular necrosis was seen predominantly in "shock" patients.[13] It is fortunate that the liver has tremendous regenerative capacity, but this may be hindered in patients with hepatitis or extensive fibrosis.

## Pathologic Findings in the Central Nervous System

The consideration of pathologic conditions of the central nervous system (CNS) starts with review of the neurologic history and imaging to identify potential focal lesions. Common CNS sources of sepsis include meningitis (see Fig. 15-241) and brain abscesses or infections (see Figs. 15-242 through 15-245).

Meningitis and brain abscesses erupting to the surface of the brain are conducive to culture. Patients with MODS often have generalized altered mental status due to the effects of SIRS on brain microvasculature; effects of metabolic, renal, and hepatic derangements; and effects of hypotensive episodes. Anatomic changes include edema and hypoxic changes to neurons, particularly well seen in the hippocampus. While the skull is open, consider nasal sinus sampling through the base of the skull, particularly if there is a history suggestive of sinusitis or a purulent nasal discharge.

## Pathologic Findings in Other Organs

The prostate and female reproductive organs can be potent sources of sepsis. Acute prostatitis is obvious on histologic sections of the prostate, making it important to submit a prostate section routinely. The sources of sepsis in female reproductive organs are usually due to pelvic inflammatory disease and abscess formation, which should be obvious grossly.

The pancreas is usually autolyzed at autopsy, often leading to flecks of postmortem fat necrosis, along with reddening from postmortem oozing of blood. Yet it is still possible to diagnose pancreatitis by finding abundant neutrophils intermixed with abundant fat necrosis. Be sure to check antemortem tests for serum amylase and lipase if entertaining the diagnosis of acute pancreatitis.

With severe hypotensive episodes, the adrenal gland shows necrosis particularly of the zona reticularis. Once again, this may be masked if autolysis is extensive. Bilateral acute adrenal hemorrhage (see Fig. 15-206) is described in meningococcal sepsis but may be seen rarely in other forms of sepsis in the hospital setting.

The bone marrow in sepsis often shows an increased myeloid-to-erythroid ratio and increased numbers of myeloid progenitors, but in severe cases of MODS there may be marrow suppression with decreased cellularity.

There has been much discussion about the spleen in sepsis. Gross softening of the spleen, particularly in comparison with other solid organs, is a fairly nonspecific finding associated with SIRS and sepsis, but it appears to be of little clinical value.[14] Likewise, increased numbers of splenic neutrophils were not found to be associated with sepsis in hospitalized, treated patients.[15] It is speculated that sepsis-associated acute splenitis was seen more commonly in the preantibiotic era, consistent with a recent report of acute splenitis being associated with septic patients who died early without antibiotic treatment.[16] Gross examination of the spleen often reveals opaque capsular plaque, unfortunately termed *perisplenitis*, which is merely nonspecific capsular fibrosis unrelated to sepsis.

## The Autopsy Report

In the autopsy report for patients with MODS, SIRS, or sepsis, the pathologist should provide a clinical history that accounts for initial presentation, medical history, and hospital course, including management decisions made regarding end-of-life care. Particular emphasis should be placed on function of

major organs leading up to death, therapeutic measures taken, and clinically important test results. The gross and microscopic descriptions should provide enough details to convey clearly all relevant findings, including the relative severity of anatomic findings associated with MODS. The outline of anatomic diagnoses should be organized so that the reader is aware of the most important findings and their causal relationships. The case summary narrative should be clear about the underlying cause, sequence of events leading to MODS, and role of concurrent pathologic conditions in organ failure.

## REFERENCES

1. Thomas L: Germs, *N Engl J Med* 287:553-555, 1972.
2. Dombrovsky VY, Martin AA, Sunderram J, Paz HL: Rapid increase in hospitalization and mortality rates for severe sepsis in the United States: A trend analysis from 1993 to 2003, *Crit Care Med* 35:1244-1250, 2007.
3. Angus DC, Linde-Zwirble WT, Lidicker J, et al: Epidemiology of severe sepsis in the United States: Analysis of incidence, outcome, and associated costs of care, *Crit Care Med* 29:1303-1310, 2001.
4. Bone RC Balk RA, Cerra FB, et al: Definitions for sepsis and organ failure and guidelines for the use of innovative therapies in sepsis. The American College of Chest Physicians/Society of Critical Care Medicine Consensus Conference, *Chest* 101:1644-1655, 1992.
5. Levy MM, Fink MP, Marshall JC, et al: 2001 SCCM/ESICM/ACCP/ATS/SIS International Sepsis Definitions Conference, *Crit Care Med* 31:1250-1256, 2003.
6. Rangel-Frausto MS, Pittet D, Costigan M, et al: The natural history of the systemic inflammatory response syndrome, *JAMA* 273:117-123, 1995.
7. Bochud PY, Glauser MP, Calandra T. Antibiotics in sepsis, *Intensive Care Med* 27(Suppl 1):S33-S48, 2001.
8. Vincent JL, Moreno R, Takala J, et al: The SOFA (sepsis-related organ failure assessment) score to describe organ dysfunction/failure, *Intensive Care Med* 22:707-710, 1996.
9. Tsokos M: Postmortem diagnosis of sepsis, *Forensic Sci Int* 165:155-164, 2007.
10. Mazuchowski EL, Meier PA: The modern autopsy: What to do if infection is suspected, *Arch Med Res* 36:713-723, 2005.
11. Watson RS, Carcillo JA, Linde-Zwirble WT, et al: The epidemiology of severe sepsis in children in the United States, *Am J Resp Crit Care Med* 167:695-701. 2003.
12. Solez K, Morel-Maroger L, Sraer JD. The morphology of "acute tubular necrosis" in man: Analysis of 57 renal biopsies and a comparison with the glycerol model, *Medicine* (Baltimore) 58:362-376, 1979.
13. Arcidi JM, Moore GW, Hutchins GM: Hepatic morphology in cardiac dysfunction: A clinicopathologic study of 1000 subjects at autopsy, *Am J Path* 104:159-166, 1981.
14. Wise R: The "septic spleen"—a critical evaluation, *J Clin Pathol* 29:228-230, 1976.
15. Feig JA, Cina SJ: Evaluation of characteristics associated with acute splenitis (septic spleen) as markers of systemic infection, *Arch Pathol Lab Med* 125:888-891, 2001.
16. Arismendi-Morillo GJ, Briceño-García AE, Romero-Amaro ZR, et al: Acute non-specific splenitis as indicator of systemic infection: Assessment of 71 autopsy cases, *Invest Clin* 45:131-135, 2004.

# 13

# Death Certification

*"Death finally comes, as it must to all, and the necessity of specifying a cause on the death certificate initiates somewhat of a scramble."*

Alan E. Treloar[1]

Death certificates (Fig. 13-1) serve two primary purposes: legal and statistical. Legally, death certificates contribute to the record of death and are commonly used in medicolegal, interment, insurance, and inheritance matters. Statistically, death certificates are widely used in epidemiologic and public health studies. However, as autopsy rates decline, the value of these data is dubious. Inaccuracies stem primarily from three situations: deaths without postmortem examinations, deaths in which death certificates are based exclusively on clinical data despite the availability of information from postmortem examination, and finally incorrect completion of death certificates leading to misinterpretation of the cause-of-death information regardless of whether a postmortem examination was obtained. The factors that contribute to these problems include lack of training in death certification during medical education, inertia on the part of physicians in amending the originally filed certificate, and failure of governmental agencies to query physicians regarding inadequate diagnoses.

Retrospective comparisons of autopsy findings and death certificates reveal major inaccuracies in recorded causes of death or contributing factors in approximately one half of cases.[2-10] In many countries, death certificates are filed before completion of autopsies, a practice that contributes significantly to this problem. Histologic typing of malignancies and causative infectious organisms are recorded infrequently.[11] Irrespective of any discrepancies between clinical, laboratory, and autopsy diagnoses, significant problems exist in the semantics of completed death certificates.[12] Jordan and Bass[13] found major errors in 32% and minor errors in 23% of death certificates at a Canadian teaching hospital. Analysis attributed many of the discrepancies to inadequate training of physicians in proper death certification, a deficiency that extended to the local coroner's office. In a survey of physicians in Vermont, Freedman and colleagues[14] found that more than one third of physicians reported difficulty in completing death certificates for their patients. Physicians pointed to confusion about the format of the certificate, inability to list multiple causes of death, and difficulty in accurately determining the cause of death in elderly people

or in patients that they were attending only while on call. A study by James and Bull[15] found that pathologists also have difficulty properly stating the cause of death. Pathologists failed to list or incoherently formulated the underlying cause of death in 11% of cases, compared with a rate of 16% for clinicians.

## THE DEATH CERTIFICATE

The United States and other countries provide the World Health Organization (WHO) with information including cause-of-death data for use in international comparisons of death statistics. Through worldwide cooperation and political agreement, there is a uniform approach to death certification and coding of disease.[16,17] The standard death certificate is revised periodically, but generally not more frequently than every 7 to 10 years, and the need for international acceptance restricts the extent to which the forms are modified.[18] Nevertheless, currently an effort is under way to overhaul the reporting system and develop a computer-based format that will facilitate interactive help and allow electronic filing. The most recent revision of the U.S. Standard Certificate of Death anticipates this eventuality with some changes related to format and confidentiality.[19]

In the United States, cause-of-death information recorded on death certificates is collected through a cooperative system of registration areas that includes the 50 states, New York City, the District of Columbia, Puerto Rico, the Virgin Islands, American Samoa, Guam, and the Trust Territory of the Pacific Islands. In exchange for federal funds, the registration areas must provide the National Center for Health Statistics (NCHS) with cause-of-death information in formats consistent with the U.S. Standard Certificate of Death (see Fig. 13-1) and the U.S. Standard Certificate of Fetal Death forms (Fig. 13-2). Thus, the NCHS, in addition to collecting and publishing the data, issues recommendations for laws, regulations, and forms related to reporting cause of death.

Most states or jurisdictions require filing of death certificates with the local registration agency within 48 to 72 hours.

# U.S. STANDARD CERTIFICATE OF DEATH

LOCAL FILE NO.                                                                 STATE FILE NO.

**NAME OF DECEDENT** — For use by physician or institution

**To Be Completed/Verified By: FUNERAL DIRECTOR:**

1. DECEDENT'S LEGAL NAME (Include AKA's if any) (First, Middle, Last) | 2. SEX | 3. SOCIAL SECURITY NUMBER

4a. AGE-Last Birthday (Years) | 4b. UNDER 1 YEAR — Months / Days | 4c. UNDER 1 DAY — Hours / Minutes | 5. DATE OF BIRTH (Mo/Day/Yr) | 6. BIRTHPLACE (City and State or Foreign Country)

7a. RESIDENCE-STATE | 7b. COUNTY | 7c. CITY OR TOWN

7d. STREET AND NUMBER | 7e. APT. NO. | 7f. ZIP CODE | 7g. INSIDE CITY LIMITS? ☐ Yes ☐ No

8. EVER IN US ARMED FORCES? ☐ Yes ☐ No | 9. MARITAL STATUS AT TIME OF DEATH ☐ Married ☐ Married, but separated ☐ Widowed ☐ Divorced ☐ Never Married ☐ Unknown | 10. SURVIVING SPOUSE'S NAME (If wife, give name prior to first marriage)

11. FATHER'S NAME (First, Middle, Last) | 12. MOTHER'S NAME PRIOR TO FIRST MARRIAGE (First, Middle, Last)

13a. INFORMANT'S NAME | 13b. RELATIONSHIP TO DECEDENT | 13c. MAILING ADDRESS (Street and Number, City, State, Zip Code)

14. PLACE OF DEATH (Check only one: see instructions)

IF DEATH OCCURRED IN A HOSPITAL: ☐ Inpatient ☐ Emergency Room/Outpatient ☐ Dead on Arrival | IF DEATH OCCURRED SOMEWHERE OTHER THAN A HOSPITAL: ☐ Hospice facility ☐ Nursing home/Long term care facility ☐ Decedent's home ☐ Other (Specify):

15. FACILITY NAME (If not institution, give street & number) | 16. CITY OR TOWN, STATE, AND ZIP CODE | 17. COUNTY OF DEATH

18. METHOD OF DISPOSITION: ☐ Burial ☐ Cremation ☐ Donation ☐ Entombment ☐ Removal from State ☐ Other (Specify): | 19. PLACE OF DISPOSITION (Name of cemetery, crematory, other place)

20. LOCATION-CITY, TOWN, AND STATE | 21. NAME AND COMPLETE ADDRESS OF FUNERAL FACILITY

22. SIGNATURE OF FUNERAL SERVICE LICENSEE OR OTHER AGENT | 23. LICENSE NUMBER (Of Licensee)

---

**ITEMS 24-28 MUST BE COMPLETED BY PERSON WHO PRONOUNCES OR CERTIFIES DEATH** | 24. DATE PRONOUNCED DEAD (Mo/Day/Yr) | 25. TIME PRONOUNCED DEAD

26. SIGNATURE OF PERSON PRONOUNCING DEATH (Only when applicable) | 27. LICENSE NUMBER | 28. DATE SIGNED (Mo/Day/Yr)

29. ACTUAL OR PRESUMED DATE OF DEATH (Mo/Day/Yr) (Spell Month) | 30. ACTUAL OR PRESUMED TIME OF DEATH | 31. WAS MEDICAL EXAMINER OR CORONER CONTACTED? ☐ Yes ☐ No

**To Be Completed By: MEDICAL CERTIFIER**

### CAUSE OF DEATH (See instructions and examples)

32. PART I. Enter the chain of events--diseases, injuries, or complications--that directly caused the death. DO NOT enter terminal events such as cardiac arrest, respiratory arrest, or ventricular fibrillation without showing the etiology. DO NOT ABBREVIATE. Enter only one cause on a line. Add additional lines if necessary.

Approximate interval: Onset to death

IMMEDIATE CAUSE (Final disease or condition --------> resulting in death) a._____

Due to (or as a consequence of):

Sequentially list conditions, if any, leading to the cause listed on line a. Enter the **UNDERLYING CAUSE** (disease or injury that initiated the events resulting in death) **LAST**

b._____

Due to (or as a consequence of):

c._____

Due to (or as a consequence of):

d._____

PART II. Enter other significant conditions contributing to death but not resulting in the underlying cause given in PART I | 33. WAS AN AUTOPSY PERFORMED? ☐ Yes ☐ No

34. WERE AUTOPSY FINDINGS AVAILABLE TO COMPLETE THE CAUSE OF DEATH? ☐ Yes ☐ No

35. DID TOBACCO USE CONTRIBUTE TO DEATH? ☐ Yes ☐ Probably ☐ No ☐ Unknown | 36. IF FEMALE: ☐ Not pregnant within past year ☐ Pregnant at time of death ☐ Not pregnant, but pregnant within 42 days of death ☐ Not pregnant, but pregnant 43 days to 1 year before death ☐ Unknown if pregnant within the past year | 37. MANNER OF DEATH ☐ Natural ☐ Homicide ☐ Accident ☐ Pending Investigation ☐ Suicide ☐ Could not be determined

38. DATE OF INJURY (Mo/Day/Yr) (Spell Month) | 39. TIME OF INJURY | 40. PLACE OF INJURY (e.g., Decedent's home; construction site; restaurant; wooded area) | 41. INJURY AT WORK? ☐ Yes ☐ No

42. LOCATION OF INJURY: State: | City or Town:

Street & Number: | Apartment No.: | Zip Code:

43. DESCRIBE HOW INJURY OCCURRED: | 44. IF TRANSPORTATION INJURY, SPECIFY: ☐ Driver/Operator ☐ Passenger ☐ Pedestrian ☐ Other (Specify)

45. CERTIFIER (Check only one):
☐ Certifying physician-To the best of my knowledge, death occurred due to the cause(s) and manner stated.
☐ Pronouncing & Certifying physician-To the best of my knowledge, death occurred at the time, date, and place, and due to the cause(s) and manner stated.
☐ Medical Examiner/Coroner-On the basis of examination, and/or investigation, in my opinion, death occurred at the time, date, and place, and due to the cause(s) and manner stated.

Signature of certifier:_____

46. NAME, ADDRESS, AND ZIP CODE OF PERSON COMPLETING CAUSE OF DEATH (Item 32)

47. TITLE OF CERTIFIER | 48. LICENSE NUMBER | 49. DATE CERTIFIED (Mo/Day/Yr) | 50. **FOR REGISTRAR ONLY**- DATE FILED (Mo/Day/Yr)

**To Be Completed By: FUNERAL DIRECTOR**

51. DECEDENT'S EDUCATION-Check the box that best describes the highest degree or level of school completed at the time of death.
☐ 8th grade or less
☐ 9th - 12th grade; no diploma
☐ High school graduate or GED completed
☐ Some college credit, but no degree
☐ Associate degree (e.g., AA, AS)
☐ Bachelor's degree (e.g., BA, AB, BS)
☐ Master's degree (e.g., MA, MS, MEng, MEd, MSW, MBA)
☐ Doctorate (e.g., PhD, EdD) or Professional degree (e.g., MD, DDS, DVM, LLB, JD)

52. DECEDENT OF HISPANIC ORIGIN? Check the box that best describes whether the decedent is Spanish/Hispanic/Latino. Check the "No" box if decedent is not Spanish/Hispanic/Latino.
☐ No, not Spanish/Hispanic/Latino
☐ Yes, Mexican, Mexican American, Chicano
☐ Yes, Puerto Rican
☐ Yes, Cuban
☐ Yes, other Spanish/Hispanic/Latino (Specify) _____

53. DECEDENT'S RACE (Check one or more races to indicate what the decedent considered himself or herself to be)
☐ White
☐ Black or African American
☐ American Indian or Alaska Native (Name of the enrolled or principal tribe) _____
☐ Asian Indian
☐ Chinese
☐ Filipino
☐ Japanese
☐ Korean
☐ Vietnamese
☐ Other Asian (Specify) _____
☐ Native Hawaiian
☐ Guamanian or Chamorro
☐ Samoan
☐ Other Pacific Islander (Specify) _____
☐ Other (Specify) _____

54. DECEDENT'S USUAL OCCUPATION (Indicate type of work done during most of working life. DO NOT USE RETIRED).

55. KIND OF BUSINESS/INDUSTRY

**Figure 13-1** The U.S. Standard Certificate of Death represents a typical death certificate.
(From Centers for Disease Control and Prevention, National Center for Health Statistics: *2003 revisions of the U.S. standard certificates of live birth and death and the fetal death report*, http://www.cdc.gov/nchs/vital_certs_rev.htm [accessed October 2, 2008].)

# US STANDARD REPORT OF FETAL DEATH

LOCAL FILE NO. _____    STATE FILE NUMBER: _____

## MOTHER

| 1. NAME OF FETUS (optional-at the discretion of the parents) | 2. TIME OF DELIVERY (24hr) | 3. SEX (M/F/Unk) | 4. DATE OF DELIVERY (Mo/Day/Yr) |

5a. CITY, TOWN, OR LOCATION OF DELIVERY

7. PLACE WHERE DELIVERY OCCURRED (Check one)
- ☐ Hospital
- ☐ Freestanding birthing center
- ☐ Home Delivery: Planned to deliver at home? ☐ Yes ☐ No
- ☐ Clinic/Doctor's office
- ☐ Other (Specify)_____

8. FACILITY NAME (If not institution, give street and number)

5b. ZIP CODE OF DELIVERY

6. COUNTY OF DELIVERY

9. FACILITY ID. (NPI)

10a. MOTHER'S CURRENT LEGAL NAME (First, Middle, Last, Suffix)

10b. DATE OF BIRTH (Mo/Day/Yr)

10c. MOTHER'S NAME PRIOR TO FIRST MARRIAGE (First, Middle, Last, Suffix)

10d. BIRTHPLACE (State, Territory, or Foreign Country)

11a. RESIDENCE OF MOTHER-STATE

11b. COUNTY

11c. CITY, TOWN, OR LOCATION

11d. STREET AND NUMBER

11e. APT. NO.

11f. ZIP CODE

11g. INSIDE CITY LIMITS? ☐ Yes ☐ No

## FATHER

12a. FATHER'S CURRENT LEGAL NAME (First, Middle, Last, Suffix)

12b. DATE OF BIRTH (Mo/Day/Yr)

12c. BIRTHPLACE (State, Territory, or Foreign Country)

## DISPOSITION

13. METHOD OF DISPOSITION:
☐ Burial   ☐ Cremation   ☐ Hospital Disposition   ☐ Donation   ☐ Removal from State   ☐ Other (Specify)_____

## ATTENDANT AND REGISTRATION INFORMATION

14. ATTENDANT'S NAME, TITLE, AND NPI

NAME: _____

NPI:_____

TITLE: ☐ MD ☐ DO ☐ CNM/CM ☐ OTHER MIDWIFE

☐ OTHER (Specify)_____

15. NAME AND TITLE OF PERSON COMPLETING REPORT

Name _____

Title _____

16. DATE REPORT COMPLETED
_____/_____/_____
MM    DD    YYYY

17. DATE RECEIVED BY REGISTRAR
_____/_____/_____
MM    DD    YYYY

## CAUSE OF FETAL DEATH

# 18. CAUSE/CONDITIONS CONTRIBUTING TO FETAL DEATH

**18a. INITIATING CAUSE/CONDITION**

(AMONG THE CHOICES BELOW, PLEASE SELECT THE ONE WHICH MOST LIKELY BEGAN THE SEQUENCE OF EVENTS RESULTING IN THE DEATH OF THE FETUS)

Maternal Conditions/Diseases (Specify) _____

Complications of Placenta, Cord, or Membranes
- ☐ Rupture of membranes prior to onset of labor
- ☐ Abruptio placenta
- ☐ Placental insufficiency
- ☐ Prolapsed cord
- ☐ Chorioamnionitis
- ☐ Other Specify)_____

Other Obstetrical or Pregnancy Complications (Specify) _____

Fetal Anomaly (Specify) _____

Fetal Injury (Specify) _____

Fetal Infection (Specify) _____

Other Fetal Conditions/Disorders (Specify) _____

☐ Unknown

**18b. OTHER SIGNIFICANT CAUSES OR CONDITIONS**

(SELECT OR SPECIFY ALL OTHER CONDITIONS CONTRIBUTING TO DEATH IN ITEM 18b)

Maternal Conditions/Diseases (Specify) _____

Complications of Placenta, Cord, or Membranes
- ☐ Rupture of membranes prior to onset of labor
- ☐ Abruptio placenta
- ☐ Placental insufficiency
- ☐ Prolapsed cord
- ☐ Chorioamnionitis
- ☐ Other Specify)_____

Other Obstetrical or Pregnancy Complications (Specify) _____

Fetal Anomaly (Specify) _____

Fetal Injury (Specify) _____

Fetal Infection (Specify) _____

Other Fetal Conditions/Disorders (Specify) _____

☐ Unknown

18c. WEIGHT OF FETUS (grams preferred, specify unit)
_____   ☐ grams   ☐ lb/oz

18d. OBSTETRIC ESTIMATE OF GESTATION AT DELIVERY
_____ (completed weeks)

18e. ESTIMATED TIME OF FETAL DEATH
- ☐ Dead at time of first assessment, no labor ongoing
- ☐ Dead at time of first assessment, labor ongoing
- ☐ Died during labor, after first assessment
- ☐ Unknown time of fetal death

18f. WAS AN AUTOPSY PERFORMED?
☐ Yes   ☐ No   ☐ Planned

18g. WAS A HISTOLOGICAL PLACENTAL EXAMINATION PERFORMED?
☐ Yes   ☐ No   ☐ Planned

18h. WERE AUTOPSY OR HISTOLOGICAL PLACENTAL EXAMINATION RESULTS USED IN DETERMINING THE CAUSE OF FETAL DEATH? ☐ Yes   ☐ No

Mother's Name _____

Mother's Medical Record No. _____

**Figure 13-2** For legend see page 150.

**MOTHER**

**19. MOTHER'S EDUCATION** (Check the box that best describes the highest degree or level of school completed at the time of delivery)

- ☐ 8th grade or less
- ☐ 9th - 12th grade, no diploma
- ☐ High school graduate or GED completed
- ☐ Some college credit but no degree
- ☐ Associate degree (e.g., AA, AS)
- ☐ Bachelor's degree (e.g., BA, AB, BS)
- ☐ Master's degree (e.g., MA, MS, MEng, MEd, MSW, MBA)
- ☐ Doctorate (e.g., PhD, EdD) or Professional degree (e.g., MD, DDS, DVM, LLB, JD)

**20. MOTHER OF HISPANIC ORIGIN?** (Check the box that best describes whether the mother is Spanish/Hispanic/Latina. Check the "No" box if mother is not Spanish/Hispanic/Latina)

- ☐ No, not Spanish/Hispanic/Latina
- ☐ Yes, Mexican, Mexican American, Chicana
- ☐ Yes, Puerto Rican
- ☐ Yes, Cuban
- ☐ Yes, other Spanish/Hispanic/Latina

(Specify)_____

**21. MOTHER'S RACE** (Check one or more races to indicate what the mother considers herself to be)

- ☐ White
- ☐ Black or African American
- ☐ American Indian or Alaska Native (Name of the enrolled or principal tribe)_____
- ☐ Asian Indian
- ☐ Chinese
- ☐ Filipino
- ☐ Japanese
- ☐ Korean
- ☐ Vietnamese
- ☐ Other Asian (Specify)_____
- ☐ Native Hawaiian
- ☐ Guamanian or Chamorro
- ☐ Samoan
- ☐ Other Pacific Islander (Specify)_____
- ☐ Other (Specify)_____

**22. MOTHER MARRIED?** (At delivery, conception, or anytime between) ☐ Yes ☐ No

**23a. DATE OF FIRST PRENATAL CARE VISIT**
_____ /_____ / _____  ☐ No Prenatal Care
M M     D D     YYYY

**23b. DATE OF LAST PRENATAL CARE VISIT**
_____ /_____ / _____
M M     D D     YYYY

**24. TOTAL NUMBER OF PRENATAL VISITS FOR THIS PREGNANCY** _____ (If none, enter "0".)

**25. MOTHER'S HEIGHT** _____ (feet/inches)

**26. MOTHER'S PREPREGNANCY WEIGHT** _____ (pounds)

**27. MOTHER'S WEIGHT AT DELIVERY** _____ (pounds)

**28. DID MOTHER GET WIC FOOD FOR HERSELF DURING THIS PREGNANCY?** ☐ Yes ☐ No

**29. NUMBER OF PREVIOUS LIVE BIRTHS**

**29a. Now Living**
Number _____
☐ None

**29b. Now Dead**
Number _____
☐ None

**30. NUMBER OF OTHER PREGNANCY OUTCOMES** (spontaneous or induced losses or ectopic pregnancies)

**30a. Other Outcomes**
Number (Do not include this fetus) _____
☐ None

**31. CIGARETTE SMOKING BEFORE AND DURING PREGNANCY**
For each time period, enter either the number of cigarettes or the number of packs of cigarettes smoked. IF NONE, ENTER "0".

Average number of cigarettes or packs of cigarettes smoked per day.

|  | # of cigarettes |  | # of packs |
|---|---|---|---|
| Three Months Before Pregnancy | _____ | OR | _____ |
| First Three Months of Pregnancy | _____ | OR | _____ |
| Second Three Months of Pregnancy | _____ | OR | _____ |
| Third Trimester of Pregnancy |  | OR |  |

**29c. DATE OF LAST LIVE BIRTH**
_____ /_____
MM     Y Y Y Y

**30b. DATE OF LAST OTHER PREGNANCY OUTCOME**
_____ /_____
MM     Y Y Y Y

**32. DATE LAST NORMAL MENSES BEGAN**
___ /___ /___
MM     D D     Y Y Y Y

**33. PLURALITY** - Single, Twin, Triplet, etc.
(Specify)_____

**34. IF NOT SINGLE BIRTH-** Born First, Second, Third, etc.
(Specify)_____

**35. MOTHER TRANSFERRED FOR MATERNAL MEDICAL OR FETAL INDICATIONS FOR DELIVERY?** ☐ Yes ☐ No
IF YES, ENTER NAME OF FACILITY MOTHER TRANSFERRED FROM: _____

**MEDICAL AND HEALTH INFORMATION**

**36. RISK FACTORS IN THIS PREGNANCY** (Check all that apply):

Diabetes
- ☐ Prepregnancy (Diagnosis prior to this pregnancy)
- ☐ Gestational (Diagnosis in this pregnancy)

Hypertension
- ☐ Prepregnancy (Chronic)
- ☐ Gestational (PIH, preeclampsia)
- ☐ Eclampsia

- ☐ Previous preterm birth

- ☐ Other previous poor pregnancy outcome (Includes perinatal death, small-for-gestational age/intrauterine growth restricted birth)

- ☐ Pregnancy resulted from infertility treatment-If yes, check all that apply:

    - ☐ Fertility-enhancing drugs, Artificial insemination or Intrauterine insemination

    - ☐ Assisted reproductive technology (e.g., in vitro fertilization (IVF), gamete intrafallopian transfer (GIFT))

- ☐ Mother had a previous cesarean delivery
    If yes, how many _____

- ☐ None of the above

**37. INFECTIONS PRESENT AND/OR TREATED DURING THIS PREGNANCY** (Check all that apply)

- ☐ Gonorrhea
- ☐ Syphilis
- ☐ Chlamydia
- ☐ Listeria
- ☐ Group B Streptococcus
- ☐ Cytomegalovirus
- ☐ Parvovirus
- ☐ Toxoplasmosis
- ☐ None of the above
- ☐ Other (Specify)_____

**38. METHOD OF DELIVERY**

A. Was delivery with forceps attempted but unsuccessful?
☐ Yes ☐ No

B. Was delivery with vacuum extraction attempted but unsuccessful?
☐ Yes ☐ No

C. Fetal presentation at delivery
- ☐ Cephalic
- ☐ Breech
- ☐ Other

D. Final route and method of delivery (Check one)
- ☐ Vaginal/Spontaneous
- ☐ Vaginal/Forceps
- ☐ Vaginal/Vacuum
- ☐ Cesarean
    If cesarean, was a trial of labor attempted?
    - ☐ Yes
    - ☐ No

E. Hysterotomy/Hysterectomy
☐ Yes ☐ No

**39. MATERNAL MORBIDITY** (Check all that apply)
(Complications associated with labor and delivery)

- ☐ Maternal transfusion
- ☐ Third or fourth degree perineal laceration
- ☐ Ruptured uterus
- ☐ Unplanned hysterectomy
- ☐ Admission to intensive care unit
- ☐ Unplanned operating room procedure following delivery
- ☐ None of the above

**40. CONGENITAL ANOMALIES OF THE FETUS**
(Check all that apply)

- ☐ Anencephaly
- ☐ Meningomyelocele/Spina bifida
- ☐ Cyanotic congenital heart disease
- ☐ Congenital diaphragmatic hernia
- ☐ Omphalocele
- ☐ Gastroschisis
- ☐ Limb reduction defect (excluding congenital amputation and dwarfing syndromes)
- ☐ Cleft Lip with or without Cleft Palate
- ☐ Cleft Palate alone
- ☐ Down Syndrome
    - ☐ Karyotype confirmed
    - ☐ Karyotype pending
- ☐ Suspected chromosomal disorder
    - ☐ Karyotype confirmed
    - ☐ Karyotype pending
- ☐ Hypospadias
- ☐ None of the anomalies listed above

**NOTE:** This recommended standard fetal death report is the result of an extensive evaluation process. Information on the process and resulting recommendations as well as plans for future activities is available on the Internet at: http://www.cdc.gov/nchs/vital_certs_rev.htm.

**Figure 13-2** The U.S. Standard Certificate of Fetal Death.
(From Centers for Disease Control and Prevention, National Center for Health Statistics: *2003 revisions of the U.S. standard certificates of live birth and death and the fetal death report*, http://www.cdc.gov/nchs/vital_certs_rev.htm [accessed October 2, 2008].)

If additional time is required to determine the cause of death, the certificate may be filed pending further investigation. The time interval before a pending investigation must be completed is subject to the laws of individual jurisdictions. To facilitate coding, state or local registrars may initiate queries to the individual certifying the death. These queries are initiated according to guidelines for death registration and coding published by the NCHS.[20] Queries may lead to significant revision of a death certificate. For example, querying physicians in Oregon regarding submitted death certificates resulted in new underlying-cause-of-death data in nearly 6% of deaths.[21]

The death certifier may amend a death certificate whenever corrected or more specific information regarding a death or decedent becomes available—for example, after completion of all autopsy studies. In this situation, the original certifier should notify the local registrar, who then initiates the amendment process. Regrettably, amendments are made only infrequently, most likely because interest wanes and this avenue is forgotten.[22]

To complete death certificates correctly, a physician must be familiar with a number of terms.[23] The *immediate cause of death* is the final disease, injury, or complication directly causing death. It precedes death as a consequence of the underlying cause or causes. In the case of a sudden, traumatic death, the violent act or accident is antecedent to an injury entered, although these two events are often almost simultaneous.

The immediate cause of death does not refer to the *mechanism (mode) of death*. The mechanism of death is a physiologic derangement or biochemical disturbance that is a complication of the underlying cause of death or a disturbance through which the underlying cause ultimately exerts its lethal effect. Thus, the mechanism of death may have more than one possible cause, and "it is not an etiologically specific or criteria-defined disease, injury, or poisoning event."[24] Defined as such, mechanisms of death include terminal events such as cardiopulmonary arrest, nonspecific physiologic derangements such as vital organ failures, or nonspecific anatomic processes such as infarction, inflammation, or hemorrhage. Except in special circumstances (as discussed in the following section), mechanisms of death are not listed on death certificates.

*Intervening cause(s) of death* includes other conditions that stem from the underlying cause. They precede and ultimately culminate in the immediate cause of death. On the death certificate, these are listed in pathophysiologic sequence. The U.S. Standard Certificate of Death (see Fig. 13-1) provides lines for the inclusion of two intervening causes of death, although more can be added (see later). The *underlying (proximate) cause of death* is defined for public health and legal purposes as "the disease or injury that initiated the train of events leading to death."[16] In other words, without an underlying cause, the death would not have happened. Finally, the *manner of death*, either natural or unnatural (accident, suicide, or homicide), explains how the cause of death arose.

As can be seen in Figure 13-1, the death certificate also provides a section for listing other significant conditions contributing to death. Although significant conditions may have adversely affected the health of the decedent, they need not

be related to the immediate or underlying causes of death. However, these listings should be conditions that hastened death from the underlying cause.[25] Risk factors such as smoking, alcohol, or drug abuse or concurrent diseases such as hypertension, diabetes mellitus, or cancer are often examples of contributing conditions.

Although the format of death certificates allows a physician to record a series of diseases leading to death, it may be difficult for the death certifier to list the immediate cause of death or to determine the underlying cause of death when two or more parallel processes contribute equally to death. For example, multiple factors often cause the death of a patient with a chronic illness or an elderly individual suffering from several degenerative diseases.[26,27] Similarly, the forensic pathologist is often faced with cases in which multiple intoxications or multiple traumatic injuries led to death.[28]

The analysis of mortality statistics based on a single underlying cause of death also has a number of shortcomings. Chief among these is that data tabulated from underlying cause of death necessarily exclude the effects of other conditions present at the time of death.[29] Compared with multiple-cause-of-death analysis, data based on a single underlying cause of death lead to underrepresentation of diseases and conditions such as diabetes,[30,31] dementia,[32] hypertension,[33] nosocomial infections,[34] and injury among elderly people.[35] Conventional cause-elimination life tables based on a single underlying cause of death may also overestimate the gains in life expectancy that might be expected from eradication of a given disease.[36] Thus, a number of epidemiologists favor a multiple-cause approach for death certification. In fact, the NCHS has presented summary data with multiple-cause statistics.[37] Although not yet a replacement for traditional underlying-cause-of-death data, multiple-cause data do provide information pertaining to disease associations, injuries leading to death, and diseases that are often associated with death even though they might not be the underlying cause. However, refinements in the methods of certifying and coding deaths are necessary before multiple-cause-of-death analysis can be used to full advantage.[38-40]

## COMPLETING A DEATH CERTIFICATE

The physician completing a death certificate must adhere to a few specific rules. Death certificates must be typed or printed in black ink only. One should not use any abbreviations but should also avoid excess verbiage. A rational determination of what led to the individual's death should be made on the basis of the data at hand. One should consider the circumstances surrounding the death, the decedent's clinical symptoms and pertinent medical history, laboratory and radiologic studies, surgical pathologic and cytologic examinations, and, of course, the findings at autopsy when formulating death certificates. The pathologist should avoid reporting mechanisms of death, and in describing the cause of death, he or she should use only the applicable terms contained in the appropriate version of the *International Classification of Diseases*.[41,42] When listing an infection, one should include the site and the causal organism. With neoplasms, the histopathologic type, the anatomic site, and whether the neoplasm is primary or metastatic should be included. One should record time intervals—minutes, hours, days, months, or years—as suitable and state the time interval as unknown only when the time of onset is entirely unknown and a reasonable estimate cannot be made.

There must always be an entry on the line for the immediate cause of death, "Part I, line a." The immediate cause of death may be a single underlying disease process if only one condition was present at death. To satisfy these conditions, a single condition listed as both the immediate and the underlying cause of death must have directly caused death or led to death through mechanisms that were complex, poorly understood, or both (Box 13-1).[25]

The death certificate provides space ("Part I, lines b to d") for listing up to three conditions in a pathophysiologic sequence that led to the immediate cause of death (Box 13-2). The initiating condition (i.e., the underlying cause of death) is listed last. If there are more than three stages in the sequence leading to death, additional lines may be added. For purposes of death certification, the length of time between the underlying cause of

death and the immediate cause of death may be short or long, but in either case there must be a continuous etiologic or pathologic relationship between them. Medical interventions such as operations or treatments should not be listed in this section of the death certificate unless they were directly related to the train of morbid events (see later).

As explained previously, mechanisms of death include nonspecific anatomic processes, terminal events, and nonspecific physiologic derangements (Box 13-3). Nonspecific anatomic processes are complications of the underlying cause of death resulting in an anatomic abnormality that has more than one possible cause. Terminal events are the fatal (without medical intervention) and final complications of the underlying cause of death. Nonspecific physiologic derangements are complications of the underlying cause of death not defined as a terminal event or nonspecific anatomic process. Box 13-4 lists two principles for the use of mechanisms of death as immediate or intermediate causes of death.[24] Box 13-5 contains several examples of mechanisms of death as immediate and intermediate causes of death.

When disease processes or events are present but unrelated to the underlying cause of death, they should be listed in order of importance under "Part II, Other Significant Conditions" of the cause-of-death section of the death certificate. This part may contain all other diseases or conditions that have unfavorably influenced the course of events and contributed to the fatal outcome but were not directly related to the sequence of events that directly caused death. Thus, these listings should be significant conditions that hastened death from the underlying cause (Box 13-6). Among individuals with complex medical conditions, the sequences of conditions resulting in death may be multiple. In these cases, the death certifier must choose the sequence that he or she feels had the greatest impact. Conditions from the alternative sequence should be listed as other significant conditions.

## MEDICOLEGAL ISSUES

In addition to formulating cause-of-death statements as just described, a pathologist working as a medical examiner must determine the manner of death. Although the autopsy is useful in determining the cause and mechanism of death, it alone generally does not determine the manner of death.[43] The death certificate allows for several possibilities—*natural, unnatural (homicide, suicide, accidental), pending investigation,* or *could not be determined* (Table 13-1). It should be noted that these classifications are primarily for statistical purposes; thus, the most probable manner of death is listed. Therefore, the death certificate has no direct bearing on criminal prosecution or insurance settlements. Box 13-7 includes a number of cause-of-death statements in which death was from unnatural causes.

In a small percentage of cases, the cause of death or manner of death, or both, cannot be determined following postmortem examination and investigation. In such situations and only after all efforts have been made to determine the cause of death, the death certifier may classify the cause or manner of death, or both, as "unknown." In a review of one county's records over a 10-year period, Murphy[44] found that a ruling of unknown or undetermined was made in 1.73%

---

| **Box 13-1** | Examples of single underlying causes of death |
| --- | --- |

The cause of death may be a single underlying disease process if only one condition was present at death and was the underlying and immediate cause of death.

| Cause of death | Interval |
| --- | --- |
| a. Anencephaly | Birth |
| **Cause of death** | |
| a. Ruptured middle cerebral artery aneurysm | Minutes |
| **Cause of death** | |
| a. Pneumococcal meningitis | 3 days |
| **Cause of death** | |
| a. Osteogenic sarcoma of the left leg with metastases | 1 year |

---

| **Box 13-2** | Immediate causes of death with underlying causes of death |
| --- | --- |

Space is provided for listing up to three intermediate causes of death on U.S. death certificates. Adding intermediate causes is not specifically prohibited.

| Cause of death | Approximate interval |
| --- | --- |
| a. Ruptured thoracic aortic aneurysm | Minutes |
| *due to, or as a consequence of:* | |
| b. Atherosclerotic cardiovascular disease | Years |
| **Cause of death** | **Approximate interval** |
| a. Acute pancreatitis | 5 days |
| *due to, or as a consequence of:* | |
| b. Choledocholithiasis | 2 weeks |
| **Cause of death** | **Approximate interval** |
| a. Disseminated aspergillosis | 2 weeks |
| *due to, or as a consequence of:* | |
| b. Acquired immunodeficiency syndrome | 4 years |
| *due to, or as a consequence of:* | |
| c. Human immunodeficiency virus infection | 6 years |

**Box 13-3**  Some examples of terminal events, nonspecific physiologic derangements, and nonspecific anatomic processes that are not underlying causes of death

| Terminal event* | Nonspecific physiologic derangements[†] | Nonspecific anatomic processes[†] |
|---|---|---|
| Asystole | Arrhythmia/dysrhythmia | Acute organ infarction or tissue necrosis |
| Cardiac arrest | Coma | Anoxic encephalopathy |
| Cardiopulmonary arrest | Dehydration | Bowel obstruction |
| Electromechanical dissociation | Edema (cerebral, pulmonary, etc.) | Cirrhosis (unless specific, e.g., primary biliary cirrhosis) |
| Respiratory arrest | Encephalopathy (hepatic, metabolic) | Hematoma (epidural, subdural) |
| Ventricular fibrillation | Exsanguinations | Hemorrhage (gastrointestinal, intracranial, subarachnoid, etc.) |
| | Hypotension | Hemorrhage into body cavity (hemopericardium, hemothorax, etc.) |
| | Ketoacidosis | Peritonitis |
| | Multiorgan failure | Pneumonia (usually has underlying cause) |
| | Organ failure (heart, liver, lung, kidney, etc.) | Pulmonary embolism |
| | Pneumothorax | |
| | Portal hypertension | |
| | Seizures | |
| | Sepsis | |
| | Serum electrolyte disturbances (hypercalcemia, hyperkalemia, etc.) | |
| | Shock (cardiogenic, hypovolemic, septic, etc.) | |

*Seldom, if ever, reported on death certificate.
[†]Reported on death certificate based on applications of the principles (see Box 13-4).
Data from Hanzlick R: Principles for including or excluding 'mechanisms' of death when writing cause-of-death statements, *Arch Pathol Lab Med* 121:377-380, 1997; and Hanzlick R, editor: *Cause of death and the death certificate. Important information for physicians, coroners, medical examiners, and the public,* Northfield, Ill, 2006, College of American Pathologists.

**Box 13-4**  Guidelines for the use of mechanisms of death as immediate and intermediate causes of death in death certification

| Principle 1 | Terminal events (see Box 13-3) should not be listed on the death certificate. |
|---|---|
| Principle 2 | A nonspecific anatomic process or nonspecific physiologic derangement is included in the cause-of-death statement if it meets the following criteria: |
| | 1. It is a recognized, potentially fatal complication of the underlying cause of death; |
| | 2. It constitutes part of the sequence of conditions that led to death as judged by clinical presentation, the historical sequence of events, or anatomic or laboratory findings; |
| | 3. It is not a symptom or sign; |
| | 4. Its existence in the patient would not be apparent unless explicitly stated in the cause-of-death statement; |
| | 5. Its inclusion does not represent an oversimplification of the facts; or |
| | 6. An etiologically specific underlying cause of death is also reported, when possible. |
| Principle 3 | If the existence in the patient of a nonspecific process or derangement (i.e., complication) is obvious on the basis of the underlying cause of death or another reported condition or complication, it need not be reported. |

Adapted from Hanzlick R, editor: *Cause of death and the death certificate. Important information for physicians, coroners, medical examiners, and the public,* Northfield, Ill, 2006, College of American Pathologists.

**Box 13-5**  Mechanisms of death as immediate and intermediate causes of death

| Cause of death | Approximate interval |
|---|---|
| a. Pulmonary thromboembolism | Minutes |
| *due to, or as a consequence of:* | |
| b. Deep venous thrombosis | Days |
| *due to, or as a consequence of:* | |
| c. Immobilization | 1 month |
| *due to, or as a consequence of:* | |
| d. Fracture of right femur | 1 month |
| **Cause of death** | **Approximate interval** |
| a. Upper gastrointestinal hemorrhage | 1 hour |
| *due to, or as a consequence of:* | |
| b. Esophageal varices | 2 years |
| *due to, or as a consequence of:* | |
| c. Macronodular cirrhosis of liver | Years |
| *due to, or as a consequence of:* | |
| d. Hepatitis B infection | 10 years |
| **Cause of death** | **Approximate interval** |
| a. Dysrhythmia | 1 hour |
| *due to, or as a consequence of:* | |
| b. Hyperkalemia | 2 hours |
| *due to, or as a consequence of:* | |
| c. Tumor lysis syndrome | 12 hours |
| *due to, or as a consequence of:* | |
| d. Burkitt's lymphoma | Months |

| Box 13-6 | Listing of other significant conditions |
|---|---|

When disease processes or events are present but unrelated to the underlying cause of death, they may be listed under other conditions. However, these listings should be significant conditions that hasten death from the underlying cause or risk factors contributing to the development of underlying disease.

| Cause of death | Approximate interval |
|---|---|
| a. Mesothelioma | 18 months |
| *due to, or as a consequence of:* | |
| b. Occupational asbestos exposure | 20 years |
| Other significant conditions: Chronic tobacco use | |

| Cause of death | Approximate interval |
|---|---|
| a. Aspiration pneumonia | 1 week |
| *due to, or as a consequence of:* | |
| b. Alzheimer disease | Approximately 8 years |
| Other significant conditions: Remote cerebral infarct, right frontal lobe | |

| Cause of death | Approximate interval |
|---|---|
| a. Myocardial infarct | 1 hour |
| *due to, or as a consequence of:* | |
| b. Atherosclerotic coronary artery disease | 10 years |
| Other significant conditions: Risk factors: essential hypertension; diabetes mellitus; obesity | |

| Box 13-7 | Medical examiner cases |
|---|---|

| Cause of death | Approximate interval |
|---|---|
| a. Cardiac tamponade | Minutes |
| *due to, or as a consequence of:* | |
| b. Hemopericardium | 15 minutes |
| *due to, or as a consequence of:* | |
| c. Stab wound of thorax | 15 minutes |
| Manner of death: Homicide | |

| Cause of death | Approximate interval |
|---|---|
| a. Massive hepatic necrosis | 5 days |
| *due to, or as a consequence of:* | |
| b. Acetaminophen toxicity | 5 days |
| Other significant conditions: Depression | |
| Manner of death: Suicide | |

| Cause of death | Approximate interval |
|---|---|
| a. Hemoperitoneum | Minutes |
| *due to, or as a consequence of:* | |
| b. Laceration of the aorta | Minutes |
| *due to, or as a consequence of:* | |
| c. Blunt thoracic trauma | Minutes |
| *due to, or as a consequence of:* | |
| d. Motor vehicle accident | Minutes |
| Manner of death: Accident | |

| Table 13-1 | Description of the various manners of death | |
|---|---|---|
| **Manner** | **Definition** | |
| Natural | Death resulting from disease | |
| Accident | Death as the result of an environmental influence | |
| Suicide | Death intentionally self-inflicted | |
| Homicide | Death resulting from the deliberate action of another | |

| Box 13-8 | Cause-of-death statements in examples of therapeutic complications |
|---|---|

| Cause of death | Approximate interval |
|---|---|
| a. Congestive heart failure | Months |
| *due to, or as a consequence of:* | |
| b. Doxorubicin cardiotoxicity | 1 year |
| Other significant conditions: Invasive ductal carcinoma of the right breast | |

| Cause of death | Approximate interval |
|---|---|
| a. Right hemothorax | 30 minutes |
| *due to, or as a consequence of:* | |
| b. Perforation of right subclavian artery by catheter | 30 minutes |
| *due to, or as a consequence of:* | |
| c. Attempted right subclavian vein catheterization | |
| Other significant conditions: Ulcerative colitis | |

of cases. The most common (34.8%) cases falling into this category were deaths resulting from known trauma but without reliable evidence on which to rule on the manner of death. Drug-related deaths with undetermined manner of death (25%), deaths in which autopsy and history failed to reveal a cause of death (21.7%), decomposed bodies with inadequate history and without obvious cause of death (8.7%), and premature birth and death without significant findings (6.5%) accounted for the vast majority of the remaining cases in which the cause or manner of death could not be determined.

## THERAPEUTIC COMPLICATIONS AND THE DEATH CERTIFICATE

Medical interventions (diagnostic procedures, medical or surgical treatments) should not be listed on the death certificate unless they were directly related to the train of morbid events (Box 13-8). In these cases, it may be difficult to certify whether the manner of death is natural or accidental.

However, when death is related to high-risk procedures for potentially fatal diseases or to a known complication of a procedure or treatment, the manner of death is considered natural. In contrast, when unexpected errors beyond the known complications or calculated risks of a procedure lead to death, the manner of death may be considered accidental.[45] These so-called therapeutic misadventures may result in civil litigation for wrongful death. In and of itself, this classification does not indicate medical malpractice, a judgment that is left to the courts. However, Hirsch and coauthors[46] feel that "therapeutic misadventure" is inflammatory and recommend an alternative, "therapeutic complication."

## FETAL DEATH CERTIFICATES

The U.S. Standard Certificate of Fetal Death (see Fig. 13-2) is similar to the birth certificate. However, like the U.S. Standard Certificate of Death, it includes a section on cause of death. Immediate, intervening, and underlying causes of death, as well as other significant conditions, should be listed as described previously. Approximate time intervals are not queried; however, space is also provided for indicating whether these causes were fetal or maternal. Items 36 and 37 (on reverse side of form shown) provide checkboxes for maternal risk factors, and item 40 adds a checkbox for congenital anomalies. The form includes a space for recording whether the fetus died before labor, during labor, or during delivery. Box 13-9 provides some examples of fetal death certification.

## CONCLUSION

Death certification requires special attention, but it is not difficult if given careful thought. In this chapter, we have summarized some basic guidelines and provided a few pertinent examples. Although it is often the responsibility of the clinician to contribute accurate cause-of-death information, the pathologist is in an advantageous position to provide guidance and education. The hospital office charged with completing the death certificate can also provide expertise. A number of publications available free from the NCHS provide instructions for writing cause-of-death statements.[47-49] *Cause of Death and the Death Certificate,*[50] published by the College of American Pathologists, is particularly recommended for its thoroughness and instructive examples. Online training

in the writing of cause-of-death statements is available at the National Association of Medical Examiners' website.[51]

## REFERENCES

1. Treloar AE: The enigma of cause of death, *JAMA* 162:1376-1379, 1956.
2. Cameron HM, McGoogan E: A prospective study of 1152 hospital autopsies: I. Inaccuracies in death certification, *J Pathol* 133:273-283, 1981.
3. Kircher T, Nelson J, Burdo H: The autopsy as a measure of accuracy of the death certificate, *N Engl J Med* 313:1263-1269, 1985.
4. Nielsen GP, Björnsson J, Jonasson JG: The accuracy of death certificates. Implications for health statistics, *Virchows Arch A Pathol Anat Histopathol* 419:143-146, 1991.
5. Hunt R, Barr P: Errors in the certification of neonatal death, *J Paediatr Child Health* 36:498-501, 2000.
6. Smith Sehdev AE, Hutchins GM: Problems with proper completion and accuracy of the cause-of-death statement, *Arch Intern Med* 161:277-284, 2001.
7. Swift B, West K: Death certification: An audit of practice entering the 21st century, *J Clin Pathol* 55:275-279, 2002.
8. Santoso JT, Lee CM, Aronson J: Discrepancy of death diagnosis in gynecology oncology, *Gynecol Oncol* 101:311-314, 2006.
9. Ravakhah K: Death certificates are not reliable: Revivification of the autopsy, *South Med J* 99:728-733, 2006.
10. Biggs MJP, Brown LJR, Rutty GN: Can cause of death be predicted from the pre-necropsy information provided in coroners' cases? *J Clin Pathol* 61:124-126, 2008.
11. James DS, Bull AD: Information on death certificates: Cause for concern? *J Clin Pathol* 49:213-216, 1995.
12. Leadbeatter S: Semantics of death certification, *J R Coll Physicians Lond* 20:129-132, 1986.
13. Jordan JM, Bass MJ: Errors in death certificate completion in a teaching hospital, *Clin Invest Med* 16:249-255, 1993.
14. Freedman MA, Rushford GA, McQuillen EN, Baron KP: Issues related to the medical certification of death: A physician survey, *N Y State J Med* 88:522-525, 1988.
15. James DS, Bull AD: Death certification: Is correct formulation of cause of death related to seniority or experience? *J R Coll Physicians Lond* 29:424-428, 1995.
16. World Health Organization: *Medical certification of cause of death,* Geneva, 1979, World Health Organization.
17. World Health Organization: *International statistical classification of diseases and related health problems,* rev 10, Geneva, 1992-1994, World Health Organization.
18. Hanzlick R: Death certificates: The need for further guidance, *Am J Forensic Med Pathol* 14:249-252, 1993.
19. Davis GG, Onaka AT: Report on the 2003 revision of the U.S. standard certificate of death, *Am J Forensic Med Pathol* 22:38-42, 2001.
20. Hanzlick R: The relevance of queries and coding procedures to the writing of cause-of-death statements, *Am J Forensic Med Pathol* 17:319-323, 1996.
21. Hopkins DD, Grant-Worley JA, Bollinger TL: Survey of cause-of-death query criteria used by state vital statistics programs in the US and the efficacy of the criteria used by the Oregon Vital Statistics Program, *Am J Public Health* 79:570-574, 1989.
22. Hanzlick R: Improving accuracy of death certificates, *JAMA* 269:2850, 1993.
23. Kircher T, Anderson RE: Cause of death: Proper completion of the death certificate, *JAMA* 258:349-352, 1987.

| Box 13-9 | Cause-of-death statements for fetal deaths |
|---|---|
| **Cause of death** | **Specify fetal or maternal** |
| a. Intrauterine fetal demise | Fetal |
| *due to, or as a consequence of:* | |
| b. Retroplacental bleeding (abruptio placentae) | Maternal |
| *due to, or as a consequence of:* | |
| c. Pregnancy-induced hypertension | Maternal |
| Other significant fetal or maternal conditions: Maternal diabetes mellitus | |
| **Cause of death** | **Specify fetal or maternal** |
| a. Severe prematurity | Fetal |
| *due to, or as a consequence of:* | |
| b. Premature labor | Maternal |
| *due to, or as a consequence of:* | |
| c. Acute *Escherichia coli* chorioamnionitis | Maternal |
| Other significant fetal or maternal conditions: Maternal urinary tract infection | |
| **Cause of death** | **Specify fetal or maternal** |
| a. Intrauterine fetal demise | Fetal |
| *due to, or as a consequence of:* | |
| b. Idiopathic (nonimmune) hydrops fetalis | Fetal |

24. Hanzlick R: Principles for including or excluding "mechanisms" of death when writing cause-of-death statements, *Arch Pathol Lab Med* 121:377-380, 1997.
25. Klatt EC, Noguchi TT: Death certification: Purposes, procedures, and pitfalls, *West J Med* 151:345-347, 1989.
26. Weiner L, Bellows MT, McAvoy GH, Cohen EV: Use of multiple causes in the classification of deaths from cardiovascular-renal disease, *Am J Public Health* 45:492-501, 1955.
27. Dorn HF, Moriyama IM: Uses and significance of multiple cause tabulations for mortality statistics, *Am J Public Health* 54:400-406, 1964.
28. Petty CS: Multiple causes of death: The viewpoint of a forensic pathologist, *J Forensic Sci* 10:167-178, 1965.
29. Goodman RA, Manton KG, Nolan TF Jr, et al: Mortality data analysis using a multiple-cause approach, *JAMA* 247:793-796, 1982.
30. Olson FE, Norris FD, Hammes LM, Shipley PW: A study of multiple causes of death in California, *J Chronic Dis* 15:157-170, 1962.
31. White MC, Selvin S, Merrill DW: A study of multiple causes of death in California: 1955 and 1980, *J Clin Epidemiol* 42:355-365, 1989.
32. Newens AJ, Forster DP, Kay DWK: Death certification after a diagnosis of presenile dementia, *J Epidemiol Community Health* 47:293-297, 1993.
33. Wing S, Manton KG: A multiple cause of death analysis of hypertension-related mortality in North Carolina, 1968-1977, *Am J Public Health* 71:823-830, 1981.
34. White MC: Mortality associated with nosocomial infections: Analysis of multiple cause-of-death data, *J Clin Epidemiol* 46:95-100, 1993.
35. Fife D: Injuries and deaths among elderly persons, *Am J Epidemiol* 126:936-941, 1987.
36. Mackenbach JP, Kunst AE, Lautenbach H, et al: Competing causes of death: An analysis using multiple-cause-of-death data from The Netherlands, *Am J Epidemiol* 141:466-475, 1995.
37. National Center for Health Statistics: Multiple causes of death in the United States, *Mon Vital Stat Rep* 32(Suppl 2):1-5, 1984.
38. Guralnick L: Some problems in the use of multiple causes of death, *J Chronic Dis* 19:979-990, 1966.
39. Wong O, Rockette HE, Redmond CK, Heid M: Evaluation of multiple causes of death in occupational mortality studies, *J Chronic Dis* 31:183-193, 1978.
40. Israel RA, Rosenberg HM, Curtin LR: Analytical potential for multiple cause-of-death data, *Am J Epidemiol* 124:161-179, 1986.
41. World Health Organization: *International classification of diseases (ICD)*, http://www.who.int/classifications/icd/en/, WHO, 2007.
42. National Center for Health Statistics: *International classification of diseases*, rev 9, Clinical Modification (ICD-9-CM). http://www.cdc.gov/nchs/about/otheract/icd9/abticd9.htm, NCHS, 2008.
43. Wetli CV, Mittleman RE, Rao VJ: *Practical forensic pathology*, New York, 1988, Igaku-Shoin.
44. Murphy GK: The "undetermined" ruling: A medicolegal dilemma, *J Forensic Sci* 24:483-491, 1979.
45. Murphy GK: Therapeutic misadventure. An 11-year study from a metropolitan coroner's office, *Am J Forensic Med Pathol* 7:115-119, 1986.
46. Hirsch CS, Morris RC, Moritz AR: *Handbook of legal medicine*, ed 5, St. Louis, 1979, Mosby.
47. U.S. Department of Health and Human Services PHS, Centers for Disease Control and Prevention, National Center for Health Statistics: *Hospitals' and physicians' handbook on birth registration and fetal death reporting* (DHHS Publication No. [PHS] 87-1107), Hyattsville, Md, 1987, USDHHS. Also available at www.cdc.gov/nchs/data/misc/hb_birth.pdf.
48. Department of Health and Human Services, Centers for Disease Control and Prevention, National Center for Health Statistics: *Medical examiners' and coroners' handbook on death registration and fetal death reporting, 2003 revision* (DHHS Publication No. [PHS] 2003-1110), Hyattsville, Md, 2003, USDHHS. Also available at www.cdc.gov/nchs/vital_certs_rev.htm.
49. Department of Health and Human Services, Centers for Disease Control and Prevention, National Center for Health Statistics: *Physicians' handbook on medical certification of death. 2003 revision* (DHHS Publication No. [PHS] 2003-1108), Hyattsville, Md, 2003, USDHHS. Also available at www.cdc.gov/nchs/vital_certs_rev.htm.
50. Hanzlick R, editor: *Cause of death and the death certificate. Important information for physicians, coroners, medical examiners, and the public*, Northfield, Ill, 2006, College of American Pathologists.
51. Hanzlick R: *Writing cause-of-death statements*, http://thename.org/index.php?option=com_content&task=view&id=108&Itemid=58, National Association of Medical Examiners.

# 14

# Medical Quality Improvement and Quality Assurance of the Autopsy

*"I like to ask this question, and you might find it helpful also, 'How do you assess the quality of care given to your sickest patients, the ones who die?' Unless the A word (autopsy) comes out right away, they flunk."*

George D. Lundberg[1]

*"In all cases of interest, therefore, the physician should feel it a duty which he owes to himself and the profession at large, to seek permission to make a post-mortem examination; but in order that the fullest benefit be derived from the same, he must know how to look for what he is in search of, and how to recognize it when found."*

A. R. Thomas[2]

Even in an era of declining autopsy rates, the autopsy continues to play a prominent role in medical quality improvement, particularly in health care facilities that support educational or academic programs. These sites remain the bastion for preserving and improving autopsy performance and perhaps someday restoring it as one of the principal methods of medical quality assurance. In the future, only vigorous efforts by pathologists to extend traditional excellence in clinicopathologic correlation by incorporating technologic advances in autopsy practice will ensure continued use of the autopsy in the medical audit.

## THE AUTOPSY AND MEDICAL QUALITY IMPROVEMENT

Despite advances in imaging techniques and laboratory diagnosis, an autopsy is still the most accurate way to identify the cause or causes of death. In fact, even as medicine becomes more advanced technologically, the autopsy continues to disclose undiagnosed conditions contributing to the cause of death. A survey of discrepancies between clinical and postmortem findings reported since the early twentieth century is shown in Table 14-1. Although the methods used by the investigators vary, the studies indicate that the autopsy continues to be a useful tool for quality assessment, a statement supported by a systematic comparison of clinical errors detected by autopsy from published studies, including many of those listed.[36]

Postmortem examinations help identify misdiagnosis or unexpected findings in patients dying from trauma,[37] cancer,[38-40] or sudden death[41]; after surgery[42-46]; during the perinatal period[47-55] or when elderly[56,57]; or while receiving care in the emergency department,[58-61] intensive care unit,[62,63] or psychiatric hospital.[64] The data from autopsy studies may have direct and indirect effects on the living. Faye-Petersen and colleagues[65] found that fetal and perinatal autopsies altered genetic counseling and recurrence risk estimates in 26% of cases in which an autopsy was performed. The autopsy remains the standard for assessing the diagnostic accuracy of imaging studies.[66] In addition, in studies too numerous to cite, postmortem examination continues to play an important role in identifying or evaluating therapeutic complications.

In relation to its role in the medical audit, the autopsy complements clinical and laboratory medicine by providing definitive diagnoses. It follows, therefore, that the autopsy should play a significant role in hospital quality improvement programs. In fact, postmortem examination provides the framework for assessing not only the quality of clinical diagnoses but also the effects of a chosen therapy. The coding system of Goldman and coworkers[9] as modified by Battle and associates[24] (Table 14-2) can be used effectively in autopsy-based quality assessment programs.[67-69]

**Table 14-1**    Survey of some clinical-postmortem discrepancies reported since the early twentieth century

| Year(s) of study | Number of cases studied | Cases with significant clinical-postmortem discrepancies (%) | Reference |
|---|---|---|---|
| ~1912 | 3000 | 5 | 3 |
| 1919 | 600 | 8 | 4 |
| 1949 | 1000 | 12 | 5 |
| 1947-1953 | 1106 | 9 | 6 |
| 1958 | 265 | 7 | 7 |
| 1959 | 100 | 7 | 8 |
| 1960 | 100 | 22 | 9 |
| 1961-1970 | 4688 | 23 | 10 |
| 1969 | 100 | 12 | 8 |
| 1970 | 200 | 8 | 11 |
| 1970 | 100 | 23 | 9 |
| 1970-1971 | 383 | 14 | 12 |
| 1972-1974 | 1000 | 36 | 13 |
| 1973 | 252 | 12 | 14 |
| 1973-1982 | 2537 | 10 | 15 |
| 1974-1978 | 1076 | 9 | 16 |
| 1977-1978 | 1455 | 27 | 17 |
| 1975-1977 | 1152 | 39 | 18 |
| 1976-1977 | 1096 | 19 | 19 |
| 1978-1987 | 7028 | 18 | 10 |
| 1979 | 100 | 12 | 8 |
| 1979-1982 | 100 | 13 | 20 |
| 1981-1984 | 2145 | 29 | 21 |
| 1983 | 111 | 13 | 22 |
| 1983-1988 | 1000 | 32 | 23 |
| 1980 | 100 | 21 | 9 |
| 1984 | 2067 | 36 | 24 |
| 1984-1985 | 233 | 12 | 25 |
| 1986 | 60 | 20 | 26 |
| 1987-1988 | 1436 | 22 | 17 |
| 1988 | 108 | 44 | 27 |
| 1988-1991 | 213 | 12 | 28 |
| 1989 | 100 | 11 | 8 |
| 1993 | 2479 | 40 | 29 |
| 1994 | 176 | 45 | 30 |
| 1994-1995 | 91 | 19 | 31 |
| 1996-1998 | 88 | 34 | 32 |
| 1998-2001 | 38 | 39 | 33 |
| 1999-2005 | 291 | 17 | 34 |
| 1999-2005 | 86 | 26 | 35 |

## QUALITY ASSURANCE OF THE AUTOPSY

The Autopsy Committee of the College of American Pathologists (CAP) has published practice guidelines for autopsy pathology.[70-73] The committee promotes improvement in autopsy diagnosis through its performance improvement program for participating laboratories.[74] Recently, the College has assembled a program for quality management in anatomic pathology that includes recommendations for autopsy performance improvement.[75] Others[27,76-78] have also outlined quality control and assurance programs for autopsies. However, the accuracy of autopsy diagnosis has rarely come under serious scrutiny. From a survey of hospital clinicians, Fowler and colleagues[13] found that with respect to answering physicians' questions, autopsies were judged satisfactory in 83%, partially satisfactory in 12%, and unsatisfactory in 2% of the examinations, respectively. A prospective audit of autopsy performance revealed that in 3 of 99 cases in which a clinician's questions were not answered definitively, the root cause was failure of the prosector to do a thorough postmortem dissection.[22] In a study of 125 autopsies performed at a university teaching hospital, Bayer-Garner and colleagues[79] found that the tasks most frequently asked of the autopsy pathologists by the clinical staff were to identify the pathologic conditions responsible for the clinical picture, to confirm a suspected diagnosis, and to determine the cause of death. Of 100 questions asked before these autopsies, 78.6% were answered in the final anatomic diagnosis, 9.7% were addressed in some part of the autopsy report, 9.7% were not addressed at all, and 1.9% could not be answered by the autopsy report. Veress and colleagues[80] compared intraobserver variability among four pathologists at the same institution with respect to macroscopic diagnoses and immediate cause of death. Although they found a high level of agreement on major diagnoses, there were moderate discrepancies in assigning the immediate cause of death and in identification of minor diseases.

Zarbo and coworkers[81] reviewed completeness of information on autopsy consent forms, time intervals between patients' deaths and postmortem examination, and turnaround time of reports listing preliminary autopsy diagnoses. Although their study identified fairly consistent documentation on autopsy permit forms and greater than 80% compliance with the CAP's laboratory standards for completion of preliminary or provisional autopsy reports, a wide range of time intervals was found between patients' deaths and start of the postmortem examination. A similar study of final autopsy report turnaround time revealed that 47.6% were completed in 30 days or less, 28.8% in 31 to 60 days, 12.2% in 61 to 90 days, and 11.5% in more than 90 days.[82] Thus, even if all these cases were to be considered complicated, an astonishingly high number of cases exceeded the 60-day (Joint Commission on Accreditation of Healthcare Organizations; JCAHO) and even the 90-day (CAP) guidelines of the two major laboratory certifying organizations of the United States.

It is unlikely that autopsy practice will receive any additional financial support or direct reimbursement by third-party payers. Furthermore, reinstatement of minimal autopsy requirements for hospital, residency, and managed care plan accreditation is not on the horizon. Thus, impetus for improving autopsy practice will remain exclusively the responsibility of pathology departments and pathologists who practice in the community, at a medical college, or at the local coroner's or medical examiner's office. Fortunately, autopsy pathologists and their institutions can accomplish significant quality assurance by following straightforward guidelines and ensuring adequate communication with clinicians, next of kin, and hospital quality-of-care committees (Boxes 14-1, 14-2, and 14-3; Table 14-3).

The first step in performing an autopsy is the review of the medical record. The pathologist must obtain a clear understanding of the patient's present and past medical history,

**Table 14-2**     Classification of diagnostic errors: premortem and postmortem diagnostic discrepancies and their etiology*

| Classification of premortem and postmortem diagnostic discrepancies | | Types of error by etiology | | |
|---|---|---|---|---|
| **Major** | | | **Type of error** | **Definition** |
| Class I | Discrepancy of a primary[†] diagnosis with adverse impact on survival | Category A | Imperfect medical knowledge | Unavoidable. Limitations in contemporary capability |
| Class II | Discrepocal of a primary[†] diagnosis with equivocal impact on survival | Category B | Necessary fallibility | Unavoidable. Patient, physician, environmental variables |
| **Minor** | | Category C | Practitioner error | Personal limitation of knowledge or skill; inaccurate technical data |
| Class III | Discrepancy of a secondary[†] diagnosis not directly related to the cause of death but either (1) was symptomatic and should have been treated or (2) would have eventually affected prognosis | Category D | Willful or malicious error | Negligent or willful disregard of accepted norms |
| Class IV | Discrepancy of a secondary[†] diagnosis that could not have been recognized before death | Category E | No discrepancy | |
| Class V | Nondiscrepant diagnosis | | | |

*Diagnostic errors are classified by both class and category.
[†]Primary diagnoses are those involving the principal underlying cause of death and major contributors thereto; secondary diagnoses are antecedent conditions, related diagnoses, contributing causes, or other important conditions.
Modified from Anderson RE, Hill RB, Gorstein F: A model for the autopsy-based quality assessment of medical diagnostics, *Hum Pathol* 21:174-181, 1990; and Gorovitz S, MacIntyre A: Toward a theory of medical fallibility. In Engelhardt HT, Callahan D, editors: *Science, ethics, and medicine*, Hastings-on-Hudson, NY, 1976, Hastings Center, pp 1149-1156.

therapeutic interventions, and the terminal events leading to the patient's death. Review of the medical record should include a review of relevant laboratory data, reports of imaging studies, and surgical pathology or cytopathology reports or material. Before beginning the prosection, the pathologist must attempt to get in touch with the patient's primary physician or physicians. The clinician usually has extensive knowledge of the patient developed over days, weeks, or even years of contact. It cannot be overemphasized how useful a brief discussion of the case with the treating clinicians can be in clarifying the clinical thought processes during the management of the patient's care. Discussion of the case with the clinician is part of the role of the pathologist as consultant. This provides the pathologist with an opportunity to ask the clinician about unresolved issues and concerns that arose during the patient's illness.

A thorough understanding of the clinical issues and questions allows the pathologist to anticipate the need for special studies that might elucidate anatomic diagnoses or best demonstrate pathologic findings. Is there a need for electron microscopy or immunofluorescence? Should any tissues or fluids be submitted for microbiologic cultures or collected for biochemical analysis? Should the pathologist alter his or her usual prosection technique or dissect an anatomic site not

**Box 14-1**     Items that should be included in an autopsy policy and procedure manual

Handling of the body
Written policies related to the autopsy permit and
  consent process
Accessioning of autopsies
Duties of the autopsy assistants
Biosafety and hygiene policies
Equipment maintenance

**Box 14-2**     Some important components of the Commission on Laboratory Accreditation of the College of American Pathologists autopsy performance quality control and assurance checklists

Are all autopsies performed, or directly supervised, by a
  pathologist qualified in anatomic pathology?
Is a documented preliminary report of the gross pathologic
  diagnoses submitted to the attending physician and the
  institutional record within a reasonable time (2 working days)?
Are the majority of autopsy final reports produced within
  30 days?
For all cases, is the final autopsy report produced within 60 days?
Are gross and microscopic descriptions clear and concise, and are
  all pertinent findings adequately described?
If microscopic descriptions are included in the report, do they
  support the diagnoses?
Does the final autopsy report contain sufficient information in
  an appropriate format to ascertain the patient's major disease
  processes and probable cause of death?
Are autopsy records organized and readily available for review?
Are major diagnoses indexed and recorded for retrieval?

Modified from Commission on Laboratory Accreditation: *Laboratory accreditation program. Anatomic pathology checklist*, Northfield, Ill, 2001, College of American Pathologists.

**Box 14-3** Improving autopsy performance through communication

Carefully review the decedent's clinical history and terminal clinical events and make contact with the primary clinician(s) before performing the autopsy. Identify the pertinent clinical questions and concerns. Assess the need for supplemental autopsy procedures.

Communicate effectively with clinicians following the prosection, following the microscopic evaluation, and if necessary during the preparation of the final report. Upon completion of the autopsy, invite the clinician to review the gross pathologic findings.

Ensure timeliness in the delivery of an accurate and thorough autopsy report that addresses the concerns of the clinicians, correlates the pathology findings with the clinical events, and identifies the cause(s) of death.

Ensure that there is a mechanism of communication between family members receiving autopsy reports and the primary clinician or autopsy pathologist.

Communicate effectively with clinical departments and participate regularly in quality improvement programs.

**Table 14-3** Recommendations for retention of materials related to the autopsy

| Item | Minimal recommended length of storage |
|---|---|
| Autopsy consent and accession records | 5 years |
| Quality assurance documentation | 2 years |
| Wet tissue | 6 months |
| Gross photographs | 5 years |
| Paraffin blocks | 5 years |
| Histologic sections | 20 years |
| Autopsy reports | 20 years |

Data from Travers H: *Quality improvement manual in anatomic pathology,* Northfield, Ill, 1993, College of American Pathologists.

normally examined? Would radiography or angiography enhance the examination? The pathologist and his or her staff can make ready needed equipment and supplies before beginning the case.

After completing the prosection, the pathologist should communicate his or her findings to the patient's clinicians. The clinical team should be invited to visit the autopsy suite during or after the autopsy. Regrettably, attendance of clinicians at autopsies is often prohibited by other demands on their time.[83] Recognizing this, the pathologist should be flexible in meeting with the clinical staff. Active dialogue with the physicians who cared for the patient during life allows the autopsy pathologist to make a greater contribution. Questions remaining after the gross autopsy can be addressed by engaging the clinicians again during a review of the microscopic findings

and reassessment of the case as a whole. The clinician's knowledge of the pathophysiology of a specific case can help the pathologist interpret the morphologic findings more accurately.

The autopsy pathologist is a consultant specialist. As such, the pathologist must report the anatomic findings to the responsible clinician in a timely manner. The preliminary or provisional autopsy report should be available within 48 hours; however, sooner—for example, the same day—is better. We feel that the final autopsy report, including neuropathologic findings, should be completed in 30 calendar days or less. This falls under both CAP and Joint Commission guidelines and regulations for routine cases. For a few rare cases requiring special studies that delay the autopsy report, we suggest that an interim report (including a statement specifying pending studies or consultations, or both) be completed by 30 days and that the subsequent findings and additional interpretations be communicated as soon as possible.

The clinician is in the best position to interpret the autopsy for the family, taking the anatomic data and placing them in a clinical context. Many clinicians meet with the family to explain the autopsy report. Nevertheless, some families contact the pathology department directly. If so, send a copy of the report together with a cover letter encouraging the family to reach the clinician to discuss the contents. At the same time, we notify the attending clinician and supply him or her with an additional copy of the autopsy report and the address and telephone numbers of the next of kin so that contact can be initiated. An example of a letter to the next of kin or other individual authorizing the autopsy is shown in Figure 14-1.[84]

Peer review can serve as an easy check on autopsy quality. At academic medical centers this is part of the teaching program; autopsy faculty review findings at a daily or weekly gross conference, or "organ recital." Periodic conferences held at a multiheaded teaching microscope corroborate, elucidate, or correct gross pathologic specimen interpretations and provide a forum for discussion of the most significant clinicopathologic correlations. In the community, pathology groups can identify an appropriate time for peer review of difficult autopsy cases.

## QUALITY IMPROVEMENT OF THE AUTOPSY

### Continuing Medical Education

Continued quality improvement of the autopsy relies on the efforts of the pathologist to stay abreast of current issues in medicine. Reading the current medical literature, researching specific topics pertinent to a specific autopsy, and seeking appropriate consultations from experts are the keys to developing and maintaining competence. Attending continuing medical education courses and seminars covering autopsy technique, diagnosis, and reporting that are given at national and international meetings and participating in quality improvement programs offered by the various pathology societies are important components of autopsy quality improvement. The CAP provides a number of outstanding educational programs and autopsy-related diagnostic and laboratory performance improvement subscription programs.

Dear (Name of Individual Who Authorized the Autopsy):


This letter is an expression of our sympathy at the recent death of your [Relationship of the

Deceased to the Letter Recipient]. We want to thank you for allowing the physicians of [Name of

Health Care Institution] to perform an autopsy.


The autopsy examination is performed by certified pathologists in [Name of Health Care

Institution]. This examination enables us to make a detailed analysis of the cause of death, the

nature of the disease(s), and the effects of treatment. The information that this examination

provides is essential for the advancement of medical science.


Enclosed you will find the final autopsy report of your [relationship of the Deceased to the

Letter Recipient]. A report of the autopsy findings has also been sent to your physician

[Physician's Name, Address and Office Telephone Number]. The results of the autopsy can be

discussed with your physician or, if you desire, with us.


Sincerely,


[Signature]

**Figure 14-1**  Example of a letter to an individual authorizing an autopsy.
(Modified from Travers H: *Quality improvement manual in anatomic pathology,* Northfield, Ill, 1993, College of American Pathologists.)

## Autopsy Report Turnaround Time

The autopsy pathologist earns the respect of his or her clinical colleagues by providing accurate consultative reports in a timely fashion. Autopsies do not require months to complete. Clinicians should receive the autopsy report while the clinical issues of the case are still fresh in their minds. Timeliness in the academic medical center takes on greater importance because the house staff is likely to rotate to other services or even other hospitals before a tardy autopsy report is completed. Several pathologists have suggested ways to speed the completion of the final autopsy report.[85-87]

## Improving Autopsy Rates

Perhaps the most effective way to improve the rate of autopsies is through a decedent affairs office fully staffed by individuals trained in obtaining autopsy consents.[88,89] Unfortunately, in this age of cost containment, in which hospital administrations are focused primarily on cutting costs and reducing hospital staff, such services are being cut. Enlisting and training nursing personnel to play a greater role in obtaining autopsy consents remains one option. The autopsy can be discussed at the same time that families are offered the opportunity to donate the organs or tissues of the deceased. McPhee[90] provides advice on the announcement of a death and request for autopsy (Table 14-4).

In many health care settings, the physician, as the individual who most often discusses the deaths of patients with the families, remains the most obvious individual to obtain permission for postmortem examination. However, regardless of which group of health care workers seeks to obtain autopsy consent, the process is improved by developing programs that train health care workers in postmortem and other decedent affairs.[91,92] Clearly, when clinicians who are adept at approaching families for autopsy consent are motivated to obtain autopsy consents as part of their clinical research programs, high autopsy rates are the usual result.[93,94] Although pathologists may not be able to provide the incentives for clinicians to increase their rate of obtaining autopsy consents, the

**Table 14-4** Methods of announcing a death and requesting an autopsy

| Announcing a death | Requesting an autopsy |
| --- | --- |
| Decide who should announce the death (primary care, attending, or house staff physician) | Decide who should request the autopsy (primary care, attending, or house staff physician; nurse; chaplain; or social worker) |
| Arrange in-person conference, avoid telephone | State autopsy request simply and directly |
| Announce death briefly and explicitly | Explain rationale |
| Express sympathy, support | Discuss potential family benefits |
| Review illness, mode of death | Mention particular expectations |
| Answer questions, concerns | Explain use, training of pathologists |
| Allow time for ventilation | Address possible concerns (e.g., disfigurement, delay of funeral, or cost) |
| Address emotional needs | Discuss organ or tissue donation |
| Accompany family to the bedside | Address possible restrictions |
| | Discuss reporting of results |
| | Make a commitment to ensure follow-up |

From McPhee SJ: Maximizing the benefits of autopsy for clinician and families: What needs to be done, *Arch Pathol Lab Med* 120:743-748, 1996. (Reprinted with permission from Archives of Pathology & Laboratory Medicine, copyright College of American Pathologists.)

pathologists or their advocates on the clinical staff of their respective hospitals can certainly promote programs designed to help physicians obtain autopsy consent. Nowhere is this more important than in medical schools and teaching hospitals, where training in this aspect of medicine is often inadequate or even absent.[95,96]

## Regional Autopsy Centers

Ultimately, the autopsy pathologist will succeed in promoting the autopsy only by demonstrating its value in clinicopathologic correlation, thereby instilling a positive attitude regarding autopsies in the clinical staff.[97] The most visionary idea to improve autopsy quality is the proposal to establish regional autopsy centers with well-trained pathologists and assistants.[98-100] Regional centers of excellence in autopsy pathology would serve both small and large health care institutions. They could be located at regional medical examiners' offices, university medical centers, or other teaching hospitals. Given the limited resources made available for autopsy services, creating autopsy centers of excellence might allow the autopsy pathologist to incorporate the technological advances,

**Box 14-4** A schedule for training the specialist in autopsy pathology

Anatomic pathology (24-30 months, unless no clinical pathology, then 36 months)
  Basic autopsy pathology (4 months)
  Surgical pathology (10 months)
  Cytology (4 months)
  Postmortem neuropathology (2 months)
  Electives (4-10 months)
Clinical pathology (18-24 months)
Autopsy-related fellowship (12-24 months)
  Forensic pathology, or
  Pediatric pathology, or
  Autopsy pathology fellowship, or
  Specialized fellowship (e.g., cardiovascular, pulmonary, renal pathology, neuropathology) that includes additional training in postmortem methods

such as postmortem imaging and molecular diagnostics, so badly needed to invigorate this venerable procedure.

## Autopsy Training

Improved autopsy quality depends on pathologists with specialized expertise in the discipline of postmortem pathology. If regional autopsy centers ever become reality, residency and fellowship training in pathology could be tailored to better prepare the autopsy pathologist. One possible schedule of specialized training is listed in Box 14-4. Others have also been suggested.[101]

## CONCLUSION

The case for the value of the postmortem examination should not be based solely on studies demonstrating that the autopsy uncovers unexpected causes of death or untreated conditions in a high percentage of cases. The pathologist must demonstrate skill in all aspects of autopsy performance: prosection, correlation of clinical medicine with pathologic findings, and communication of final results in a coherent and vital autopsy report. An accurate and instructive autopsy report must be communicated in a timely manner. The report must help the clinical team correlate clinical impressions, diagnostic studies, and therapeutic management of the case with the final outcome. As the treating physician uses all the technology available for clinical diagnosis, the autopsy pathologist should likewise incorporate into autopsy performance whatever technology is appropriate. Finally, just as the clinician asks the autopsy pathologist to investigate an unsuccessful clinical outcome, the pathologist must critically evaluate his or her own work with the goal of improving the practice of autopsy pathology.

## REFERENCES

1. Lundberg GD: College of American Pathologists Conference XXIX on Restructuring Autopsy Practice for Health Care Reform. Let's make this autopsy conference matter, *Arch Pathol Lab Med* 120:736-738, 1996.

2. Thomas AR: *A practical guide for making post-mortem examinations, and for the study of morbid anatomy, with directions for embalming the dead, and for the preservation of specimens of morbid anatomy,* New York, 1873, Boericke & Tafel.

3. Cabot RC: Diagnostic pitfalls identified during a study of three thousand autopsies, *JAMA* 59:2295-2298, 1912.

4. Karsner HT, Rothschild L, Crump ES: Clinical diagnosis as compared with necropsy findings in 600 cases, *JAMA* 80:737-740, 1919.

5. Munck W: Autopsy finding and clinical diagnosis. A comparative study of 1,000 cases, *Acta Med Scand* 266:775-781, 1952.

6. Gruver RH, Freis ED: A study of diagnostic errors, *Ann Intern Med* 47:108-120, 1957.

7. Wilson RR: In defense of the autopsy, *JAMA* 196:1011-1012, 1966.

8. Kirch W, Schafii C: Misdiagnosis at a university hospital in 4 medical eras: Report on 400 cases, *Medicine (Baltimore)* 75:29-40, 1996.

9. Goldman L, Sayson R, Robbins S, et al: The value of the autopsy in three medical eras, *N Engl J Med* 308:1000-1005, 1983.

10. Grundmann E, Menke GG: Autopsy diagnosis versus clinical diagnosis, particularly in malignant disease, comparison of two periods: 1961-70 and 1978-87. In Riboli E, Delendi M, editors: *Autopsy in epidemiology and medical research.* Lyon, France, 1991, International Agency for Research on Cancer, pp 81-90.

11. Holler JW, De Morgan NP: A retrospective study of 200 postmortem examinations, *J Med Educ* 45:168-170, 1970.

12. Britton M: Diagnostic errors discovered at autopsy, *Acta Med Scand* 196:203-210, 1974.

13. Fowler EF, Nicol AG, Reid IN: Evaluation of a teaching hospital necropsy service, *J Clin Pathol* 30:575-578, 1977.

14. Burrows S: The postmortem examination: Scientific necessity or folly? *JAMA* 233:441-443, 1975.

15. Friederici HHR, Sebastian M: Autopsies in a modern teaching hospital, *Arch Pathol Lab Med* 108:518-521, 1984.

16. Clark MA: The value of the hospital autopsy: Is it worth the cost? *Am J Forensic Med Pathol* 2:231-237, 1981.

17. Veress B, Alafuzoff I: Clinical diagnostic accuracy audited by autopsy in a university hospital in two eras, *Qual Assur Health Care* 5:281-286, 1993.

18. Cameron HM, McGoogan E: A prospective study of 1152 hospital autopsies: II. Analysis of inaccuracies in clinical diagnoses and their significance, *J Pathol* 133:285-300, 1981.

19. Sandritter W, Staeudinger M, Drexler H: Autopsy and clinical diagnosis, *Pathol Res Pract* 168:107-114, 1980.

20. Scottolini A, Weinstein SR: The autopsy in clinical quality control, *JAMA* 250:1192-1194, 1983.

21. Stevanovic G, Tucakovic G, Dotlic R, Kanjuh V: Correlation of clinical diagnoses with autopsy findings: A retrospective study of 2,145 consecutive autopsies, *Hum Pathol* 17:1225-1230, 1986.

22. Schned AR, Mogielnicki RP, Stauffer ME: A comprehensive quality assessment program on the autopsy service, *Am J Clin Pathol* 86:133-138, 1986.

23. Sarode VR, Datta BN, Banerjee AK, et al: Autopsy findings and clinical diagnoses: A review of 1,000 cases, *Hum Pathol* 24:194-198, 1993.

24. Battle RM, Pathak D, Humble CG, et al: Factors influencing discrepancies between premortem and postmortem diagnoses, *JAMA* 258:339-344, 1987.

25. Landefeld CS, Chren M-M, Myers S, et al: Diagnostic yield of the autopsy in a university hospital and a community hospital, *N Engl J Med* 318:1249-1254, 1988.

26. Peacock SJ, Machin D, Duboulay CE, Kirkham N: The autopsy: A useful tool or an old relic? *J Pathol* 156:9-14, 1988.

27. Harrison M, Hourihane DOB: Quality assurance programme for necropsies, *J Clin Pathol* 42:1190-1193, 1989.

28. Mitchell ML: Interdepartmental quality assurance using coded autopsy results, *Mod Pathol* 6:48-52, 1993.

29. Zarbo RJ, Baker PB, Howanitz PJ: The autopsy as a performance measurement tool—diagnostic discrepancies and unresolved clinical questions, *Arch Pathol Lab Med* 123:191-198, 1999.

30. Nichols L, Aronica P, Babe C: Are autopsies obsolete? *Am J Clin Pathol* 110:210-218, 1998.

31. Tai DYH, El-Bilbeisi H, Tewari S, et al: A study of consecutive autopsies in a medical ICU: A comparison of clinical cause of death and autopsy diagnosis, *Chest* 119:530-536, 2001.

32. Durning S, Cation L: The educational value of autopsy in a residency training program, *Arch Intern Med* 160:997-999, 2000.

33. Perkins GD, McAuley DF, Davies S, Gao F: Discrepancies between clinical and postmortem diagnoses in critically ill patients: An observational study, *Crit Care* 7:R129-R132, 2003 (doi 10.1186/cc2359; http://ccforum.com/content/7/6/R129 [accessed October 6, 2008].)

34. Tavora F, Crowder CD, Sun C-C, Burke A: Discrepancies between clinical and autopsy diagnoses: A comparison of university, community and private autopsy practices, *Am J Clin Path* 129:102-109, 2008.

35. Pastores SM, Dulu A, Voigt L, et al: Premortem clinical diagnoses and postmortem autopsy findings: Discrepancies in critically ill cancer patients, *Crit Care* 11:R48, 2007. (doi:10.1186/cc5782; http://ccforum.com/content/11/2/R48 [accessed October 6, 2008].).

36. Shojania KG, Burton EC, McDonald KM, Goldman L: Changes in rates of autopsy-detected diagnositic errors over time: A systematic review, *JAMA* 289:2849-2856, 2003.

37. Stuart RD: The autopsy, *J Pathol* 175:453-460, 1995.

38. Koszyca B, Moore L, Toogood I, Byard RW: Is postmortem examination useful in pediatric oncology? *Pediatr Pathol* 13:709-715, 1993.

39. dePangher Manzini V, Revignas MG, Brollo A: Diagnosis of malignant tumor: Comparison between clinical and autopsy diagnosis, *Hum Pathol* 26:280-283, 1995.

40. Sirkiä K, Saarinen-Pihkala UM, Hovi L, Sariola H: Autopsy in children with cancer who die while in terminal care, *Med Pediatr Oncol* 30:284-289, 1998.

41. Lundberg GD, Voigt GE: Reliability of a presumptive diagnosis in sudden unexpected death in adults. The case for the autopsy, *JAMA* 242:2328-2330, 1979.

42. Stothert JC Jr, Gbaanador G: Autopsy in general surgery practice, *Am J Surg* 162:585-588, 1991.

43. Shanks JH, Anderson NH, McCluggage G, Toner PG: Use of the autopsy in Northern Ireland and its value in perioperative deaths. In Riboli E, Delendi M, editors: *Autopsy in epidemiology and medical research,* Lyon, France, 1991, International Agency for Research on Cancer, pp 115-124.

44. Barendregt WB, de Boer HHM, Kubat K: The results of autopsy of patients with surgical diseases of the digestive tract, *Surg Gynecol Obstet* 175:227-232, 1992.

45. Zehr KJ, Liddicoat JR, Salazar JD, et al: The autopsy: Still important in cardiac surgery, *Ann Thorac Surg* 64:380-383, 1997.

46. Acosta S, Krantz P: Trends in prevalence of fatal surgical diseases at forensic autopsy, *ANZ J Surg* 77:718-721, 2007.

47. Valdés-Dapena M, Arey JB: The causes of neonatal mortality: An analysis of 501 autopsies on newborn infants, *J Pediatr* 77:366-375, 1970.

48. Gau G: The ultimate audit, *Br Med J* 1:1580-1581, 1977.

49. Craft H, Brazy JE: Autopsy: High yield in neonatal population, *Am J Dis Child* 140:1260-1262, 1986.

50. Meier PR, Manchester DK, Shikes RH, et al: Perinatal autopsy: Its clinical value, *Obstet Gynecol* 67:349-351, 1986.

51. Rushton DI: West Midlands perinatal mortality survey, 1987. An audit of 300 perinatal autopsies, *Br J Obstet Gynaecol* 98:624-627, 1991.

52. Hägerstrand I, Lundberg L-M: The importance of postmortem examinations of abortions and perinatal deaths, *Qual Assur Health Care* 5:295-297, 1993.

53. Husain AN, O'Conor GT: The perinatal autopsy: A neglected source of discovery. In Riboli E, Delendi M, editors: *Autopsy in epidemiology and medical research*, Lyon, 1991, International Agency for Research on Cancer, pp 151-162.

54. Bosman C, Boldrini R, Falcocchio G: Role of necropsy at neonatal and infantile ages. In Riboli E, Delendi M, editors: *Autopsy in epidemiology and medical research*, Lyon, France, 1991, International Agency for Research on Cancer, pp 163-175.

55. Criscuolo M, Migaldi M, Botticelli AR, Losi L: Pathological findings in perinatal autopsies. In Riboli E, Delendi M, editors: Autopsy in epidemiology and medical research, Lyon, France, 1991, International Agency for Research on Cancer, pp 177-181.

56. Puxty JAH, Horan MA, Fox RA: Necropsies in the elderly, *Lancet* 1:1262-1264, 1983.

57. Bauco C, Arabia A, Salza MC, et al: Autopsy study of very old hospitalized patients, *Arch Gerontol Geriatr Suppl* 5:437-440, 1996.

58. Burke MC, Aghababian RV, Blackbourne B: Use of autopsy results in the emergency department quality assurance plan, *Ann Emerg Med* 19:363-366, 1990.

59. Whitehouse SR, Kisoon N, Singh N, Warren D: The utility of autopsies in a pediatric emergency department, *Pediatr Emerg Care* 10:72-75, 1994.

60. Vanbrabant P, Dhondt E, Sabbe M: What do we know about patients dying in the emergency department? *Resuscitation* 60:163-170, 2004.

61. Mushtaq F, Ritchie D: Do we know what people die of in the emergency department? *Emerg Med J* 22:718-721, 2005.

62. Papadakis MA, Mangione CM, Lee KK, Kristof M: Treatable abdominal pathologic conditions and unsuspected malignant neoplasms at autopsy in veterans who received mechanical ventilation, *JAMA* 265:885-887, 1991.

63. Blosser SA, Zimmerman HE, Stauffer JL: Do autopsies of critically ill patients reveal important findings that were clinically undetected? *Crit Care Med* 26:1332-1336, 1998.

64. Ferencic Z, Belicza M: Autopsy and clinical diagnoses in a psychiatric hospital. In Riboli E, Delendi M, editors: *Autopsy in epidemiology and medical research*, Lyon, France, 1991, International Agency for Research on Cancer, pp 109-113.

65. Faye-Petersen OM, Guinn DA, Wenstrom KD: Value of perinatal autopsy, *Obstet Gynecol* 94:915-920, 1999.

66. Jonasson JG: Autopsy: Clinicopathological concordance and imaging techniques. In Riboli E, Delendi M, editors: *Autopsy in epidemiology and medical research*, Lyon, France, 1991, International Agency for Research on Cancer, pp 91-98.

67. Boers M: The prospects of autopsy: Mortui vivos docuerunt? [Have the dead taught the living? *Am J Med* 86:322-324, 1989.

68. Anderson RE, Hill RB, Gorstein F: A model for the autopsy-based quality assessment of medical diagnostics, *Hum Pathol* 114:174-181, 1990.

69. Saracci R: Is necropsy a valid monitor of clinical diagnosis performance? *Br Med J* 303:898-900, 1991.

70. Hutchins GM: Practice guidelines for autopsy pathology: Autopsy performance. Autopsy Committee of the College of American Pathologists, *Arch Pathol Lab Med* 118:19-25, 1994.

71. Hutchins GM, Berman JJ, Moore GW, Hanzlick R: Practice guidelines for autopsy pathology: Autopsy reporting. Autopsy

Committee of the College of American Pathologists, *Arch Pathol Lab Med* 123:1085-1092, 1999.

72. Powers JM: Practice guidelines for autopsy pathology: Autopsy procedures for brain, spinal cord, and neuromuscular system. Autopsy Committee of the College of American Pathologists, *Arch Pathol Lab Med* 119:777-783, 1995.

73. Bove KE: Practice guidelines for autopsy pathology: The perinatal and pediatric autopsy. Autopsy Committee of the College of American Pathologists, *Arch Pathol Lab Med* 121:368-376, 1997.

74. Derman H, Wagner LR: The College of American Pathologists, 1946-1996: Anatomic and consultative pathology practice, *Arch Pathol Lab Med* 121:1214-1222, 1997.

75. Nakhleh RE, Fitzgibbons PL: *Quality management in anatomic pathology: Promoting patient safety through systems improvement and error reduction*, Northfield, Ill, 2005, College of American Pathologists.

76. Travers H: Quality assurance indicators in anatomic pathology, *Arch Pathol Lab Med* 114:1149-1156, 1990.

77. Young NA, Naryshkin S: An implementation plan for autopsy quality control and quality assurance, *Arch Pathol Lab Med* 117:531-534, 1993.

78. Association of Directors of Anatomic and Surgical Pathology, Nakhleh R, Coffin C, Cooper K: Recommendations for quality assurance and improvement in surgical and autopsy pathology, *Am J Clin Pathol* 126:337-340, 2006.

79. Bayer-Garner IB, Fink LM, Lamps LW: Pathologists in a teaching institution assess the value of the autopsy, *Arch Pathol Lab Med* 126:442-447, 2002.

80. Veress B, Gadaleanu V, Nennesmo I, Wikstrom BM: The reliability of autopsy diagnostics: Inter-observer variation between pathologists: a preliminary report, *Qual Assur Health Care* 5:333-337, 1993.

81. Zarbo RJ, Baker PB, Howanitz PJ: Quality assurance of autopsy permit form information, timeliness of performance, and issuance of preliminary report: A College of American Pathologists Q-probes study of 5434 autopsies from 452 institutions, *Arch Pathol Lab Med* 120:346-352, 1996.

82. Zarbo RJ: Quality assessment in anatomic pathology in the cost-conscious era, *Am J Clin Pathol* 106(Suppl 1):S3-S10, 1996.

83. Friederici HHR, Sebastian M: An argument for the attendance of clinicians at autopsy, *Arch Pathol Lab Med* 108:522-523, 1984.

84. Travers H, editor: *Quality improvement manual in anatomic pathology*, Northfield, Ill, 1993, College of American Pathologists, 1993.

85. Benbow EW, Howard JC: Speeding up necropsy histology reports in a teaching hospital, *J Clin Pathol* 46:567-568, 1993.

86. Adickes ED, Sims KL: Enhancing autopsy performance and reporting: A system for a 5-day completion time, *Arch Pathol Lab Med* 120:249-253, 1996.

87. Rosai J: The posthumous analysis (PHA): An alternative to the conventional autopsy, *Am J Clin Pathol* 106(Suppl 1):S15-S17, 1996.

88. Haque AK, Cowan WT, Smith JH: The Decedent Affairs Office: A unique centralized service. *JAMA* 266:1397-1399, 1991.

89. Haque AK, Patterson RC, Grafe MR: High autopsy rates at a university medical center. What has gone right? *Arch Pathol Lab Med* 120:727-732, 1996.

90. McPhee SJ: Maximizing the benefits of autopsy for clinicians and families: What needs to be done, *Arch Pathol Lab Med* 120:743-748, 1996.

91. Smith RD, Zumwalt RE: One department's experience with increasing the autopsy rate, *Arch Pathol Lab Med* 108:455-457, 1984.

92. Clayton SA, Sivak SL: Improving the autopsy rate at a university hospital, *Am J Med* 92:423-428, 1992.

93. King EM, Smith A, Jobst KA: Autopsy: Consent, completion and communication in Alzheimer's disease research, *Age Ageing* 22:209-214, 1993.

94. Fillenbaum GG, Huber MS, Beekly D, et al: The Consortium to Establish a Registry for Alzheimer's Disease (CERAD). Part XIII, *Neurology* 46:142-145, 1996.

95. Katz JL, Gardner R: The intern's dilemma: The request for autopsy consent, *Psychol Med* 3:197-203, 1972.

96. Chana J, Rhys-Maitland R, Hon P, et al: Who asks permission for an autopsy? *J R Coll Physicians Lond* 24:185-188, 1990.

97. Champ C, Tyler X, Andrews PS, Coghill SB: Improve your hospital autopsy rate to 40-50 percent: A tale of two towns, *J Pathol* 166:405-407, 1992.

98. Hutchins GM: Whither the autopsy? . . . To regional autopsy centers, *Arch Pathol Lab Med* 120:718, 1996.

99. Trelstad RL, Amenta PS, Foran DJ, Smilow PC: The role for regional autopsy centers in the evaluation of covered deaths: Survey of opinions of US and Canadian chairs of pathology and major health insurers in the United States, *Arch Pathol Lab Med* 120:753-758, 1996.

100. Horowitz RE, Naritoku WY: The autopsy as a performance measure and teaching tool, *Hum Pathol* 38:688-695, 2007.

101. Roberts WC: The autopsy: Its decline and a suggestion for its revival, *N Engl J Med* 299:332-338, 1978.

# 15

# Atlas of Autopsy Pathology

*Remember, then, that the great bulk of our knowledge of the origin and progression of most diseases has been slowly acquired by painstaking observations.*

Howard W. Florey[1]

## EXTERNAL FINDINGS

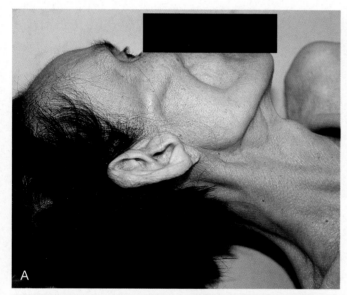

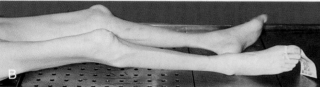

**Figure 15-1** Cachexia. The general state of nourishment of the deceased should be assessed at autopsy. **A,** In this individual with cachexia from colon cancer, the skin is thin, dry, sallow, and drawn tight over bony prominences. The eyes are sunken, and the temporal regions and cheeks are hollowed. **B,** The extremities show generalized loss of subcutaneous fat and wasting of skeletal muscle.

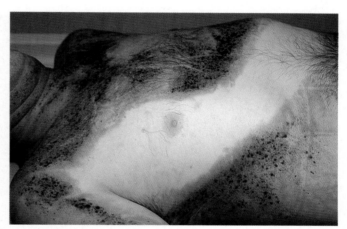

**Figure 15-2** Livor mortis (lividity). Violaceous livor mortis develops in dependent areas of the body as blood pools in small vessels after the circulation ceases. Areas of the body resting against firm surfaces remain pale in contrast to surrounding areas of lividity. This individual was found dead in a prone position, his right arm underneath him, preventing postmortem hypostasis. Lividity develops in 30 minutes to 2 hours. It reaches its maximum from 8 to 18 hours, depending on local conditions. After a somewhat variable time period dependent on environment, livor becomes "fixed" and does not blanch to applied pressure or change on repositioning of the body. Sometimes, the pressure of the pooling blood can even rupture small vessels, resulting in postmortem purpura or petechial-type hemorrhages know as Tardieu spots, such as those seen in this decedent. Note that the Tardieu spots are not present where the arm was compressed against the chest.

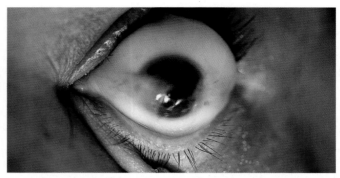

**Figure 15-3** Pterygia. Generally found in middle-aged or elderly individuals, these are localized, elevated, yellow-white areas that develop on the conjunctiva and cornea. Located most often nasally but sometimes temporally, pterygia are generally bilateral. In this example there are both nasal and temporal lesions. The conjunctival component of pterygium is identical histologically to pingueculae, lesions that involve only the conjunctiva.

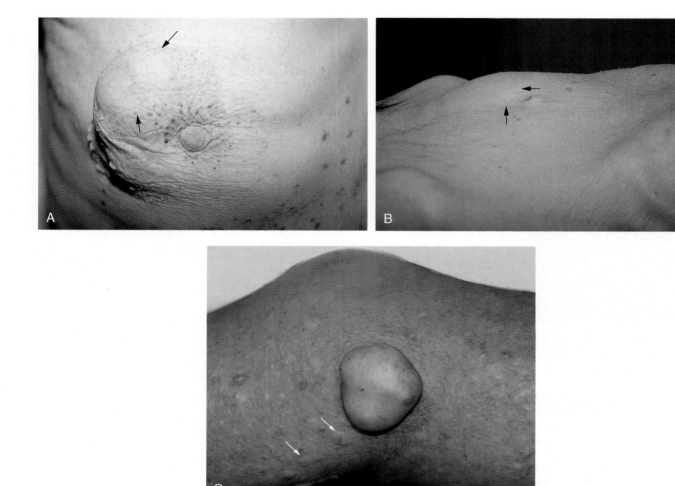

**Figure 15-4** Visible or palpable masses. Before beginning the prosection, the body regions should be inspected and palpated in order to detect masses or other abnormalities. **A,** A mass *(arrows)* is visible in the superolateral quadrant of the right breast. **B,** A mass *(arrows)* can be seen in the right lower quadrant of the abdomen. **C,** This patient with neurofibromatosis, type 1 has hundreds of small cutaneous neurofibromas *(arrows)* and several large, pedunculated lesions such as this one present on his leg. Café au lait macules were also present (see Figure 15-7, B).

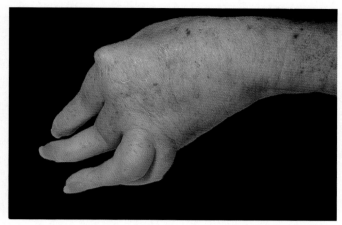

**Figure 15-5** This patient with rheumatoid arthritis had ulnar deviation of the phalanges from subluxations of the metacarpophalangeal joints.

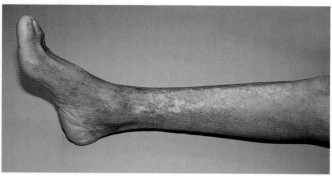

**Figure 15-8** Stasis dermatitis. This common condition begins as red, scaly patches that become vesicular and crusted. Hyperpigmentation or atrophic scarring, or both, follows healing. Varying degrees of stasis dermatitis affect virtually the entire right lower leg of this elderly patient.

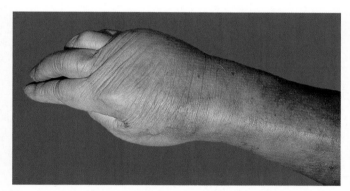

**Figure 15-6** Edema. Examination of the hand of a patient who died of septic shock from infective endocarditis shows peripheral edema.

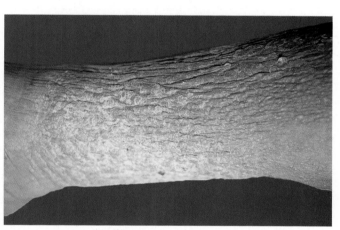

**Figure 15-9** Lymphedema. Lymphatic obstruction related to metastatic prostate carcinoma has led to chronic lymphedema with brawny induration. This lower extremity has a scaly, irregular surface.

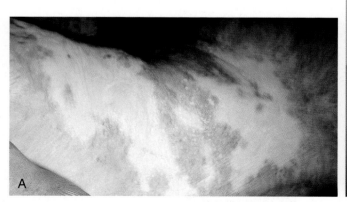
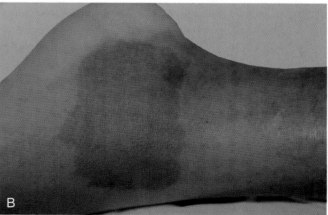

**Figure 15-7** Abnormalities of pigmentation. **A,** Vitiligo appears as irregular areas of depigmented skin with occasional hyperpigmented borders. **B,** Café au lait spots are round to ovoid, hyperpigmented macules often lying over nerve trunks. They may be seen in normal individuals; however, the presence in an adult of six or more macules greater than 1.5 cm indicates neurofibromatosis type 1.

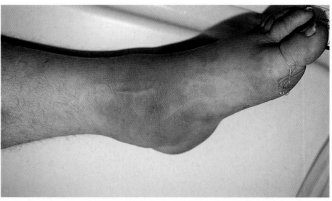

**Figure 15-10** Cellulitis. Marked erythema of the skin and swelling of the subcutaneous tissues are present overlying an infected ankle joint.

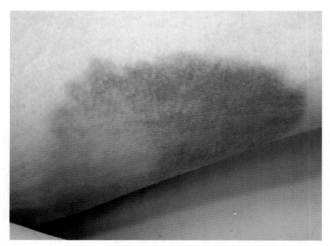

**Figure 15-11** Contusions (bruises) indicate hemorrhage into the skin or subcutaneous tissues, or both. Contusions change color from blue-red to dark purple, green, yellow, and brown over time, the exact length dependent on the extent and depth of the contusion and the local circulation.

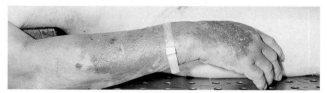

**Figure 15-12** Ecchymoses are often seen in patients receiving long-term corticosteroid therapy and in elderly persons after minor trauma (senile purpura). The numerous ecchymoses seen on the hand and arm of this elderly individual were associated with trauma from placement of intravenous catheters.

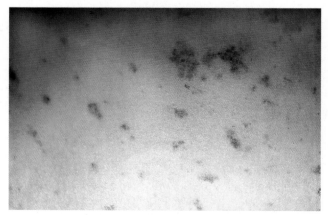

**Figure 15-13** Petechiae and purpural hemorrhages related to disseminated intravascular coagulation in meningococcemia.

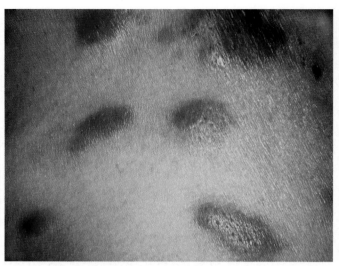

**Figure 15-14** Kaposi's sarcoma. Multiple red-purple, slightly raised nodules associated with herpesvirus type 8 infection in an individual with acquired immunodeficiency syndrome (AIDS).

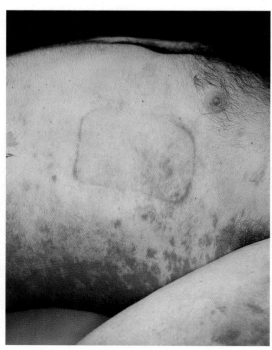

**Figure 15-15** Rectangular "paddle" marks from an attempted defibrillation.

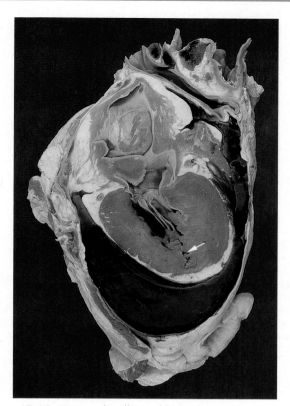

**Figure 15-16** Hemopericardium. This specimen demonstrates massive hemopericardium, the basis for cardiac tamponade in this patient with a ruptured transmural infarct of the apex of the left ventricle. A narrow tract *(arrow)* through the necrotic muscle indicates the point at which cardiac rupture occurred.

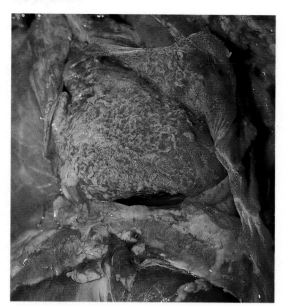

**Figure 15-18** Suppurative pericarditis. Suppurative pericarditis follows infection of the pericardial space by bacterial, fungal, or parasitic organisms and (rarely) viral infections. Infections reach the pericardial sac by direct extension, hematogenous or lymphatic spread, or direct inoculation after regional trauma or surgery. The pericardial surfaces are red, granular, and coated with exudate, and the pericardial cavity contains purulent fluid. In this case of infective *(Staphylococcus aureus)* pericarditis that followed open heart surgery, the thick parietal pericardium has been reflected to show the purulent exudate covering the epicardial surface in the fresh specimen. After fixation of the heart, the exudate can appear much less impressive, but the abnormal dullness of the epicardial surface that remains is key.

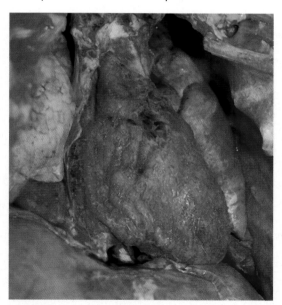

**Figure 15-17** Fibrinous and serofibrinous pericarditis. The most common forms of pericarditis, fibrinous pericarditis and serofibrinous pericarditis, are typically caused by uremia, radiation to the thorax, rheumatic fever, systemic lupus erythematosus, trauma, cardiac surgery, and myocardial infarcts (Dressler syndrome). With or without a pericardial effusion, pericarditis is readily identified at the autopsy table. The parietal pericardium is thick because of edema, inflammatory cells, fibrin, and other components of active inflammation. This is visible in the epicardium as loss of the shiny, smooth appearance. In this example of acute fibrinous pericarditis, the surface of the heart is covered by a shaggy coat of inflammatory debris.

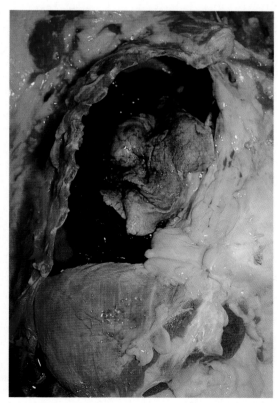

**Figure 15-19** Noninflammatory collections of fluid in the pleural cavities may consist of serous fluid, lymph (chylothorax), or blood (hemothorax). Hemothorax such as shown here is usually a complication of traumatic injury.

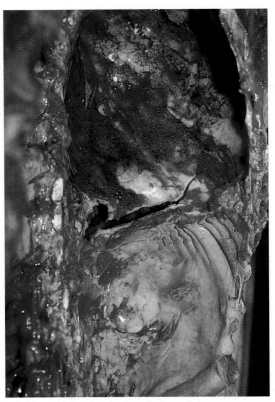

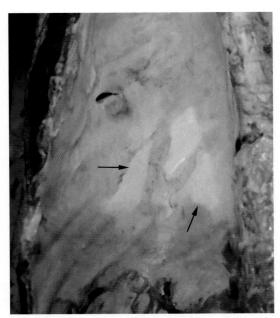

**Figure 15-22** Pleural plaques. Pleural plaques *(arrows)* are raised fibrous lesions on the superior surface of the diaphragm or the parietal pleura found in the lower lung zones, such as shown here. They are found in association with asbestos exposure but also occur after resolution of hemothorax, empyema, or traumatic injury.

**Figure 15-20** Acute serofibrinous pleuritis related to pneumonia. The serous, serofibrinous, and fibrinous forms of pleuritis develop in the setting of inflammation from pneumonia, pulmonary infarcts, collagen vascular disease, uremia, radiation, or malignant neoplasms metastatic to the pleura.

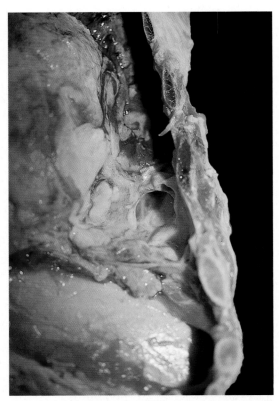

**Figure 15-21** Suppurative pleuritis (empyema). Empyema usually develops from spread of bacterial or fungal infections of the lung parenchyma. Rarely, empyema develops after subdiaphragmatic infections, more commonly on the right side from liver abscesses. In this example of empyema developing as a complication of bacterial pneumonia of the left lower lobe of the lung, the inferior left pleural cavity is filled with yellow pus.

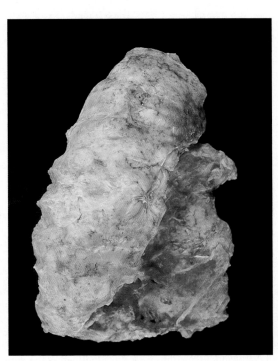

**Figure 15-23** Malignant mesothelioma. A thick rind of tumor totally encases this left lung. These neoplasms are usually associated with exposure to fibrous minerals, asbestos, or erionite; however, some cases lack a definable cause. Other neoplasms that involve the pleura include soft tissue sarcomas generally arising from the chest wall and lymphomas.

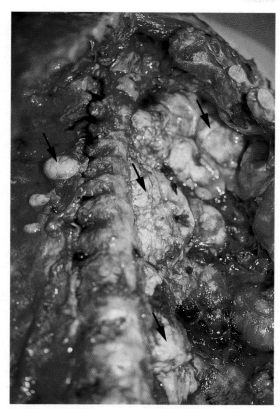

**Figure 15-24** Metastatic malignant melanoma involving the parietal pleura *(arrows)*. The most common type of tumor to involve the pleura is carcinoma, either as a distant metastasis or by direct extension from a peripheral lung carcinoma, usually adenocarcinoma.

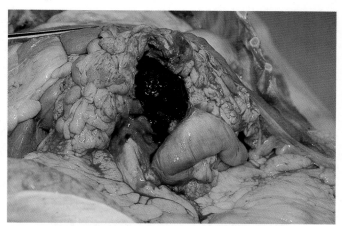

**Figure 15-26** Hemoperitoneum. As in the pleural cavities, collections of serous, serosanguineous, and lymph fluid may accumulate in the peritoneal cavity. Hemoperitoneum may result from rupture of blood vessels. In this patient, retroperitoneal hemorrhage developed after perforation of a posterior gastric ulcer.

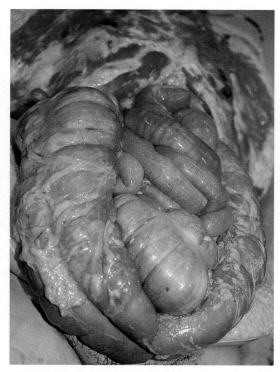

**Figure 15-25** Dilation of the small and large intestines. Dilation of the intestines is a common finding at autopsy. It is generally due to adynamic ileus caused by a variety of infectious and inflammatory processes, the postoperative state, or electrolyte abnormalities. Dilated bowel may also be seen in association with mechanical obstruction or bowel ischemia. This photograph shows dilated loops of small and large bowel in a patient with *Clostridium perfringens* enterocolitis.

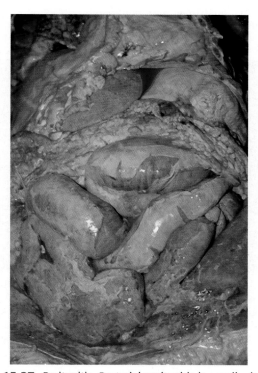

**Figure 15-27** Peritonitis. Bacterial peritonitis is usually due to rupture of a hollow viscus or extension of bacteria through the wall of the gastrointestinal tract, gallbladder, or fallopian tube. Although the exact mechanism is not understood, spontaneous bacterial peritonitis may also develop in patients with chronic ascites. In this patient with peritonitis, virtually the entire serosal surface of the intestines, as well as the liver capsule, is covered with a shaggy, fibrinous exudate.

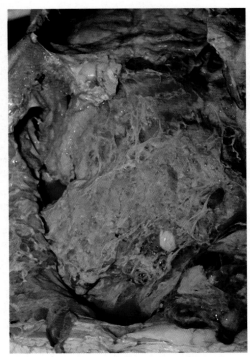

**Figure 15-28** Peritonitis may also occur in response to chemical irritation (e.g., from bile or material from ruptured dermoid cysts), abrasion of serosal surfaces during surgery, introduction of foreign material (e.g., surgically introduced talc), or blood from peritoneal implants of endometriosis. In this patient with bile leakage after biliary tract surgery, fibrinous exudate associated with peritonitis obscures the intraabdominal anatomy.

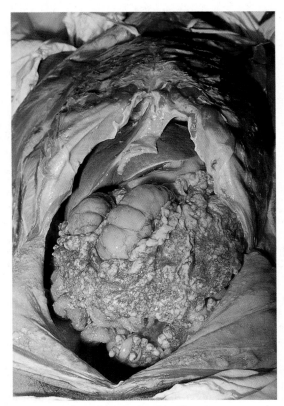

**Figure 15-30** Tuberculous peritonitis. The omentum and serosal surfaces of the abdominal organs demonstrate numerous caseating granulomas.

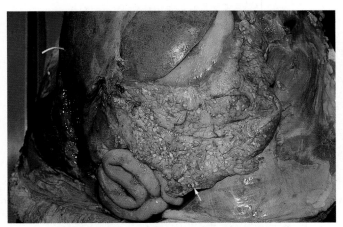

**Figure 15-29** Omentum with fat necrosis. Pancreatitis resulting in the release of pancreatic enzymes has produced multifocal areas of necrosis *(arrow)* of the omental fat. Enzymatic digestion of fat results in chalky white precipitates from fatty acid precipitation of calcium. This patient also had terminal liver failure, causing the generalized yellow appearance.

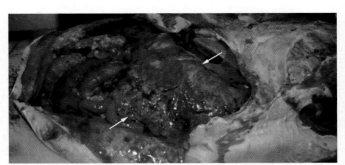

**Figure 15-31** Carcinoma metastatic to peritoneum. Primary malignant mesotheliomas and tumors arising from the peritoneal mesenchymal tissues are quite rare; however, extension of tumors from abdominal organs and metastatic seeding of the peritoneum are common. Diffuse metastatic seeding of the peritoneum (peritoneal carcinomatosis) occurs most commonly from carcinomas of the ovary and pancreas. The extensive peritoneal metastasis shown here *(arrows)* arose from an esophageal primary.

## CARDIOVASCULAR SYSTEM

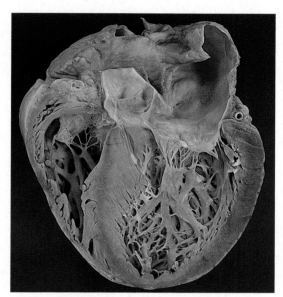

**Figure 15-32** Dilated cardiomyopathy. The left ventricular long-axis cut of this enlarged heart shows a portion of the mitral valve, the left ventricular inlet and outlet, and a portion of the aortic valve; the right ventricle is also in the view. Both ventricular cavities are dilated, and hypertrophy is present, denoted by increased thickness of the free walls and septum. The myocardium is homogeneously dark red; there is no visible scar. Atrial dilation in this case of cardiomyopathy is not well illustrated in this view.

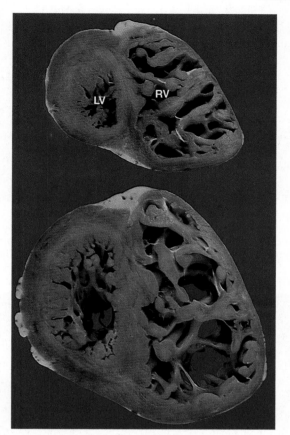

**Figure 15-34** Right ventricular hypertrophy. These short-axis cuts of the heart from an adult with a congenital ventricular septal defect show the right ventricular hypertrophy and marked cavity dilation that are associated with long-standing pulmonary hypertension. In the normal heart, the right ventricular apex does not quite reach the apex of the heart, so in this specimen the apical cut (top) is particularly revealing. The left ventricle is relatively normal. *RV,* Right ventricle; *LV,* left ventricle.

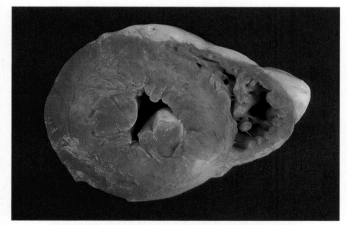

**Figure 15-33** Left ventricular hypertrophy. The short-axis plane of section shows the cavities and entire circumference of the ventricular walls to good advantage. In this patient with hypertension, the left ventricular cavity is small because of concentric hypertrophy of the walls and papillary muscles.

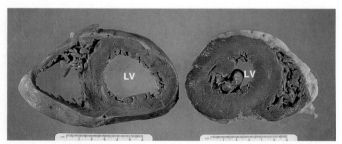

**Figure 15-35** Concentric and eccentric hypertrophy. The difference between concentric hypertrophy and eccentric hypertrophy is illustrated in these two short-axis cuts from two different hearts of approximately the same weight (*left,* 575 g; *right,* 600 g). In the specimen on the left, the left ventricular cavity *(LV)* is dilated and the walls appear nearly normal in thickness. In contrast, the heart on the right has very thick left ventricular walls that diminish the cavity. Both specimens showed histopathologic features of hypertrophy.

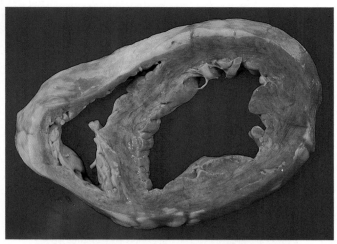

**Figure 15-36** Dilated cardiomyopathy. The short-axis cut of a heart with dilated cardiomyopathy shows enlarged left and right ventricular cavities, as well as septum and walls of relatively normal thickness. The mottled myocardium was firm, consistent with fibrosis.

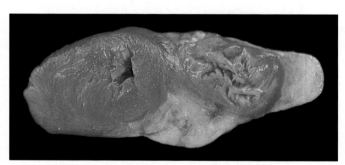

**Figure 15-37** Right ventricular hypertrophy and dilation. Normally, the right ventricular apex does not quite reach the apex of the heart. This apical cut of a heart from a patient with chronic liver disease shows the right ventricular cavity, consistent with pulmonary hypertension.

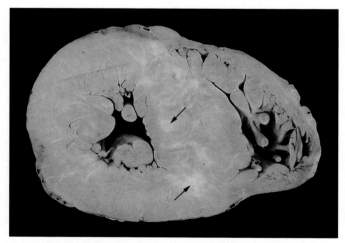

**Figure 15-38** Hypertrophic cardiomyopathy. This short-axis cut comes from the heart of an adolescent patient who died suddenly. Although there is generalized hypertrophy (including small ventricular cavities), the septum of this heart is disproportionately thick (defined as a ratio of septum to left ventricular free wall greater than 1.3). In addition, the septum contains numerous scars *(arrows)* indicative of healed ischemic damage. No significant coronary artery atherosclerosis was seen, and the ischemic damage resulted from demand-perfusion mismatch in this massively hypertrophied heart.

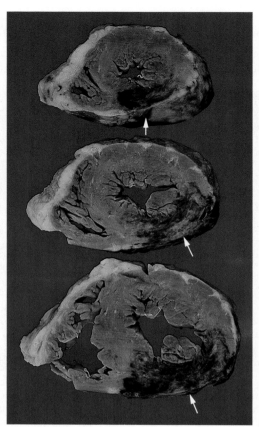

**Figure 15-39** These short-axis cuts demonstrate a transmural hemorrhagic infarct *(arrows)* from ischemic damage that occurred 2 or 3 days before death. Segmental in distribution, this infarct in the posterolateral left ventricle was correlated with an occlusion of the right coronary artery.

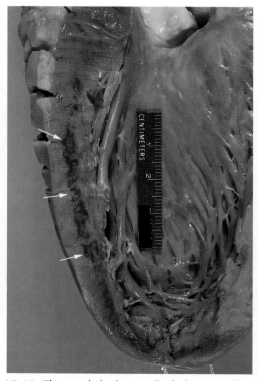

**Figure 15-40** The mottled, abnormally dark myocardium *(arrows)* of this left ventricle indicates a recent infarct. The ischemic damage is located in the inner one-half of the wall—defined as *subendocardial* as compared with *transmural*.

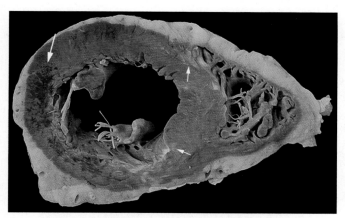

**Figure 15-41** This short-axis cut disclosed several infarcts of different ages. The dark myocardium in the posterolateral left ventricle *(large arrow)* denotes a recent large infarct less than a week old. In the posterior and anterior septum, scars *(small arrows)* associated with healed infarcts from ischemic damage months to years before death can be seen. Because scars contract over time, it is impossible to be certain of the true extent of the damage during the acute phase.

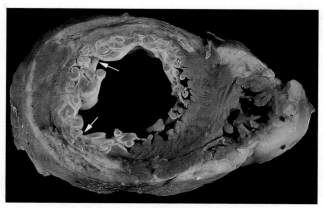

**Figure 15-43** The short-axis cut of this specimen demonstrates several areas of scarring denoting healed ischemic damage. There is extensive subendocardial infarct *(arrows)*, as well as two areas in which the damage is present throughout the entire wall, from endocardium to epicardium. The variegated appearance of the scars suggests surviving myocardium within the area of healed infarct. The fibrotic endocardium overlying the infarct may reflect a response to increased wall stress in this region.

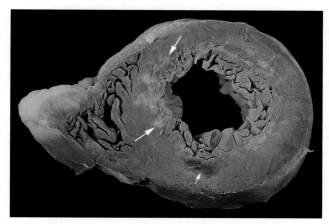

**Figure 15-44** This heart has several subendocardial infarcts of different ages. The patch of dark myocardium *(small arrow)* denotes a recent infarct from ischemic damage occurring several days before death. Numerous scars *(large arrows)* indicate healed damage from much older insults. This patient had atherosclerosis markedly narrowing all the major extramural coronary arteries.

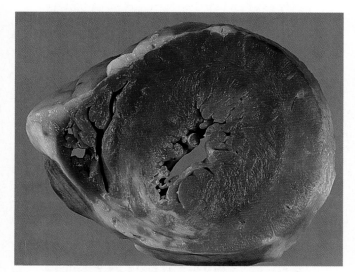

**Figure 15-42** This short-axis slice demonstrates a transmural lesion localizing ischemic damage that occurred months or years before death. The scar *(arrow)* indicates a healed infarct. The posteroseptal lesion correlated with an occlusion of the right coronary artery. Undoubtedly, there was hypertrophy in the remaining viable myocardium (because of loss of muscle); however, part of the massive concentric hypertrophy must be attributed to uncontrolled hypertension in this case.

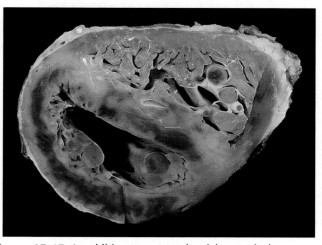

**Figure 15-45** In addition to spectacular right ventricular hypertrophy, this short-axis cut of the heart from a patient with repaired congenital heart defects demonstrates extensive hemorrhagic infarct. The generalized subendocardial distribution is consistent with a low-output state that led to underperfusion of the coronary arteries 2 to 3 days before death.

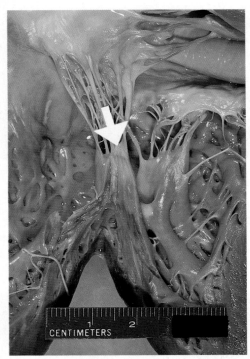

**Figure 15-46** Even in patients without clinical evidence of mitral valve dysfunction, the tips of the papillary muscles should be examined for signs of ischemic damage *(arrow)*. Considered subendocardium, this part of the myocardium is at greatest risk for ischemic damage in any number of settings. In this specimen there is scar signifying a healed infarct from remote injury.

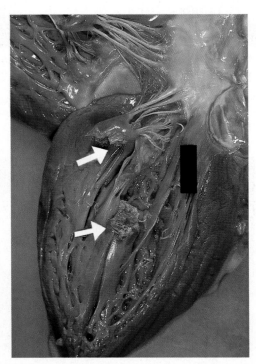

**Figure 15-47** Cardiac rupture may be a consequence of a transmural myocardial infarct and almost always leads to serious morbidity with high mortality. In the patient whose heart is pictured here, acute transmural infarction led to papillary muscle rupture *(arrows)*, the basis for heart failure related to mitral insufficiency. Another site of rupture is shown in Figure 15-16.

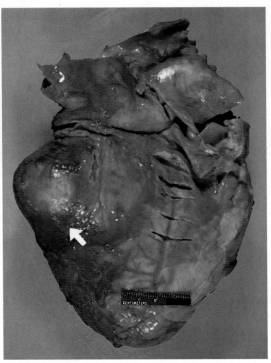

**Figure 15-48** From the diaphragmatic surface, an aneurysm related to a posteroinferior left ventricular infarct is indicated by the localized bulge of the heart *(arrow)*.

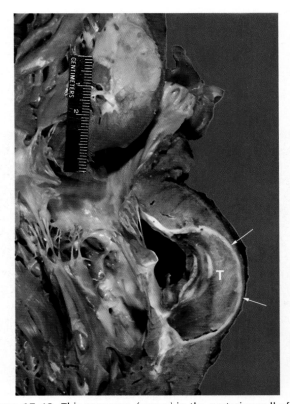

**Figure 15-49** This aneurysm *(arrows)* in the posterior wall of the left ventricle represents a healed transmural infarct. The endocardium is fibrotic, and the scar is very thin. This region had been dyskinetic, and there is an organizing thrombus *(T)* filling the aneurysm.

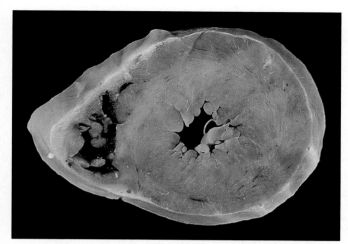

**Figure 15-50** Myocarditis. The heart with myocarditis may appear normal or dilated with hypertrophy, depending on the duration of the inflammatory process before death. As shown here, the myocardium may appear mottled with pale foci or small hemorrhages signifying active inflammation. With chronicity of the myocarditis, hypertrophy may develop, although confounding preexisting conditions such as hypertension must be considered.

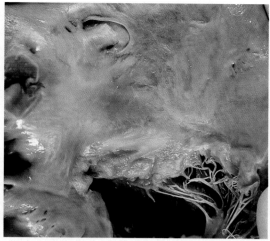

**Figure 15-52** The heart with significant deposits of amyloid is firm and rubbery. This specimen demonstrates subendocardial amyloid, with irregular gray atrial lesions after fixation. The cut surface of an amyloid-infiltrated heart appears smooth and glassy.

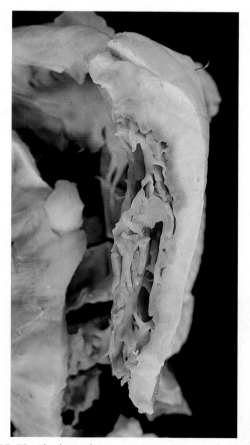

**Figure 15-53** The heart from a patient with arrhythmogenic right ventricular dysplasia often exhibits a unique gross appearance with fibro-fatty tissue replacing muscle in the right ventricular apex, free wall of the right ventricle adjacent to the diaphragm, or anterior infundibulum (the so-called triangle of dysplasia). In this heart from a young man who died suddenly, a cross section of the right ventricular free wall demonstrates several areas in which the muscle has been replaced by fibro-fatty tissue. Although the left ventricle may show a similar change, the right ventricle is characteristically the more severely affected chamber.

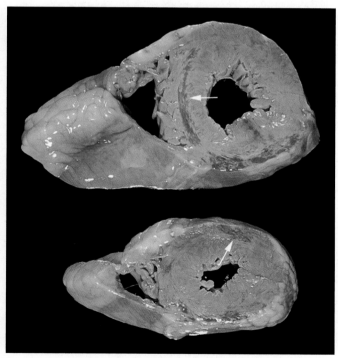

**Figure 15-51** Giant cell myocarditis. This type of rapidly progressive myocarditis has a poor prognosis and generally shows widespread areas of hemorrhage and necrosis *(arrows)*.

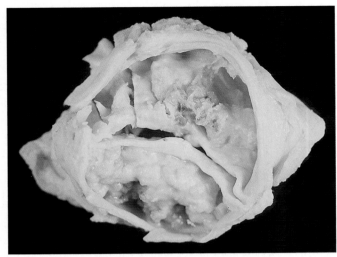

**Figure 15-54** The congenitally bicuspid aortic valve is hemodynamically imperfect and develops degenerative change at an accelerated rate as compared with the trileaflet aortic valve. Viewed from the aortic aspect, this specimen from a middle-aged patient with aortic stenosis demonstrates fibrosis of both leaflets, as well as large irregular nodular deposits of calcified tissue protruding into the sinuses of Valsalva.

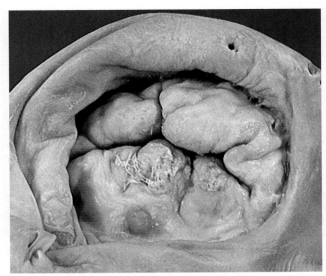

**Figure 15-56** Acquired mitral stenosis is almost always due to rheumatic heart disease. In a specimen viewed from the atrial aspect, this mitral valve shows the "fishmouth" configuration characteristic of long-standing mitral stenosis. The leaflets of this valve are thickened and deformed by fibrosis, making the leaflets much less mobile.

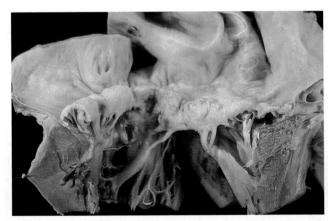

**Figure 15-57** In the atrioventricular view of an enlarged heart from a patient with mitral stenosis, the mitral valve leaflets are deformed by fibrosis, signifying years of damage, and fibrosis has resulted in shortening and fusion of the chordae tendineae.

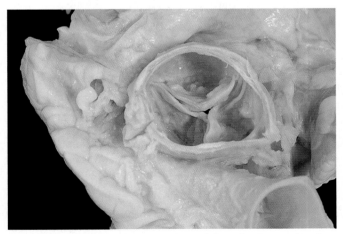

**Figure 15-55** The semilunar leaflets of the trileaflet aortic valve may eventually become less mobile because of wear-and-tear degenerative change. In this heart from an elderly patient with aortic stenosis, all three aortic valve leaflets are thickened by fibrosis and contain nodular calcified lesions extending into the sinuses.

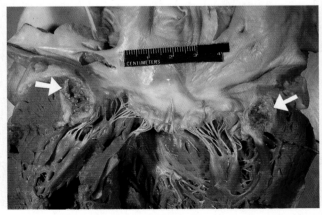

**Figure 15-58** Mitral annular calcification is usually an incidental finding in an older patient. In the atrioventricular view, the calcified tissue *(arrows)* is seen in cross section, and the leaflets show mild irregular fibrosis associated with aging.

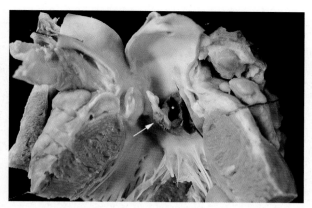

**Figure 15-59** Ring (annular) abscess may be a consequence of infective endocarditis and lead to further complications. In this specimen from a 6-year-old patient with congenitally bicuspid aortic valve, a vegetation *(arrow)* can be identified on the ventricular aspect. The cutaway view demonstrates infective necrotic debris in the sinus of Valsalva *(*)*, as well as an abscess involving the annulus and eroding the adjacent myocardium, which was the basis for rupture into the pericardial space.

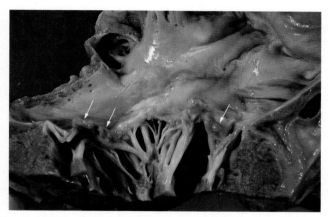

**Figure 15-60** Typically, infective endocarditis arises on valve leaflets that are subjected to hemodynamic injury. This mitral valve is deformed by leaflet fibrosis and thick, fused chordae tendineae characteristic of chronic rheumatic heart disease. Superimposed infective endocarditis is identified by the presence of numerous friable red-gray vegetations on the atrial aspect of the valve leaflets *(arrows)*.

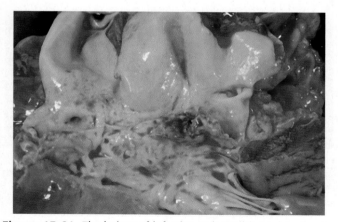

**Figure 15-61** The lesions of infective endocarditis tend to develop on the side of the valve exposed to lower pressures (atrial side of an atrioventricular valve or ventricular side of an arterial valve). This aortic valve in a patient with chronic rheumatic heart disease contains a single friable red-black ulcerated vegetation on the ventricular aspect. A lesion such as this may embolize, resulting in cerebrovascular accident or other organ infarct.

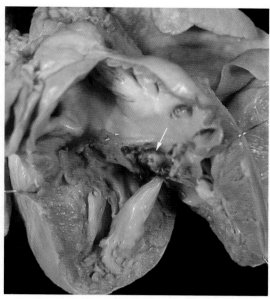

**Figure 15-62** Foreign material can be a nidus for infection. The heart from this infant with a repaired congenital heart defect demonstrates a large red-tan vegetation *(arrow)* on the atrial aspect of the tricuspid valve. A lesion such as this could be the origin of a thromboembolus that results in a pulmonary infarct or lung abscess.

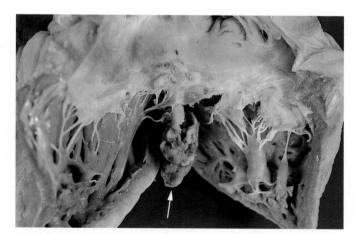

**Figure 15-63** This large red-tan lesion *(arrow)* on the tricuspid valve of an intravenous drug user was easily identified as a mobile pedunculated vegetation by echocardiography. The anterosuperior leaflet is ruptured because of necrosis, and the nodular appearance of the valve surface at the commissure alludes to an extension of the infective process into the adjacent myocardium. In this case, a myocardial abscess eroded the specialized muscle of the conduction tissue, explaining the patient's heart block.

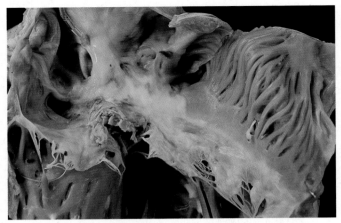

**Figure 15-64** This vegetation eroded a portion of the tricuspid valve in an intravenous drug user. The infective process extended into the adjacent myocardium, and the resulting abscess destroyed specialized muscle of the conduction system, resulting in complete heart block. The lung also contained several abscesses.

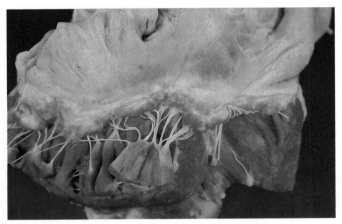

**Figure 15-65** Nonbacterial thrombotic endocarditis affects primarily debilitated patients and elderly persons. Resembling the lesions of infective endocarditis, these nodules are composed of sterile platelet-fibrin material. This mitral valve shows a linear array of small vegetations along the edges of the leaflets.

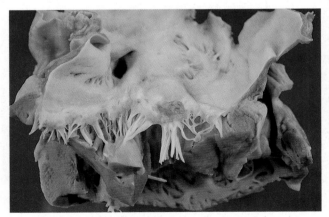

**Figure 15-66** Most often, the lesions of nonbacterial thrombotic endocarditis are small and inconspicuous along the lines of valve closure. In this example, however, a relatively large tan, ulcerated vegetation arises on the atrial aspect of the septal leaflet of the mitral valve in the heart of a cancer patient who died from noncardiac disease.

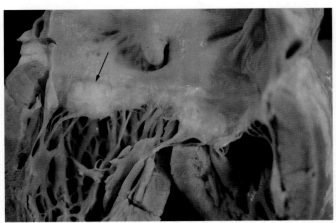

**Figure 15-67** The anatomic correlate of mitral valve prolapse reflects the long-standing abnormal movement of the posterior leaflet into the left atrium during systole. This specimen demonstrates "hooding" or arching of the leaflet *(arrow)*, with the convex aspect facing the atrium to give the leaflet a festooned appearance. The leaflet tissue is thickened by myxoid change. The chordae tendineae may be elongated and attenuated, predisposing to rupture.

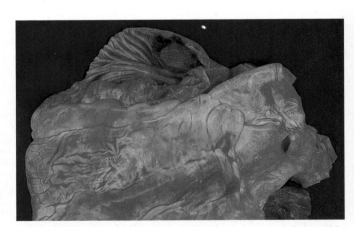

**Figure 15-68** The atrial appendages may harbor mural thrombi that can embolize. The autopsy pathologist is often confronted with the question of whether a clot represents real thrombus present during life or postmortem coagulum. The latter is usually rubbery and does not stick to the endocardial surface; a true thrombus may demonstrate lines of Zahn, is brittle, and is more difficult to remove. The pectinate muscles of the atrial appendages, however, may trap even postmortem clots; often only a histologic section establishes the nature of the lesion. A large organized thrombus is obvious in this right atrial appendage, but many other thrombi are smaller and less conspicuous.

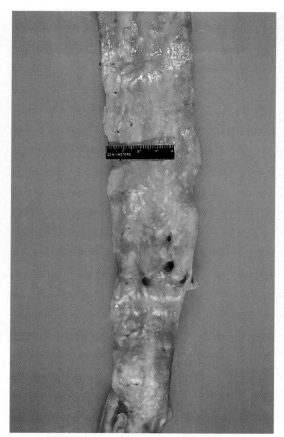

**Figure 15-69**  This abdominal aorta contains many fatty streaks (flat yellow discolorations of the intimal surface) and early plaques (raised yellow lesions).

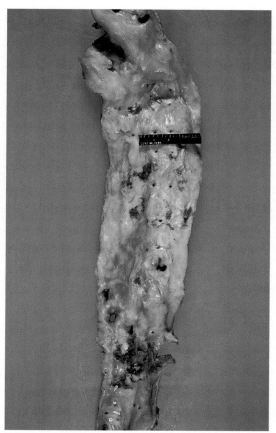

**Figure 15-70**  The abdominal aorta below the origins of the large arteries supplying the alimentary tract or kidneys is the usual site of the most severe aortic atherosclerosis. In this example, the entire aorta shows atherosclerosis characterized by widespread plaques, but the portion below the origins of the larger arteries shows larger plaques, as well as complicated plaques with thrombus and ulceration.

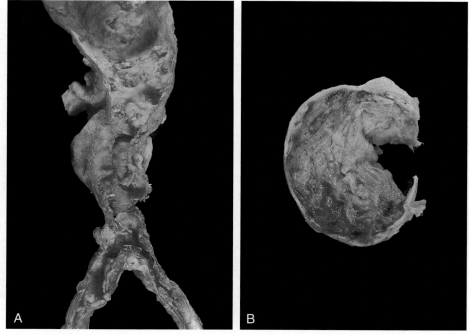

**Figure 15-71**  In areas where atherosclerosis is most severe, the aortic wall may be weakened to the extent that the blood pressure deforms the vessel, creating an aneurysm. **A,** This specimen shows severe atherosclerosis in the abdominal aorta and iliac arteries. There is a saccular aneurysm above the bifurcation. **B,** Cross section through the aneurysm revealing extensive organizing thrombus.

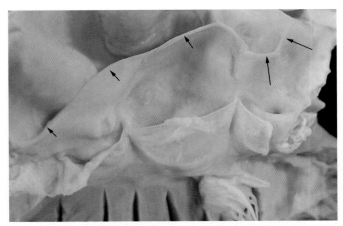

**Figure 15-72** In this heart with a bicuspid aortic valve, aortic stenosis over the years weakened the ascending aorta, facilitating dissection. Beyond the flap *(small arrows)*, the false lumen extended virtually throughout the aorta. The dissection occurred over months and shows evidence of healing *(large arrows)*.

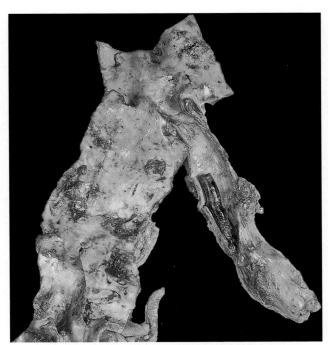

**Figure 15-74** Systemic thromboembolism to the superior mesenteric artery. Approximately 80% of systemic thromboemboli arise from intracardiac mural thrombi, as did this embolus to the superior mesenteric artery. Other sources of systemic thromboemboli include aortic aneurysms, thrombi associated with ulcerated atherosclerotic plaques, and vegetations of the cardiac valves.

## RESPIRATORY SYSTEM

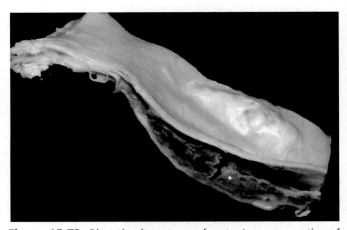

**Figure 15-73** Dissecting hematoma of aorta. In a cross section of the opened aorta, the false lumen *(\*)* is filled with organizing thrombus. Typically, the dissection propagates in the outer portion of the media. In addition to the extent and consequences of dissection, the autopsy pathologist should identify the entrance tear and the distal point of rupture; the substrate for dissection (basis for medial weakening) is usually diagnosed by microscopy.

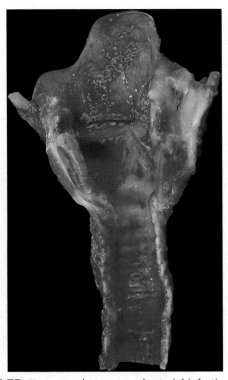

**Figure 15-75** Upper respiratory tract bacterial infection. Laryngitis may be due to allergens, chemicals, or infections. In this larynx and trachea, a bacterial infection caused diffuse mucosal hyperemia and multifocal purulent exudates.

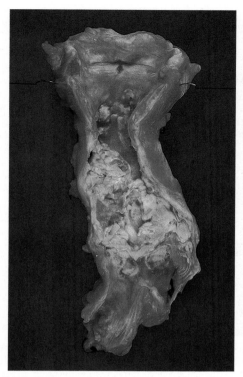

**Figure 15-76** Upper respiratory tract fungal infection. The larynx and trachea show large, yellow exophytic exudates caused by invasive aspergillosis.

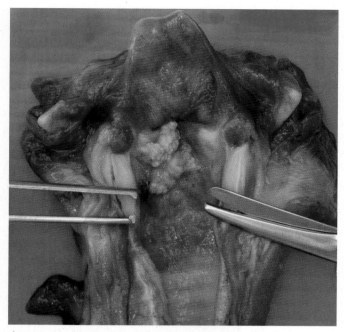

**Figure 15-78** Upper respiratory tract with papillomatosis. Caused by human papillomavirus types 6 and 11, squamous papillomas usually occur on the true vocal cords. Typically single in adults, they may be multiple in children (juvenile laryngeal papillomatosis). Although they rarely exceed 1 cm in diameter, when left untreated these warty excrescences may sometimes obstruct the airway and lead to death, as occurred in this young child. (Courtesy of Gregory Reiber, MD.)

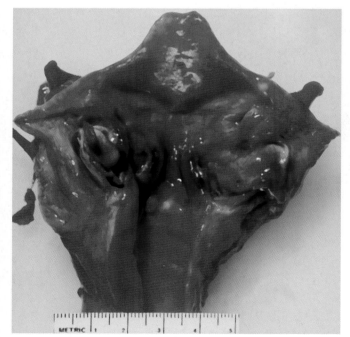

**Figure 15-77** Laryngeal edema. The mucosal and submucosal tissues of the larynx may swell dramatically in anaphylactic reactions, in infections, or after trauma. This larynx shows marked edema and focal necrosis resulting in obstruction after traumatic intubation.

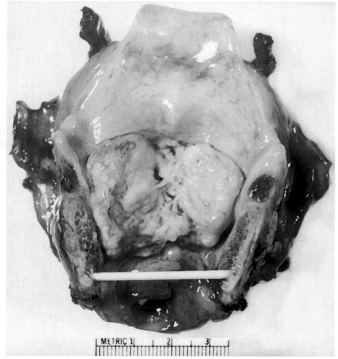

**Figure 15-79** Squamous cell carcinoma of the larynx. The vast majority of laryngeal cancers are squamous cell carcinomas. This large fungating lesion involves the vocal cords and pyriform sinuses.

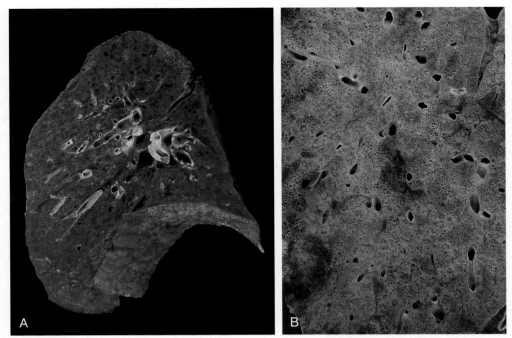

**Figure 15-80** Diffuse alveolar damage (adult respiratory distress syndrome). The lung is susceptible to diffuse alveolar epithelial and capillary endothelial damage from direct injury and systemic disorders. **A,** In the acute exudative stage of diffuse alveolar damage, the lungs are heavy, with firm, boggy, red parenchyma. **B,** Patients who die during the later proliferative stage have lungs with widespread organization including alveolar remodeling, interstitial fibrosis, and occasional cyst formation.

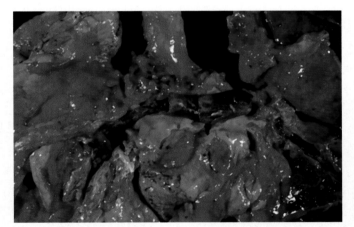

**Figure 15-81** Pulmonary saddle thromboembolus. Pulmonary thromboembolism remains a common cause of death in hospitalized patients, although only about one third are diagnosed premortem. The incidence of thromboemboli discovered at autopsy varies depending on underlying conditions but is quite high in patients who die after severe burns, trauma, or fractures. Large thromboemboli may lodge at the bifurcation of the main pulmonary artery, so-called saddle emboli, usually leading to sudden death.

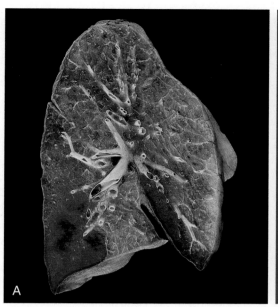 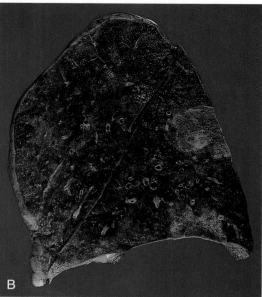

**Figure 15-82** Pulmonary infarcts. **A,** In this specimen two thromboemboli lodged in pulmonary artery branches *(small arrows)* have resulted in acute pulmonary infarcts *(large arrows)*. Acute infarcts are hemorrhagic, may appear slightly raised, and extend to the pleura, where a fibrinous exudate usually develops. The beginning of such an exudate can be seen here on the diaphragmatic visceral pleura. **B,** As the infarcts age, they become paler and eventually red-brown as increased amounts of hemosiderin accumulate. Finally, as fibrous replacement ensues, the margins show a gray-white zone that eventually incorporates the entire infarct, converting it to a contracted scar.
(**A** and **B** from Finkbeiner WE: Respiratory pathology. In Gold WM, Murray JF, Nadel JA, editors: *Atlas of procedures in respiratory medicine,* Philadelphia, 2002, WB Saunders, pp 75-154.)

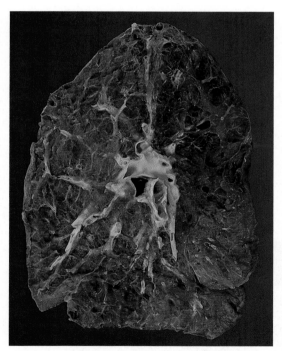 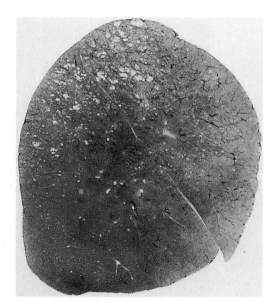

**Figure 15-83** Centriacinar (centrilobular) emphysema. Centriacinar emphysema, primarily a complication of smoking, involves the upper two thirds of the lungs. Early in the disease the gross findings may not be impressive, detectable only by subtle loss of parenchyma and inward collapse of the pleura evident on routinely prepared cut lung sections. As shown here, as the disease progresses, dilation of air spaces and destruction of alveolar parenchyma become more generalized.

**Figure 15-84** Centriacinar emphysema, paper mounted, lung (Gough-Wentworth) section. This section from a lung of a chronic smoker shows enlarged air spaces in the upper zones of the upper and lower lobes of the left lung.
(From Finkbeiner WE: Respiratory pathology. In Gold WM, Murray JF, Nadel JA, editors: *Atlas of procedures in respiratory medicine,* Philadelphia, 2002, WB Saunders, pp 75-154.)

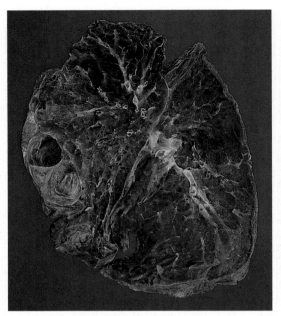

**Figure 15-85** Panacinar emphysema. In its severe form, this type of emphysema is associated with $\alpha_1$-antitrypsin deficiency. The anterior margins and lower zones of the lung are most severely affected. In its mild form, it occurs with advancing age.

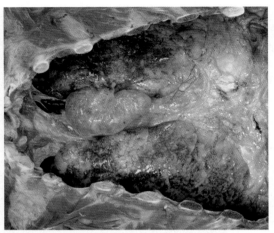

**Figure 15-86** Emphysematous bullae. These are thin-walled emphysematous spaces greater than 1 cm in diameter. A large bulla is seen in situ along the medial edge of the left upper lobe.

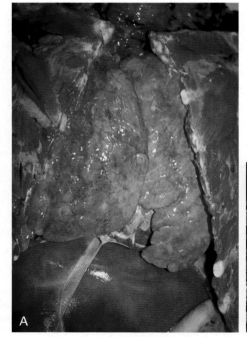

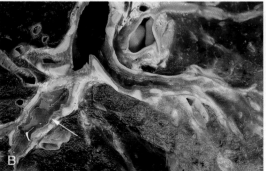

**Figure 15-87** Sudden death in a patient with asthma. Patients who die suddenly of asthma usually show a combination of lung hyperinflation and atelectasis along with airways occluded by mucus plugs. **A,** Markedly expanded lungs fill the pleural cavities, obscuring the heart. **B,** Mucous plugs *(arrow)* fill and occlude the bronchi.

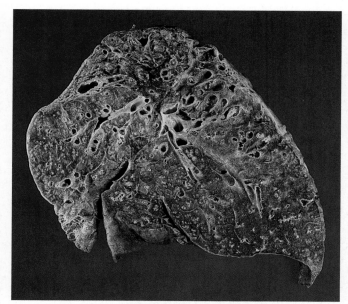

**Figure 15-88** Bronchiectasis. Bronchiectasis has numerous causes, including bronchial obstruction, inherited propensity to develop airway infection (cystic fibrosis, immunoglobulin A deficiency, ciliary dyskinesia syndrome), and necrotizing pneumonia with subsequent bronchial damage. In each case, the development of bronchiectatic airways involves a vicious cycle of airway obstruction, recurrent infection, and progressive airway dilation. This specimen is from a patient who died of cystic fibrosis. It shows diffuse, purulent bronchiectasis, worse in the upper lobes. Note that the dilated airways may extend to the subpleural region.

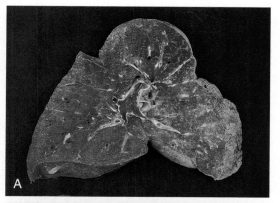

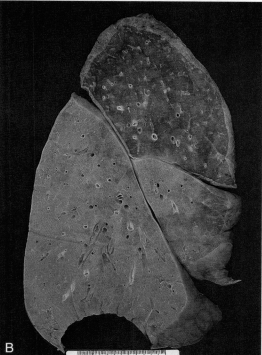

**Figure 15-89** Bacterial pneumonia. Bacterial organisms cause intraalveolar exudation, resulting in consolidation of the lung parenchyma. Traditionally, bacterial pneumonias have been classified anatomically according to whether the infection involves an entire lobe or segment of the lung diffusely (lobar pneumonia) or the infection is centered around the airways in a patchy distribution (bronchopneumonia). **A,** In this case of lobar pneumonia in the stage of red hepatization, the entire right lower lobe is inflamed, hyperemic, and consolidated. **B,** As the inflammation of lobar pneumonia organizes (gray hepatization stage), the involved lung becomes gray-brown, dry, and firm, as seen in the right middle and lower lobes in this case.
(**B** from Finkbeiner WE: Respiratory pathology. In Gold WM, Murray JF, Nadel JA, editors: *Atlas of procedures in respiratory medicine,* Philadelphia, 2002, WB Saunders, pp 75-154.)

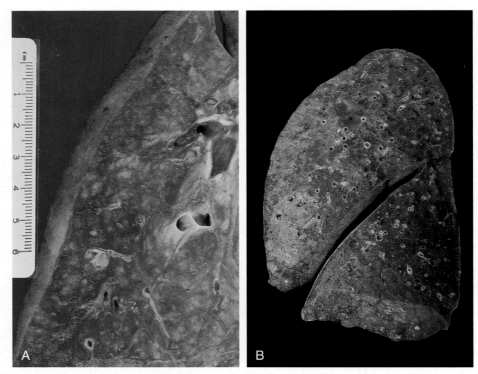

**Figure 15-90** Bronchopneumonia. **A,** Patchy consolidation around small bronchi and bronchioles can be seen. The lesions are slightly elevated, dry, granular, and gray-red to yellow. **B,** Some species of bacteria cause a necrotizing bronchopneumonia, seen here as the confluent gray areas.
(**A** from Finkbeiner WE: Respiratory pathology. In Gold WM, Murray JF, Nadel JA, editors: *Atlas of procedures in respiratory medicine,* Philadelphia, 2002, WB Saunders, pp 75-154.)

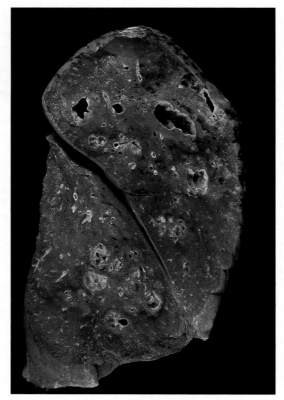

**Figure 15-91** Lung abscess. Among the pulmonary complications of pneumonia are pleuritis, empyema, abscess formation, organization of the exudates (organizing pneumonia), and diffuse alveolar damage. The lung shown here shows necrotizing bronchopneumonia with multiple abscess cavities caused by *Staphylococcus aureus*. The occurrence rate of lung abscesses associated with pneumonia varies with the etiologic agent.

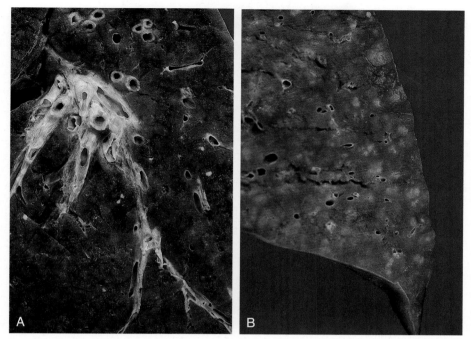

**Figure 15-92** Viral pneumonias. Mild viral pneumonias cause patchy consolidation of the lungs or mild diffuse interstitial inflammation along with acute congestion. Severe or fatal pneumonias result in more extensive lung injury that may be patchy or diffuse. Superimposed bacterial infection may modify the process. **A,** Organizing diffuse alveolar damage in cytomegalovirus pneumonia. **B,** Patchy necrosis related to *Herpes simplex* virus pneumonia.

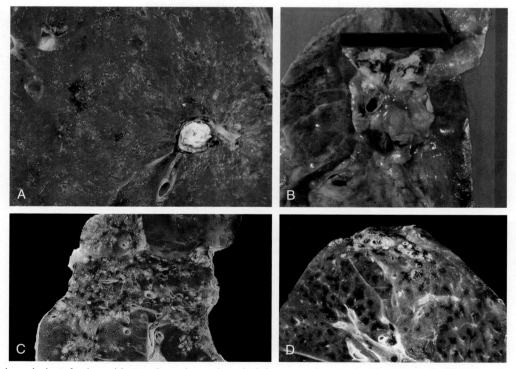

**Figure 15-93** Tuberculosis. Infection with *Mycobacterium tuberculosis* has several recognizable stages and variations. **A,** Inhaled bacilli implant in distal air spaces of the lower part of the upper lobe or the upper part of the lower lobe. Following a nonspecific inflammatory reaction, delayed hypersensitivity (type IV) to the bacillus develops 2 to 4 weeks after the initial infection. At this point, the primary infection appears as a 1- to 1.5-cm gray-white area of caseous necrosis called the Ghon focus. **B,** Drainage of bacilli, either free or within macrophages, to regional lymph nodes forms secondary areas of infection, and caseous necrosis develops in regional hilar lymph nodes. With resolution, these lesions become fibrocalcific scars that may harbor viable organisms for years. The combination of the Ghon focus and nodal involvement is referred to as the Ghon complex. **C,** This example shows a localized area of tuberculous pneumonia in a case of progressive primary tuberculosis. **D,** Secondary tuberculosis is localized to the apices of upper lobes and typically consists of 1- to 2-cm areas of consolidation with central caseation and peripheral fibrotic reaction and cavitation.

(From Finkbeiner WE: Respiratory pathology. In Gold WM, Murray JF, Nadel JA, editors: *Atlas of procedures in respiratory medicine,* Philadelphia, 2002, WB Saunders, pp 75-154.)

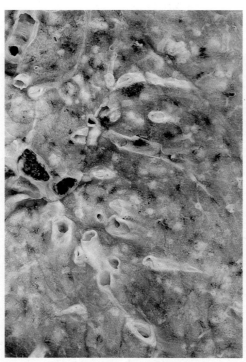

**Figure 15-94** *Mycobacterium avium* complex (MAC). Numerous small light-colored foci of caseous necrosis caused by miliary spread in a case of MAC infection as a complication of AIDS.

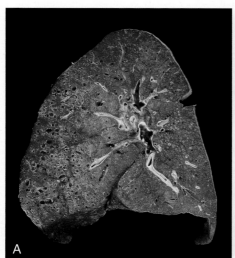

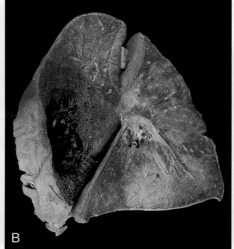

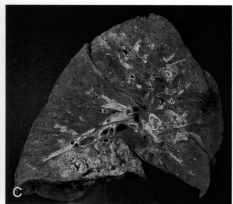

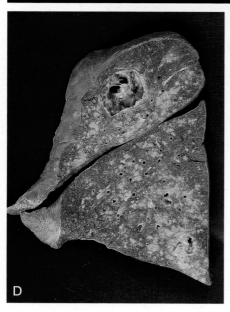

**Figure 15-95** The gross pathologic findings in fungal infections of the lung in immunocompetent persons may be indistinguishable from tuberculosis. In those who are immunocompromised, fungal infections of the lung are severe and associated with necrosis or diffuse alveolar damage, or both. **A,** Disseminated coccidioidomycosis causing miliary-like lesions, diffuse alveolar damage, and cyst formation. **B,** Localized necrotizing infection related to zygomycosis (mucormycosis). **C,** Invasive aspergillosis causing necrotizing pneumonia and diffuse alveolar damage. **D,** Necrotizing and cavitating infection with *Pneumocystis carinii* in a child with congenital AIDS. (**A** from Finkbeiner WE: Respiratory pathology. In Gold WM, Murray JF, Nadel JA, editors: *Atlas of procedures in respiratory medicine,* Philadelphia, 2002, WB Saunders, pp 75-154.)

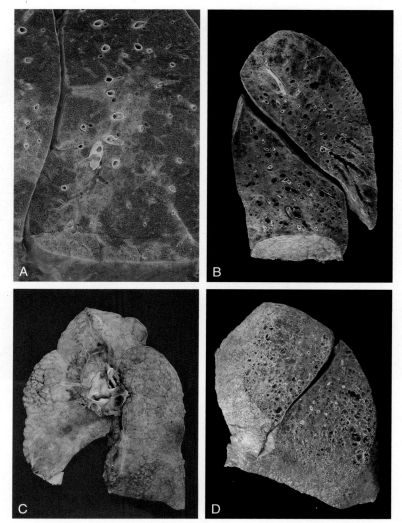

**Figure 15-96** The appearance of lungs with idiopathic pulmonary fibrosis (usual interstitial pneumonia) and other restrictive lung diseases varies according to the specific disease and stage of the disease. **A,** In the early stages, the lungs show alternating areas of light-colored fibrosis and normal lung. **B,** As the disease advances, the degree of fibrosis increases and small subpleural cysts appear. **C,** During this stage the visceral pleural surface becomes progressively more irregular. **D,** The late stage is marked by progressive cyst formation (honeycomb lung).

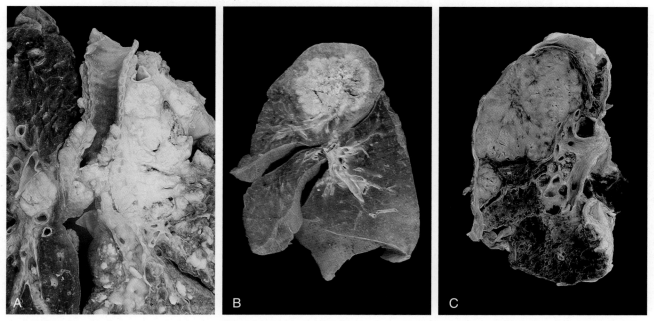

**Figure 15-97** Lung carcinoma. **A,** Squamous cell carcinoma. Posterior view. A large central squamous cell carcinoma has completely obstructed the lumen of the right main-stem bronchus. Metastatic tumor deposits are evident in both lungs. **B,** Adenocarcinomas of the lung arise most commonly in the periphery. **C,** A small cell neuroendocrine (oat cell) carcinoma developed in an asbestosis-scarred lung.

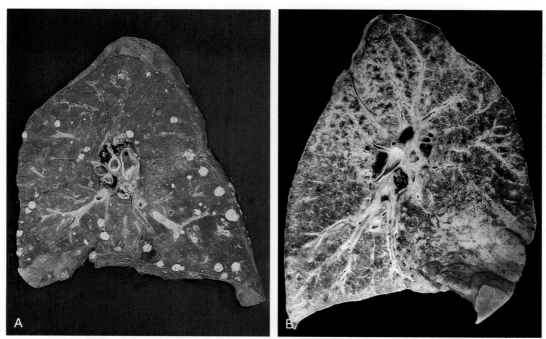

**Figure 15-98** Metastatic tumors. The lung is a common site of metastases. **A,** Generally, metastatic tumors form multiple discrete nodules scattered throughout all lobes, as this hepatocellular carcinoma has. **B,** Metastases to the lung may also spread through the lung lymphatics, diffusely infiltrating the lung parenchyma (lymphangitic spread).

## GASTROINTESTINAL SYSTEM

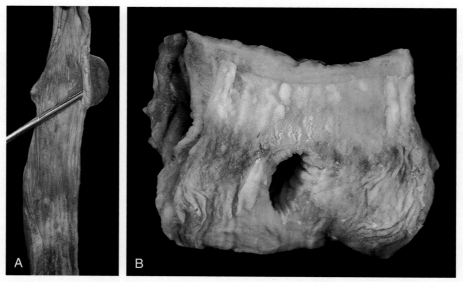

**Figure 15-99** Esophageal diverticula. Diverticula develop in three regions of the esophagus: above the upper esophageal sphincter (Zenker diverticulum), near the midpoint of the esophagus (traction diverticulum), and just above the lower esophageal sphincter (epiphrenic diverticulum). **A,** Zenker diverticulum. **B,** Epiphrenic diverticulum.

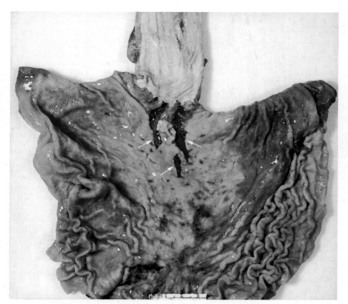

**Figure 15-100** The lacerations *(arrows)* present in the mucosa of this esophagus and stomach occurred during a prolonged bout of vomiting (Mallory-Weiss syndrome). Most commonly encountered in chronic alcoholics, these lacerations are irregularly linear and oriented in the longitudinal axis of the esophagus. Typically, they develop at the esophagogastric junction or in the proximal portion of the stomach. They may involve only the mucosa or may extend completely through the wall of the organ (Boerhaave syndrome).

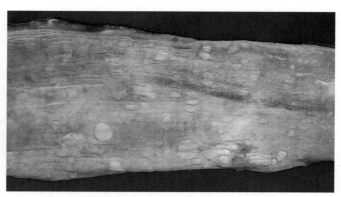

**Figure 15-101** Glycogenic acanthosis. These asymptomatic, superficial, plaquelike lesions of the squamous epithelium of the esophagus are often identified at autopsy.

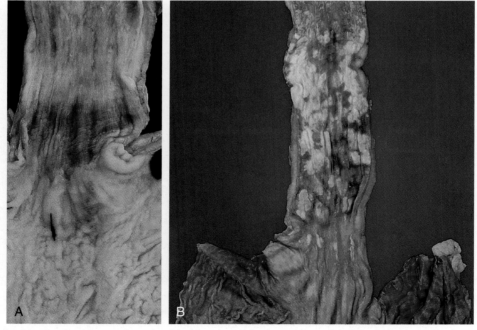

**Figure 15-102** Esophagitis. Esophagitis may be caused by chemical irritation or bacterial, fungal, or viral infections. The gross pathologic changes associated with esophagitis range from mere hyperemia to frank ulceration and necrosis. **A,** This fixed specimen shows hyperemia and loss of a distinct gastroesophageal junction associated with reflux of gastric acid. **B,** This example of esophageal candidiasis shows the distal esophagus covered by adherent gray and yellow pseudomembranes that contain numerous fungi.

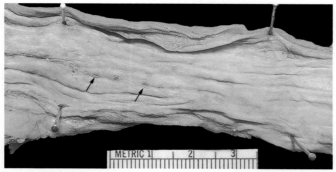

**Figure 15-103** Viral esophagitis. The most common viruses to infect the esophagus, cytomegalovirus and herpesvirus, typically cause mucosal ulcerations *(arrows)* such as those seen in this example of herpesvirus infection.

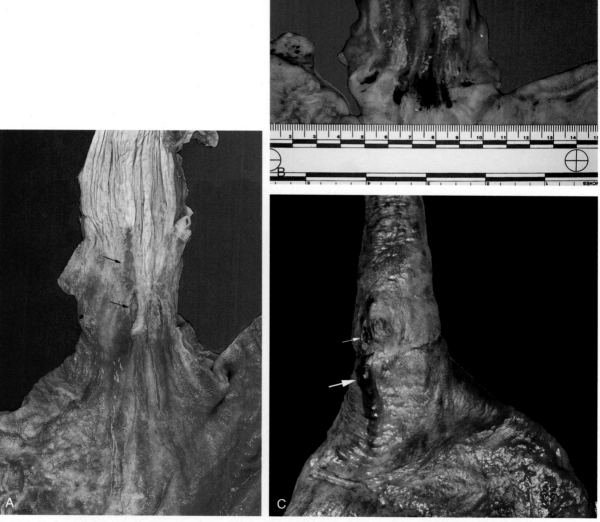

**Figure 15-104** Varices. Esophageal varices consisting of dilated and tortuous submucosal veins produced by chronic portal hypertension are often difficult to visualize after death because they collapse. **A,** In this specimen, the mucosa overlying the varices is inflamed and eroded *(arrows)*. **B,** The varices in this esophagus contain thrombi, indicating previous rupture. **C,** Demonstration of varices may be aided by inverting the specimen by pulling the proximal end of the esophagus through the pylorus. In this specimen a large varix *(large arrow)* with an area of rupture *(small arrow)* is demonstrated to best advantage.
(**B** courtesy of Robert M. Anthony, MD, PhD.)

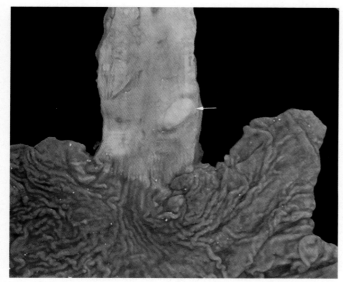

**Figure 15-105** Leiomyoma. A number of benign tumors generally arising from stromal elements and appearing as solid, gray-white intramural masses occur in the esophagus. This esophagus contains a leiomyoma *(arrow)*, the most common type of benign intramural tumor, which was discovered incidentally during an autopsy.

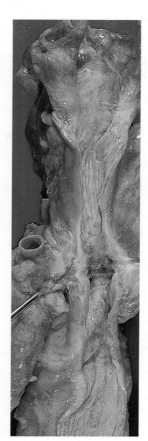

**Figure 15-106** Carcinoma of the esophagus. Squamous cell carcinomas are the most common malignant tumors of the esophagus. Although they develop at all levels, there is some regional predilection, with 20% located in the upper third, 50% in the middle third, and 30% in the lower third of the esophagus. This ulcerating tumor is associated with thickening of the esophageal wall and narrowing of the esophageal lumen.

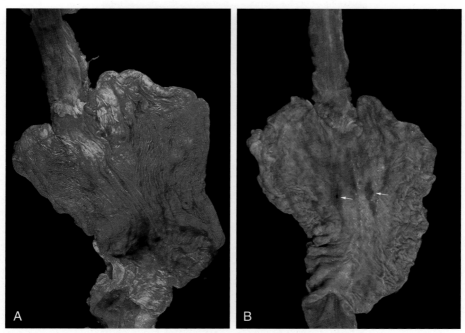

**Figure 15-107** Acute gastritis. The pathogenesis of acute gastritis is unclear, but it is associated with nonsteroidal antiinflammatory drugs, excessive consumption of alcohol, uremia, trauma, shock, burns, systemic infections, and chemical injury. The appearance of acute gastritis may vary from hyperemia and mucosal edema to diffuse hemorrhage and erosive sloughing of the mucosa. **A,** This specimen shows primarily marked mucosal hyperemia, although the darker foci represent areas of mucosal denudation and hemorrhage. **B,** This stomach shows acute erosive gastritis, characterized by red areas *(arrows)* representing superficial mucosal denudation.

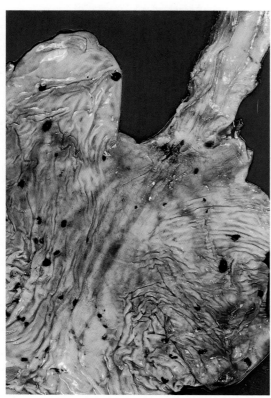

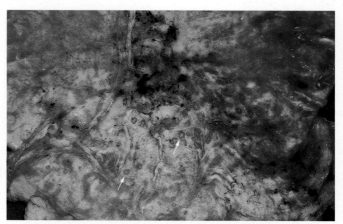

**Figure 15-109** Gastric candidiasis. Ulcers of the gastric mucosa may develop as a consequence of fungal infections. This immunosuppressed patient had multiple ulcers *(arrows)* with hyperemic margins at sites of infection with *Candida albicans*.

**Figure 15-108** An extension of acute gastritis, acute gastric ulcers (stress ulcers) are seen in patients with massive trauma, extensive burns, sepsis, increased intracranial pressure, or shock. This stomach shows numerous ulcers that developed in a patient with hypovolemic shock. Stress ulcers develop in all regions of the stomach, are generally less than 1 cm in diameter, and have a dark brown base with indistinct margins.

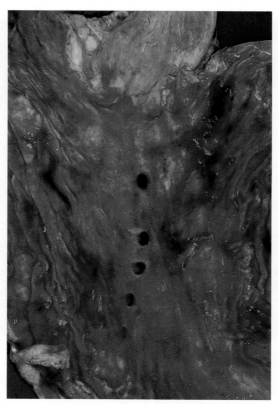

**Figure 15-110** Iatrogenic ulceration of the stomach is sometimes seen with therapeutic nasogastric suction. This specimen shows multiple superficial mucosal ulcers of uniform diameter corresponding to the diameter of a nasogastric tube.

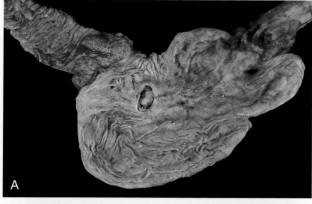

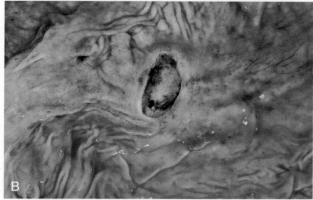

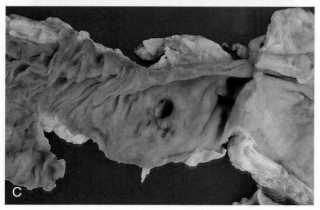

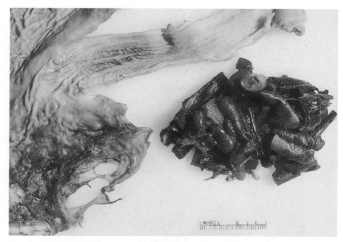

**Figure 15-112**  Bezoars. Indigestible material may form concretions within the stomach lumen. Trichobezoars (hairballs) consist of ingested hair and decaying foodstuff. Phytobezoars are made up of indigestible plant matter. This phytobezoar caused a localized chronic gastritis. The gastric wall *(left)* became focally atrophic and eventually perforated.

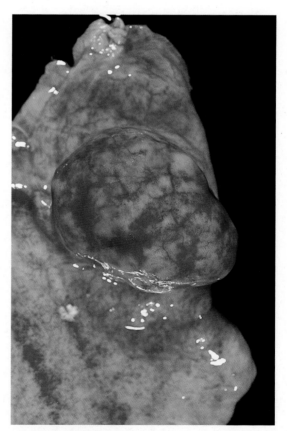

**Figure 15-111**  Peptic ulcers. Peptic ulcers develop anywhere in the gastrointestinal tract in contact with acid-pepsin secretion. Thus, the vast majority are found in the duodenum or stomach. In the stomach, peptic ulcers are most commonly found in the antrum or along the lesser curvature. Peptic ulcers of the stomach are generally solitary; however, 10% to 20% of patients have an associated duodenal ulcer. Although they may become quite large, most are less than 2 cm in diameter and they rarely exceed 4 cm. **A,** Peptic ulcers such as this one located in the antrum are round to oval defects with straight walls and margins that are level with or just slightly elevated above the adjacent mucosa. **B,** Peptic digestion of any exudates keeps the base of a peptic ulcer relatively smooth and clean. **C,** Peptic ulcer in the first portion of the duodenum.

**Figure 15-113**  Leiomyoma. The most common mesenchymal neoplasms to arise in the stomach are of smooth muscle origin, such as this leiomyoma.

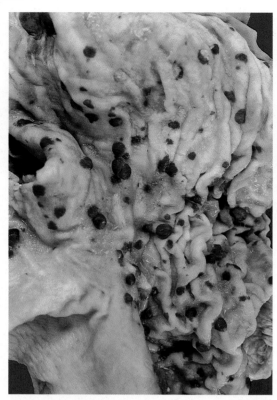

**Figure 15-114** Kaposi sarcoma. In disseminated Kaposi sarcoma, the stomach may show dark red to purple mucosal nodules.

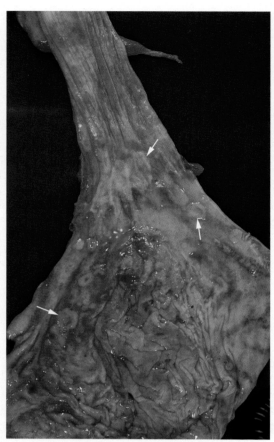

**Figure 15-116** Lymphoma. Upper gastrointestinal lymphomas may produce plaquelike lesions, polypoid or fungating masses, or full-thickness mural expansion, as in this specimen, in which there are multifocal infiltrates of tumor *(arrows)* in the mucosa and submucosa of the esophagus and stomach diffusely.

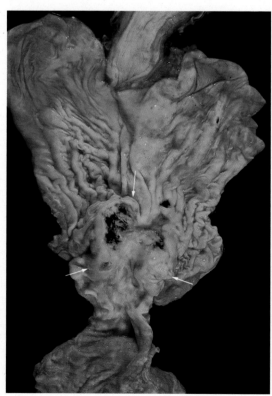

**Figure 15-115** Carcinomas are the most common type of malignant tumor found in the stomach, accounting for 90% to 95%, in comparison with lymphomas (4%), carcinoids (3%), and malignant stromal tumors (2%). Gastric carcinomas may occur throughout the stomach and take the form of flat mucosal lesions, ulcerated craters, or exophytic masses such as the one shown here *(arrows)*.

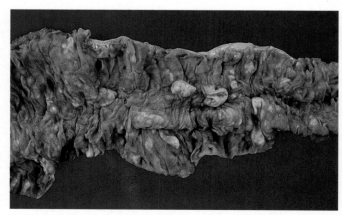

**Figure 15-117** Lacteals. Examination of the small intestines during autopsy often reveals dilated lacteals. These thin-walled lymphatic channels are filled with chylous fluid and protrude on the mucosal surface.

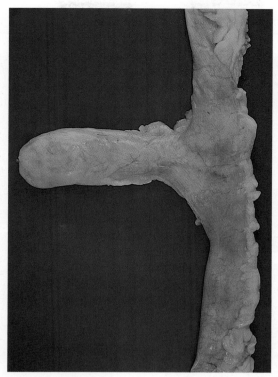

**Figure 15-118** The solitary Meckel diverticulum develops from the vestigial omphalomesenteric duct, usually within 12 inches of the ileocecal valve but sometimes up to 2 to 3 feet proximally. Heterotopic islands of gastric mucosa may be found in up to 50% of Meckel diverticula, and release of acid from these sites may produce peptic-type ulcers of the adjacent small intestinal mucosa. Meckel diverticula such as the one depicted occur at the antimesenteric side of the ileal wall.

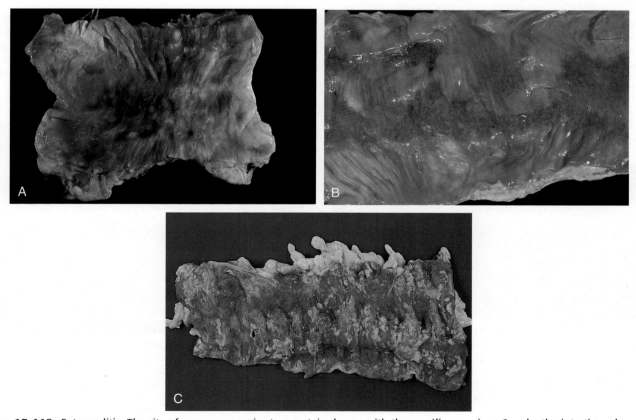

**Figure 15-119** Enterocolitis. The site of occurrence varies to a certain degree with the specific organism. Grossly, the intestines show hyperemia and a variable amount of mucosal damage and exudate. **A,** Cytomegalovirus colitis in an immunosuppressed patient. Diffuse hyperemia and multiple circular ulcerations are seen. **B,** Colon showing mucosal hyperemia and submucosal edema caused by *Clostridium perfringens*. **C,** Antibiotic-associated (pseudomembranous) colitis caused by *Clostridium difficile* shows characteristic yellow plaques of fibrin, mucus, and inflammatory debris.

*Continued*

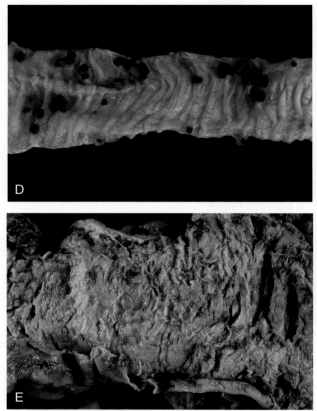

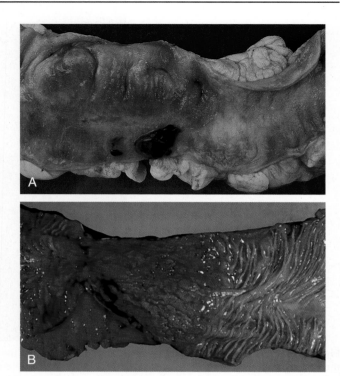

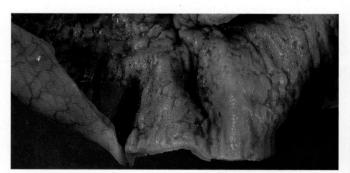

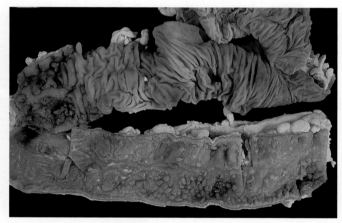

**Figure 15-119—Cont'd D,** Fungal enteritis related to invasive aspergillosis in an immunosuppressed patient with lymphoma results in numerous dark red-brown fungal abscesses involving the mucosa and submucosa. **E,** Fixed specimen showing severe ulcerating colitis caused by *Entamoeba histolytica* (amebic dysentery).

**Figure 15-121** Crohn disease. Crohn disease may involve any part of the gastrointestinal tract but most commonly affects the small intestine alone (40%), the small and large intestines (30%), or the large intestines alone (30%). The lesions are generally discontinuous. **A,** Early lesion of the ileum showing hyperemia and focal ulceration. **B,** Chronic lesion involving the ileum. There is a sharp demarcation between the normal area on the right and the involved area on the left. Narrowing of the lumen, thickening of the intestinal wall, and coarsely textured ("cobblestone") mucosa with fissures are seen.

**Figure 15-120** AIDS enteropathy. Patients infected with human immunodeficiency virus (HIV) may experience a malabsorptive syndrome with intestinal villous atrophy. Although some have attributed the disease directly to HIV-induced mucosal damage, other microbial organisms may contribute. This small intestine shows mucosal flattening and marked wall thickening.

**Figure 15-122** Ulcerative colitis. The disease begins in the rectum and extends proximally without skip lesions. In this specimen, broad-based ulceration of the colonic mucosa of the distal colon can be seen. Regenerating mucosa adjacent to areas of ulceration creates pseudopolyps.

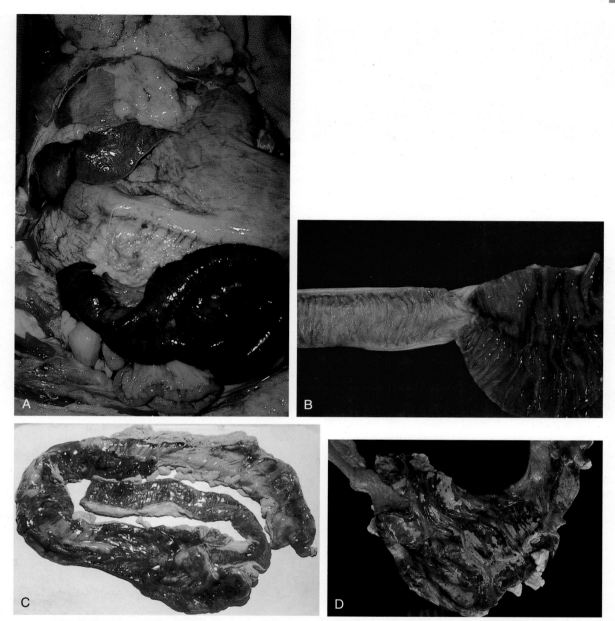

**Figure 15-123**  Ischemic bowel disease. Transmural infarction of the intestines may result from thrombosis of or embolism to the superior or inferior mesenteric arteries and their branches; stenosis of the arterial supply, usually secondary to atherosclerotic disease; thrombosis of the mesenteric venous system; or severe hypotension. Initially the necrotic bowel becomes purple-red from intense congestion. During the first 24 hours, the bowel wall becomes thickened and hemorrhagic. The lumen contains blood or bloody mucus. Over 1 to 4 days, intestinal bacteria produce gangrene, and perforation of the bowel may occur. **A,** Dark purple serosa of necrotic small intestines. **B,** Transmural infarct of small intestines due to arterial thrombosis of a branch of the superior mesenteric artery. A distinct demarcation can be seen between the viable and nonviable tissue. **C,** Multifocal mucosal hemorrhagic infarcts in the small and large bowel. **D,** Transmural infarct of the cecum. Yellow exudates overlie the necrotic purple-red mucosa.

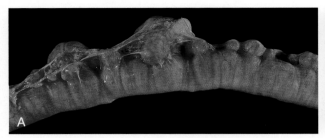
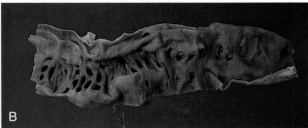

**Figure 15-124** Acquired diverticular disease of the intestines. **A,** Diverticula occur less commonly in the small intestines than in the large intestines. They develop at the points where the mesenteric vessels and nerves enter the jejunal and ileal walls, points of weakness from which the mucosa and submucosa can herniate into mesentery. This jejunum shows multiple wide-based diverticula along its mesenteric border. **B,** Greater than 90% of colonic diverticula occur in the sigmoid region. The sacs are small (usually 1 cm or less in diameter) and located along the margins of the taenia coli. They have soft, compressible walls filled with feces.

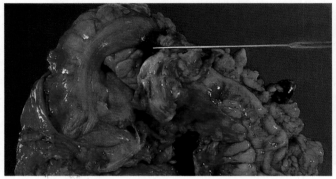

**Figure 15-125** Rupture of diverticula leads to inflammation (diverticulitis). Chronic inflammation may lead to thickening and fibrosis of the colonic wall sufficient to mimic carcinoma. Serious complications also include pericolonic abscess formation, development of sinus tracts, and sometimes peritonitis. The probe demonstrates a perforated diverticulum that resulted in fatal peritonitis.

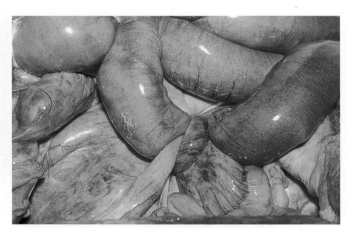

**Figure 15-127** Volvulus, the complete twisting of a loop of bowel about its mesentery, generally occurs in redundant loops of sigmoid colon or cecum but may also involve the transverse colon, small intestines, or stomach. Here, adhesions resulted in both herniation and complex volvulus of the small intestines.

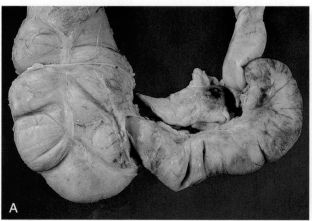
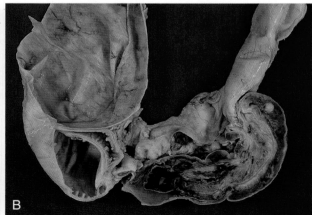

**Figure 15-126** Intussusception. Approximately 80% of intestinal obstructions are caused by nonneoplastic disease, including hernias, intestinal adhesions, volvulus, and intussusception. Intussusception occurs when peristalsis propels one segment of bowel and its mesentery into the immediately distal segment. In adults this generally signifies an intraluminal mass at the point of traction. **A,** In this case lung adenocarcinoma metastatic to the small intestines caused intussusception of the terminal ileum. **B,** Cross section of the same specimen showing the telescoped segment of bowel.

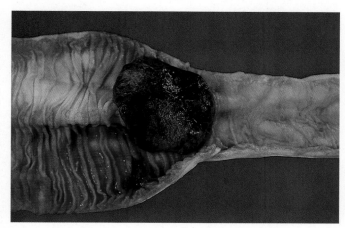

**Figure 15-128** Tumor metastatic to small intestines. Melanoma metastatic to the small intestines resulted in obstruction with dilation of the proximal bowel.

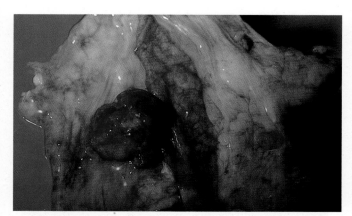

**Figure 15-129** Colonic polyps. Thorough washing of the bowel facilitates detection of colonic polyps.

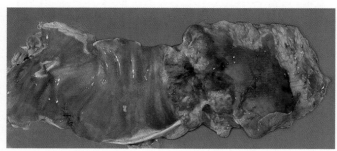

**Figure 15-130** Carcinoma of the colon. Nearly all (98%) cancers of the colon and rectum are adenocarcinomas. Carcinomas of the proximal colon grow as nonobstructing polypoid, exophytic masses. Shown here, carcinomas of the distal colon are often annular, ulcerated lesions that produce narrowing of the bowel lumen.

## HEPATOBILIARY SYSTEM

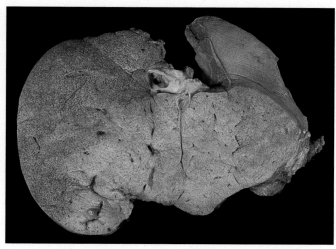

**Figure 15-131** Steatosis. Steatosis or fatty change imparts a yellow to orange cast to the liver parenchyma. The tissue is also greasy to touch. It may result from a variety of toxic insults to the liver. This case was associated with morbid obesity.

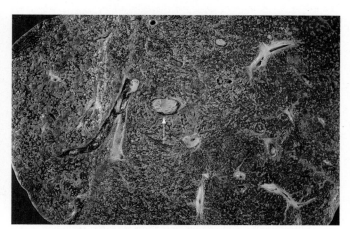

**Figure 15-132** Cholestasis. With cholestasis, the liver becomes green. This color is accentuated after fixation. In addition to cholestasis, this liver shows hepatic vein thrombosis (Budd-Chiari syndrome) *(arrow)* and early cirrhosis.

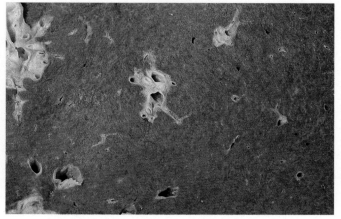

**Figure 15-133** Hemochromatosis. The accumulation of iron results in a rusty brown liver such as is seen in this case of primary (genetic) hemochromatosis.

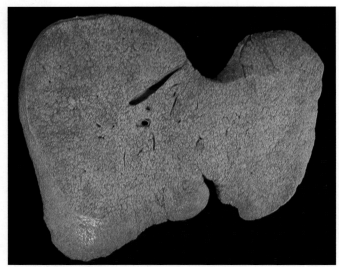

**Figure 15-134** Micronodular cirrhosis of the liver. In micronodular cirrhosis, nodules are less than 0.3 cm in diameter. Causes of micronodular cirrhosis include alcoholic liver disease (shown here), primary and secondary biliary cirrhosis, glycogenosis type IV, Indian childhood cirrhosis, galactosemia, and cardiac sclerosis.

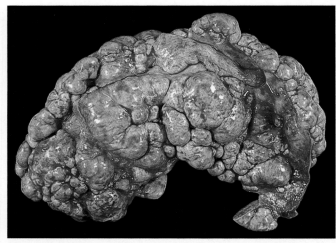

**Figure 15-137** Cystic fibrosis. About 5% of patients with cystic fibrosis have cirrhosis characterized by diffuse hepatic nodularity.

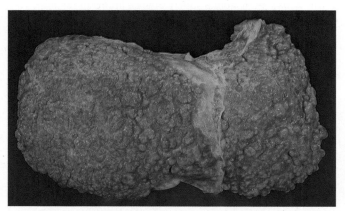

**Figure 15-135** Macronodular cirrhosis. In macronodular cirrhosis, the nodules show marked variation in size but are greater than 0.3 cm. Macronodular cirrhosis is typically seen in cases of viral hepatitis, drug-induced injury, and various hereditary diseases, including Wilson disease, hereditary tyrosinemia, and $\alpha_1$-antitrypsin deficiency. Cirrhosis developed in this case of chronic infection with hepatitis C virus.

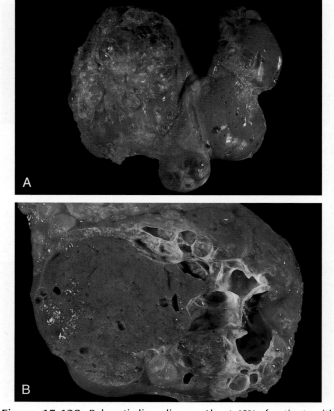

**Figure 15-138** Polycystic liver disease. About 40% of patients with autosomal dominant polycystic kidney disease have cysts in the liver. These thin-walled cysts are derived from the biliary epithelium.
**A,** Liver surface showing scattered cysts. The cysts contain clear fluid.
**B,** Cut section showing multiple cysts of varying sizes.

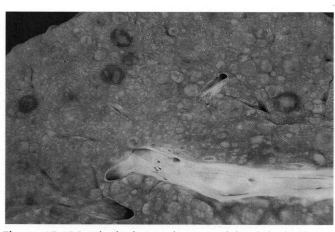

**Figure 15-136** Mixed micro- and macronodular cirrhosis. The mixed type of cirrhosis has approximately equal numbers of micronodules and macronodules. The differential diagnosis includes alcoholic cirrhosis and causes of macronodular cirrhosis.

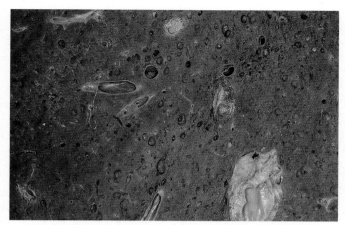

**Figure 15-139** Peliosis hepatis. This rare condition occurs as a result of primary dilation of the liver sinusoids. It is associated with use of anabolic steroids and oral contraceptives and is a component of bacillary angiomatosis, the cause in this case.

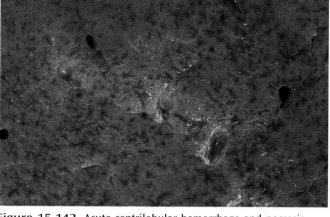

**Figure 15-142** Acute centrilobular hemorrhage and necrosis. Shock from acute blood loss or sepsis causes centrilobular hemorrhage and necrosis and accentuation of the lobular architecture of the liver.

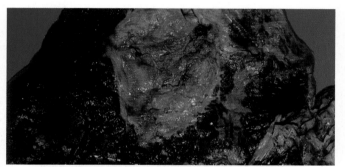

**Figure 15-140** Hepatic abscess. Hepatic abscesses occur in bacterial, fungal, parasitic, and helminthic infections and are usually pyogenic. This bacterial abscess developed as a complication of ascending cholangitis and contained both *Escherichia coli* and enterococcus organisms.

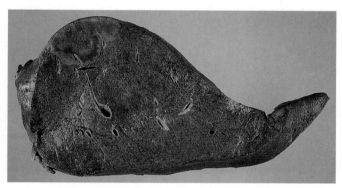

**Figure 15-143** Liver infarct. Hepatic infarcts are rare because of the liver's dual blood supply but may occur after thrombosis or compression of the hepatic arterial system. The infarct is initially pale with a hyperemic border. It yellows as organization takes place.

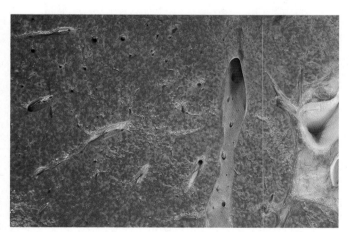

**Figure 15-141** Chronic passive congestion and centrilobular necrosis (nutmeg liver). With acute congestion from right-sided heart failure or obstruction of the inferior vena cava or hepatic vein, the liver becomes enlarged and tense, and its edges become rounded rather than sharp. On sectioning, blood oozes from the cut surface, and the central veins show prominence. With chronic congestion, centrilobular necrosis and hemorrhage lead to variegated, mottled red hepatic parenchyma.

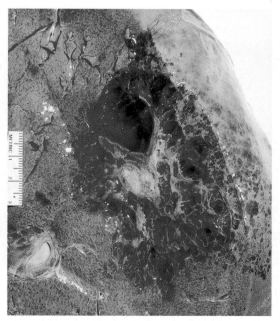

**Figure 15-144** Hemangioma. Hemangiomas, the most common tumors of the liver, are usually less than 5 cm in diameter and found only incidentally at autopsy. Large (>10 cm) hemangiomas may cause symptoms of pain related to thrombosis and infarction.

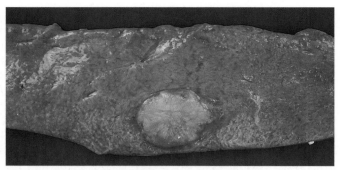

**Figure 15-145** Focal nodular hyperplasia. These pale to yellow nodules are poorly encapsulated but well demarcated from adjacent liver parenchyma. They occur most commonly in young to middle-aged women.

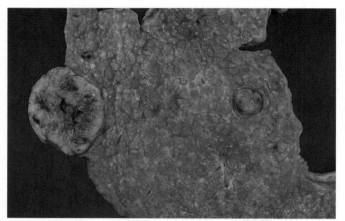

**Figure 15-146** Carcinoma. There are two major types of carcinoma of the liver. Hepatocyte-derived hepatocellular carcinomas such as the one depicted in this cirrhotic liver account for 90% of all primary liver tumors. In the example pictured here the multicentric tumors show evidence of bile. Cholangiocarcinomas, which arise from bile duct epithelium, account for nearly all the remainder.

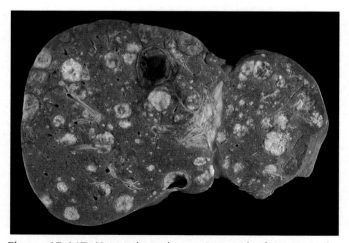

**Figure 15-147** Metastatic carcinoma. Metastasis of tumors to the liver occurs more often than primary hepatic malignancies. Breast, lung, and colon carcinomas are the most common primaries producing liver metastasis, but virtually any cancer may spread to the liver. This liver is widely replaced by metastatic small cell carcinoma of the lung. Some of the metastatic tumors show central necrosis or depressed centers (umbilication) after outgrowing their blood supply.

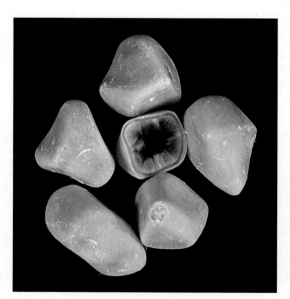

**Figure 15-148** Cholesterolosis in gallbladder. Yellow flecks visible on the mucosa represent accumulations of cholesterol within macrophages. In the extreme case, these accumulations can form cholesterolosis polyps.

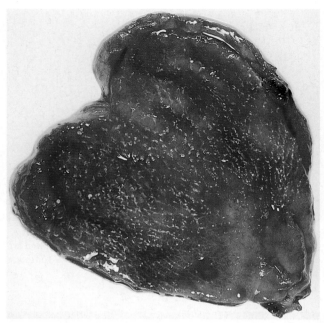

**Figure 15-149** Cholelithiasis. Gallstones range from the pure cholesterol type, which is pale yellow and semitransparent, to the brown and black pigment type. Cholesterol stones contain from 50% to 100% cholesterol. When pure, they are pale yellow. With increasing amounts of calcium carbonate, phosphates, and bilirubin, they become lamellated and have dark centers because of accumulation of calcium bilirubinate in this region. The multifaceted stones here are representative of this mixed type. Cholesterol stones form in type IV hyperlipidemia, obesity, pregnancy, or diabetes mellitus; during ileal disease or resection and estrogen therapy; and after intestinal bypass surgery.

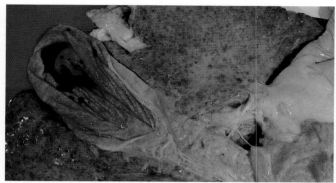

**Figure 15-150** Cholelithiasis. Pigment stones may be black (calcium bilirubinate, phosphate, and carbonate; very little cholesterol within a glycoprotein matrix) or brown (cholesterol along with calcium salts of bilirubin and fatty acids within a glycoprotein matrix). Black pigment stones such as those depicted in this gallbladder are generally small and easily crushed. They occur in conditions associated with increased concentrations of unconjugated bilirubin (hemolysis, cirrhosis, pancreatitis, advanced age, or parenteral nutrition). Brown pigment stones occur in the setting of biliary tract infection.

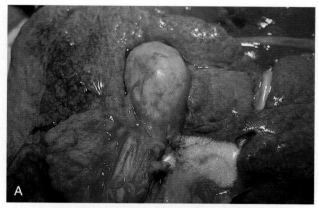

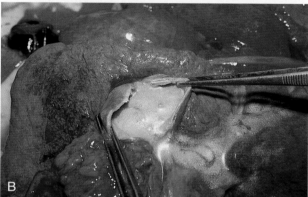

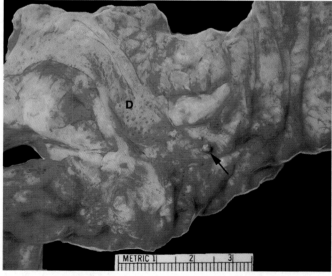

**Figure 15-152** Chronic cholecystitis. The morphologic changes of chronic cholecystitis may be quite minimal or may consist only of thickening of the gallbladder wall. The serosa may be smooth and glistening or, if there has been previous acute cholecystitis, covered by dense fibrous adhesions. Stones are generally present. **A,** In some cases, such as the one shown here, chronic cholecystitis leads to extensive dystrophic calcification, the so-called porcelain gallbladder, which is associated with an increased risk of carcinoma. **B,** The gallbladder lumen is filled with viscous, lipid-rich mucus, crystals, and small cholesterol stones (not seen).

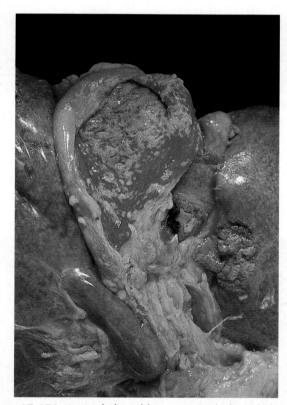

**Figure 15-151** Acute cholecystitis. In acute calculous cholecystitis, the gallbladder becomes distended and its mucosal surface blotchy red or violaceous because of subserosal hemorrhage. In most cases, a stone obstructs the neck of the gallbladder or the cystic duct. In severe cases, suppurative exudate covers the mucosal surface and the lumen contains frank pus. This case of acute necrotizing cholecystitis was associated with ascending cholangitis and hepatic abscess formation.

**Figure 15-153** Common bile duct *(D)* containing gallstones *(arrow)*. The biliary tract has been dissected and the common bile duct opened, revealing the presence of cholesterol-type gallstones at the ampulla of Vater.

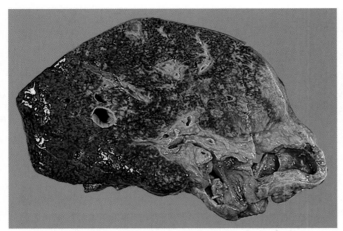

**Figure 15-154** Gallbladder with adenocarcinoma. Carcinomas, usually adenocarcinomas, may be found in the biliary tract in the gallbladder, ampulla of Vater, common bile duct, hepatic duct, or junction of the hepatic and common ducts, in that order of frequency. This adenocarcinoma of the gallbladder has extended to the liver by local invasion and metastatic spread.

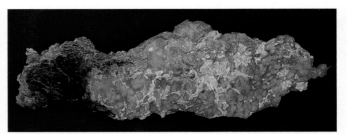

**Figure 15-157** Acute pancreatitis. The pancreas shows dark red to black hemorrhage and chalky white necrosis of interstitial and peripancreatic fat.

## PANCREAS

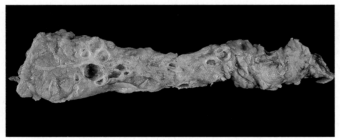

**Figure 15-155** Pancreatic cysts. Thin-walled, serous, fluid-filled cysts may be found in the pancreas in some patients with autosomal-dominant polycystic kidney disease.

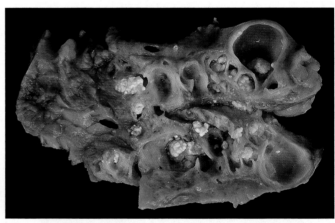

**Figure 15-158** Chronic pancreatitis. The pancreas becomes hard and gray and contains numerous areas of mineralization. Ducts are cystically dilated and contain scattered calculi.

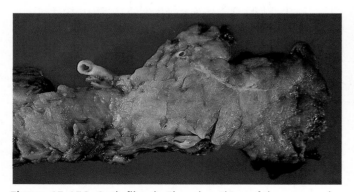

**Figure 15-156** Cystic fibrosis. The acinar tissue of the pancreas has been replaced by adipose tissue.

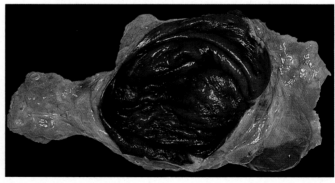

**Figure 15-159** Pseudocyst of the pancreas. Pseudocysts of the pancreas develop after inflammation from pancreatitis. Typically located within or adjacent to the tail of the pancreas, they may reach 10 cm in size. The cyst wall varies in thickness, and the cyst fluid is usually serous and turbid, occasionally containing organizing blood clot, calcium precipitates, and cholesterol crystals.
(Courtesy of Robert M. Anthony, MD, PhD.)

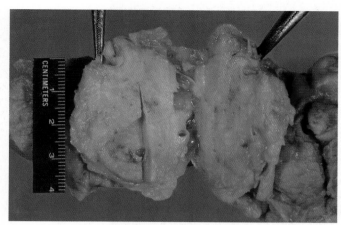

**Figure 15-160** Pancreas with adenocarcinoma. Adenocarcinoma of the pancreas may arise in the head (60%), body (15%), or tail (5%) of the pancreas; in 20% of cases there is involvement of more than one segment. This specimen shows a large tumor infiltrating the head of the pancreas.

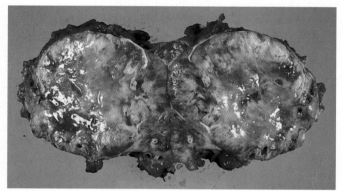

**Figure 15-161** Pancreatic endocrine tumor. Derived from islet cells, pancreatic endocrine tumors may produce insulin, glucagon, somatostatin, gastrin, or other hormones and active neuropeptides. The tumors vary from soft to firm and gray-white or gray-yellow to mottled or deep red.

## URINARY TRACT SYSTEM

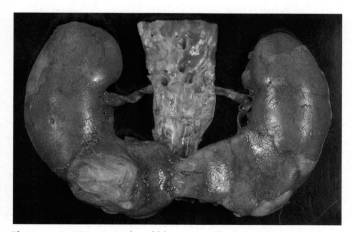

**Figure 15-162** Horseshoe kidney. Usually an incidental finding at autopsy, horseshoe kidney, resulting from fusion of the lower (90%) or upper poles (10%), has an incidence of 1 in 500 to 1 in 1000 autopsies. This posterior view shows fusion at the lower poles and a simple renal cyst of the left kidney.

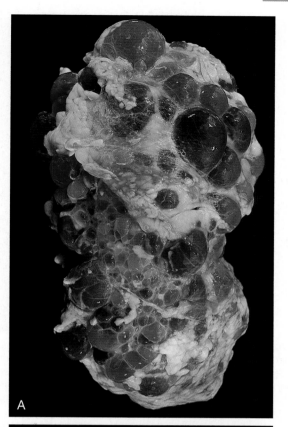

A

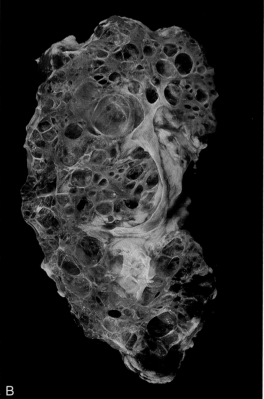

B

**Figure 15-163** Autosomal-dominant polycystic kidney disease. Affected kidneys may show massive enlargement. **A,** The external surface of the intact specimen shows numerous cysts without obvious intervening parenchyma. The cysts reach 3 to 4 cm in diameter and are filled with serous or turbid red-brown fluid. **B,** Bisected specimen showing diffuse nature of cysts and deformation of the renal calyces and pelvis.

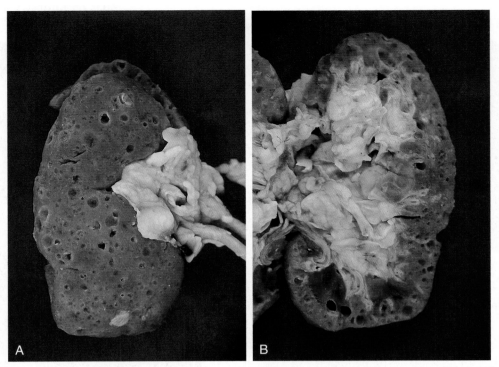

**Figure 15-164** Kidney with acquired cysts related to chronic renal dialysis. The kidneys of patients undergoing dialysis may develop numerous cortical and medullary cysts that typically range from 0.5 to 2 cm in diameter. Complications of acquired cystic disease include hemorrhage into the cysts or development of tumors, adenomas, or occasionally adenocarcinomas within their walls. This end-stage kidney shows marked cortical atrophy and scattered cortical and medullary cysts. **A,** Cortical surface after removal of capsule. **B,** Cut section.

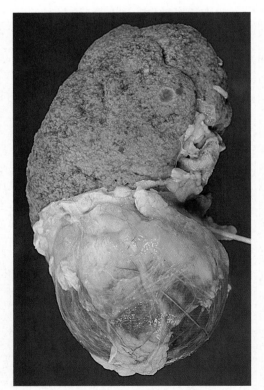

**Figure 15-165** Benign nephrosclerosis and simple cysts. Long-standing hypertension or diabetes mellitus, or both, lead to hyaline arteriolosclerosis associated with fine granular scarring. The kidneys may be normal or moderately reduced in size. Simple (urinary retention) cysts are common findings at autopsy. Filled with serous fluid, these cystic spaces typically range from 1 to 5 cm in diameter but may reach a larger size. Single or few in number, they generally involve only the cortex, as did this large cyst in the inferior pole of the kidney.

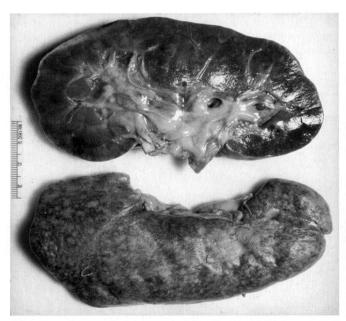

**Figure 15-166** Malignant nephrosclerosis. Accelerated or malignant hypertension causes petechial hemorrhages in the cortex because of rupture of arterioles and glomerular capillaries, imparting a "flea-bitten" appearance.

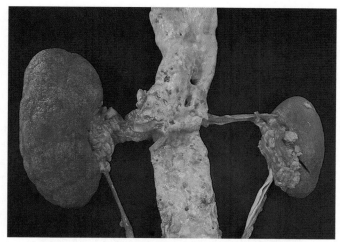

**Figure 15-167**  Renal artery stenosis. Caused by either atherosclerosis or fibromuscular dysplasia, renal artery stenosis leads to a marked reduction in the size of the kidney. This specimen consists of the aorta, opened longitudinally along its posterior aspect, and both kidneys. Atherosclerotic plaque at the origin of the right renal artery has led to marked atrophy of the right kidney (so-called Goldblatt kidney). Exposed to the full impact of hypertension, the left kidney shows evidence of nephrosclerosis.

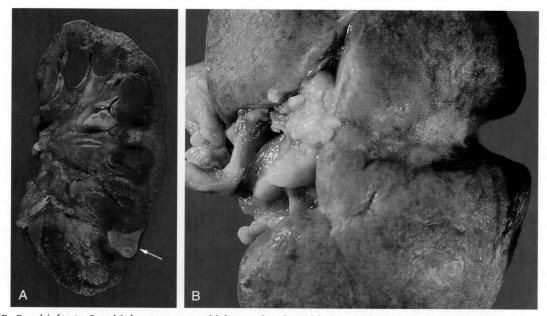

**Figure 15-168**  Renal infarcts. Renal infarcts are pyramidal or wedge-shaped lesions with the base at the cortical surface and the apex pointing to the medullary origin of the arterial supply. Beginning as pale areas of necrosis with hyperemic borders, they progress to yellow-gray lesions that ultimately become depressed V-shaped gray-white furrows. **A,** Acute renal infarct *(arrow).* **B,** Corticomedullary scar from healed infarct (fixed specimen).

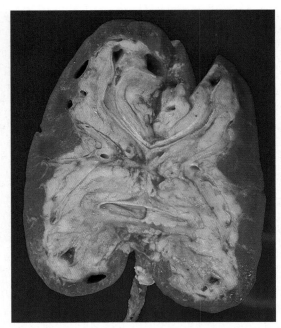

**Figure 15-169** Kidneys with chronic end-stage glomerulonephritis of varying causes are reduced in size and have diffusely granular cortical surfaces. The cortex is thinned, and the peripelvic fat is prominent.

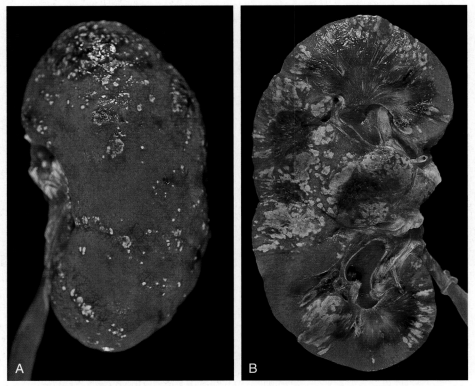

**Figure 15-170** Acute bacterial pyelonephritis. A hematogenous route of infection leads to scattered infective foci in the cortex. In contrast, ascending infection from the lower urinary tract affects the medulla first with secondary extension to the cortex in a segmental manner. **A,** Cortical surface. **B,** Bisected specimen. The relative sparing of the medulla as shown in the cut section suggests a hematogenous route.

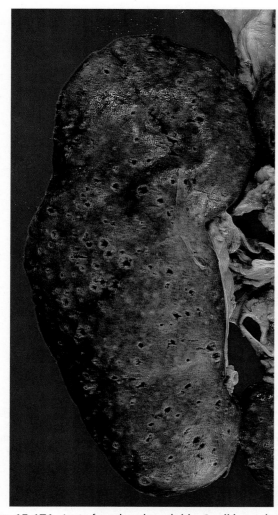

**Figure 15-171** Acute fungal pyelonephritis. *Candida tropicalis* infection in a patient with alcoholic cirrhosis and liver failure. There are numerous cortical abscesses.

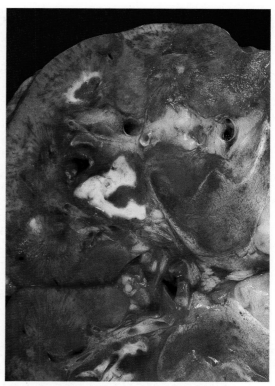

**Figure 15-172** Kidney with papillary necrosis. A complication of acute pyelonephritis most commonly seen in patients with diabetes and those with urinary tract obstruction, papillary necrosis generally involves the tips or distal portion of the pyramid. The area of necrosis is gray-white or yellow and is separated from the preserved proximal pyramid by a zone of hyperemia.

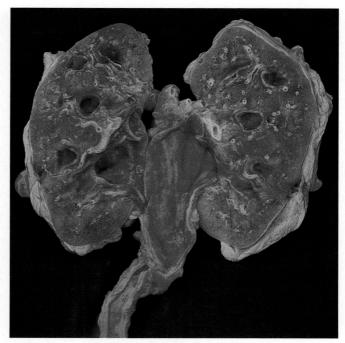

**Figure 15-173** Chronic pyelonephritis. The most common forms of chronic pyelonephritis are associated with chronic obstruction and chronic reflux (reflux nephropathy). In this case, a stricture of the ureter led to chronic pyelonephritis. Thinning of the renal cortex, blunting and dilation of the calyces, and dilation of the renal pelvis and ureter are present.

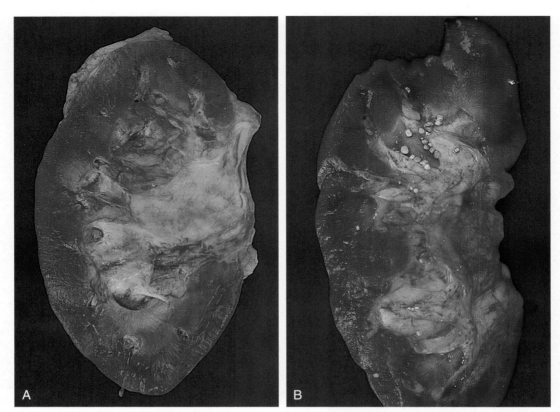

**Figure 15-174** Obstructive nephropathy. Obstruction to urinary flow may be due to calculi, tumors, strictures of the urinary tract from kidney to urethra, or extrinsic compression from extraurinary masses or may be secondary to functional disturbances such as vesicoureteral reflux or neurogenic bladder. Early on there is dilation of the calyces, pelvis, and ureter proximal to the obstruction. Later, there is progressive blunting of the apices of the pyramids, which eventually become cup shaped. Finally, as cortical parenchyma atrophies, the kidney is converted into a cystic structure. **A,** Obstruction related to prostate cancer causing dilation of the pelvis and calyces. **B,** Late-stage hydronephrosis from urolithiasis.

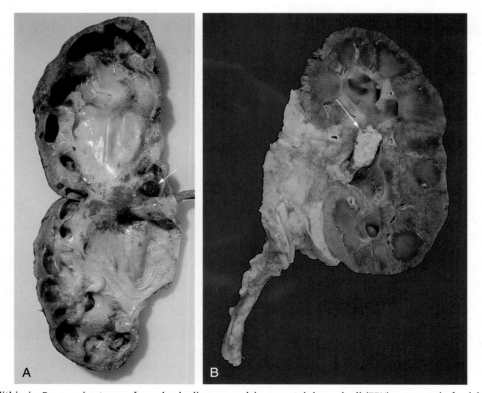

**Figure 15-175** Urolithiasis. Four major types of renal calculi occur: calcium-containing calculi (75%) composed of calcium oxalate or calcium oxalate and calcium phosphate, struvite or "triple stones" (15%) composed of magnesium ammonium phosphate, uric acid stones (6%), and cystine stones (1% to 2%). **A,** Most stones *(arrow)* are small and spherical. **B,** Occasionally, progressive precipitation may lead to the formation of staghorn calculi *(arrow)* that assume the shape of the pelvis and calyces.

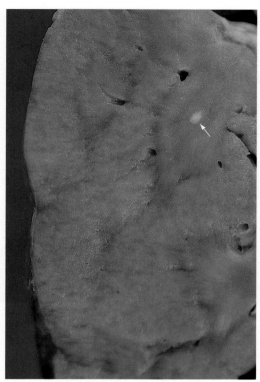

**Figure 15-176** Renal fibroma (hamartoma). These small gray-white lesions *(arrow)* are found incidentally at autopsy.

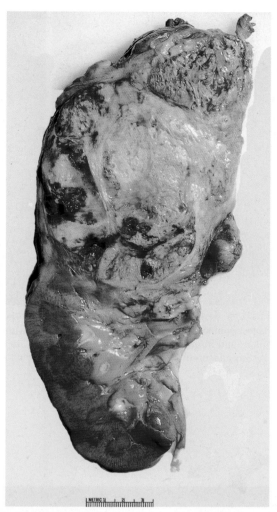

**Figure 15-178** Renal cell adenocarcinoma. Renal cell adenocarcinomas generally arise at one of the renal poles, more often the superior one. They grow as large spherical masses of moderately firm, yellow to gray-white tissue that can reach 15 cm in diameter. As they grow, foci of hemorrhage, softening, and necrosis develop. With enlargement, the tumor may extend into the collecting portion of the kidney or may invade the renal vein, eventually extending into the inferior vena cava. Peripheral extension may involve the renal capsule. Satellite lesions may also develop.

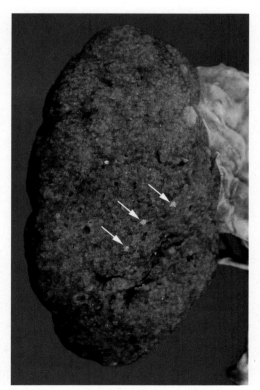

**Figure 15-177** Renal papillary adenoma. These are small, usually less than 0.5 cm in diameter, yellow-gray cortical tumors *(arrows)* commonly found at autopsy after the renal capsule is removed. Histologically, they resemble low-grade papillary carcinomas, and, in fact, the benign lesion cannot be clearly differentiated from its malignant counterpart.

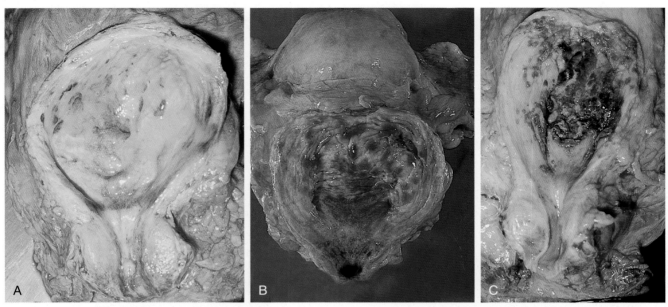

**Figure 15-179** Acute and chronic cystitis. Acutely, infection of the bladder results in hyperemia of the mucosa that may be accompanied by hemorrhage, suppurative exudates, mucosal ulcers, or polypoid epithelial growth. With chronicity, the bladder mucosa becomes red, friable, and granular, and fibrosis within the tunica propria leads to thickening of the bladder wall. **A,** Acute purulent bacterial cystitis. **B,** Acute and chronic cystitis and urethritis. **C,** Necrotizing fungal (candida species) cystitis in an immunosuppressed patient.

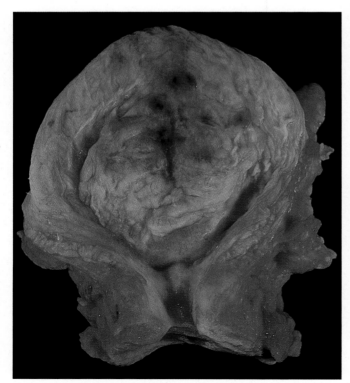

**Figure 15-180** Focal hemorrhage from indwelling catheter. Discrete linear and roughly circular areas of acute hemorrhage are often found in patients with Foley catheters.

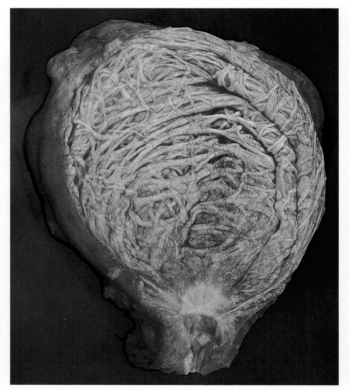

**Figure 15-181** Smooth muscle hypertrophy. In response to chronic obstruction, the bladder dilates and the smooth muscle undergoes hypertrophy and trabeculation. Eventually, crypts may form, producing acquired diverticula. This specimen shows smooth muscle hypertrophy and trabeculation secondary to partial urethral obstruction from nodular hyperplasia of the prostate.

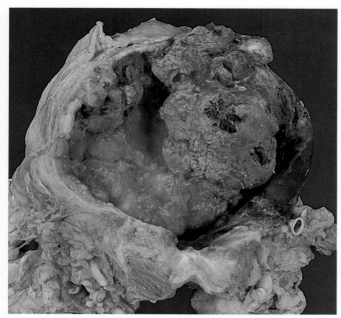

**Figure 15-182** Malignant tumors of the bladder take on various gross appearances depending on the histopathologic type and pattern of growth. Approximately 90% are transitional cell (urothelial) carcinomas. Transitional cell carcinomas may be papillary, flat, or a mixture of the two. This large exophytic tumor that nearly fills the bladder cavity is a high-grade transitional cell carcinoma.

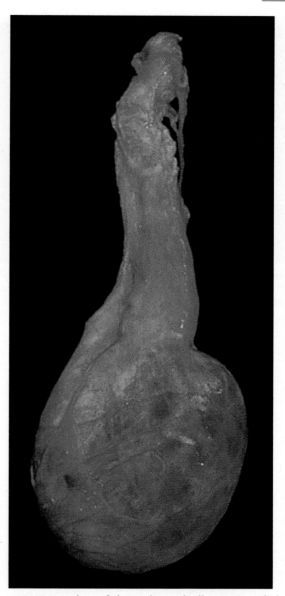

**Figure 15-184** Lesions of the tunica vaginalis. Hematocele is associated with direct trauma to the testis or torsion of the testis. Chylocele occurs in the setting of severe lymphatic obstruction. Hydrocele (depicted here) occurs spontaneously and is found quite often at autopsy.

# REPRODUCTIVE SYSTEM (MALE)

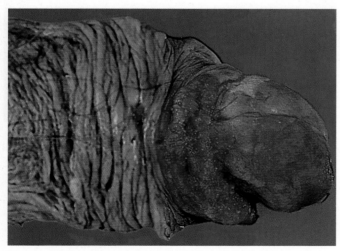

**Figure 15-183** Squamous cell carcinoma of the penis. Squamous cell carcinoma of the penis begins on the glans or the inner surface of the prepuce. It is rare after circumcision. In this specimen, the red tumor tissue involves most of the glans and prepuce.

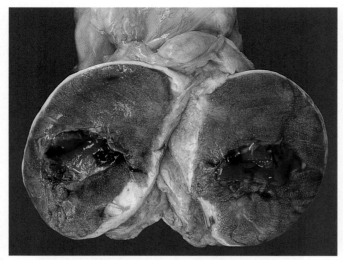

**Figure 15-185** Infarcts. Twisting of the spermatic cord with resultant interruption of the venous drainage of the testis results in marked vascular congestion followed by infarction. The infarct of the testis shown here occurred in association with vasculitis.

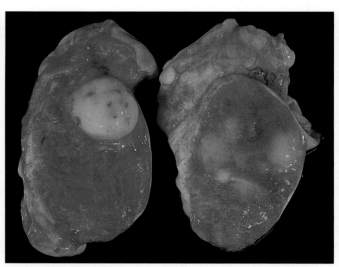

**Figure 15-187** Testicular lymphoma. Testicular lymphomas, usually as part of disseminated disease, account for 5% of testicular neoplasms in men 60 years of age and older. Diffuse large cell lymphomas are most common. In this case, both testes contained multiple nodules of tumor.

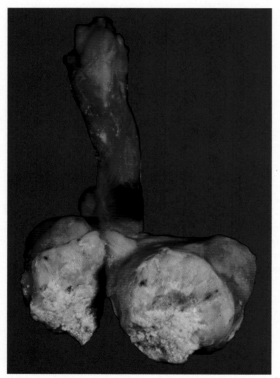

**Figure 15-186** Primary testicular neoplasms. A wide variety of germ cell and nongerminal cell (stroma or sex cord) tumors originate in the testis. This teratocarcinoma, primarily solid, has a variegated appearance.

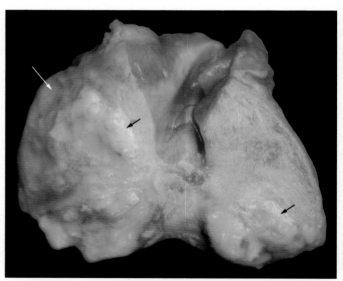

**Figure 15-188** Prostatitis. Prostatitis is divided into three main categories: acute and chronic bacterial prostatitis, chronic abacterial prostatitis, and granulomatous prostatitis. This is a case of acute bacterial prostatitis due to drug-resistant *Staphylococcus aureus*. Areas of necrosis *(white arrow)* and purulent abscesses *(black arrows)* are evident.

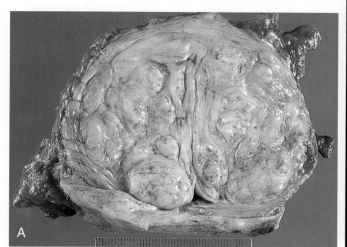

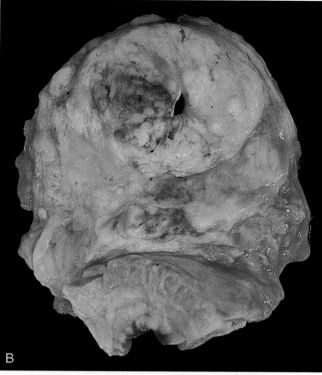

**Figure 15-189** Growth disorders of the prostate. **A,** Nodular hyperplasia (benign prostatic hypertrophy) of the prostate is characterized by well-defined, yellow-gray nodules of variable size. This cross section of a large gland demonstrates how the tumor may obstruct the urethra. **B,** Prostate adenocarcinoma. The majority (70%) of prostate adenocarcinomas arise in the periphery of the gland, most often in a posterior location. On cross section, the tumors are yellow-white masses that can be difficult to discern from the adjacent prostate parenchyma. (**A** courtesy of Werner Rosenau, MD, University of California, San Francisco.)

## REPRODUCTIVE SYSTEM (FEMALE)

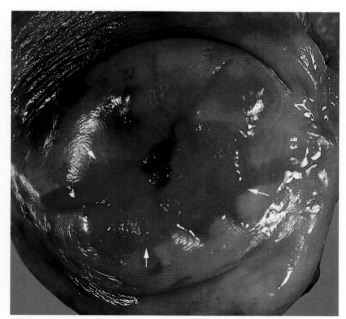

**Figure 15-190** Squamous cell carcinoma of the cervix. These tumors may exhibit exophytic ulcerating or infiltrating patterns grossly. This exophytic keratinizing (well-differentiated) squamous cell carcinoma *(arrows)* surrounds the lower half of the cervical os and extends across the exocervix.

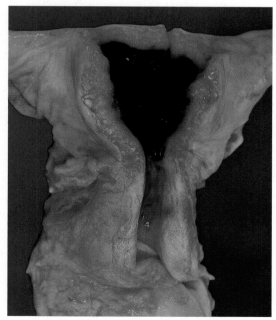

**Figure 15-191** Acute agonal endometrial hemorrhage. With profound hypotension, there may be variable amounts of endometrial hemorrhage. The uterine cavity is filled with hematoma.

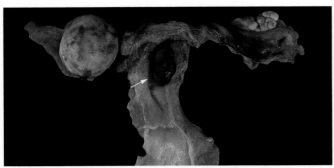

**Figure 15-192** Endometrial polyp. These variable-sized circumscribed masses bulge into the endometrial cavity. They are relatively common (25% prevalence) and occasionally (25%) multiple. This large endometrial polyp *(arrow)* has a hemorrhagic surface. Note the ovarian mass, a mature teratoma.

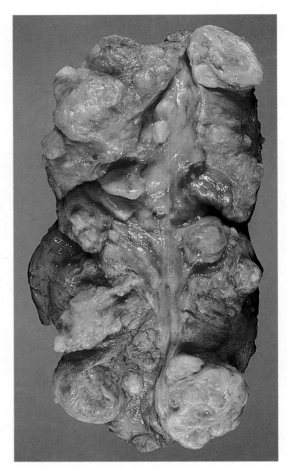

**Figure 15-194** Leiomyomas. The most common tumors in women, these gray-white masses are sharply circumscribed and distinct from the adjacent myometrium. They can develop within the myometrium (intramural), just beneath the endometrium (submucosal), or beneath the serosa (subserosal). There are often multiple tumors and, as seen in this bivalved uterus, marked distortion of the normal anatomy.

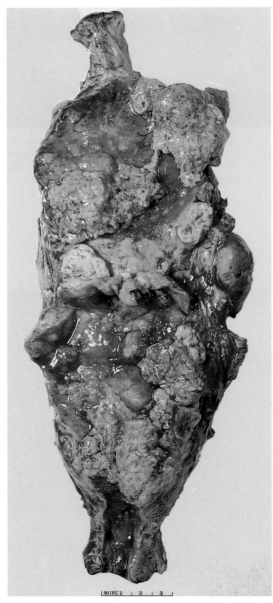

**Figure 15-193** Endometrial carcinoma. In this bivalved uterus, endometrial carcinoma forms large polypoid masses of friable, gray-tan tissue that histologically not only involved the endometrial surface but also invaded the myometrium.

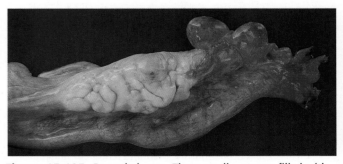

**Figure 15-195** Paratubal cysts. These small cysts are filled with serous fluid. Those occurring near the fimbria are called hydatids of Morgagni.

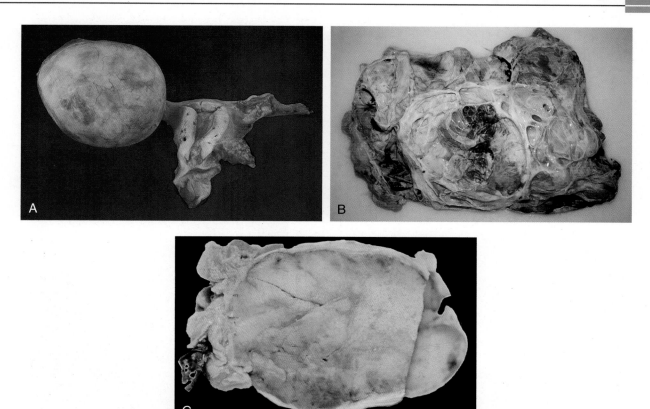

**Figure 15-196** Ovarian tumors. The classification of ovarian tumors is extensive, including a variety of benign and malignant neoplasms of epithelial, stromal, and germ cell origin. **A,** Serous epithelial tumors consist of one or a few fibrous-walled cysts with variable amounts of solid or papillary growth correlating with malignancy. This right ovarian mass is a single-walled serous cystadenoma. **B,** Mucinous epithelial tumors may become quite large, such as this complex mucinous cystadenoma that weighed 10 kg. **C,** Thecomas are benign tumors, generally unilateral solid masses. Their cut surface may be yellow due to the presence of lipids.

## ENDOCRINE SYSTEM

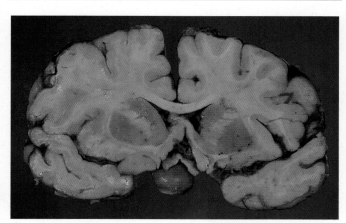

**Figure 15-197** Pituitary adenoma. Nearly all pituitary neoplasms arise in the anterior pituitary. Malignant tumors are extremely rare. Pituitary adenomas are common lesions; some are found only at autopsy, often recognized first on microscopic examination. Pituitary adenomas are well circumscribed and soft. This pituitary was markedly enlarged by a prolactin cell adenoma.

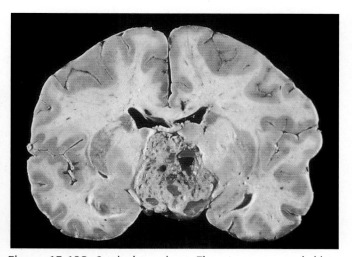

**Figure 15-198** Craniopharyngioma. These tumors are probably derived from vestigial remnants of Rathke's pouch. Generally cystic and multiloculated but occasionally solid and encapsulated, craniopharyngiomas encroach on the optic chiasm and bulge into the floor of the third ventricle, as depicted in this example.
(From Davis RL: Pathological lesions of the third ventricle and adjacent structures. In Apouzzo MLJ, editor: *Surgery of the third ventricle,* Baltimore, 1987, Williams & Wilkins, pp 235-252; and the permission of the Armed Forces Institute of Pathology, Washington, DC.)

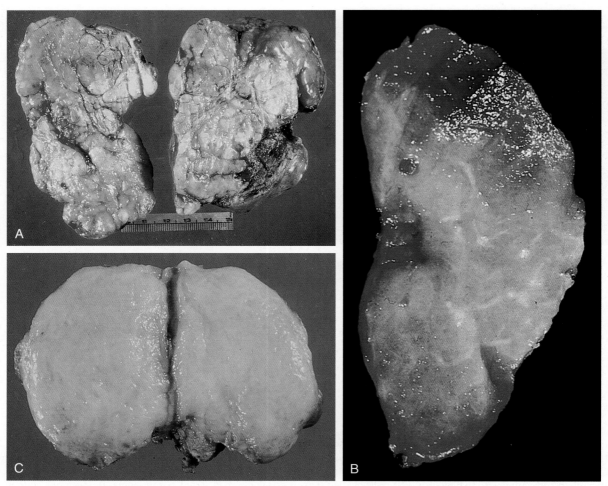

**Figure 15-199** Thyroiditis. Thyroiditis refers to a number of different disorders associated with inflammation of the thyroid and includes infective thyroiditis, granulomatous thyroiditis, subacute lymphocytic thyroiditis, fibrous (Riedel) thyroiditis, and Hashimoto thyroiditis. The appearance of the thyroid varies among these conditions. It appears relatively normal in subacute lymphocytic thyroiditis but enlarged, pale, and gray-tan in Hashimoto or granulomatous thyroiditis. Fibrous thyroiditis may spare parts of the gland but when present results in firm, white hyalinized tissue with effacement of the lobules. **A,** Hashimoto thyroiditis. **B,** Granulomatous thyroiditis. **C,** Riedel thyroiditis. (Courtesy of Werner Rosenau, MD, University of California, San Francisco.)

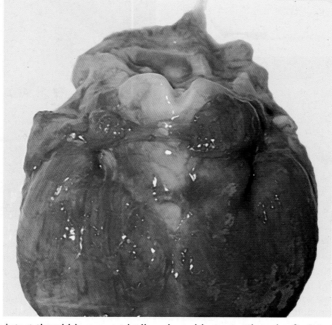

**Figure 15-200** Graves disease. The intact thyroid is symmetrically enlarged but smooth and soft. Cut section showed homogenous beefy red parenchyma.

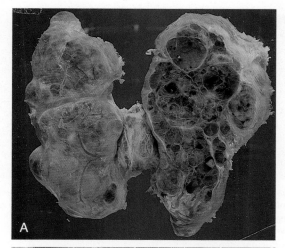

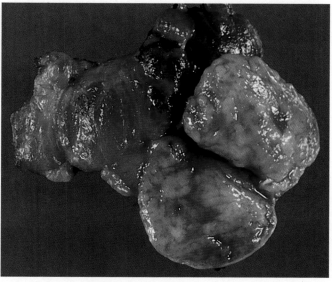

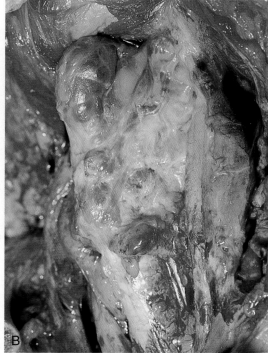

**Figure 15-202** Thyroid neoplasms. Common neoplasms of the thyroid include adenomas and carcinomas (papillary, follicular, and medullary types). Follicular carcinomas tend to occur as single nodules, such as the one shown here. Often well circumscribed, they can be difficult to distinguish from follicular adenomas on gross examination alone.
(Courtesy of Henry Sanchez, MD, and Werner Rosenau, MD, University of California, San Francisco.)

**Figure 15-201** Diffuse nontoxic (simple) and multinodular goiter. The hyperplastic thyroid of diffuse nontoxic goiter is enlarged symmetrically, but, as it involutes, its cut surface shows brown, glassy, colloid-rich areas. **A,** Multinodular goiters are asymmetrically enlarged and multilobulated, brown, and gelatinous on cut section, as in this fixed specimen. The enlarging goiter may expand against the adjacent neck and even thoracic structures. **B,** This view of the fresh thyroid in situ demonstrates enlargement of the right lobe.

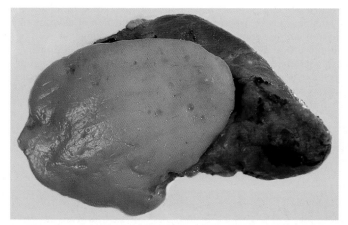

**Figure 15-203** Parathyroid adenoma. Parathyroid adenomas are usually single well-circumscribed nodules of soft, tan tissue covered with a thin, delicate capsule. The remaining glands are normal or decreased in size. In this surgical specimen, a portion of thyroid was also removed.

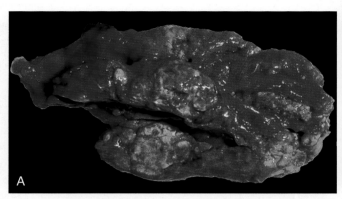
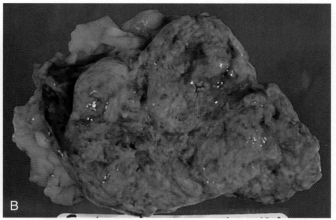

**Figure 15-204** Hypercortisolism (Cushing syndrome). Hypercortisolism originating in the adrenal gland is due to diffuse hyperplasia and functional neoplasms (cortical adenomas or carcinomas). **A,** With diffuse hyperplasia, both adrenal glands are enlarged and the adrenal cortex is thickened and yellow. Nodularity, seen here, is often present. **B,** Adrenocortical adenomas are circumscribed but not encapsulated. Color varies from yellow to orange with variegated tan, brown, or even black areas. Their gross appearance, however, is generally not distinctive enough to separate them from nonfunctional or aldosterone-producing adenomas.

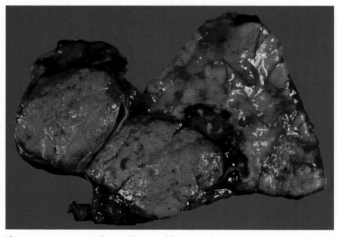

**Figure 15-205** Primary hyperaldosteronism caused by an adrenal adenoma. As with hypercortisolism, overproduction of aldosterone may be due to adrenocortical hyperplasia or functional adrenocortical neoplasms. Approximately 80% of cases of primary hyperaldosteronism (Conn syndrome) are caused by an aldosterone-secreting adenoma in one adrenal gland. The tumors are generally solitary and less than 2 cm in diameter, more common on the left than the right, and yellow to yellow-orange on cut section.

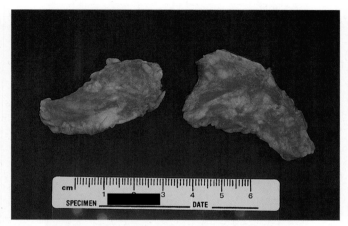

**Figure 15-207** Adrenal atrophy. Chronic adrenocortical insufficiency may be primary (Addison disease) or secondary. Addison's disease results from damage to the adrenal cortex by primary and metastatic neoplasms, amyloidosis, sarcoidosis, hemochromatosis, infections, and autoimmune adrenalitis. Secondary adrenocortical insufficiency occurs in the setting of disorders of the hypothalamus and pituitary that reduce adrenocorticotropic hormone production or with prolonged therapy with glucocorticoids. These very small adrenal glands developed after postpartum necrosis of the pituitary (Sheehan syndrome).

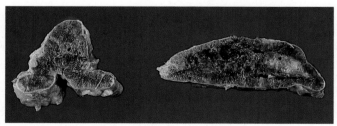

**Figure 15-206** Bilateral acute adrenal hemorrhage from a patient with Waterhouse-Friderichsen syndrome. Overwhelming bacterial infection classically associated with *Neisseria meningitidis* septicemia and shock, disseminated intravascular coagulation with purpura, and rapidly progressive adrenocortical insufficiency related to bilateral adrenal hemorrhage are the hallmarks of the Waterhouse-Friderichsen syndrome (fixed specimen).

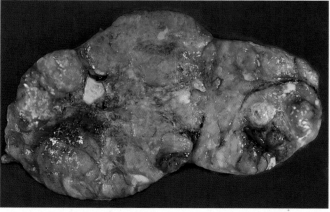

**Figure 15-208** Adrenocortical carcinoma. These tumors are poorly encapsulated yellow to yellow-brown masses with areas of hemorrhage, necrosis, and cyst formation. They are often quite large at the time of diagnosis, commonly exceeding 20 cm in diameter.

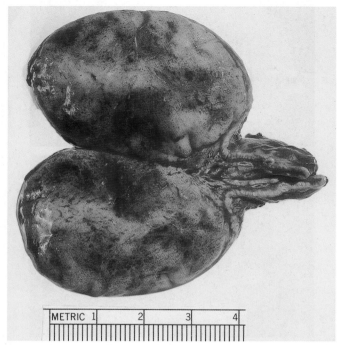

**Figure 15-209** Pheochromocytoma. These uncommon tumors vary from small to quite large. Composed of gray to pale red tissue, larger lesions may show extensive areas of hemorrhage, necrosis, and cystic degeneration.

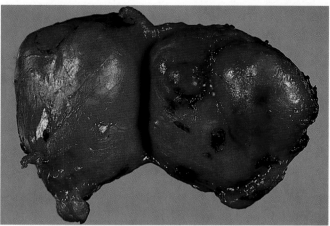

**Figure 15-211** Thymic neoplasms. The thymus may be the primary site of lymphomas, germ cell tumors, neuroendocrine tumors, and tumors of thymic epithelial cells (thymomas). Benign thymomas are lobulated, firm, gray-white masses that may show calcification, necrosis, and cystic degeneration. Type I malignant thymomas have gross and cytologic features identical to those of benign thymomas; however, they show microscopic evidence of capsular penetration and local invasion. Type II malignant thymomas (thymic carcinoma) are characteristically fleshy masses (as shown here) that readily invade adjacent structures.

## LYMPHORETICULAR SYSTEM

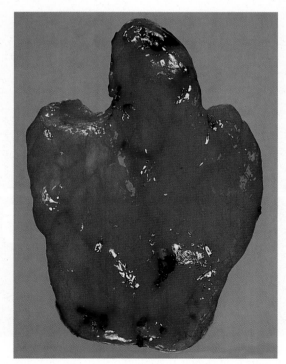

**Figure 15-210** Thymic hyperplasia. Thymic hyperplasia is seen in a number of immunologic states including Graves disease, collagen vascular disorders, and, most commonly, myasthenia gravis, where it occurs in about 75% of cases. This greatly enlarged thymus was removed from a patient with myasthenia gravis.

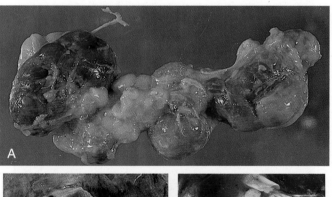

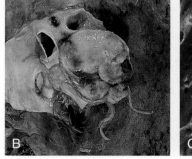
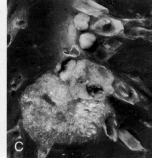

**Figure 15-212** Lymphadenopathy. The specific causes of lymphadenopathy are many but in broad categories include acute and chronic nonspecific lymphadenitis, primary lymphoid neoplasms, and metastatic cancer. **A,** Chain of axillary and infraclavicular lymph nodes enlarged by non-Hodgkin lymphoma. **B,** Hilar lymph nodes replaced by gray-white non-Hodgkin's lymphoma. **C,** Hilar lymph nodes replaced by spread of non–small cell lung carcinoma.

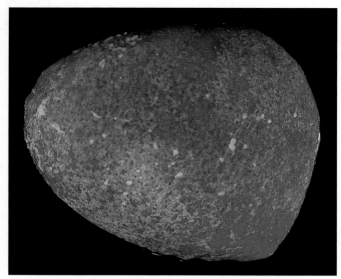

**Figure 15-213** Perisplenitis. In this view of the surface of the spleen, the gray-white areas represent patchy fibrosis of the splenic capsule (perisplenitis) developing in the setting of chronic ascites.

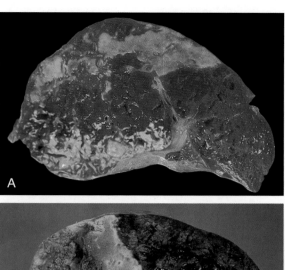

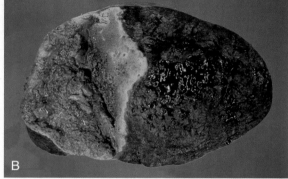

**Figure 15-215** Splenic infarcts. **A,** Infarcts of the spleen are typically wedge shaped. Initially pale with a hemorrhagic border, the infarct turns pale yellow-gray as it undergoes organization, eventually contracting into a depressed scar. **B,** Septic infarcts undergo liquefactive necrosis, shown here in an infarct caused by an embolus from the mitral valve in a case of bacterial endocarditis (fixed specimen).

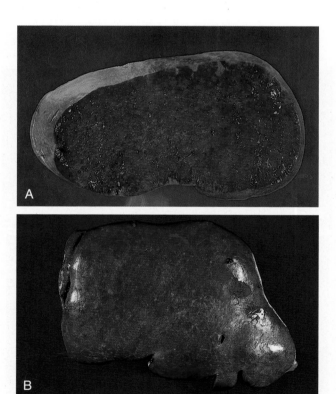

**Figure 15-214** Splenomegaly. Numerous conditions result in splenomegaly, but major disease categories associated with splenic enlargement include infections, passive congestion, lymphohematogenous disorders, immunologic disorders, and disorders of metabolism resulting in abnormal storage. **A,** Enlarged spleen from a patient with AIDS. Marked extramedullary hematopoiesis was seen. Note also the small acute infarcts. **B,** Splenomegaly, often massive, is sometimes the only abnormal physical finding in hairy cell leukemia.

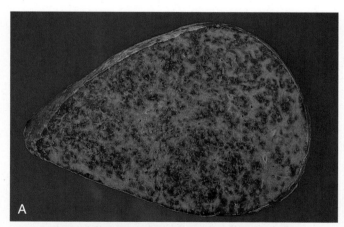

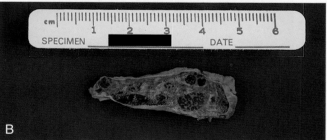

**Figure 15-216** Sickle cell anemia. **A,** Early in the disease, splenomegaly from chronic congestion is seen. The sinusoids dilate, and collagen deposits in the basement membrane. There is increased destruction of sequestered red blood cells (hypersplenism) and hemorrhage. Hemorrhages organize, and the connective tissue foci become encrusted with iron and calcium salts (Gandy-Gamna nodules). **B,** Eventually the spleen becomes progressively fibrotic and nonfunctional (autosplenectomy), resulting in a minute spleen.

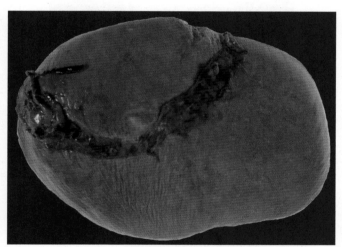

**Figure 15-217** Accessory spleens. Small spherical accessory spleens (spleniculi) are found in approximately 20% of autopsies.

## MUSCULOSKELETAL SYSTEM

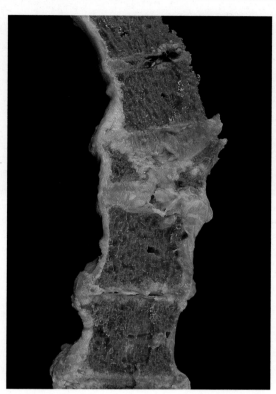

**Figure 15-220** Osteoporosis. Associated with a number of primary and secondary conditions, osteoporosis may be generalized or localized to a certain bone or skeletal region. In this segment of the thoracic vertebral column from an elderly female with postmenopausal osteoporosis, marked osteopenia and an associated compression fracture can be seen.

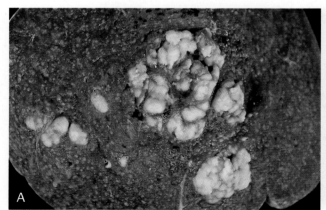

**Figure 15-218** Splenic rupture. Blunt-force trauma to the abdomen may result in splenic lacerations. Spontaneous, nontraumatic rupture may occur in association with infectious mononucleosis, malaria, typhoid fever, and leukemia. The lacerations shown here were from abdominal trauma sustained in a motor vehicle accident and led to massive hemoperitoneum and death.

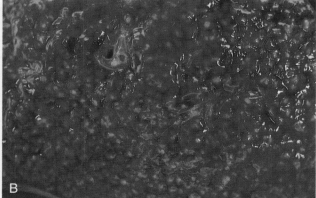

**Figure 15-219** Lymphoma involving the spleen. **A,** Lymphoma consisting of multiple large masses and prominent white pulp. **B,** Lymphoma causing expansion of white pulp but no discrete mass.

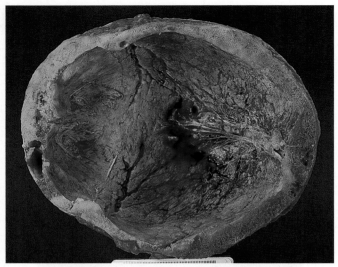

**Figure 15-221**  Paget's disease (osteitis deformans). In this view of the opened calvarium, the bone is markedly thickened, and there is loss of diploic architecture.

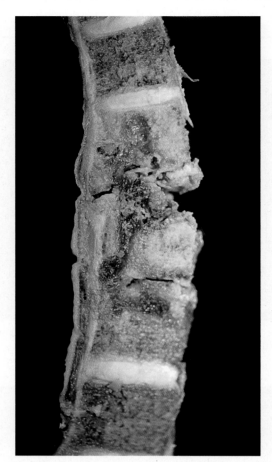

**Figure 15-223**  Pyogenic osteomyelitis. The appearance of pyogenic osteomyelitis depends on the stage and location of infection. Initial osteonecrosis is followed by subperiosteal abscesses. With healing, there is deposition of reactive bone around the devitalized bone tissue. The process can be quite destructive, as seen in this example of osteomyelitis involving three vertebral bodies (fixed specimen).

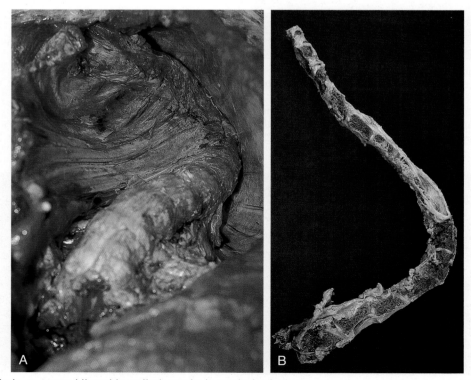

**Figure 15-222**  Scoliosis. **A,** Severe idiopathic scoliosis results in marked spinal curvature, as seen in this photograph of the thorax and abdominal cavities after organ evisceration. **B,** Vertebral column removed demonstrating distortion of vertebral bodies and joints.

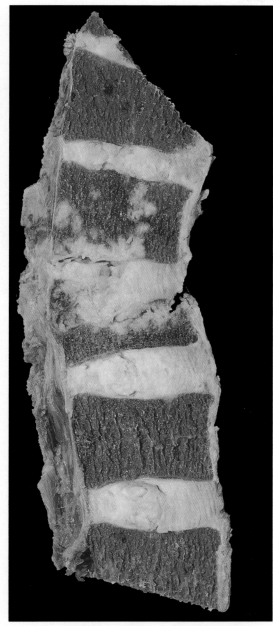

**Figure 15-224** Tuberculous osteomyelitis. The thoracic and lumbar vertebrae (Pott disease), knees, and hips are the most common sites affected by tuberculous osteomyelitis. Note the severe bone destruction, the basis for pathologic fracture.

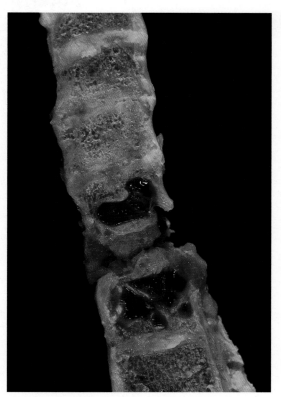

**Figure 15-225** Multiple myeloma. Diffuse infiltration of red, gelatinous-appearing tumor and associated lytic lesions can be seen.

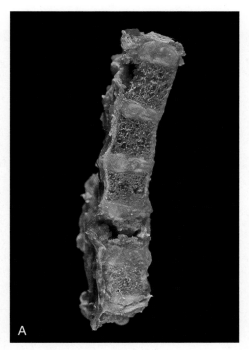

**Figure 15-226** Metastatic cancer. Metastatic tumors are the most common form of skeletal malignancy. The metastases are generally multiple, although thyroid and renal carcinomas often produce solitary metastatic deposits. Bone metastasis may produce lytic, blastic, or mixed lytic and blastic lesions. Most metastases result in mixed lesions. However, carcinomas of the thyroid, lung, gastrointestinal tract, and kidney and melanoma may produce lytic lesions, and metastatic prostate and breast carcinomas often produce a blastic or sclerotic response. **A,** Metastatic small cell carcinoma of the lung to the spine resulting in destruction and collapse of a vertebral body.

*Continued*

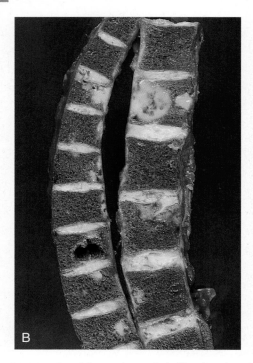

**Figure 15-226—Cont'd  B,** Metastatic infiltrating ductal carcinoma of the breast to the spine creating predominantly osteoblastic lesions.

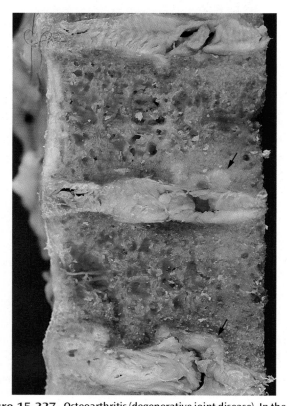

**Figure 15-227**  Osteoarthritis (degenerative joint disease). In the early stages of osteoarthritis the joint cartilage is degraded, evident as softening and surface granularity. Progression results in sloughing of the cartilage, and the exposed bone surface is smoothed by constant friction (eburnation). Subchondral regions develop fibrous-walled cysts, and bony outgrowths (osteophytes) develop at the articular surfaces. With spinal osteoarthritis, articular disk tissue often herniates into the vertebral body (Schmorl nodule, *arrows*), a common finding at autopsy.

## CENTRAL NERVOUS SYSTEM

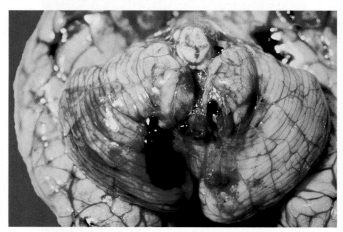

**Figure 15-228**  Cerebellar tonsillar herniation, recent. Cerebellar tonsillar herniation is a relatively rare but often fatal complication of any mass lesion, especially in the posterior fossa. Less commonly it may result from a supratentorial mass-increasing lesion. Note the swollen, partially hemorrhagic appearance of the molded tonsils. Grossly, they are softened and compress the medulla oblongata, the latter being the mechanism of death in afflicted patients.

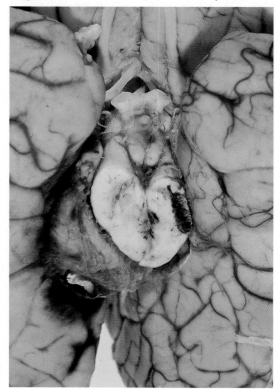

**Figure 15-229**  Transtentorial herniation. Transtentorial herniation is the most common herniation phenomenon, complicating any form of supratentorial mass-increasing lesion within or outside of the brain itself. This is a complex phenomenon with a variety of symptom complexes that result from one or more of the following anatomic distortions: stretching of one or both third nerves, compression of one or both cerebral crura against tissue or the tentorial edge, compression of one or both posterior cerebral arteries, and hemorrhage into the midbrain or upper pons related to arterial stretching. The compression of the crus cerebri contralateral to the mass lesion against the edge of the tentorium results in hemorrhagic necrosis of the crus; this lesion is called "Kernohan notch." Also present is contralateral hippocampal transtentorial herniation.

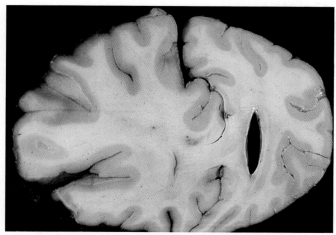

**Figure 15-230** Subfalcial herniation. The herniation of the cingulate gyrus and adjacent tissue under the edge of the falx cerebri results from hemispheric shift related to a unilateral mass lesion. This may be an intraaxial or extraaxial tumor, a subdural or extradural hematoma, a large infarct, or any other space-occupying lesion that is unihemispheric.

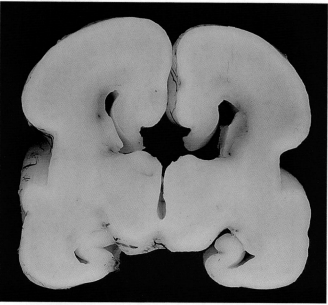

**Figure 15-232** Absence of the corpus callosum. The absence of any structure is often easily overlooked, particularly if it is a symmetrical absence. Here, along with evidence of earlier periventricular hemorrhage, the anterior horns of the lateral ventricles are "turned up," and the cingulate gyri appear to be rotated laterally. A prominent Probst bundle, a mass of anterior-posterior intracerebral fibers, is also present.

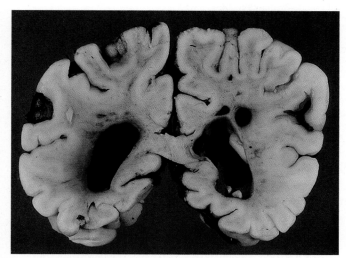

**Figure 15-231** Periventricular hemorrhage with intraventricular extension and periventricular leukomalacia. Periventricular hemorrhage is a common finding in perinatal deaths, often with some degree of intraventricular extension. This is most often a recent event, although occasionally evidence of earlier bleeding is seen. The leukomalacia, resulting in cystic small lesions, is due to necrosis of the periventricular white matter, the exact mechanism or mechanisms of which are still in dispute. Chalky lesions caused by mineralization (calcification) of the necrotic tissues may be seen grossly.

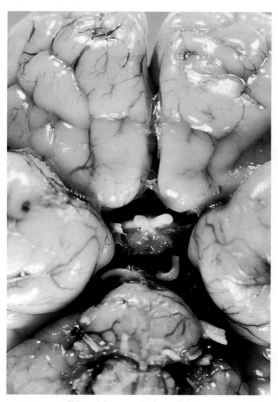

**Figure 15-233** Mild arrhinencephaly. Mild degrees of the complex malformation of arrhinencephaly can be easily missed. Unilateral or bilateral absence of the first nerve is the mildest form of this malformation and is illustrated here. Obviously, it is important to be certain that these delicate nerves have not been lost in dissection. Absence of the olfactory sulci and therefore of a defined gyrus rectus accompanies this malformation.

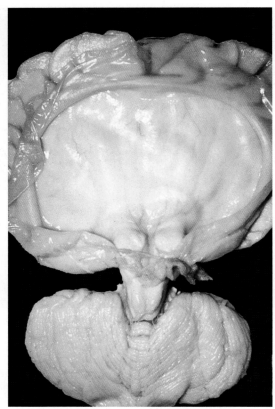

**Figure 15-234** Lobar holoprosencephaly (severe arrhinencephaly). The posterior fossa contents appear quite normal, as does the midbrain. However, the third ventricle is a midline crease on the floor of the markedly enlarged single ventricle, with the basal ganglia bulges seen on both sides of this crease. There is marked hydrocephalus with loss of white matter and cortical mantle thinning. There is some lobulation of cortex; in the alobar form, this "gyration" is absent.

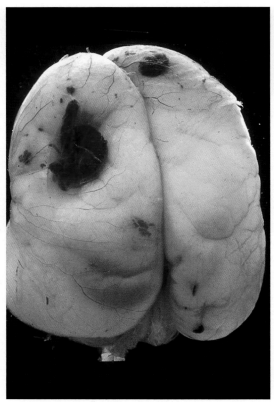

**Figure 15-236** Agyria (lissencephaly). In order to recognize this rare and severe abnormality, it is essential to know the developmental stage and the size of the fetus or newborn. Because this brain was that of a near-term infant, the lack of any gyration aside from suggestive creases is significant. The focal subarachnoid hemorrhages were sustained during delivery. Note that the terms *agyria* and *lissencephaly* (smooth brain) are interchangeable. (Reproduced with permission from the Armed Forces Institute of Pathology, Washington, DC.)

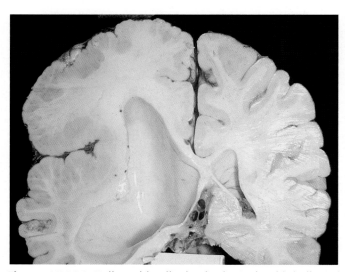

**Figure 15-235** Unilateral localized polymicrogyria with ipsilateral hydrocephalus. The zone of markedly small gyri with shallow sulci is clear when compared with the contralateral hemisphere; local loss of white matter and a markedly enlarged adjacent ventricle are also seen. Although it may be asymptomatic, the lesions are usually accompanied by some neurologic deficit.

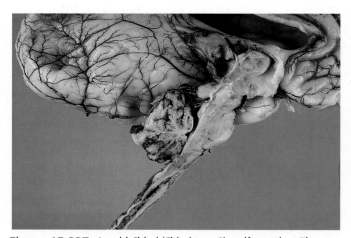

**Figure 15-237** Arnold-Chiari (Chiari type 2) malformation. The Arnold-Chiari malformation is one of the most common central nervous system lesions seen in the neonate. It is almost universally associated with lumbar meningomyelocele. This midline section of the cerebrum, cerebellum, and brainstem shows many of the commonly seen features of this complex. There is "beaking" of the posterior midbrain, as well as elongation and anterior-posterior narrowing of the fourth ventricle, downward shifting and narrowing of the medulla oblongata and superior cervical cord, a funnel shape of the inferior cerebellum, and hemorrhage in and softening of the inferior cerebellar gyri.

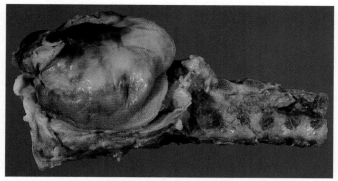

**Figure 15-238** Meningomyelocele. This gross dissection illustrates the bulging mass of meninges and spinal cord tissue in the lower lumbar region of the back. The herniated mass of tissue is covered by attenuated thinned skin, often showing local breakdown, with a surrounding "cuff" of more normal-appearing skin. This mass is in continuity with the midline defect in the lumbar vertebrae and, although not illustrated here, with the intravertebral superior spinal cord. The commonly accompanying skin ulcers readily explain why coliform bacteria gain access to the cerebrospinal fluid, causing the purulent meningitis so often seen in these patients.

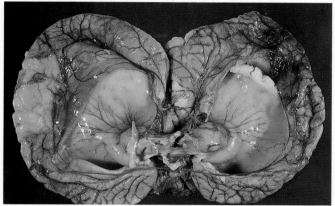

**Figure 15-239** Severe hydrocephalus. The marked ventricular dilation is diagnostic of hydrocephalus. The cause is often obscure; the appearance here is of a noncommunicating hydrocephalus, although it may not be possible to identify the obstruction.

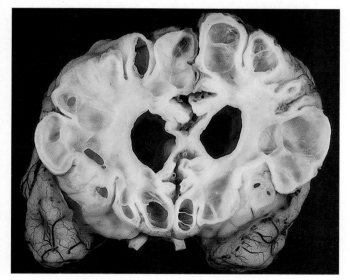

**Figure 15-240** Polycystic encephalopathy. This appearance, with multiple cysts in the cerebrum involving the cortex and superficial white matter, is relatively rare. Although the exact mechanism is unclear, it is generally agreed that the cause is late gestational, severe symmetrical anoxia, with resulting cystic "infarcts." It is commonly most severe in the middle and anterior cerebral artery distributions. It is important to recognize this abnormality; this case presented as possible child abuse, but these lesions do not support such a diagnosis.

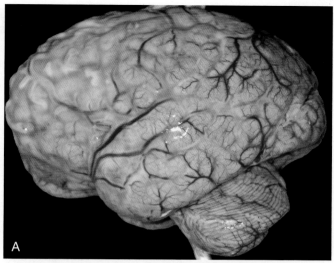

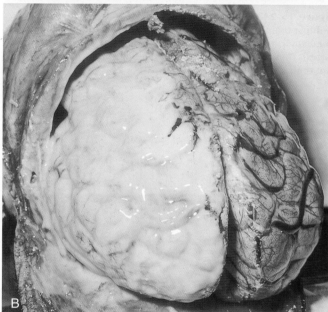

**Figure 15-241** Purulent meningitis. **A,** The gross appearance of opaque creamy-appearing exudate most prominent in the sulci over the cerebrum is typical of purulent meningitis. The most common bacterial agents responsible vary with the age of the patient and the clinical setting. The exudate most often is also concentrated at the base of the brain, extending down to the medulla oblongata and with less obvious involvement lower down. **B,** Pneumococcal meningitis, most commonly associated with a pale green exudate, may involve only the cerebral convexities or may even be unilateral.

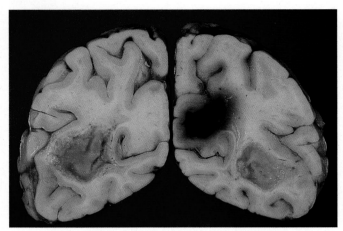

**Figure 15-242** Bilateral purulent abscesses. This brain shows multiple brain abscesses, one of which has been drained surgically (the hemorrhagic lesion in the white matter just above the visual cortex). These abscesses are in mid-evolution, with well-defined walls and central necrosis.

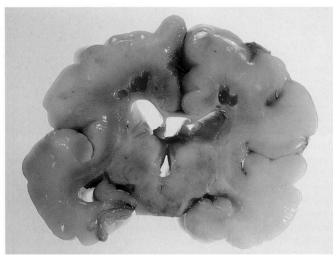

**Figure 15-244** Infant brain with TORCH infection (toxoplasma, other agents, rubella virus, cytomegalovirus, and herpes simplex virus). This infant brain shows cystic centrum semiovale lesions, as well as linear chalky-appearing cortical lesions. The white matter lesions alone could be due to periventricular leukomalacia but, in concert with the cortical lesions, are more suggestive of a TORCH infection; both may present with similar clinical and pathologic findings.

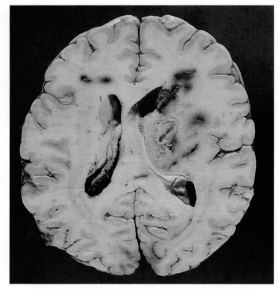

**Figure 15-243** Deep purulent abscess with intraventricular rupture. This purulent abscess, which developed after a dental extraction, was due to nocardia species. It shows prominent surrounding edema and herniation toward the contralateral side. The cause of death was rupture into the ventricles, which were filled with purulent material at autopsy. Note the needle tracts. Computed tomography and magnetic resonance imaging methods have greatly aided diagnosis of this type of lesion in the modern era.

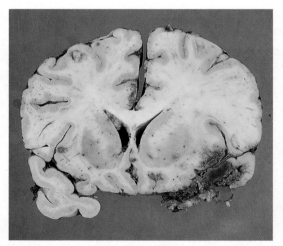

**Figure 15-245** Herpes simplex encephalitis. The hemorrhagic destruction of one temporal lobe and the adjacent inferior frontal cortex is typical of a fulminating herpes infection in an adult. Bilateral involvement is most common, but unilateral examples are seen. The cingulate gyrus may also be involved.

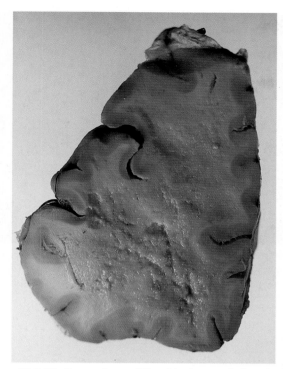

**Figure 15-246** Progressive multifocal leukoencephalopathy (of Ästrom, Mancall, and Richardson). This frontal lobe lesion shows the somewhat defined granular-appearing zone of white matter, one of several such lesions found in this brain. The lesions are most prominent in the white matter, vary greatly in size and shape, and occasionally extend into the adjacent gray. Most commonly they are seen in immunosuppressed individuals.

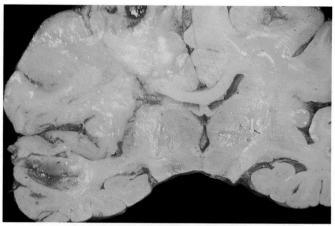

**Figure 15-248** Massive recent infarct. The cerebrum on the left side of this photograph shows a large, mostly pale infarct in the middle cerebral artery distribution. (In the superior temporal lobe at the periphery, there is a zone of hemorrhagic infarct, a common accompanying feature of these large pale infarcts.) Note the mass effect, with compression of the contralateral cerebrum. A linear "cystic" change can be seen adjacent to the necrotic area. This is in part artifact and in part a reflection of early removal of tissue at the periphery of the infarct.
(Reproduced with permission from the Armed Forces Institute of Pathology, Washington, DC.)

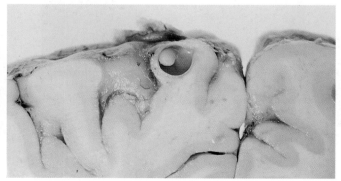

**Figure 15-247** Cysticercosis. This is an "incidental" cysticercal cyst. These lesions are most commonly seen in persons from or visiting in areas of the world where this illness is endemic: Mexico, Central America, and Eastern Europe.

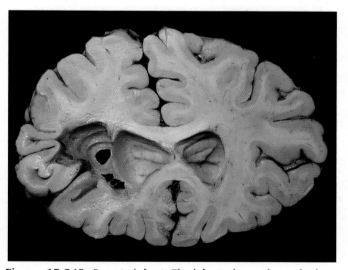

**Figure 15-249** Remote infarct. The left cerebrum shows the large cystic defect of a remote infarct. Note the loss of deep cortex in one area of this lesion. Fine strands line the periphery of this cyst, and the ependymal lining is intact. Infarcts typically spare the ependymal lining and the subpial membrane; both are most commonly disrupted if hemorrhage is the cause. The apparent "shift" seen here is an artifact.

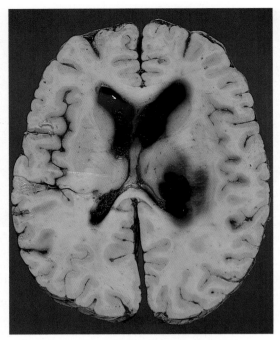

**Figure 15-250** Recent intracerebral hemorrhage with intraventricular extension. The primary hemorrhage is in the right thalamus with massive extension into the ventricles. There is a slight right-to-left shift.

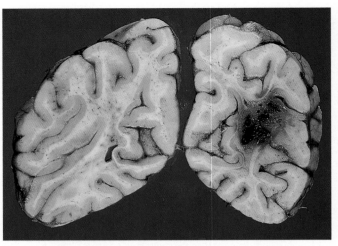

**Figure 15-252** Deep arteriovenous malformation. One occipital lobe shows a deep arteriovenous malformation. In one area it came to the surface like the "tip" of an iceberg. This patient died of uncontrolled seizures caused by this lesion.

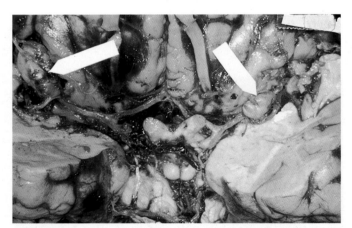

**Figure 15-251** Bilateral berry aneurysm *(arrows)*. Bilateral berry aneurysms are present; the larger one, that on the right, has recently ruptured. Among patients diagnosed with berry aneurysm, 16% will have a "mirror-image" berry aneurysm. More than one aneurysm is present in as many as 20% of cases.

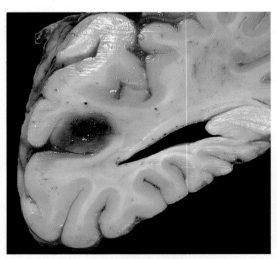

**Figure 15-253** Cavernous venous vascular malformation. This temporoparietal cortical lesion showed markedly ectatic venous channels histologically. It was associated with Jacksonian seizures.

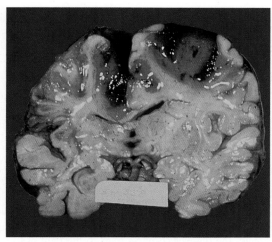

**Figure 15-254** Bilateral hemorrhagic infarcts related to sagittal sinus thrombosis. The presence of bilateral hemorrhagic infarcts with or without subarachnoid or intracortical hemorrhage should raise the possibility of the presence of superior sagittal sinus thrombosis. This is a difficult clinical diagnosis and may be missed pathologically, if care is not taken. The sinus should always be examined for thrombosis.
(Reproduced with permission from the Armed Forces Institute of Pathology, Washington, DC.)

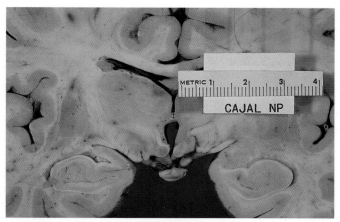

**Figure 15-256** Remote Wernicke encephalopathy (Wernicke-Korsakoff disease). Bilateral small mammillary bodies are very suggestive of remote damage due to Wernicke encephalopathy. Involvement of thalamic nuclei almost always occurs, but this is not evident grossly.

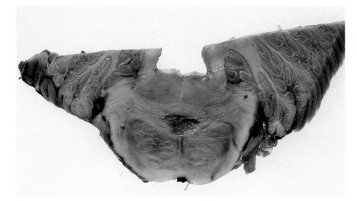

**Figure 15-257** Central pontine myelinopathy. The wedge- or diamond-shaped cystic zone in the center of the dorsal basis pontis is almost diagnostic of central pontine myelinopathy. Note that the lesion crosses the midline, unlike small vascular lesions, which do not violate this boundary. The lesion is most commonly seen in chronic alcohol abusers but may be seen in others who have had rapid correction of hyponatremia.

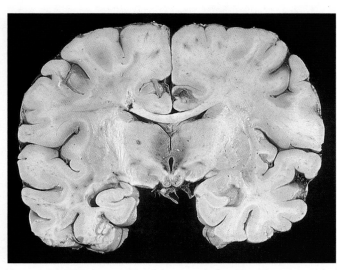

**Figure 15-255** Recent Wernicke encephalopathy. The symmetrical hemorrhagic involvement of the mammillary bodies and wall of the third ventricle is quite typical of acute Wernicke encephalopathy. In this case the periaqueductal zone and floor of the fourth ventricle had similar changes. Such extensive involvement is commonly fatal.

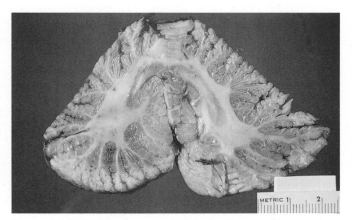

**Figure 15-258** Superior vermal sclerosis. The superior vermal cortex appears to have lost its separation and is gray and firm. This lesion is more commonly defined histologically rather than grossly and should always be confirmed with histologic examination.

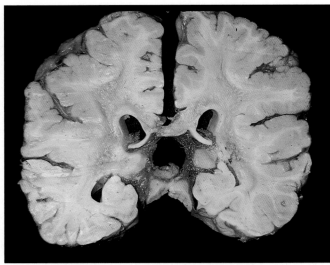

**Figure 15-259** Leukodystrophy, type uncertain. Prominent symmetrical loss of myelin of the deep white matter is seen. Note the sparing of the U fibers, the subcortical-intracortical connections. The unmyelinated tracts appear gray rather than white because of the myelin loss; grossly, they are often firm. Once called "Schilder disease," the lesion has now been divided into a number of entities on the basis of biochemical and other studies.

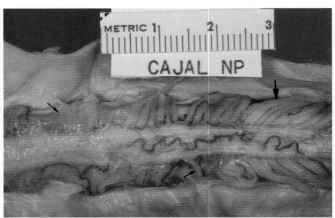

**Figure 15-261** Amyotrophic lateral sclerosis (ALS). In this spinal cord segment, the uninvolved nerve roots to the right of the photograph are full and pale cream in color *(large arrow)*. Small, gray atrophic nerve roots *(small arrows)* are present primarily on the left, but a few roots to the right also show the gray appearance of Wallerian degeneration. Atrophy of the spinal cord itself is not evident in this photograph. Though not illustrated, a cross section of cord may show atrophy of the anterior horns and gray discoloration in the area of the lateral columns. Frank "sclerosis" to palpation in the area of the columns is unusual except in very advanced cases.

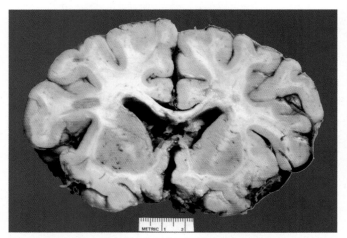

**Figure 15-260** Multiple sclerosis. Multiple gray-appearing zones in the white matter of both frontal lobes can be seen. They are present in the centrum semiovale on the right side, and farther out in the subcortical white matter on the left.

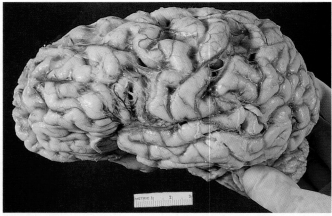

**Figure 15-262** Alzheimer disease. Marked frontal cortical atrophy with prominent widening of the subarachnoid space is seen in the older individual with dementia. The ventricles are also usually enlarged, but this is a common nonspecific change of aging. The diagnosis must be confirmed histologically. More subtypes of dementia seen in older individuals are being defined, and careful clinicopathologic correlation is essential for proper diagnosis, so appropriate family counseling can be provided.

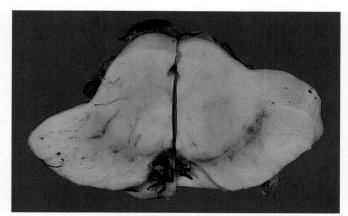

**Figure 15-263** Paired sections of midsagittally sectioned midbrain: Parkinson disease *(left)* and normal *(right)*. The right section is normal grossly, with a sharply defined, linear, densely black zone of substantia nigra and a small (normal) aqueduct. The left section shows diffusion of the nigral pigment into the surrounding anatomic areas with decrease of pigment; an enlarged Sylvian aqueduct is also present, reflecting the loss of brain substance. With the degeneration of nigral neurons, the neuromelanin pigment is phagocytosed by macrophages that migrate into surrounding areas, causing the loss of crisp definition of the pigmented zone. With time, the areas appear brown.

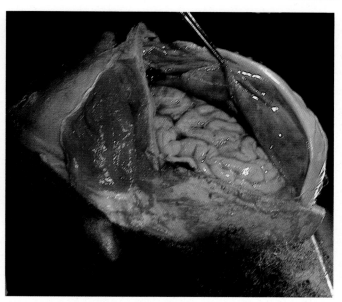

**Figure 15-265** Evolving subdural hematoma. The semiliquid membrane-bound mass of blood in the subdural space is typical of an evolving subdural hematoma. Unfortunately, these curable lesions are missed even with the availability of modern imaging methods. This patient had experienced head trauma as a passenger in a vehicular accident months earlier. She had not been symptomatic at that time. Clinically, she was thought to have had a recent infarct.

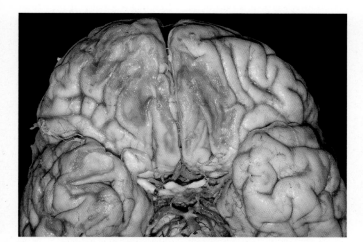

**Figure 15-264** Remote orbital surface contusions. Bilateral brown zones of cortical loss of the orbital surfaces of the frontal lobes can be seen. These are the result of remote contrecoup contusions involving these areas. This type of lesion is typical of old healed damage from trauma.

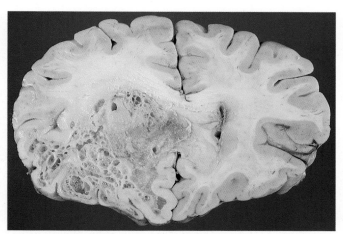

**Figure 15-266** Glioblastoma multiforme. This inferior frontal lobe mass lesion shows some of the variety of gross features that may be seen in glioblastomas. It is multicystic, has zones of necrosis, shows evidence of a mass effect, involves both gray and white matter, and already involves the corpus callosum. This is typically a tumor of adults.

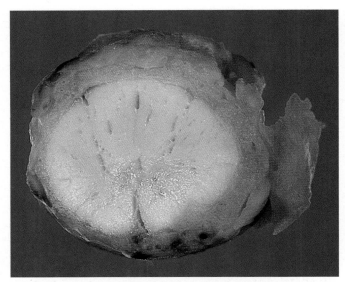

**Figure 15-267** Spinal subarachnoid tumor seeding. Spinal subarachnoid seeding can be seen with a variety of primary central nervous system tumors. Although most commonly seen in childhood medulloblastoma, any infiltrating tumor may spread by cerebrospinal fluid pathways. In this case, a cerebral glioblastoma was the source of the seeding.

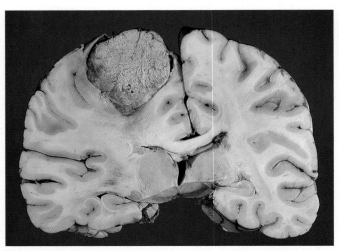

**Figure 15-269** Parasagittal meningioma. This sharply defined extraaxial mass in the parasagittal area is typical of meningioma. Note the cortical atrophy adjacent to the mass lesion. This is usually a tumor of adults.

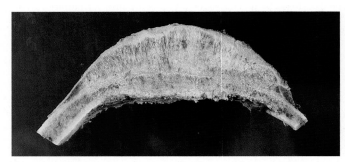

**Figure 15-270** Intraosseous meningioma. This meningioma has preferentially grown within bone, expanding it greatly. It presented as an enlarged area of skull. An intracranial mass may be present as well; some meningiomas produce thickening of the adjacent bone without infiltration by tumor. This, too, is a lesion seen in adults.

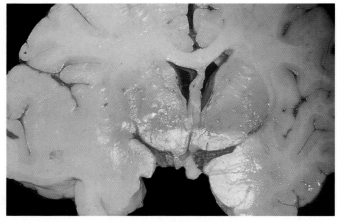

**Figure 15-268** Diffusely infiltrating astrocytoma. This coronal section shows extensive infiltration of the left cerebral hemisphere by astrocytoma. A diffuse increase in mass and loss of gray-white demarcation is seen, and the consistency would typically be firm. Even relatively low-grade (grade 2) tumors may show this extensive infiltration at presentation. Such tumors may be seen in children or in adults.

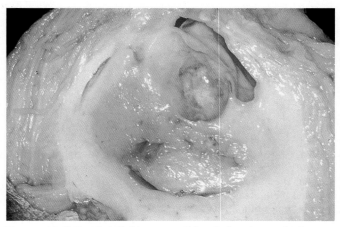

**Figure 15-271** Medulloblastoma. This soft fourth ventricular lesion arising in the cerebellar vermis is typical of medulloblastoma. These tumors are most commonly seen in children. In the past they were more common in males, but there has been some shift in sex ratio in recent decades. They commonly seed through cerebrospinal fluid pathways.

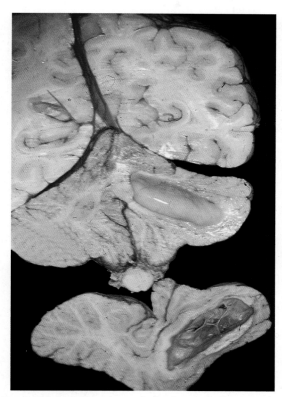

**Figure 15-272** Juvenile pilocytic astrocytoma. This largely cystic cerebellar hemispheric tumor is typical of the juvenile pilocytic (or pilocytic) astrocytoma classically found in this site. The same tumor is also common in the third ventricle and optic nerve. These tumors may have a mural nodule of tumor, but only histologic examination can determine whether the remainder of the cyst wall is also neoplastic. These tumors are most common in children and usually grow quite slowly. (Reproduced with permission from the Armed Forces Institute of Pathology, Washington, DC.)

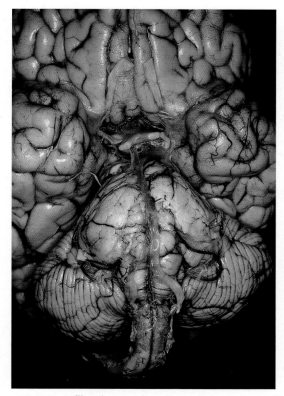

**Figure 15-273** Infiltrating pontine glioma (astrocytoma). The illusion of pontine "hypertrophy" is due to the diffusely infiltrating tumor causing enlargement of the mass of the pons and the upper medulla oblongata. There is also a nodular appearance of the pontine surface. Occasionally, the basilar artery may be "buried" in a tunnel of tumor, although that is not present here. The astrocytomas may be either grade 2 or 3, or even glioblastoma. They are most commonly seen in children and young adults.

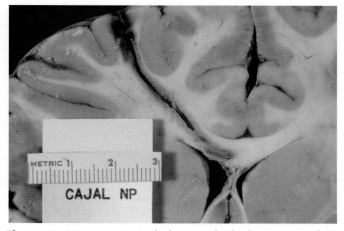

**Figure 15-274** Recent ventriculostomy site (catheter removed). This coronal section of cerebrum through the heads of the caudate nuclei shows a linear brown-stained cavity extending from the surface toward the anterior horn of the lateral ventricle.

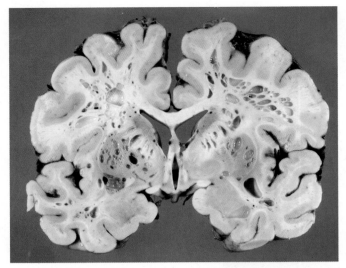

**Figure 15-275** Postmortem cystic artifact. This coronal section of brain through the mammilothalamic tracts shows multiple cystic lesions in the deep white matter and cortex. The cysts are sharply delimited and vary in size. This "Swiss cheese" appearance is typically the result of postmortem growth of gas-forming bacteria during decomposition or inadequate fixation. Histological sections show bacterial growth in vessels and surrounding tissue without evidence of a cellular reaction.

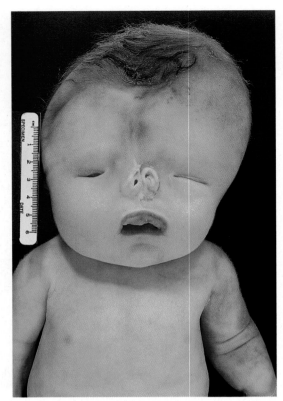

**Figure 15-277** Holoprosencephaly sequence with amniotic band syndrome. The complicated facial defects seen in this infant delivered at 34 weeks' gestation include anophthalmia of the right eye and microphthalmia of the left eye. The deformed nose is associated with choanal atresia. The palate is high and arched.

## PEDIATRIC PATHOLOGY

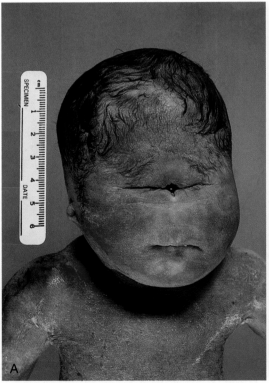
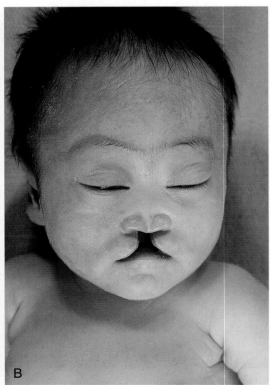

**Figure 15-276** Holoprosencephaly sequence. Holoprosencephaly includes a spectrum of cerebral (see Fig. 15-234) and facial malformations resulting from absent or incomplete division of the embryonic forebrain. Approximately 40% of cases are associated with a chromosomal abnormality, most often trisomy 13. **A,** Failure of separation of the orbits presents a spectrum of hypotelorism with cyclopia (single or fused double eye), as seen in this infant with trisomy 13, with holoprosencephaly being the extreme. Nasal structures may be absent or a proboscis may be present. **B,** This newborn with holoprosencephaly demonstrates incomplete facial development including absent nasal septum, single naris, absent philtrum, and median cleft lip/palate. There is also synophrys (midline union of the eyebrows).

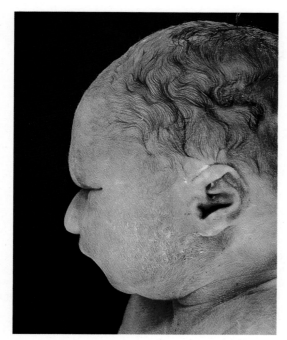

**Figure 15-278** Malformations of the nose vary widely. This infant with trisomy 13 demonstrates a beaked nose.

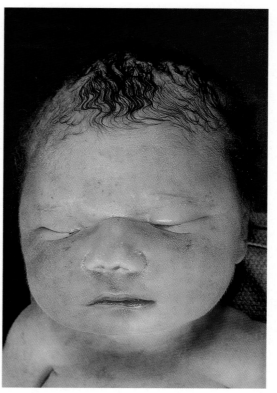

**Figure 15-280** Arthrogryposis (congenital contractures; see Fig. 15-291). Facial abnormalities associated with arthrogryposis include round face with prominent eyes, hypertelorism, telecanthus, epicanthal folds, short nose, malformed ears, and micrognathia.

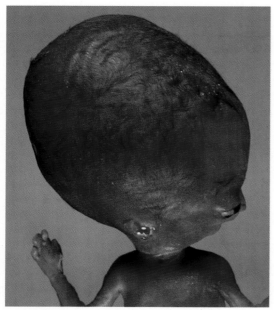

**Figure 15-279** Triploidy. A large number of facial and cranial abnormalities may be observed in triploidy. This fetus had marked hydrocephalus; low-set, severely malformed ears; and micrognathia (small mandible). The right hand shows syndactyly of digits 3 and 4 and clinodactyly.

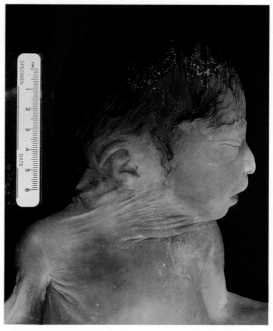

**Figure 15-281** Oligohydramnios sequence (Potter facies). Oligohydramnios sequence includes deformation of the head by the uterine wall. In this profile, the effect of this molding is manifest by the slanting forehead, blunt-tipped nose, and small chin.

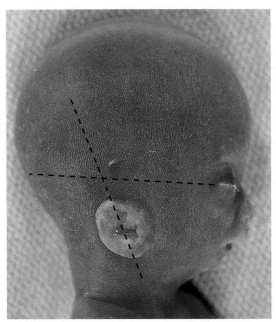

**Figure 15-282** Low-set, slanted ears in a fetus of 23 weeks' gestation with osteogenesis imperfecta. The ear is low set because the helix does not reach the line extending from the lateral canthus to the occiput. The ear is slanted because a line between the crest of the helix and the lobule deviates from the coronal (vertical) plane by greater than 15 degrees.

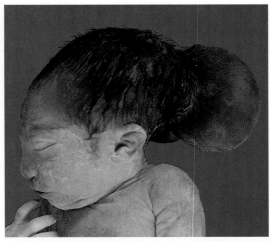

**Figure 15-284** Meningoencephalocele. A large portion of occipitoparietal brain tissue protruded through a wide posterior fontanelle in this infant with Meckel-Gruber syndrome. There was also a Dandy-Walker malformation with absent cerebellar vermis.

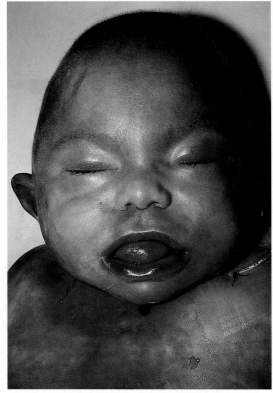

**Figure 15-283** Macroglossia. In this infant with Beckwith-Wiedemann syndrome, the enlarged tongue is not contained by the oral cavity. A variety of other conditions include macroglossia. In this case, the facies also demonstrate periorbital edema.

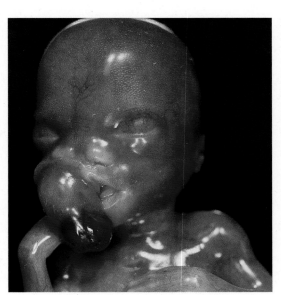

**Figure 15-285** Encephalocele. Less common than posterior lesions, an anterior encephalocele in this fetus demonstrates brain protruding through a defect in the base of the skull and the palate. Dilated blood vessels in the dependent portion give a two-tone appearance.

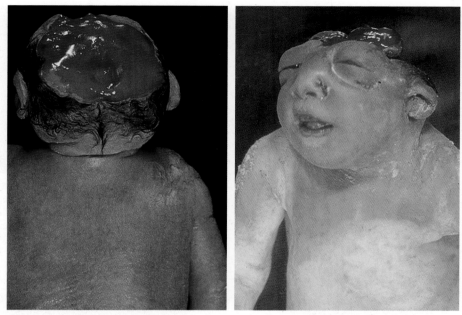

**Figure 15-286** Anencephaly. The characteristic facies of an infant with anencephaly include absent forehead that gives the eyes an appearance of bulging. The lack of cranial bones means that the cranial cavity is completely open. There is no discernible brain grossly; however, there is sometimes a small mass of neurovascular tissue (area cerebrovasculosa) in the base of the cranium.

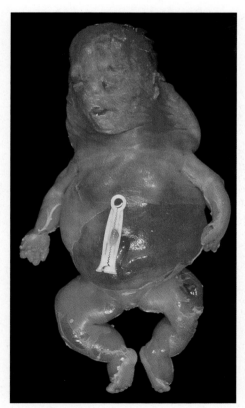

**Figure 15-287** Macerated fetus with nuchal lymphangiomas. The excess skin on either side of the neck represents residual cystic lymphangioma (hygroma) caused by a malformation of lymphatics in this abortus. Together with generalized edema, this finding is characteristic of 45,X but is also associated with several other abnormal karyotypes. Cystic lymphangioma serves as a marker for these syndromes on fetal ultrasonograms.

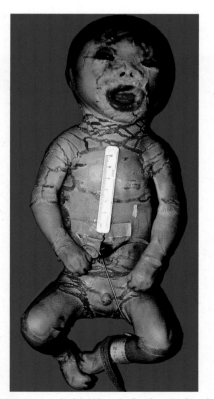

**Figure 15-288** Congenital ichthyosis (harlequin fetus). This dysmorphic small-for-gestational-age fetus demonstrates the platelike sections of skin with deep fissures denoting flexion points. The deformation is marked at the mucosal-epidermal borders, where the thick skin retracts and distorts the mouth and eyes (ectropion), ears, and scrotum.

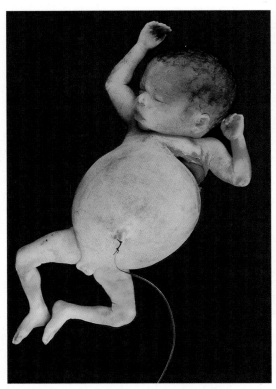

**Figure 15-289** Fetal hydrops. Several patterns of excessive extravascular fluid characterize fetal hydrops. This liveborn fetus with cardiomyopathy illustrates truncal enlargement related to ascites. In other cases, the extremities are also edematous, appearing swollen (sausagelike) with tense skin and deep creases.

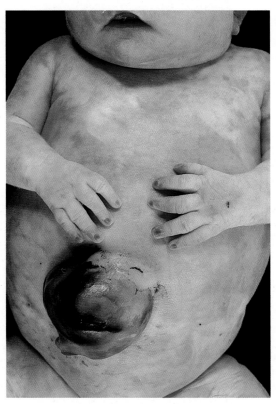

**Figure 15-290** Omphalocele in association with several malformations. The enlargement at the umbilical area contains portions of abdominal organs covered by amnion and peritoneal membrane. The umbilical cord arises from the dome of the lesion.

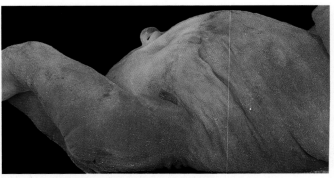

**Figure 15-291** Prune-belly syndrome. This constellation of anomalies associated with obstructive nephropathy includes deficient abdominal wall musculature and cryptorchidism. The wrinkled abdominal wall likely results from decompression of the distended lower urinary tract. Less mature fetuses with obstructive nephropathy may show a distended abdomen.

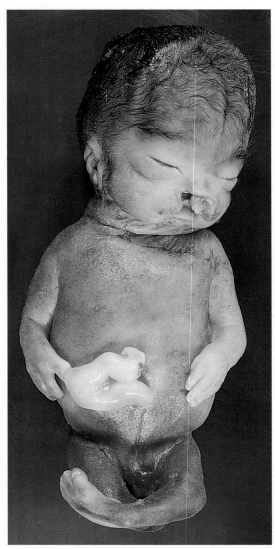

**Figure 15-292** Caudal regression sequence related to truncated spinal cord. The lower extremities are short and the musculature underdeveloped. Both feet show clubfoot deformity. Malformations of the upper extremities and cleft lip-palate are also seen in this infant. An increased incidence of caudal regression is seen in infants of diabetic mothers.

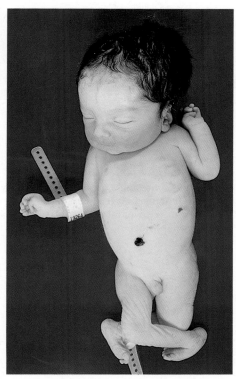

**Figure 15-293** Arthrogryposis (multiple congenital contractures). Arthrogryposis is characterized by multiple joint contractures caused by abnormalities of muscle (muscular dystrophy, congenital myopathies, congenital absence of muscle), abnormal nerve function or innervation (central nervous system malformations, congenital neuropathy, failure of nerves to form or myelinate, exposure to toxins that affect nerve function), abnormality of connective tissue, and mechanical limitation to movement in utero (uterine leiomyomas, oligohydramnios, amniotic bands, multiple gestation).

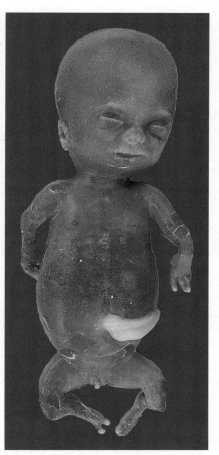

**Figure 15-294** Osteogenesis imperfecta congenita. This macerated abortus demonstrates the short limbs characteristic of the lethal form of the disease. The head is often soft and deformable because of the absence of mineralized cranial bone. The small thorax may result in lung hypoplasia.

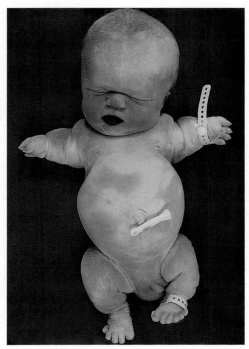

**Figure 15-295** Thanatophoric dysplasia. This infant has short limbs and digits and a relatively large cranium. The thorax is typically narrow, and there may be lung hypoplasia. The distinctive radiographic findings include short ribs and curved long bones with flared ends, among others.

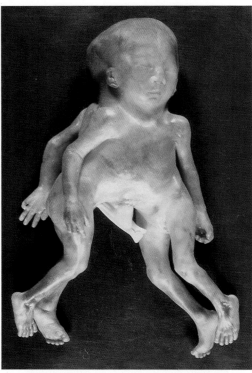

**Figure 15-296** Conjoined twins, an example of incomplete twinning. Cephalothoracopagus syncephalus, represented here, is only one type of conjoined twins, thoracopagus being the most common. The type is often the first indication of the internal anatomy, which can be very complex and bizarre. Although monozygotic, conjoined twins may have discordant malformations.

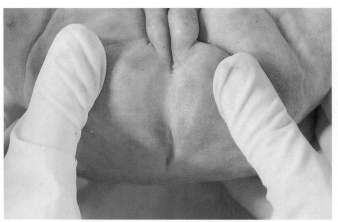

**Figure 15-298** Imperforate anus. Imperforate anus may be associated with anal or anorectal agenesis. In males there is often a rectourethral fistula or rectovesical fistula. In females there is sometimes a rectovaginal fistula.

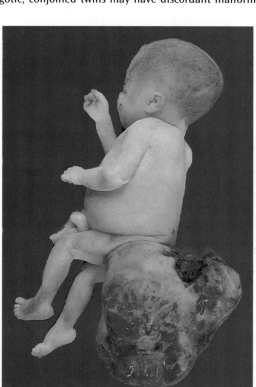

**Figure 15-297** Sacrococcygeal teratoma. Today, these tumors can be detected in the fetus. The vascular tumors may lead to high-output state and thus fetal hydrops. The large tumor pictured here is typical in that it is mainly external. In addition to the hemodynamic status of the infant, the degree of pelvic extension and its complications determines prognosis.

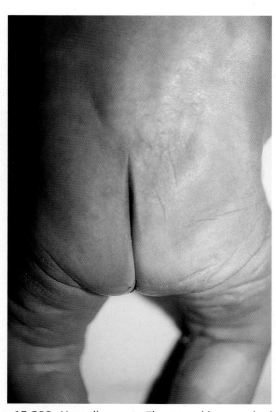

**Figure 15-299** Mongolian spots. These gray-blue macular lesions may be present over the sacrum in Asian children or children of dark-skinned parents. The spots disappear during childhood. They should not be mistaken for contusions from blunt-force trauma.

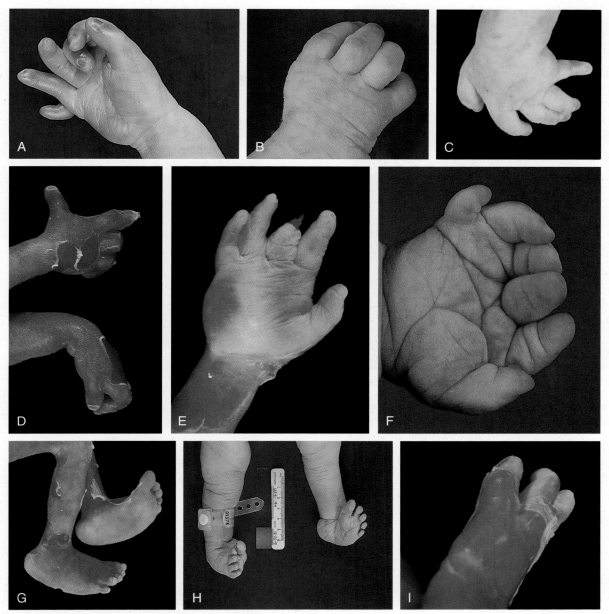

**Figure 15-300** Abnormalities of the hands and feet in the fetus and neonate are important clues to an underlying syndrome. **A,** Polydactyly. An extra digit is either medial (preaxial) or lateral (postaxial) and may or may not contain bone. **B,** Oligodactyly. Absence of a digit, in this case the right thumb, can be due to amniotic band disruption sequence. **C,** Syndactyly. Two or more fingers or toes are partially or completely adherent because of fusion of skin or of skin and bone. **D,** Camptodactyly. Flexion deformity of one or more digits. **E,** Partial amputation related to amniotic band disruption sequence. **F,** Simian crease (also polydactyly and syndactyly, digits 4 and 5). **G,** Rocker-bottom feet. **H,** Clubfoot deformity in oligohydramnios sequence. Both feet are inverted and plantar flexed ("equinovarus"). The calf muscles are underdeveloped. **I,** Split foot. In oligodactyly, a cleft exists between the deformed digits.

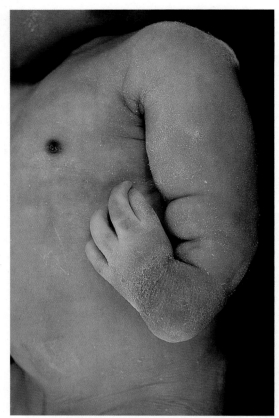

**Figure 15-301** VATER and expanded VACTERL associations. This group of anomalies clusters with greater than random frequency and includes the following: *V,* vertebral abnormalities; *A,* anal malformations; *C,* cardiac and vascular (single umbilical artery) defects; *TE,* tracheoesophageal fistula, esophageal atresia; *R,* renal defects; and *L,* limb anomalies. Among many defects, this infant with VACTERL association had agenesis of the radius and ulna. Camptodactyly of the second and third digits is also present.

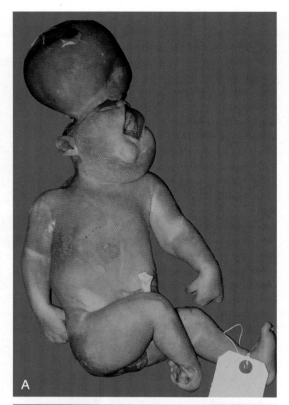

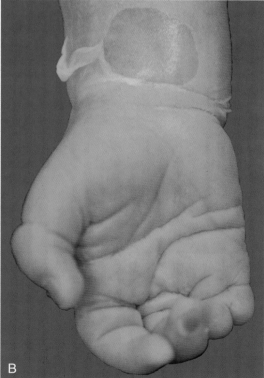

**Figure 15-302** ADAM complex (amniotic deformities, adhesions, mutilations) or amniotic band syndrome. The cause of this sporadic complex is unknown, but the leading theory suggests that it is due to a tear in the amnion followed by rupture and extrusion of parts of the developing fetus into the chorionic cavity. Defects result from strands of amnion wrapping around and constricting fetal development. Swallowing of amniotic bands may produce severe oral facial clefts and disruptions of the craniofacial structures. Amputations of parts or even entire limbs may occur. Internal anomalies are rare. **A,** Severe facial malformations, encephalocele, and abnormalities of the hands and feet in this 34-week-old fetus with ADAM complex. **B,** The fourth and fifth digits are partially amputated.

*Continued*

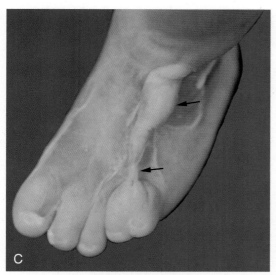

**Figure 15-302—Cont'd  C,** The left foot shows syndactyly of the fourth and fifth toes and a fibrous band of tissue *(arrows)* running from the lower leg across the dorsum of the foot to the abnormal toes. There was bilateral hydronephrosis but no other internal anomalies.

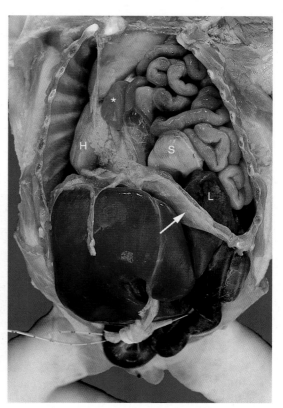

**Figure 15-304**  Diaphragmatic hernia. The left diaphragm is represented by a band of muscle anteriorly *(arrow)* that has deformed the left lobe of the liver. A portion of the intrathoracic left lobe of the liver *(L)*, the stomach *(S)*, and a portion of intestines crowd the developing left lung *(\*)* and shift the heart *(H)* and mediastinum to the right. Behind the heart in the posterior right thorax, the right lung is not visible. (See also Figure 15-317.)

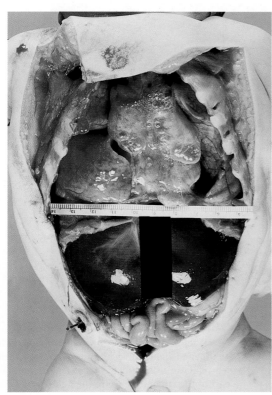

**Figure 15-303**  Pneumomediastinum. The large blebs of air over the lower thymus and upper pericardial sac resulted from ventilation of relatively noncompliant lungs associated with hyaline membrane disease in this neonate.

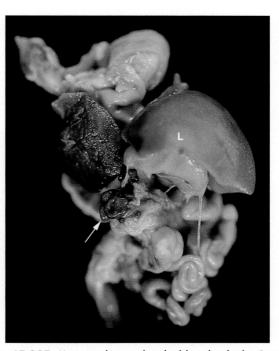

**Figure 15-305**  Heterotaxia associated with polysplenia. Complex cardiac defects and abnormalities of abdominal situs are characteristic of asplenia and polysplenia syndromes. From the right lateral oblique aspect of this induced abortus, the liver *(L)* is right sided, but there is a cluster of small spleens *(arrow)* in the right upper quadrant as well.

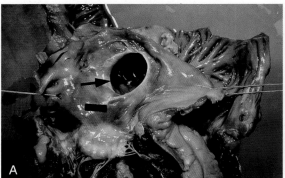

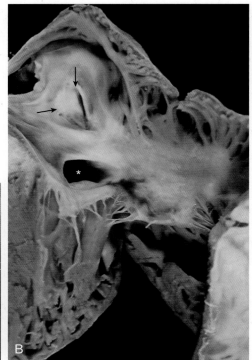

**Figure 15-306** Atrial septal defect. **A,** A large communication *(arrow)* leading to the left ventricle occupies the position of the oval fossa. Deficiency of the membrane that usually covers this part of the interatrial septum causes a secundum atrial septal defect, the most common type. **B,** Primum atrial septal defect is a more inferiorly and apically situated communication *(\*)* that is close to the tricuspid valve annulus; it does not involve the oval fossa *(arrows)*. Primum atrial septal defects are part of a constellation of defects that includes "cleft mitral valve," so the left atrioventricular connection is also abnormal. The more severe end of this spectrum is atrioventricular septal defect.

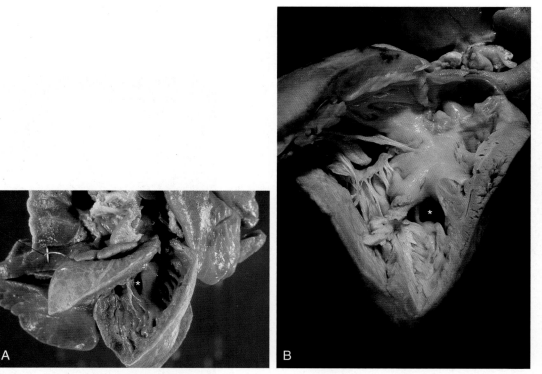

**Figure 15-307** Ventricular septal defect. There are two categories of ventricular septal defect: those that involve the membranous portion of the interventricular septum and those that are entirely within the muscular portion. **A,** The opened right ventricle shows an interventricular communication *(\*)* in the center of the heart, between the tricuspid valve and the right ventricular outflow tract. That the perimembranous ventricular septal defect involves the membranous portion of the septum means that one part of the circumference of the defect is fibrous (i.e., nonmuscular). **B,** The muscular ventricular septal defect *(\*)* is surrounded entirely by muscle. If located in the apical portion of the ventricle, the muscular ventricular septal defect may be partially covered by a trabeculum in the right ventricle, appearing larger as viewed from the left ventricle. Although the example pictured is located well toward the apex, many muscular ventricular septal defects are situated relatively high in the interventricular septum, and the prosector must look carefully to see that the rim is entirely muscular. One practical implication of the distinction between perimembranous and muscular defects is that the conduction tissues run close to the superior margin of a muscular defect and along the apical margin in a perimembranous one.

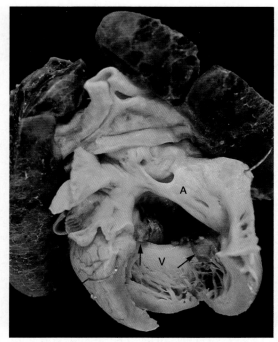

**Figure 15-308** Atrioventricular septal defect. In this view of the left side of the heart, a large defect is seen between the lower edge of the atrial septum *(A)* and the crest of the ventricular septum *(V)*. In comparison with the perimembranous type of ventricular septal defect, the atrioventricular septal defect is more inferior (closer to the diaphragmatic surface). The atrioventricular orifice is guarded by a common atrioventricular valve *(arrows)* that straddles the septum. The relative size of the ventricles depends on the position of the straddling valve—whether oriented centrally, rightward, or leftward.

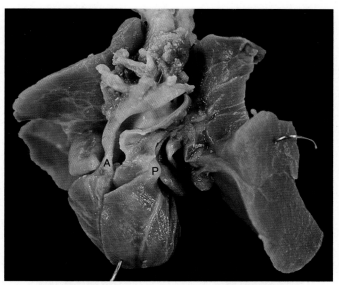

**Figure 15-310** Double-outlet right ventricle. In this close-up view of a dissected fetal heart, the aorta *(A)* and pulmonary artery *(P)* roots are side by side, with the aorta rightward. Both are situated over the right heart, as suggested by the position of the anterior descending artery, which indicates the position of the septum. The main pulmonary artery is narrow, consistent with pulmonary stenosis. Double-outlet right ventricle is subclassified according to the position of the ventricular septal defect, whether subaortic, subpulmonic, doubly committed (beneath both arterial valves), or noncommitted (at some distance from both).

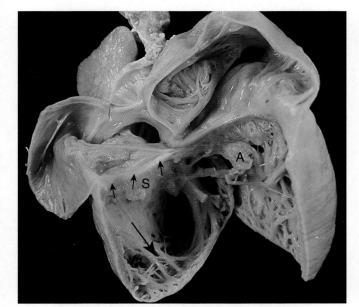

**Figure 15-309** Ebstein malformation. The opened right atrioventricular aspect demonstrates a dilated right atrium and patent foramen ovale, as well as the tricuspid valve deformity characteristic of this condition. The large anterosuperior leaflet *(A)* is dysplastic (misshapen, thick, and nodular), and the septal and posterior leaflets *(S)* are largely inseparable from the endocardial surface of the right ventricle. Normally close to the atrioventricular junction *(small arrows)*, the hinge point of the septal leaflet *(large arrow)* is displaced apically to a variable degree, depending on the severity of the defect. Because the effective valve orifice is shifted toward the apex, the portion of the ventricular free wall proximal to the new hinge point is thinned ("atrialized").

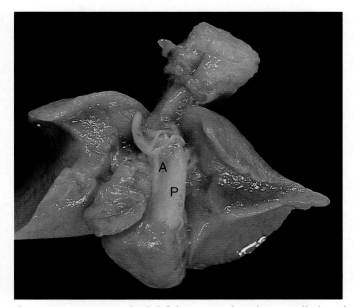

**Figure 15-311** Hypoplastic left heart complex. The constellation of anomalies constituting hypoplastic left-sided heart complex is suggested by the appearance of the heart and great vessels even before dissection. In this fetal case of aortic atresia, the ascending aorta *(A)* is very narrow as compared with the pulmonary artery *(P)*. The transverse arch (opened) is somewhat wider because of retrograde flow to the neck vessels from the arterial duct. The prosector should also pay close attention to the positions of the anterior and posterior descending coronary arteries on the epicardial surface, as these vessels delimit the septum and suggest the size and position of the left ventricle. In this specimen, the anterior descending artery appears far leftwards of its usual position, indicating a very small left ventricle.

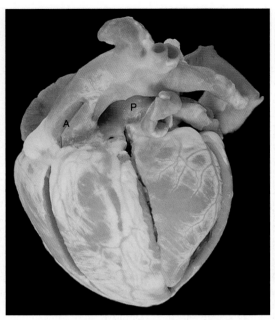

**Figure 15-312** D-transposition of the great arteries. The prosector should suspect D-transposition of the great arteries from the abnormal relationship of the vessels in situ. This heart shows the typical parallel configuration of the aorta and pulmonary artery in D-transposition of the great arteries. The root of the aorta *(A)* is rightward and anterior to that of the pulmonary artery *(P)*.

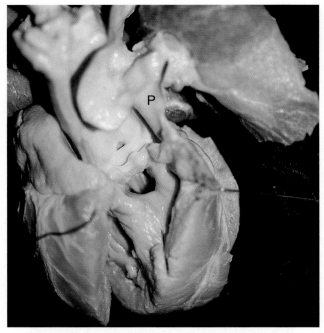

**Figure 15-314** Common arterial trunk (truncus arteriosus). From the epicardial aspect, only one great artery arises from the heart. The prosector must identify the takeoff of the pulmonary arteries *(P)* from the trunk, as the common arterial trunk is subclassified according to the position of the arteries' origin. The truncal valve usually has three semilunar leaflets as shown here, but in some cases there may be either two or more than three. Dysplastic leaflet tissue is associated with a severe hemodynamic abnormality. A subarterial ventricular septal defect is always present.

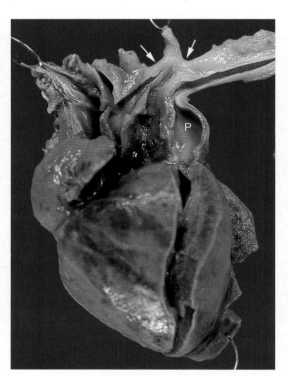

**Figure 15-313** Aortic coarctation. In this view, the transverse portion of the aortic arch *(arrows)* is abnormally narrow, constituting "tubular coarctation." The relatively large main pulmonary artery *(P)* and patent arterial duct suggest that this 2-week-old infant had a ductal-dependent lesion. The prosector could anticipate that the heart may demonstrate features of hypoplastic left-sided heart complex. Another type of aortic coarctation is due to a discrete ridge of vascular tissue that narrows the aorta at its junction with the arterial duct.

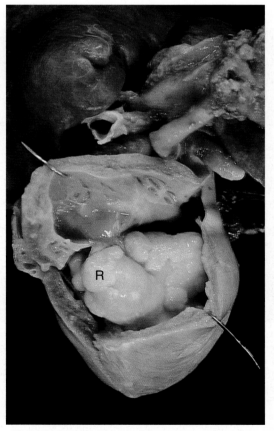

**Figure 15-315** Rhabdomyoma. This newborn with tuberous sclerosis has a large exophytic rhabdomyoma *(R)* arising from the ventricular septum to fill the right ventricle and occlude the tricuspid valve orifice. Microscopy disclosed numerous small rhabdomyomas in both ventricles.

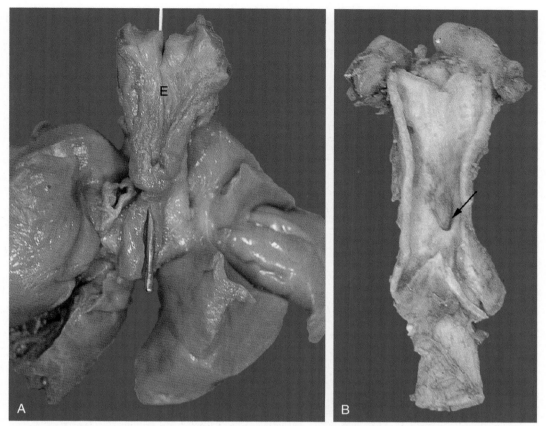

**Figure 15-316** Tracheoesophageal fistula. **A,** The trachea and esophagus must be dissected so that they retain their usual anterior-posterior relationship. In this newborn, the proximal portion of the esophagus *(E)* ends blindly. The probe is positioned in the larynx *(top of figure)*, passing into the trachea and through a defect near the carina to reach the distal esophagus *(bottom)*. **B,** The posterior aspect of the trachea discloses the malformation *(arrow)* that communicates with the distal esophagus.

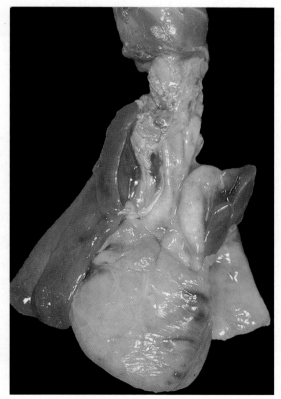

**Figure 15-317** Lung hypoplasia in association with diaphragmatic hernia. The heart-lung block demonstrates the marked lung hypoplasia, left much greater than right, that is a consequence of intrathoracic liver and gastrointestinal tract during development. (See also Figure 15-304.)

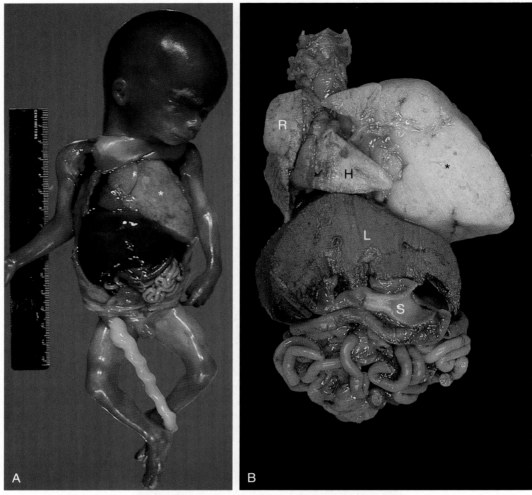

**Figure 15-318** Adenomatoid malformation of the lung. **A,** A solid mass *(*)* in the left lower lobe of lung crowds out the developing left upper lobe and shifts the heart and mediastinum to the right in this fetus of 12 weeks' gestation. **B,** Eviscerated organs (fixed) showing the large adenomatoid malformation *(*)*. *H,* Heart; *L,* liver; *R,* hypoplastic right lung; *S,* stomach.

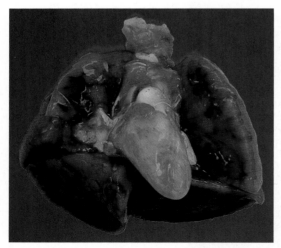

**Figure 15-319** Hyaline membrane disease of the premature neonate. Diffuse alveolar damage in the premature infant usually runs its course within a few days. In this 1-day-old infant who died with marked respiratory distress, the lungs are beefy with a lacy pattern of hemorrhage in the subpleural lymphatics. These poorly aerated lungs will sink in a container of water.

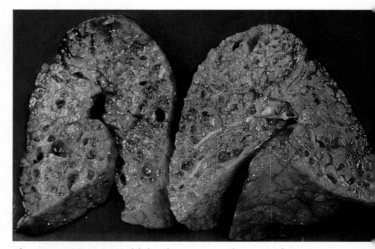

**Figure 15-320** Interstitial pulmonary emphysema. The cut surfaces of this premature neonate's lungs demonstrate extensive cleftlike spaces denoting interstitial collections of air that have dissected along airways, vessels, and interlobular septa as a consequence of ventilating noncompliant lungs.

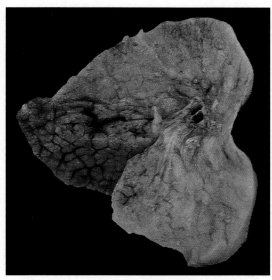

**Figure 15-321** Bronchopulmonary dysplasia. The pathology of bronchopulmonary dysplasia varies depending on the gestational age of the infant at birth, the age of the lesion, and the effect of other disease processes such as pneumonia and pulmonary interstitial emphysema. Typically, lungs with bronchopulmonary dysplasia demonstrate irregular pleural surfaces with "pseudofissures" and have firm, solid parenchyma.

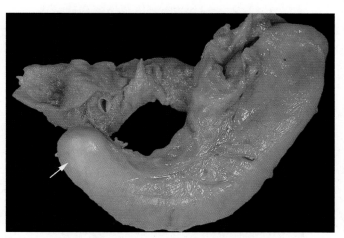

**Figure 15-323** Pyloric stenosis. An incidental finding in this 1-month-old infant was hypertrophic pyloric stenosis, denoted by the thick mass of muscle *(arrow)* at the gastric outlet. Several malformation syndromes include hypertrophic pyloric stenosis.

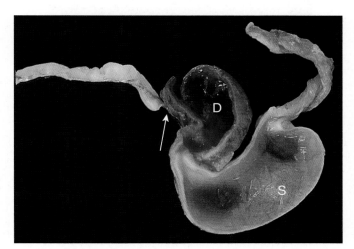

**Figure 15-324** Duodenal atresia. The stomach *(S)* and first part of the duodenum *(D)* are dilated, indicating the point of obstruction *(arrow)* caused by membranous atresia of the duodenum. A relatively common malformation, duodenal atresia often occurs with other anomalies and has a strong association with Down syndrome.

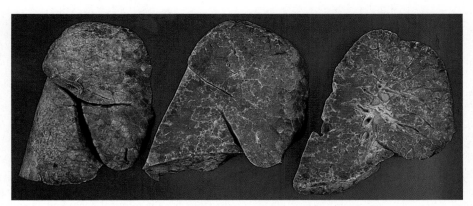

**Figure 15-322** Pulmonary alveolar proteinosis. Pulmonary alveolar proteinosis is an idiopathic chronic interstitial pneumonia characterized by accumulation of surfactant-like lipid and glycoprotein material within the alveoli. Although there may be different causes, dysfunction of alveolar macrophages plays a role in the pathogenesis. It occurs in patients of all ages, including newborns. Yellow-gray areas of consolidation are seen in a background of hyperemia from acute congestion in this infant, who died of a poorly characterized immune deficiency and pulmonary alveolar proteinosis.

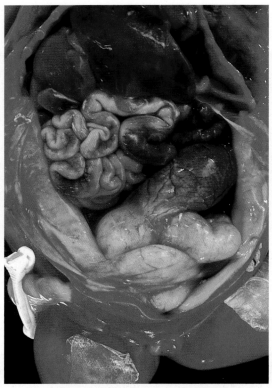

**Figure 15-325** Anorectal agenesis. The rectosigmoid colon is massively dilated as a consequence of anorectal agenesis in this macerated fetus.

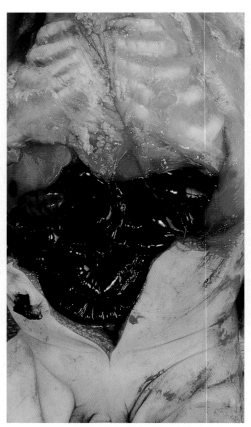

**Figure 15-327** Volvulus in a 3-day-old with malrotation. Virtually the entire small intestine is necrotic. The hemorrhagic luminal contents have been likened to currant jelly.

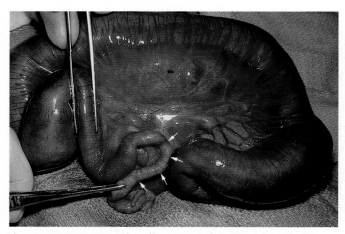

**Figure 15-326** Meconium ileus. Meconium ileus, intestinal obstruction caused by thick meconium in cystic fibrosis, may lead to small intestinal atresia, volvulus, or perforation with associated meconium peritonitis. Here, a segment of ileum is obstructed *(arrows)* and the proximal intestines are markedly dilated.

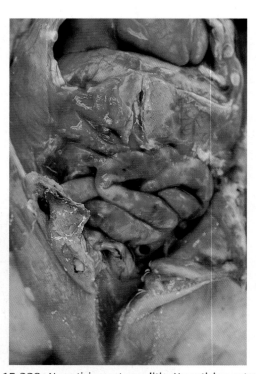

**Figure 15-328** Necrotizing enterocolitis. Necrotizing enterocolitis may develop in the premature infant. The length of bowel involved is variable, but the terminal ileum and ascending colon are generally affected. A severely involved, necrotic colon was removed prior to the death of this infant of 32 weeks' gestation. At autopsy, the small intestines are dilated and hyperemic. The mucosa was green and the bowel wall friable. Perforation, a common complication of severe cases, was not present here.

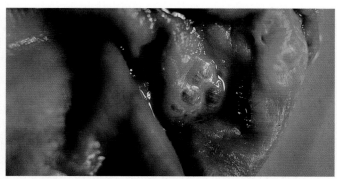

**Figure 15-329** Intestinal pneumatosis in association with necrotizing enterocolitis. Close inspection of the serosal surface of affected bowel occasionally discloses bubbles, denoting intestinal overgrowth by gas-forming organisms. In milder cases, submucosal lesions may be identified only by microscopy.

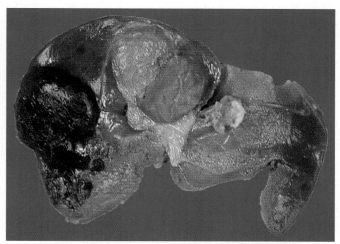

**Figure 15-332** Ruptured subcapsular hematoma in liver. Usually a consequence of manipulation during delivery, a hepatic hematoma may tamponade and resolve. This ruptured subcapsular hematoma was found at autopsy of a premature male with hemoperitoneum.

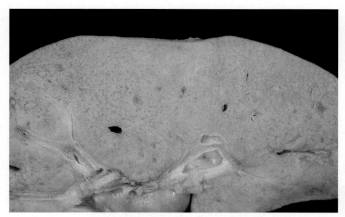

**Figure 15-330** Congenital hepatic fibrosis in association with autosomal recessive polycystic kidney disease. The cut surface of the liver shows the variegated appearance of expanded portal tracts.

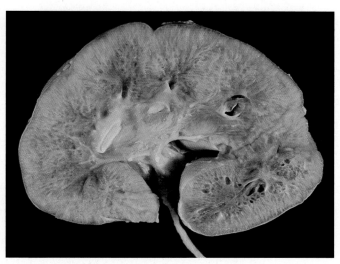

**Figure 15-333** Autosomal recessive polycystic kidney disease. The cut surface of this neonate's enlarged kidney discloses elongated, radially oriented cysts characteristic of this rare condition.

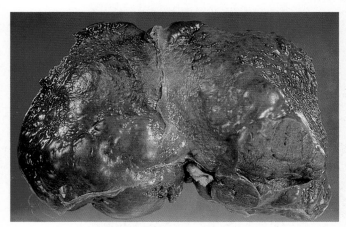

**Figure 15-331** Massive hepatic necrosis. In contrast to the finely granular capsular surface in cirrhosis, the wrinkled capsule and irregular nodularity of the generally necrotic liver is due to collapse of the parenchyma. There are several possible causes, including viral infection.

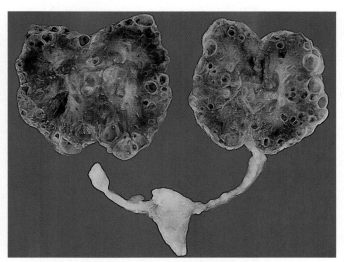

**Figure 15-334** Renal dysplasia. These small fibrotic kidneys contain peripheral cysts typical of obstructive nephropathy; however, the narrow caliber of the ureters suggests an obstructive lesion close to the kidneys, perhaps in the renal pelves.

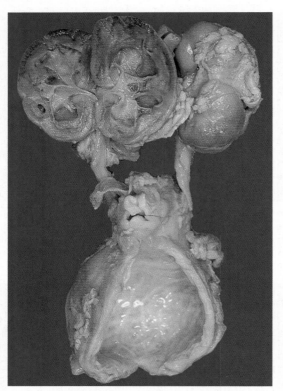

**Figure 15-335** Hydronephrosis related to neurogenic bladder. This stillborn with meningomyelocele had a dilated thick-walled bladder with hydronephrosis characterized by dilated renal calyces.

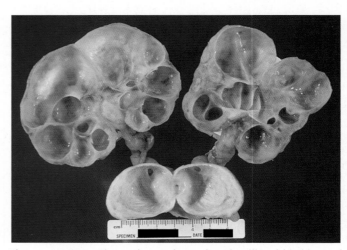

**Figure 15-336** Obstructive nephropathy. The dilated bladder and hydroureter indicate urethral obstruction, most likely caused by a membrane at the verumontanum. The reniform kidneys with dilated calices and little normal parenchyma demonstrate an extreme degree of hydronephrosis.

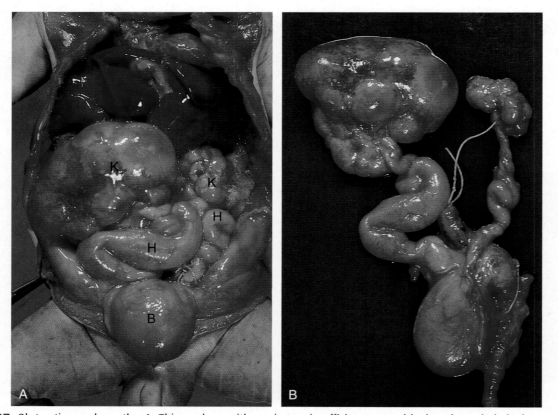

**Figure 15-337** Obstructive nephropathy. **A,** This newborn with respiratory insufficiency caused by lung hypoplasia had posterior urethral valves. This view with the intestines removed demonstrates the severity of the hydroureters *(H),* as well as the dilated bladder *(B).* The right kidney is markedly expanded by cysts, and the left is cystic but small. *K,* Kidney. **B,** Urinary system removed from abdomen.

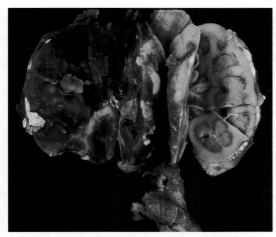

**Figure 15-338** Renal vein thrombosis. The color difference between kidneys in this newborn is the first clue to the possibility of renal vein thrombosis. The affected kidney, or renal segment, will be dark red because of extreme congestion and hemorrhagic necrosis.

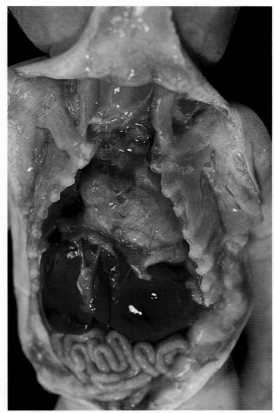

**Figure 15-340** Thymic agenesis (DiGeorge anomaly). The thymus is absent (or, in some cases, hypoplastic), resulting in severe defects in T-lymphocyte function. Anomalies of the parathyroid glands (agenesis, hypoplasia) and cardiovascular system (heart and aorta) are associated. This constellation of anomalies is responsible for DiGeorge syndrome.

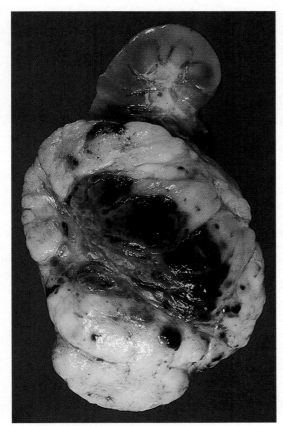

**Figure 15-339** Wilms tumor (nephroblastoma). Usually encapsulated and well circumscribed, Wilms tumor is a pale tan renal tumor with focal areas of necrosis or hemorrhage. The prosector should be aware that there are numerous malformations and syndromes associated with Wilms tumor.

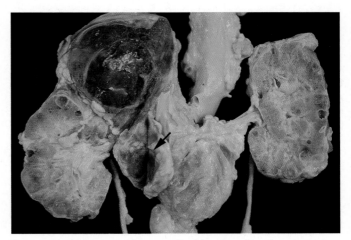

**Figure 15-341** Neuroblastoma. In this coronal section through kidney and adrenal gland, a large red-brown tumor with calcification replaces the adrenal gland. Metastatic tumor is present in a paraaortic lymph node *(arrow)*. Neuroblastoma may be a part of a neurocristopathy or a non-neural crest-associated syndrome. In this case, there was also renal dysplasia.

# PLACENTA AND UMBILICAL CORD

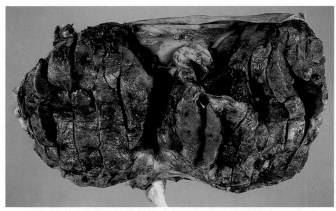

**Figure 15-342** Placental shape. Variations in placental shape include accessory lobes, bipartite (bilobed) placenta (shown here), and circumvallate placenta. Abnormalities of placental shape usually are of limited clinical significance.

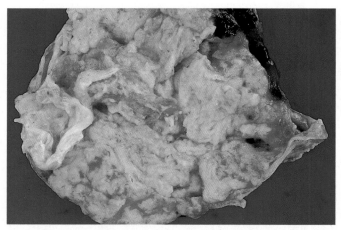

**Figure 15-343** Placental hydrops. Normally, the cotyledons are red. Parenchyma that is deep red indicates congestion. Paleness indicates anemia or, if boggy in texture, immaturity or hydrops (shown here).

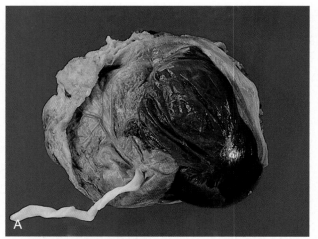

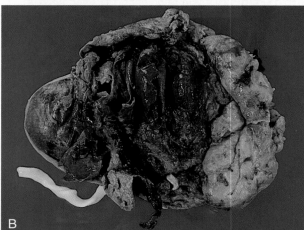

**Figure 15-344** Retroplacental hemorrhage. Retroplacental hemorrhage is present in 4.5% of placentas, but the incidence is higher among women with preeclampsia or chronic essential hypertension. The healthy placenta can withstand a loss of up to 30% of its villous surface. The recent placental hematoma is soft, red, and separable from the maternal surface. It may detach during delivery, leaving only a craterlike depression. There may be associated placental infarct. The older hematoma is brown, firm, and adherent to the maternal surface. Retroplacental hemorrhage is accompanied by the clinical syndrome of abruptio placentae in about 35% of cases. The retroplacental hemorrhage seen in this fixed specimen is recent and resulted in abruptio placentae. **A,** Fetal surface. **B,** Maternal surface.

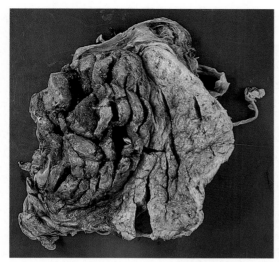

**Figure 15-345** Placental infarct. In normal-term pregnancies, about 25% of patients have placental infarcts involving less than 5% of the placental parenchyma. The frequency is increased in preeclampsia and hypertension. Extensive infarcts are present in 60% to 70% of patients with severe disease. Extensive placental infarction is associated with a high incidence of fetal hypoxia, intrauterine growth retardation, and fetal demise. Generally, there is no compromise of placental function until 30% of the placental tissue is infarcted if the remaining placenta has a normal blood supply. Diseased placentas such as those seen in preeclampsia can withstand loss of only 15% to 20% of villi. Centrally localized infarcts are of greater significance because the marginal area of the placenta is relatively poorly perfused even normally. Recent infarcts are variably to roughly triangular in shape with their base toward the basal plate of the placenta. They are well demarcated, dark red, and firm. Older infarcts are firmer and brown to yellow or white by 10 to 15 days of age. Cystic degeneration may be evident in old infarcts. This example shows an older infarct in a twin placenta in which the entire placenta on the right was necrotic.

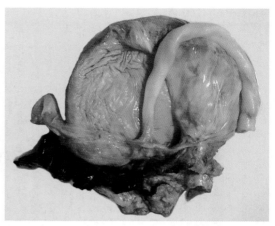

**Figure 15-347** Velamentous umbilical cord insertion. Umbilical cord insertions may be central (approximately 30%), eccentric (approximately 60%), marginal (5% to 7%), or velamentous (1% to 2%). Marginal insertions have a higher incidence of rupture and compression and are associated with fetal growth restriction, stillbirth, and neonatal death when uteroplacental blood flow is reduced. Velamentous (membranous) cord insertions, as shown here, are at higher risk for compression, thrombosis, and tears with fetal hemorrhage.

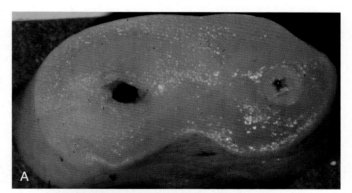

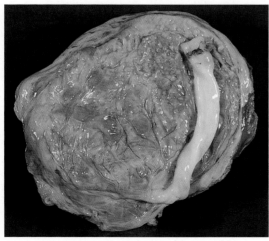

**Figure 15-346** Chorioamnionitis. Histologically, chorioamnionitis includes amnionitis, chorionitis, membranitis, funisitis, and umbilical cord vasculitis. Intense inflammation associated with *Escherichia coli* infection has resulted in cloudy, white to yellow membranes. The prosector should fix the fresh membranes in a roll and submit a slice to facilitate the histologic examination.

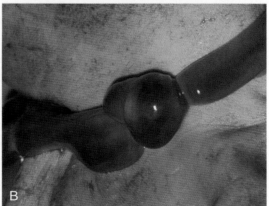

**Figure 15-348** Lesions of the umbilical cord. Various umbilical cord lesions may be seen, some of which may have adverse effects on fetal health. Abnormalities include single umbilical artery, vascular looping (pseudoknots), false knots, true knots, torsion, ulceration, aneurysms, thrombi, cysts, and tumors. **A,** Single umbilical artery. **B,** True knot of umbilical cord resulting in vascular occlusion and intrauterine fetal death.
(Courtesy of Richard Oi, MD, University of California, Davis.)

## FORENSIC PATHOLOGY

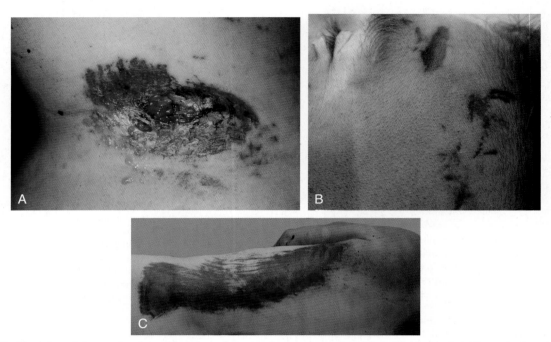

**Figure 15-349** Blunt force injury—abrasions. Blunt force injury or trauma is produced by a blunt object striking a body or the impact of a body against a blunt object or surface. Abrasions result from force applied tangentially or across the skin, resulting in removal of part of the superficial epidermis or, in deeper abrasions, removal of part of the dermis. **A,** Superficial and deep abrasions with lacerations. **B,** Impact or pressure abrasions occur when the blunt force is received perpendicular to the skin, usually over a bony prominence. **C,** Brush burn abrasion refers to scraping injuries over a large portion of the body such as occurred here during a motor vehicle accident. (Courtesy of Mark A. Super, MD, Sacramento County Coroner's Office.)

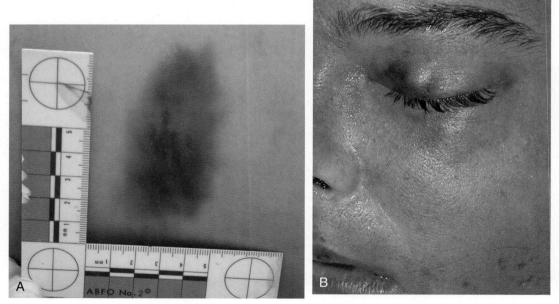

**Figure 15-350** Blunt force injury—contusions (bruises). Contusions result from rupture of blood vessels and extravasation of blood into adjacent tissues. Contusions may occur in the skin or within internal organs. Hematomas are focal collections of blood within a contusion. **A,** Homicide victim with contusion received during a fight. The overlying skin remains unbroken. **B,** This partially decomposed body found in the woods contained multiple contusions and superficial abrasions. However, the apparent periorbital contusion was not due to direct trauma but rather to the dissection of blood into the mastoid air cells and fascial planes following a basilar skull fracture. This is the so-called Battle's sign or "raccoon eyes."

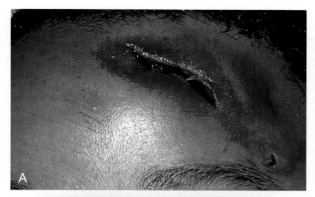

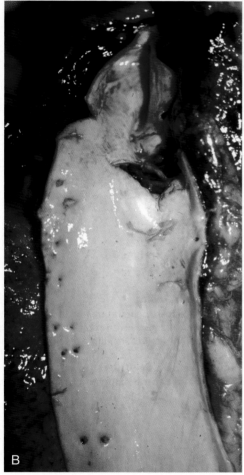

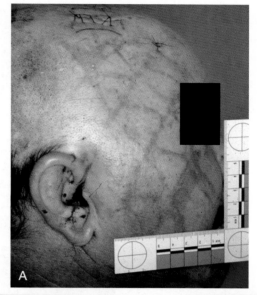

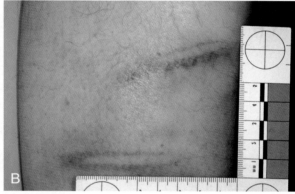

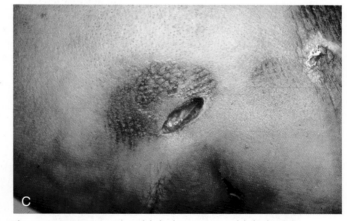

**Figure 15-351** Blunt force injury—lacerations. Lacerations may involve the skin and subcutaneous tissues or internal organs. Lacerations of the skin result from tearing of tissues. They may be located anywhere but occur more often over bone or bony prominences. **A,** Laceration on the forehead due to motor vehicle accident. Lacerations are characterized by tissue bridging and often, as in this example, have abrasions along their margins. **B,** Laceration of the aorta. Lacerations of the descending thoracic aorta just distal to the origin of the left subclavian artery are among the most common of the deceleration injuries of the thorax (the moving body decelerates rapidly as a result of an impact against stationary or relatively stationary objects). The aortic injury may be a laceration as depicted here or a complete transection.

**Figure 15-352** Patterned injuries. Patterned injuries are abrasions/contusions that imprint the pattern of the object, or in some cases, intermediary objects such as articles of clothing (buttons, zippers, etc.), on the injured. **A,** This patterned lesion was from a tire tread. **B,** Patterned contusions from an elongated object. **C,** Patterned injury from a hammer adjacent to a laceration. (Courtesy of Drs. Robert Anthony and Gregory Reiber, Northern California Forensic Pathology.)

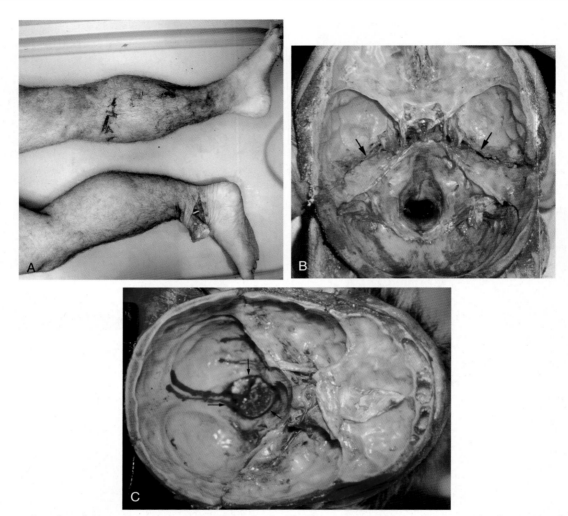

**Figure 15-353** Blunt force injury—fractures. Fractures may be caused by direct trauma (focal, crush, penetrating fractures) or indirect trauma (traction, angulation, rotational, and vertical compression fractures; combinations of angulation fractures with rotational or compression fractures). **A,** This person fell from a building construction site and has bilateral lower extremity fractures including a compound fracture and dislocation of the right tibia. **B,** Hinge fractures of the skull typically occur anterior to the petrous ridges *(arrows)*. This view of the skull base of a motor vehicle accident victim shows side-to-side bone separation in both temporal fossae. The dura should be stripped in all cases to allow identification of subtle fractures. **C,** Ring fractures of the skull on a motor vehicle accident victim encircle the foramen magnum *(arrows)*. Here there is complete dislocation of the atlantooccipital joint.

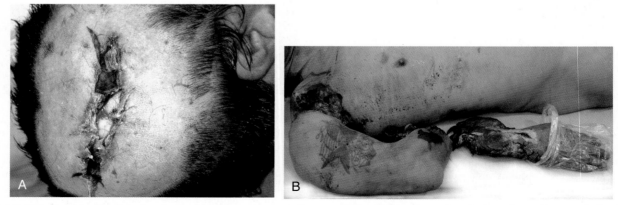

**Figure 15-354** Combination injuries. Severe blunt force trauma often results in combinations of contusions, lacerations, and abrasions. **A,** Here, a blow delivered with a pipe resulted in a scalp laceration and skull fracture. **B,** Crushing injuries are among the most devastating. This pedestrian was hit by a train, resulting in severe skull injuries (not shown), as well as partial amputation of the right arm at the shoulder and complete amputation of the lower arm.

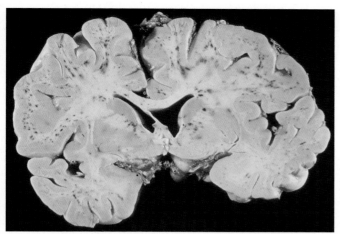

**Figure 15-355** Fat embolism, shown on a coronal section of the cerebrum at the level of the anterior basal ganglia. Multiple variously sized red-brown lesions are seen in both the white matter and less prominently in the gray matter bilaterally. Close inspection shows the lesions to be ill defined, not sharply delimited. The appearance of "brain purpura" is seen in several different conditions but is quite typical of fat embolism, classically following trauma to long bones or the pelvis. The same appearance can be present with diffuse emboli of other types and in some acute leukemias. Special stains for fat will show the intravascular fat.

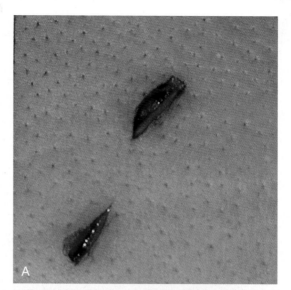

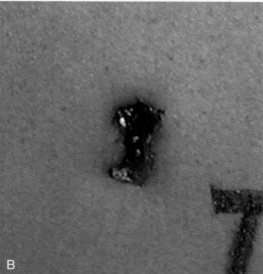

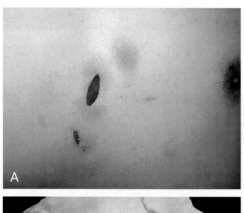

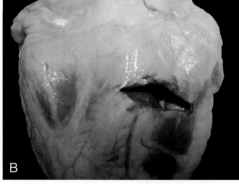

**Figure 15-356** Sharp force injury—stab wounds. Stab wounds are made with pointed instruments, and the depth of penetration of the inner wound (internal component) is typically greater than the skin wound (external component). Stab wounds lack bridging tissue, distinguishing them from lacerations. **A,** Sharp force stab wounds of the chest with a single-edge blade as shown here have a blunted margin and a V-shaped margin. Double-edged instruments produce a V-shaped margin at both ends. **B,** The internal wound from the larger of the two stab wounds depicted in **A** entered the heart.

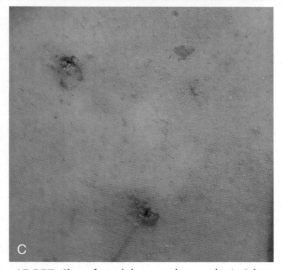

**Figure 15-357** Sharp force injury—stab wounds. **A,** Scissors leave stab wounds that are broader than a typical knife stab wound. These wounds were inflicted with open scissors. **B,** Closed scissor wounds will have a step along one or both edges due to the overlapping blades of the scissors. **C,** Stab wounds from a Phillips screwdriver leave a characteristic lesion of four abrasions or cuts spaced equally around a circular wound.

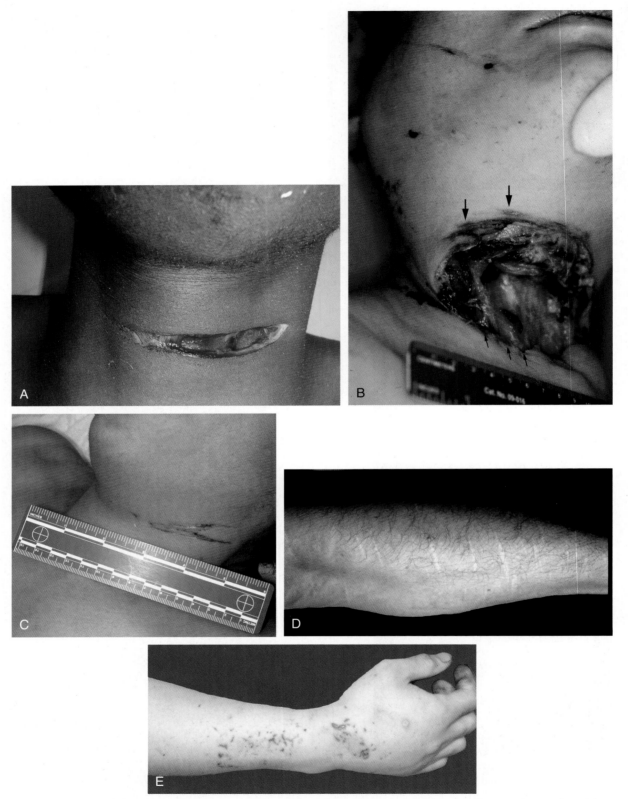

**Figure 15-358** Sharp force injury—incised wounds. Incised wounds are longer than they are deep. Similar to stab wounds and in contrast to lacerations, they lack bridging tissue within the wound. Lethal incised wounds in homicides are usually to the neck and often associated with multiple stab wounds. **A,** Incised wound of the neck. **B,** Lethal incised wound of the neck. This wound was made with a serrated blade. Subtle serrations can be seen along the inferior edge of the wound *(small arrows)*. Serrated blades may also cause curvilinear abrasions as the blade scrapes across the skin *(large arrows)*. **C,** Hesitation wounds may be caused by struggling of the victim, hesitancy on the part of the assailant, or failed suicide attempts. **D,** Multiple hesitation marks or scars on the wrist and arm generally indicate a previous suicide attempt. **E,** During motor vehicle accidents, fragmented cubes of tempered glass windows often produce these clusters of short, linear, angulated, and rectangular incised wounds known as "dicing" injuries. Dicing refers to the dice-shaped fragments of broken glass. (**A, C,** and **E** Courtesy of Mark A. Super, MD, Sacramento County Coroner's Office; **B** courtesy of Drs. Robert Anthony and Gregory Reiber, Northern California Forensic Pathology.)

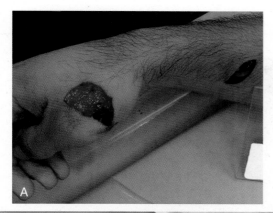

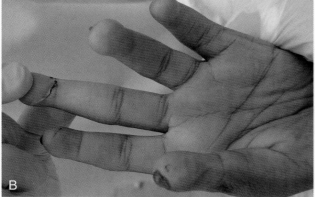

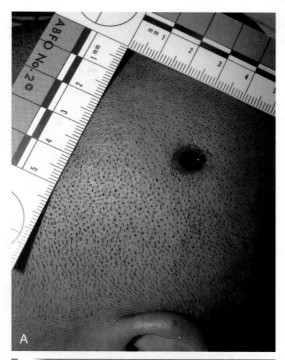

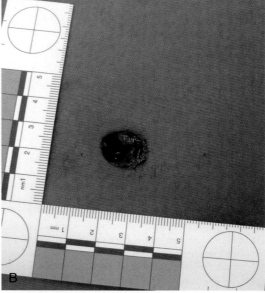

**Figure 15-359** Sharp force injury—defensive wounds. Defensive sharp force wounds typically occur on the hands, forearms, upper arms, or legs and feet if the victim tries to kick at an assailant. They may be stab wounds or incised wounds. **A,** Defensive incised wounds on the hand and forearm. **B,** Small defensive incised wounds on the fingers. (Courtesy of Mark A. Super, MD, Sacramento County Coroner's Office.)

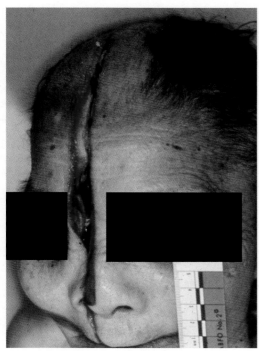

**Figure 15-360** Sharp force injury—chop wounds. Heavy weapons with a sharp or relatively sharp edge such as axes, machetes, propellers, shovels, etc. cause chop wounds. Chop wound injuries have both a sharp force and blunt force component. The injury depicted here was from a meat cleaver. (Courtesy of Drs. Robert Anthony and Gregory Reiber, Northern California Forensic Pathology.)

**Figure 15-361** Entrance gunshot wounds—indeterminate range. Entrance gunshot wounds are classified in four main categories: contact, near contact, intermediate, and indeterminate (distant). With indeterminate or distant range gunshot wounds, only the projectile reaches the target. Gunshot range may become indeterminate from distances as short as 12 inches to 2 feet with flake gunpowder and up to about 4 feet with ball powder. For handguns, indeterminate gunshot entrance wounds consist of a relatively round or elliptical defect surrounded by a ring of abraded skin (abrasion collar). **A,** Indeterminate entrance gunshot wound. **B,** The elliptical shape of this indeterminate range entrance gunshot wound is consistent with an angled path of entry. (Courtesy of Mark A. Super, MD, Sacramento County Coroner's Office.)

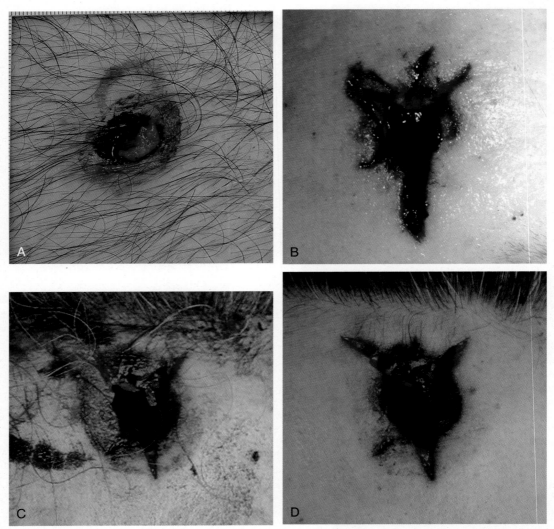

**Figure 15-362** Entrance gunshot wounds—contact range. Contact gunshot wounds may be hard or loose, but in both cases the muzzle is touching the skin when the gun is fired. With hard contact gunshot wounds, the muzzle is pushed hard against the skin, indenting it, and all the material exiting the muzzle enters the body. **A,** Hard contact range entrance gunshot wound of the chest. The gas entering the thoracic cavity has caused the chest wall to bulge out, producing a mark of the gun's muzzle. **B,** Hard contact entrance gunshot wound of the head. Contact gunshot wounds of the head may be round with blackened and seared margins. As shown here, they may also be stellate as gas from the gun penetrates between the scalp and underlying bone, tearing the skin and creating radiating lacerations. Note the slight cherry red color of the skin surrounding the wound due to a localized carbon monoxide effect. Muzzle imprinting may also occur in hard contact gunshot wounds of the head. **C,** Loose contact range entrance gunshot of the head. In loose contact gunshot wounds a slight gap develops between the gun muzzle and the skin allowing soot to be deposited around the wound. **D,** The soot of loose contact gunshot wounds is easily washed away. (**A, C,** and **D,** Courtesy of Mark A. Super, MD, Sacramento County Coroner's Office.)

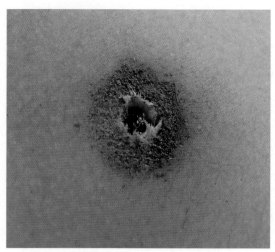

**Figure 15-363** Entrance gunshot wounds—near contact. In near contact wounds the gun muzzle is only a short distance from the skin. This results in a rim of seared, blackened skin around the defect. (Courtesy of Mark A. Super, MD, Sacramento County Coroner's Office.)

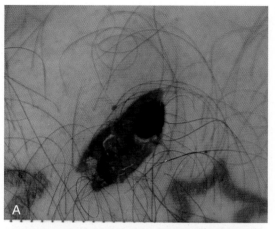

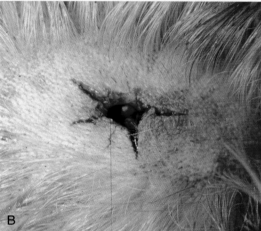

**Figure 15-365** Exit gunshot wounds. Exit gunshot wounds are quite variable, slitlike to stellate with a wide range in size. They lack the features of entrance wounds such as muzzle imprinting, searing, soot, and powder tattoo marks. Unless the skin at the exit site is supported by a firm surface, such as a wall or strong tight-fitting clothing such as a belt (shored exit wounds), typical exit wounds lack any semblance of an abrasion ring. **A,** Typical slitlike exit gunshot wound of the chest. **B,** Large, stellate exit wound of the head.

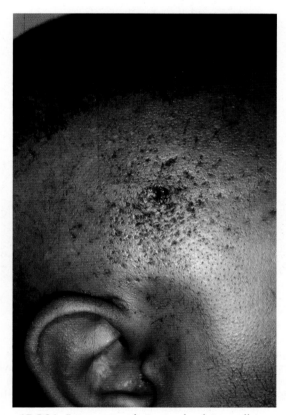

**Figure 15-364** Entrance gunshot wounds—intermediate range. The hallmark of intermediate range entrance wounds is powder tattoo marks, or stippling. This occurs when the powder grains leaving the gun impact the skin, causing punctate abrasions. Unlike gunpowder soot, these abrasions cannot be wiped or washed away.

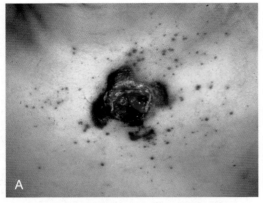

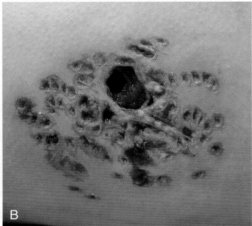

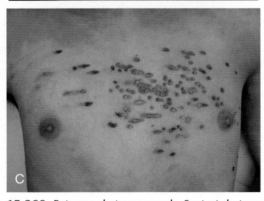

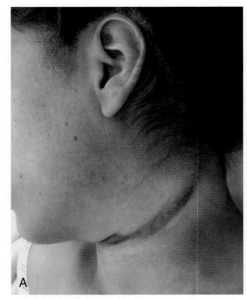

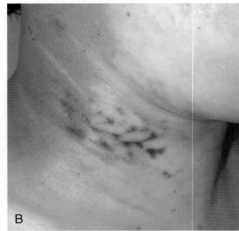

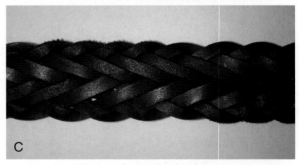

**Figure 15-366** Entrance shotgun wounds. Contact shotgun wounds of the head, like wounds from high-velocity, centerfire rifles, are explosive and cause massive injuries. **A,** From contact to distances of about 2 feet, entrance shotgun wounds of the abdomen and chest create circular defects with seared, blackened margins. In this example, the shotgun wad has also reached the victim, creating a cross mark. From a distance of about 3 feet, the size of the wound is larger and has scalloped margins from the separating shotgun pellets. **B,** Further distances are characterized by satellite pellet lesions surrounding the major defect. These satellite wounds increase in number and spread as the distance increases. **C,** Depending on the choke of the gun, the wound may consist of multiple pellet holes when fired beyond a distance of 10 feet.
(**A,** Courtesy of Drs. Robert Anthony and Gregory Reiber, Northern California Forensic Pathology; **B** and **C,** Courtesy of Mark A. Super, MD, Sacramento County Coroner's Office.)

**Figure 15-367** Asphyxia. Deaths from asphyxia include those caused by strangulation, suffocation, and chemical asphyxia. Strangulation results from occlusion of the blood vessels in the neck and may be caused by hanging, ligature strangulation, or manual strangulation. **A,** Hanging. The body weight tightens a ligature around the neck, creating an abrasion furrow on the skin. Furrows have an inverted V-shape, coursing up toward the point of suspension. Often a gap is seen at the furrow apex. Furrows may be absent with soft ligatures or if the body is cut down shortly after hanging. If the feet are suspended off the ground, the carotid arteries are often compressed and the face of the victim is pale. However, if the body is supported, then the jugular veins rather than the carotid arteries may be compressed. If this occurs, the face is congested and petechiae are often present. Other findings include a protruding tongue, Tardieu spots (see Fig. 15-2) in the lower extremities and forearms, hemorrhage in the strap muscles of the neck, and rarely fractures of the hyoid bone, thyroid cartilage, or cervical spine. **B** and **C,** The pattern of the furrow abrasion may mimic the ligature.

*Continued*

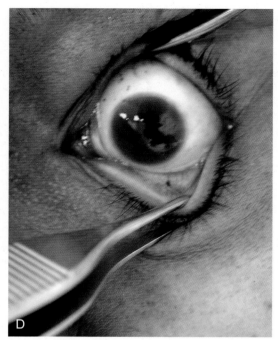

D

**Figure 15-367—Cont'd  D,** Petechial hemorrhages. With all cases of suspected strangulation, it is important to look carefully for scleral and conjunctival hemorrhages and petechiae.

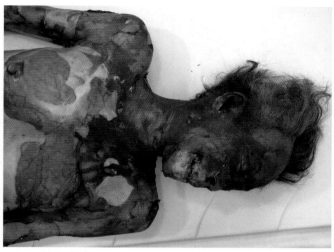

**Figure 15-369**  Thermal injury. Third (full thickness) and fourth degree (charring) burns in a house fire victim.
(Courtesy of Drs. Robert Anthony and Gregory Reiber, Northern California Forensic Pathology.)

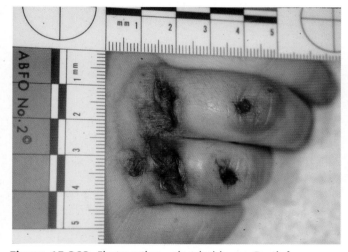

**Figure 15-368**  Electrocution—electrical burns. Death from low-voltage electrocution is usually due to lethal ventricular arrhythmias. Electrical burns may not be present in up to half of cases. In high-voltage electrocutions (greater than 1000 volts) electrical burns are almost always present. As shown in this high-voltage electrical burn, there is central charring of the tissue, pale raised borders, and a zone of hyperemia.

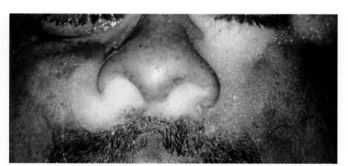

**Figure 15-370**  Drowning. Immersion of a body in water leads to softening and maceration of the skin. The hands and feet are noticeably wrinkled and pale. Examination of the body for signs of external blunt trauma should be delayed until the body is dry because saturation of the skin with water may diminish the appearance of abrasions. White or blood-tinged foam, a mixture of proteinaceous lung fluid and air, may extrude from the nose and mouth and also the cut surfaces of the lungs.
(Courtesy of Drs. Robert Anthony and Gregory Reiber, Northern California Forensic Pathology.)

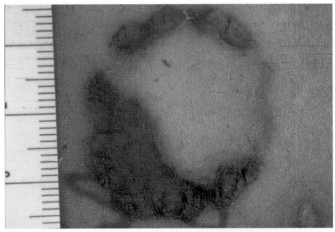

**Figure 15-371** Bite marks. This mark clearly shows a recognizable dental pattern. Bite marks should be analyzed prior to cleaning the body and starting the autopsy. Consulting a forensic odontologist may be necessary. Analysis involves swabbing for DNA, photographing the mark with an appropriate scale, and casting the mark with dental casting material.
(Courtesy of Drs. Robert Anthony and Gregory Reiber, Northern California Forensic Pathology.)

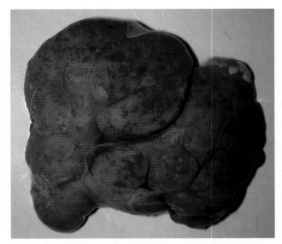

**Figure 15-372** Sudden infant death syndrome (SIDS)—thymus. Nonspecific findings in SIDS include intrathoracic (visceral pleura, epicardium, thymus) petechial hemorrhages. Thymic petechiae are most common.

## REFERENCE

1. Florey HW: The history and scope of pathology. In Florey L, editor: *General pathology*, Philadelphia, 1970, WB Saunders, pp 1-21.

# Appendix A

## Description of Gross Autopsy Findings

This appendix provides templates (adult and pediatric) that we use for recording the gross autopsy findings. Also included is a template for use in the description of traumatic injuries in forensic cases. The guide for description of gross autopsy findings is shown in the column on the left. The right-side column contains cues for observations and descriptions of both important and common findings. These are designed to help the pathologist in training develop a systematic approach to the autopsy and correlate gross findings with pathology diagnoses. Included is a template for description and diagnoses for use with examination of fragmented fetuses. This template lacks the right-side column of observations and descriptions.

Rather, the reader should refer to the listings provided with the pediatric autopsy template.

Some may find the templates too detailed; others may wish to include additional elements. In either case, these templates can form the starting point for the development of your own style and preferences. Also refer to Chapter 10 for a general discussion of the gross autopsy section of the autopsy report. Examples and further discussion of gross autopsy findings are provided in Chapter 15. In addition, consult the various general and specialized pathology textbooks for more detailed discussions of the macroscopic findings of specific disorders.

---

### ADULT AUTOPSY DESCRIPTION OF GROSS FINDINGS

**External Examination**

The decedent (length, _____ cm; weight, _____ kg) is a _well-developed, well-nourished/poorly nourished/obese/cachectic_, phenotypically _(race) male/female_ appearing _younger than/older than_ the recorded age of _____. The _unembalmed/embalmed, unclothed/clothed_ body is identified by a tag attached to the _right/left_ great toe. (_In forensic cases, describe the identification on the outside of the body bag and any security precautions preventing unauthorized opening of the bag. Describe the decedent's clothing, jewelry, pocket contents, and so forth in detail._) There is _mild/moderate/pronounced_ rigor mortis present in the jaws, neck, back, and extremities. A violaceous _posterior/anterior/other_ lividity pattern is present. The body is _cold/warm/other_.

The decedent is _normocephalic/other_ and without _apparent trauma about the face or scalp/other_. The scalp hair is _(color)_ and ____cm in average length. (_In males, describe facial hair._) The bones of the forehead, nose, cheeks, and jaw are _intact/other_ to palpation. The irides are _(color)_, and the pupils are _equal and round measuring _____ cm bilaterally/other_. The conjunctivae are _pink/other,_ and the sclerae are _clear/icteric/other_. The ears are _well-formed and symmetrical/other,_ and the external auditory canals are _without/with_ discharge. The nose is _well-formed and symmetrical/other_. The external nares are _patent/other_ and _without hemorrhage or discharge/other_. The lips are _intact/other_. The mouth contains _a small amount of seromucous secretion/other_ and _no obstructing materials or lesions/other_. The native teeth are _present/absent_ and in _good/poor_ repair. The buccal mucosa is _pink/other_ and shows _no signs of trauma/other_.

**Body as a Whole**

*General Observations*

Height; weight; nutritional status; development; apparent race, sex, and age

Postmortem changes: degree and distribution of postmortem rigidity; character and distribution of lividity; body temperature

*Specific Findings*

Obesity: generalized type involves particularly the face, neck, trunk, upper arms, thighs, and breasts; Cushing disease or corticosteroid therapy is characterized by "moon" face, thick neck with pad of fat over upper thoracic spine, abdominal obesity with purple striae, and contrasting thin extremities; obesity associated with portal hypertension involves breasts, pelvis, lower abdomen

Cachexia: gaunt face, sunken eyes, sharp tip of nose, prominent ribs, sunken flat abdomen flaring away from costal margins and iliac crests, wasting of extremities with greatest diameter at knees and elbows (camel-like limbs), hair dull and brittle

Rigor mortis: begins in the jaw muscles; proceeds to the neck, face, and arms and finally to the lower extremities, with the muscles of the ankles last; reverses in same order

Livor mortis: seen in dependent parts both externally and internally

Develops in 30 minutes to 2 hours, reaching maximum at 8 to 18 hours, depending on local conditions

Becomes "fixed" or nonblanching with time (8 to 12 hours)

*table continues*

## ADULT AUTOPSY DESCRIPTION OF GROSS FINDINGS *(continued)*

The neck is *symmetrical*. There is *no* palpable crepitus or hypermobility. The trachea is palpably *straight and in the midline/ deviated to the right or left*. The chest is *symmetrical/other* and *without palpable crepitus or bony deformity*. The breasts are *soft/ other without palpable masses, skin retraction, or nipple discharge/ other*. The abdomen appears *flat/distended* and *soft/hard without palpable evidence of organomegaly or external trauma/other*. Pubic hair is present in the *usual male/female distribution/other*. The external genitalia are *unremarkable and atraumatic*. (For males: The penis appears *circumcised/uncircumcised*. Both testes are *descended and palpable in the scrotum/other*.) There is *no palpable cervical, axillary, or inguinal lymphadenopathy/other*. The upper extremities are *symmetrical and well developed/other*. The fingernails are *thin and translucent/other*. The nail beds show *no cyanosis/other*. There is *no clubbing/other*. The lower extremities are *symmetrical and well muscled/other*. There is *no pedal edema/other*. The toenails are *thin/thickened/other* and *translucent/opaque/other*. The soles of the feet are *soft/callused/ other*. The posterior trunk shows a *symmetrical external contour/ other*. The spine appears *straight/other*. The anus is *closed and atraumatic/other*. The skin color is *white/brown/tan/yellow/pale*. The skin shows *no irregularity/poor turgor and elasticity/eruptions/ rashes/other*.

### Scars and Identifying Marks
Describe scars and identifying marks.

### Evidence of Therapeutic Intervention
The following medical paraphernalia are in place: *(Describe intravenous or intraarterial lines, Foley catheters, endotracheal tubes, recent surgical incisions, and so forth.)*

### Evidence of External Trauma
See Trauma Template, later.
Note: Specific observations described in the adult autopsy section are not necessarily repeated here.

Pressure of pooling blood may rupture small vessels, causing "Tardieu spots" (postmortem purpura or petechial-type hemorrhages)

May be difficult to see in dark-skinned decedents

Color of postmortem lividity varies

Distinctive livor mortis colors:

Blue-purple—normal

Black-green—putrefaction; hydrogen sulfide poisoning

Pink, cherry red—cyanide, carbon monoxide, or fluoroacetate poisoning; moist postmortem environment

Minimal or absent—exsanguination

Other postmortem changes:

Drying of skin in areas of abrasion, thermal injury, or ruptured vesicles within a few hours after death

Skin becomes dry, wrinkled, and eventually leathery

Hair loosens

Apparent lengthening of fingernails due to shrinkage of fingertips

Eyes dry in 1 to 2 hours; if eyelids are open, sclerae sometimes show a dark red–brown horizontal band along opening ("tache noire")

Film appears on cornea; later cornea becomes opacified

Globes become softened and flattened

### Head
### General Observations
Head size and shape; color, amount, and distribution of scalp and facial hair; fractures of skull and facial bones and swellings of soft tissues; symmetry of face; fluid or discharge coming from ears, nose, or mouth; color of irides; size and equality of pupils; color of sclerae; clarity of corneae and lens; patency of auditory canal; patency of nares; abnormal contents or lesions of oral cavity; presence, absence, and condition of teeth; abnormal size, coatings, or lesions of tongue; lesions of palate and pharynx

### Specific Findings
Loss of hair: may follow debilitating illnesses, chemotherapy, or radiation therapy

Hirsutism: virilization in women due to Cushing disease, masculinizing ovarian tumors, adrenal hyperactivity, or androgen administration

Facial edema: myxedema, superior vena cava syndrome (with upper limb edema), part of generalized anasarca

Eyelid edema: local infection, sinusitis, angioneurotic edema, renal failure, cavernous sinus thrombosis, superior vena cava syndrome

Corneal ulceration: hyperthyroidism, facial paralysis, herpes zoster infection

Corneal haziness: acute glaucoma

Corneal opacification: cataract, injury, inflammation

Corneal rings:

Arcus senilis: ill-defined gray ring just inside cornea

Kayser-Fleischer ring: green-brown ring just inside cornea, seen in Wilson's disease

Pigmented nodules of iris (Lisch nodules): neurofibromatosis type 1

Blue sclerae: Ehlers-Danlos syndrome

Subconjunctival hemorrhage from anterior cranial fossa fracture

Necrosis of nasal tip: acute bacterial endocarditis

Epistaxis: hypertension, coagulation disorder, nasal trauma, anterior cranial fossa fracture

Bloody discharge from auditory canals indicates middle fossa skull fracture

Purulent discharge from auditory canals: otitis media or meatal abscess

Creases in earlobes may indicate vascular disease

Gingival hemorrhages seen with coagulation defects, periodontitis, or trauma

Exudates and lesions of the oral cavity and tongue:

Tough, gray-white adherent membrane over red, ulcerated mucosa in diphtheria

White exudates due to candidiasis (thrush)

Vesicular lesions in herpes simplex, herpangina, and aphthous stomatitis

Severe vesicular eruptions in Stevens-Johnson syndrome, Behçet's syndrome, and pemphigus

Gray-white plaques, indurated white fissures in leukoplakia

Network of threadlike, lacy white lines in lichen planus

Hyperplastic gingiva with diphenylhydantoin use

Enlargement of the tongue in angioneurotic edema

Atrophy of tongue in pernicious anemia

## Neck

### General Observations

Symmetry, mobility, crepitus, position of trachea and thyroid, distention of neck vessels, palpable cervical lymphadenopathy or masses

### Specific Findings

Crepitus of skin: subcutaneous emphysema

Crepitus or increased mobility: cervical spine fracture or atlantooccipital dislocation (if possible, obtain confirming radiographs prior to dissection)

Masses: lymphadenopathy, thyroid tumors, goiter, other tumors

Tracheal deviation: retrosternal goiter, lymphadenopathy

Distension of neck vessels: congestive heart failure, superior vena caval obstruction

## Chest

### General Observations

Thoracic symmetry; pectus deformities; size, asymmetry, consistency, and masses of breasts; discharge or scaling/excoriation of nipples; inversion/retraction of nipples; dimpling or edema of skin

Palpate axilla for lymphadenopathy

### Specific Findings

Asymmetry of chest wall: rickets, osteomalacia, kyphoscoliosis, rib fractures

Increased anterior-posterior chest diameter: chronic obstructive lung disease

Chest deformities:

Pectus carinatum—sternum arches forward (pigeon breast)

Pectus excavatum—sternum and adjacent costal cartilages curve backward (funnel chest)

Gynecomastia—estrogen administration; estrogen, prolactin, or human chorionic gonadotropin–forming tumors; congenital syndromes with increased estrogen secretion, decreased androgen secretion, or decreased androgen activity; testicular failure; liver failure (cirrhosis); complications of various therapeutic drugs; thyrotoxicosis; idiopathic

Breast hypertrophy: pregnancy, idiopathic

Mastitis: reddening and edema of overlying skin

Nipple discharge: benign or malignant tumors, hormonal therapy

*table continues*

**ADULT AUTOPSY DESCRIPTION OF GROSS FINDINGS** *(continued)*

Galactorrhea: therapeutic drug complication, suprahypophyseal or hypophyseal tumor, ectopic prolactin production (renal or bronchogenic neoplasms), hypothyroidism, Addison's disease, adrenal carcinoma, polycystic ovarian syndrome, renal failure, liver failure

Scaling and excoriation of nipple: Paget disease

Edema *(peau d'orange),* dimpling of breast: carcinoma

Palpable breast masses: benign and malignant tumors

### Abdomen
#### General Observations
Contour, local bulges, distension, organomegaly (liver, spleen), masses, discoloration, abnormal veins, hernias

Palpate inguinal region for lymphadenopathy

#### Specific Findings
Masses: neoplasms

Distension: ileus, ascites, peritoneal carcinomatosis

### External Genitalia
#### General Observations
Development; pubic hair; edema; lesions; trauma; circumcision; palpate scrotum for testes, masses; inspect introitus; vaginal speculum examination for sexual trauma/specimen collection

#### Specific Findings
Abnormalities of urethral orifice: epispadias, hypospadias

Scrotal/vulvar edema: anasarca from any cause (e.g., cardiac or renal failure), localized edema from regional venous obstruction, portal vein obstruction, pelvic vein thrombosis

Scrotal/vulvar lymphedema: lymphatic blockage (tumors, filariasis)

Ulcers: chancroid, syphilis, lymphogranuloma venereum, herpes

Warty lesions: condyloma, carcinoma

Absent testis: maldescended (cryptorchism), surgically removed

Testicular atrophy: remote infarcts, healed mumps orchitis, syphilis, filariasis, liver failure

Scrotal swellings or testicular enlargements: hematocele, acute and chronic infections (mumps, tuberculosis, tertiary syphilis), neoplasms

Spermatic cord swellings: epididymitis, hydrocele, spermatocele, varicocele, hematoma, infections, tumors

Uterus protruding from introitus: uterine prolapse

### Extremities
#### General Observations
Symmetry (measure circumference of asymmetrical limbs), edema, muscle wasting, ulcers, masses

Check for joint deformities, swelling, subluxation, contracture, mobility (avoid interpretive errors due to rigor or refrigeration)

Inspect hands/feet; note condition of fingernails and toenails, color of nail beds (cyanosis), clubbing

#### Specific Findings
Edema of single limb or upper or lower extremities due to venous thrombosis or lymphatic obstruction

Atrophy of muscles: upper/lower motor neuron disease, muscular dystrophies

Joint swelling: connective tissue diseases, gout

Joint effusions: suppurative arthritis, connective tissue diseases

Fusiform enlargement of proximal interphalangeal joints; ulnar deviation of hand; flexion deformities in elbows/knees; subcutaneous nodules on backs of elbows, wrists, and fingers indicate rheumatoid arthritis

Tophi: gout
Clubbing of fingers without periostosis: idiopathic
Clubbing with periostosis: hypertrophic pulmonary
    osteoarthropathy

**Back**
*General Observations*
Inspect/palpate; check for symmetry, deformities; inspect anus
*Specific Findings*
Curvature of spinal column: kyphosis, lordosis, scoliosis
Ulcers: pressure sores due to immobility
Pigmented area, tuft of hair, dimple, fistula: spina bifida occulta
Dimple near anus: rectoperineal fistula
Perianal skin tags or pedunculated masses: external hemorrhoids

**Skin**
*General Observations*
Elasticity and turgor, color, pigmentation, edema (localized,
    generalized, dependent, pitting), dermatoses, tumors,
    hemorrhages
*Specific Findings*
Decreased elasticity and turgor: progressive postmortem change
Loose skin that wrinkles when pushed with finger: weight loss
Skin color:
    Pallor—exsanguinating hemorrhage
    Yellow—jaundice
    Blue—cyanosis (nail beds, lips, one limb)
Generalized hyperpigmentation: Addison disease,
    hemochromatosis, chronic malaria, cachexia
Localized hyperpigmentation:
    Chloasma (melasma)—pregnancy, oral contraceptive use,
        Addison disease
    Café au lait spots—neurofibromatosis
    Hypermelanotic papillary or verrucous excrescences—
        acanthosis nigricans (about half of adult cases have
        associated carcinoma)
    Brown to black spots around mouth, nostrils, eyelids, hands,
        feet—Peutz-Jeghers syndrome
    Depigmentation: vitiligo
Pitting, taut shiny skin in dependent areas: edema from acute
    and chronic cardiac and renal failure, hypoalbuminemia,
    allergic reactions, starvation
Hemorrhages: trauma, disseminated intravascular coagulopathy
    (petechiae), purpura (coagulopathy), senile purpura
Ulcers: varicose ulcers are generally above medial malleolus;
    arterial insufficiency; diabetic ulcers involve toes, heels, lower
    anterior surface of leg; ulcers from infections variable with
    associated cellulitis

**Scars and Identifying Marks**
Describe characteristics of scars (site, healing, surgical, traumatic);
    measure scars; describe identifying marks such as tattoos,
    body piercings

**Evidence of Therapeutic Intervention**
Inspect for evidence of recent medical therapy; describe needle
    puncture marks in reasonable detail (may be a clue to blood
    effusions in body cavities); describe remote wounds/scars;
    note presence of endotracheal or nasogastric tube, indwelling
    peripheral or central intravascular catheter, urethral catheter,
    feeding tube, and so forth
Do not remove devices until proper placement is ascertained

*table continues*

## ADULT AUTOPSY DESCRIPTION OF GROSS FINDINGS *(continued)*

### Primary Incision, Neck, and Body Cavities

A standard Y-shaped thoracoabdominal incision reveals a subcutaneous fat thickness of _____ cm at the midabdominal level. There is *no evidence of hemorrhage in the anterior muscles and soft tissues of the neck/other*. The carotid sheaths are *intact/other*. The anterior cervical spine is *palpably unremarkable/other*. *No obstructive material or lesions are present in the glottis or larynx/other*. The hyoid bone and laryngeal cartilage are *normally formed and intact without evidence of fractures or hemorrhage/other*.

The breast tissue consists of *a small amount of white stroma within yellow fat/other*. The sternum and ribs of the anterior chest are *intact/other*. The mediastinum is *midline/other*. The pericardial sac contains ____mL of serous fluid; its surfaces are *glistening and smooth/other*. The parietal pleural surfaces are *glistening and smooth except for a few easily lysed apical fibrous adhesions/other*. There is *no pleural fluid/other*. There are *no pneumothoraces/other*. The domes of the diaphragm are at the *fifth rib bilaterally/other*. Omental and mesenteric fat is *abundant/other*. The peritoneal surfaces are *glistening and smooth/other*; there are *no unusual fluid collections in the abdominal space/other*, and the organs *occupy their usual positions/other*.

### Neck

#### General Observations

Inspect soft tissues, muscles, and hyoid bone for evidence of trauma and major arteries and veins for obstruction; inspect hypopharynx, epiglottis, external larynx, and trachea for obstruction, deviation, or compression; check for trauma; inspect initial thyroid gland in situ; palpate cervical spine; recheck neck mobility

#### Specific Findings

Lymphadenopathy: hyperplasia, tuberculosis, lymphoma, metastatic carcinoma

Midline neck cysts or sinus tract anterior to trachea or proximal to thyroid: thyroglossal cyst or duct

Gray, yellow-brown homogeneous mass below angle of jaw: carotid body tumor

Thyroid and parathyroid masses: see Endocrine System, later

### Breasts

#### General Observations

From posterior aspect, serially incise female breasts (or abnormal male breast) and examine mammary tissue for tumors, cysts

#### Specific Findings

Brown to blue, semitranslucent fluid-filled cysts: fibrocystic change

Hard areas without yellow streaks or yellow-white foci: sclerosing adenosis

#### Masses

Firm, pale, sharply demarcated, sometimes with slitlike spaces: fibroadenoma

Hard, sometimes gritty, gray, with radiating edges: may be invasive ductal carcinoma (scirrhous carcinoma)

Firm, glistening, pale gray–blue, homogeneous, often well circumscribed: may be colloid (mucinous) carcinoma

Firm, rubbery, poorly circumscribed: may be lobular carcinoma

Soft, gray-white, fleshy, smooth to slightly irregular borders: may be medullary carcinoma

### Thoracic Cavity

#### General Observations

Inspect ribs, sternum for trauma, abnormalities; note height of each hemidiaphragm; check for pneumothorax prior to cutting anterior ribs; inspect mediastinum for displacement, blood

Identify/inspect thymus, aorta, esophagus, thoracic duct (if indicated); inspect pericardial sac for size, type, and character of fluid, fibrin, or adhesions; inspect pleural cavities for type and character of fluid; inspect pleura for dullness, fibrin, type and location of adhesions, plaques, masses

#### Specific Findings

Mediastinum

Crepitus: pneumomediastinum

Widening: infection, neoplasm, hemorrhage, pericardial or cardiac causes

Displacement: neoplasms, pleural effusions

Esophagus, aorta, thymus: see appropriate sections (following)

Pericardial cavity

Effusions with no adhesions

Clear or straw-colored (serous): congestive heart failure, hypoproteinemia, serous pericarditis due to nonbacterial infections, systemic lupus erythematosus, scleroderma, uremia, tumors

Pale red (serosanguineous): blunt trauma, cardiopulmonary resuscitation

Frank blood (hemopericardium): cardiac rupture, rupture of intrapericardial aorta, rarely coagulopathies

Chylous (white with lipid droplets): lymphatic obstruction (usually secondary to neoplasms)

Cholesterol (fluid with crystals, lipid droplets): myxedema, idiopathic

Effusions with adhesions (pericarditis)

Fibrinous: rubbery fibrin ("bread and butter") adhesions attaching visceral and parietal pericardium; causes— infection (generally nonbacterial), myocardial infarct, uremia, radiation, rheumatic fever, systemic lupus erythematosus, and trauma, including cardiac surgery

Fibrous: dense adhesions following organization of fibrinous adhesions

Purulent: reddened, granular serosal pericardial surfaces, creamy yellow fluid; causes—bacterial, fungal, or parasitic infection

Adhesions without fluid: healed pericarditis may yield dense fibrous adhesions with or without calcification or obliteration of pericardial space (constrictive pericarditis)

Pleural Cavity

Pneumothorax: complication of pulmonary disease (emphysema, asthma, tuberculosis), spontaneous, idiopathic (distal acinar emphysema), trauma to chest wall or lungs

Effusions without pleuritis (noninflammatory)

Clear, straw-colored, serous (hydrothorax): congestive heart failure; may be serosanguineous due to premortal pleural taps, coagulation disorders; a few fibrous adhesions possible but no loculations

Frank blood (hemothorax): ruptured aortic aneurysm, cardiac rupture, thoracic trauma

Milky white chyle (chylothorax): obstruction of lymphatics by intrathoracic malignancies

Effusions with pleuritis

Serofibrinous (serous or serosanguineous effusions with fibrinous adhesions): inflammation in adjacent lung (tuberculosis, pneumonia, lung infarcts, lung abscess, bronchiectasis) or systemic disorders (rheumatoid arthritis, systemic lupus erythematosus, uremia, radiation therapy, systemic infections)

Yellow-green, creamy pus (empyema, suppurative pleuritis): suppurative infection in adjacent lung

Bloody exudates (sanguineous effusions, hemorrhagic pleuritis): pleural neoplasms, rickettsial disease, coagulation disorders

Fibrous adhesions with or without loculated fluid: after healing, previously mentioned conditions, particularly empyema, may yield dense adhesions

Plaques: fibrous pleural plaques, primary and secondary neoplasms

Masses

Masses with pedicles, occasional cysts: solitary fibrous tumors

Spreading mass of soft, gelatinous gray tissue: malignant mesothelioma

Variable nodular and plaquelike masses: metastatic neoplasms

**Peritoneal Cavity**

*General Observations*

Inspect thickness, color of subcutaneous fat; amount of intraperitoneal fat; position/relationship of viscera; peritoneal membranes; fluid; position, thickness, color of omentum; adhesions; lesser peritoneal cavity; bladder distension

Collect urine if indicated

Identify position, mobility of appendix

*table continues*

*Specific Findings*

Abnormal situs: complete situs inversus, situs inversus limited to abdomen

Chalky, white precipitates in fat: fat necrosis from pancreatitis

Ascites: clear, straw-colored—heart failure; clear, yellow—liver failure

Purulent fluid: peritonitis from extension of bacteria through hollow viscus or viscus rupture, gynecologic infection, spontaneous bacterial peritonitis

Dull, granular peritoneal membranes (sterile peritonitis): mild leakage of bile or pancreatic enzymes

Small, firm nodular exudates: granulomatous (tuberculous) peritonitis

Purulent peritonitis—change in peritoneal membranes and fluid with time

Initial: glistening gray to dull/serous or slightly turbid fluid

Later: creamy suppurative exudate forms—may be localized by omentum, accumulate under liver or diaphragm (subhepatic/subphrenic abscesses)

Exudate may resolve or organize in delicate or dense fibrous adhesions

Walled-off abscesses may persist and reinitiate peritonitis/sepsis

Dense retroperitoneal or mesenteric fibromatosis: sclerosing retroperitonitis

Cysts (mesenteric): mostly benign; malignant usually metastatic adenocarcinoma

Nodular masses (implants) or diffuse tumor: most commonly metastatic, rarely primary (mesothelioma)

Hemorrhagic implants: endometriosis

## Cardiovascular System

The heart (_____ g) is *normally formed/other* and located *in its usual position in the left chest/other*, with its apex pointing to the *left/right/midline*. There is a *minimal/moderate/large* amount of epicardial fat. The epicardial surface is *glistening and smooth/other*. The atrial chambers are *not dilated/dilated*. The interatrial septum is *intact/other*. The atrioventricular connections are *present/other,* and the leaflets of the atrioventricular valves are *thin and delicate/other*. The chordae tendineae are *thin/other*. The interventricular septum is *intact/other*. The myocardium is *firm and red-brown/other*. The right and left ventricular free walls measure ___cm and _____ cm, respectively. The outflow tracts are *widely patent/other,* and the semilunar valves each contain *three thin and delicate/other* cusps. The pulmonary artery is of *appropriate caliber and configuration/other*; its intimal surface is *glistening and intact/other*. The coronary arteries course over the surface of the heart in the *usual fashion/other*. There is *balanced/right dominant/left dominant* coronary artery circulation. The coronary arteries are *patent/other* and *free of atherosclerosis/other*. The ascending aorta is of the *usual* caliber and arches *left/other* before descending along the *left/other* side of the vertebral column. The major arteries arise from the aortic arch and descending aorta in the *usual configuration/other* and are *patent/other*. The intimal surface of the aorta is *smooth/other*. The venae cavae and other major veins are *patent and thin walled/other*.

## Cardiovascular System

### General Observations

Heart weight

Inspect epicardium; position of apex; atrial size; atrial appendages; foramen ovale; coronary sinus; ventricular size; ventricular inflow and outflow tracts; ventricular septum; endocardium; valve leaflets; chordae tendineae; papillary muscles; myocardium (color, consistency, wall thickness); papillary muscles; coronary ostia; coronary artery anatomy and dominance; lumens and intima of coronary arteries; lumens and intima of aorta and major branches, pulmonary arteries and veins, and great veins; portal vein tributaries; and smaller vessels when indicated

### Specific Findings

Increased epicardial and subepicardial fat: obesity, aging

Increased chamber size: left atrial chamber with aging; valvular insufficiency; left-sided heart failure due to ischemic heart disease, hypertension, or aortic/mitral valve abnormalities; nonischemic myocardial diseases; isolated primary right ventricular dilation and secondary right atrial dilation due to right-sided heart failure from chronic pulmonary hypertension

Decreased size of left ventricle chamber: aging

Hypertrophy

Hypertrophy and normal or reduced cavity diameter (concentric hypertrophy): pressure overload (e.g., hypertension, aortic stenosis)

Hypertrophy with dilation: volume overload or pressure and volume overload (e.g., mitral or aortic valve insufficiency—walls of dilated hearts may be of normal thickness while still being markedly hypertrophied), valvular disease, cardiomyopathies

Myocardial disease (cardiomyopathies, myocarditis)

Hypertrophy, dilation, mural thrombi in ventricles or atrial appendages, normal valves: dilated (primary or secondary) cardiomyopathy

Left ventricle usually more involved than right ventricle; often disproportionate thickening of interventricular septum compared with left ventricular free wall (3:2 ratio); ventricular cavity becomes slitlike rather than round: hypertrophic cardiomyopathy

Firm myocardium, variably hypertrophied or normal ventricles, biatrial dilation, variably dilated ventricles: restrictive cardiomyopathies (idiopathic, radiation fibrosis, amyloidosis, sarcoidosis, metastatic tumor, inborn metabolic errors)

Waxy, rubbery myocardium and tan, waxy endocardial deposits: amyloidosis

Granulomata causing visible scars; endothelial lesions: sarcoidosis

White, thickened endocardium and subendocardium: endomyocardial fibrosis with and without eosinophilia

Left ventricular dilation and hypertrophy, gray-white myocardial scars, left ventricular aneurysms, patchy endocardial fibrous thickening, coronary artery atherosclerosis: chronic ischemic heart disease (ischemic cardiomyopathy)

Marked thinning, yellow discoloration, slight or focal dilation of right ventricle: right ventricular cardiomyopathy (arrhythmogenic right ventricular dysplasia)

Variable hypertrophy, flabby myocardium, subtle mottling with pale foci or minute hemorrhages, sometimes mural thrombi: myocarditis

### Valvular Heart Disease

Atrioventricular valves with thickened, distorted leaflets and short, thickened chordae tendineae; semilunar valves with thick, distorted and fused cusps: rheumatic valvular heart disease (chronic)

Heaped-up, irregular, calcified masses both within cusps and protruding into the sinuses of Valsalva; free margins of cusps generally uninvolved: calcific aortic stenosis, degenerative type

Calcification beginning at free margins of cusps with bicuspid valve or valve with rudimentary third cusp: calcific aortic stenosis, congenital type

"Hooding" of the leaflet; rubbery thickening of edge of the leaflet; elongation, attenuation, or even rupture of chordae tendineae: mitral valve prolapse

Irregular, hard ring of calcification at the leaflet-myocardial connection: calcification of the mitral valve annulus

Plaquelike thickenings of endocardium and valves of the right side of heart (rarely do lesions involve left-sided structures): carcinoid heart disease

### Vegetations

Small, friable, irregular, and often multiple vegetations along the lines of closure of a valve or on the chordae: acute rheumatic endocarditis

Large irregular masses overhanging free margins that extend to chordae and valve leaflets or cusps, with or without abscess, possible valve perforation: infective endocarditis

Small, bland, often single vegetations attached at the line of valve closure: nonbacterial thrombotic (marantic) endocarditis

Small to medium-sized vegetations on atrioventricular valves; may be on both sides of valve leaflets: Libman-Sacks endocarditis

*table continues*

## ADULT AUTOPSY DESCRIPTION OF GROSS FINDINGS *(continued)*

Myocardial Infarcts
Color changes with time:
Less than 4 hours: no color change
4-12 hours: occasionally dark mottling
12-24 hours: dark mottling, red-blue pallor
1-3 days: mottling with yellow-tan center
3-7 days: yellow-tan, central softening, hyperemic border
7-10 days: maximally yellow-tan, progressive softening; red-tan margins
10-14 days: pale red-gray borders
2 weeks to 2 months: replacement with firm gray-white scar

Atherosclerotic Cardiovascular Disease
Yellow, flat spots and streaks: fatty streaks
White to white-yellow plaques protruding into arterial lumen, may coalesce with neighboring plaques (sectioning reveals firm, white luminal surface with soft, white-yellow central region): atheroma
Atheromas with calcification, ulceration, hemorrhage: complicated atheroma
Dilation of vessel, often containing thrombus: aneurysm
Small spherical dilation: berry aneurysm
Large spherical dilation: saccular aneurysm
Spindle-shaped dilation: fusiform aneurysm
Hematoma extending between layers of artery: arterial dissection

### Respiratory System

The trachea is of *normal/other* caliber and courses in the *usual/other* fashion. The lungs (right, _____ g; left, _____ g) contain the *usual/other* lobes and fissures. The lungs *collapse completely/collapse only partially/do not collapse*. The visceral pleural surfaces are *slightly opaque/other* with a *small/moderate/large* amount of anthracotic pigment. The parenchyma is *soft and pale red/other*. Air spaces are *not enlarged/other*. Respiratory mucosa is *smooth and pale/other,* and the lumen *contains a small amount of clear mucus/other*. The vessels are *patent/other*.

### Respiratory System
#### General Observations

Inspect luminal contents, mucosa of larynx, trachea; weigh lungs; inspect lungs for anomalies, including lobation (complete, incomplete, abnormal); inspect visceral pleural surfaces; palpate lung parenchyma for consistency, crepitation; examine bronchi, vessels, parenchyma, lymph nodes

#### Specific Findings

Heavy lungs that do not collapse with diffuse, firm, red, boggy parenchyma: diffuse alveolar damage, exudative stage (numerous causes)
Heavy lungs that do not collapse with diffuse, firm, gray parenchyma with dilated, remodeled air spaces: diffuse alveolar damage, organizing stage
Slightly elevated, granular, firm gray-red to yellow, poorly demarcated areas (up to 4 cm) patchily distributed around airways; may be multilobar; often basilar: bronchopneumonia
Consolidation in large areas of lobe or even in entire lobe: lobar pneumonia
Stages of lobor pneumonia:
Congestion: lungs heavy and boggy
Red hepatization: lungs red, firm, airless
Gray hepatization: lungs gray-brown, dry, firm
Resolution: patchy return to normal-appearing lung parenchyma
Organization: areas of firm, gray-tan lung
Gray-white to yellow-white friable necrosis: tuberculosis, fungal (e.g., coccidioidomycosis, blastomycosis, and histoplasmosis) infection
1- to 1.5-cm gray-white, subpleural caseous lesion typically in superior portion of lower lobe with associated gray-white caseous lesion in hilar lymph nodes: primary pulmonary tuberculosis

Small foci of caseous necrosis typically in apex of one or both lungs with similar lesions in regional lymph nodes: early secondary (reactivation) tuberculosis

Cavities lined by yellow-gray caseous material: progressive secondary tuberculosis (cavitary fibrocaseous tuberculosis)

Fibrocalcific scars, cavities in lung apices: healed secondary tuberculosis

Patchy, or confluent, unilateral or bilateral consolidation and congestion: acute interstitial pneumonias due to viruses, *Mycoplasma pneumoniae, Chlamydia* species, *Coxiella* species

Patchy, firm parenchyma: interstitial lung diseases of various causes, sometimes with helpful diagnostic gross features (but these diseases usually require histologic diagnosis)

Black scars, 2 to 10 cm in diameter: may be complicated coal workers' pneumoconiosis (progressive massive fibrosis)

Hard scars with central softening and cavitation, fibrotic lesions in hilar lymph nodes and pleura: may be silicosis

Solid firm areas alternating with normal lung, subpleural cysts; worse in lower lobes: may be usual interstitial pneumonia

Cysts of varying sizes surrounded by firm, gray-tan parenchyma resembling honeycombs: honeycomb lung due to end-stage interstitial fibrosis

Heavy, red-brown consolidation and blood in airways: pulmonary hemorrhage syndromes

Dilation of air spaces: emphysema

Centriacinar emphysema: upper lobe involvement worse than lower lobe involvement

Panacinar emphysema: lower lobe involvement worse than upper lobe involvement

Paraseptal (distal acinar) emphysema: subpleural, along lobular septa

Air space enlargements 1 cm or greater in diameter: bullae

Mucus secretions filling normal-sized airways: chronic bronchitis, asthma

Mucus plugs, alternating overdistention and small areas of atelectasis: acute asthma, status asthmaticus

Dilated airways that reach pleural surface and are often filled with pus: bronchiectasis

Diffuse bronchiectasis: more likely cystic fibrosis, ciliary dyskinesia, immunodeficiency states

Localized bronchiectasis: more likely postinfection (tuberculosis, suppurative pneumonias, measles, adenovirus)

## Lung Tumors

Gray, yellow, white masses, predominantly central (90% in segmental or larger bronchi), with or without cavitation: squamous cell carcinoma

Gray or white peripheral masses, rarely with cavitation, though areas of necrosis may be present: adenocarcinoma

Single nodules or multiple diffuse or coalescing nodules with gelatinous or solid, gray-white regions resembling pneumonia: bronchioloalveolar carcinoma

Soft, gray or tan, often necrotic masses, 50% central, 50% peripheral: large cell carcinoma

Gray to white, somewhat fleshy masses, generally arising centrally: neuroendocrine carcinoma, small cell type

Polypoid masses projecting into bronchial lumen: neuroendocrine carcinoma, carcinoid type

*table continues*

## ADULT AUTOPSY DESCRIPTION OF GROSS FINDINGS *(continued)*

### Gastrointestinal System

The esophagus courses in the *usual/other* fashion to enter the stomach; its mucosal surface is *white and intact/other*. The squamocolumnar junction is *sharp/indistinct/other*. The stomach is *empty/other* and *does not contain residuals of medication/other*. An ethanol-like odor is *apparent/not apparent*. Gastric mucosa *is intact with tall rugal folds/other*. The wall is *pliable/other*. The pylorus is *contracted/other*. The small intestine is of the *usual/other* caliber, and its walls are *pliable/other*. The cecum is *freely mobile/fixed* in the right lower quadrant. The appendix is *retrocecal/other* and *not inflamed/other*. The colon contains *formed brown stool/other* and is of *generous caliber/other*. *No focal mass lesions are identified throughout the gastrointestinal tract/other*.

### Gastrointestinal System
### *General Observations*

Inspect oral cavity (contents, mucosa, teeth, gingiva, tongue), pharynx (mucosa, contents); inspect esophagus (position, contents, mucosa); look for tracheoesophageal fistula by opening esophagus before removing it from the trachea; inspect stomach (size, contents, mucosa—including rugae); inspect small intestines (contents, mucosa, serosa); identify and inspect ampulla of Vater; inspect large intestines (contents, mucosa, wall thickness, serosa); identify and note size, position, mobility of appendix

### *Specific Findings*

Esophagus

Diverticula: Zenker, traction, epiphrenic

Linear lacerations oriented along the axis of the lumen involving only mucosa or extending into the submucosa: Mallory-Weiss tears

Red, velvety mucosa at gastroesophageal junction: Barrett esophagus

Loss of sharp demarcation at gastroesophageal junction: reflux esophagitis

Gray-white to dark pseudomembranes: candidiasis

Hyperemia, small ulcers: viral (herpes simplex; cytomegalovirus) infection

Dilated esophageal veins: varices (varices are difficult to identify postmortem when collapsed; often, mucosa overlying varices is eroded—take microscopic sections from such areas)

Firm, gray-white masses within esophageal wall: gastrointestinal stromal tumors (leiomyomas)

Exophytic, infiltrative, or excavating ulcerative masses: squamous cell carcinoma

Stomach

Edema and hyperemia: mild acute gastritis

Mucosal erosion, hemorrhage into gastric wall: severe acute gastritis

Flattening of mucosa with loss of rugal folds and thinning of gastric wall: chronic gastritis

Round to oval, sharply punched-out defects with straight walls and smooth, clean bases generally located along the lesser curvature in the border zone between corpus and antrum or in the first portion of the duodenum: peptic ulcers

Small, superficial ulcers with poorly defined margins, dark brown bases, and no anatomic predilection: superficial stress ulcers

Small sessile polyps: usually hyperplastic

Exophytic, excavated, diffuse infiltrative tumors: usually gastric adenocarcinoma

Small and Large Intestines

Small blind outpouchings: diverticula; may occur anywhere in gastrointestinal tract but most commonly seen in the colon along margins of taeniae; with diverticulitis, the walls of the diverticula become firm and thickened and may cause narrowing of the wall of the colon

Solitary diverticulum on antimesenteric side of terminal ileum: Meckel diverticulum

Focal mucosal hyperemia; enlargement of lymphoid tissues; ulcerations; hemorrhagic or friable mucosal exudates; pseudomembranes; serosal surfaces unaffected or covered with serous, fibrinous, or hemorrhagic exudates: enterocolitis (however, appearance variable depending on pathogens)

Dusky purple-red discoloration of serosal and subserosal tissues; thickened, rubbery bowel wall; lumen containing sanguineous mucus or frank blood: transmural infarct (if due to arterial occlusions, there is usually a sharp demarcation from normal; in venous occlusions, no clear demarcation from adjacent normal tissue is seen)

Dark red or red-purple mucosa, multifocal or continuous with unaffected serosa: mucosal infarct

Hyperemia and focal ulceration (early lesion), coalescence of ulcers into serpentine linear ulcers and fissures along bowel axis, narrowing of the lumen, thickening of the wall, coarsely textured ("cobblestone") mucosa with fissures and intervening normal mucosa (chronic lesions): Crohn disease

Broad-based ulceration beginning in rectum and extending proximally; pseudopolyps created by regenerating mucosa adjacent to areas of ulceration: ulcerative colitis

Smooth, round, <5-mm sessile lesions on mucosal folds: hyperplastic polyps

Irregular pedunculated lesion with slender stalk; occasionally sessile, ovoid, or flat: tubular adenoma

Generally sessile polypoid lesion up to 10 cm in diameter: villous adenoma

Polypoid exophytic mass (generally in proximal and transverse colon): adenocarcinoma

Annular, encircling mass narrowing lumen (generally of distal colon): adenocarcinoma

Intramural or submucosal polypoid or elevated yellow-tan masses or bulbous swellings of the tip of appendix: carcinoid (neuroendocrine) tumor

## Hepatobiliary System

The liver (_____ g) has a *sharp/blunt/other* anterior margin; its surface is *intact, smooth and glistening/other*. The parenchyma is red-brown and firm with the *usual/accentuated/other* lobular pattern. Intrahepatic bile ducts and vessels are *patent/other*. The gallbladder is *present/other* and *contains approximately _____ mL of viscid dark green bile/other*. The wall is *thin and pliable/other* with *reticulated intact/other* mucosa. The common bile duct is *patent/other* into the duodenum.

## Hepatobiliary System
### General Observations
Liver weight

Inspect liver surface (color, capsule, lobulation, consistency) and parenchyma (color, pattern, consistency, markings, differences between right and left lobes) and intrahepatic parts of portal vein, bile ducts, hepatic ducts, hepatic artery, and hepatic vein; check patency of cystic and common bile ducts; inspect bile duct (circumference, mucosa, wall, contents), gallbladder (mucosa, contents, wall), cystic duct (circumference, contents), ampulla of Vater

### Specific Findings
Liver

Capsule: subcapsular hematomas, lacerations, calcified thrombi

Nodularity of capsular surface: cirrhosis

Firmer than usual parenchyma but without nodularity: fibrosis

Yellow-tan, greasy parenchyma: fatty change

Yellow-tan parenchyma when fresh, green after fixation: cholestasis

Firm nodules 3 cm or less in diameter: micronodular cirrhosis due to alcoholic liver disease, primary and secondary biliary cirrhosis, glycogenosis type IV, Indian childhood cirrhosis, galactosemia and congestive (cardiac) cirrhosis

Firm nodules greater than 3 cm in diameter: macronodular cirrhosis due to alcoholic liver disease; viral hepatitis; drug-induced injury; hepatotoxins; or various hereditary diseases including Wilson's disease, hereditary tyrosinemia, and $a_1$-antitrypsin deficiency

Firm nodules showing approximately equal numbers of micronodules and macronodules: mixed micro- and macronodular cirrhosis caused by alcoholic cirrhosis and diseases causing macronodular cirrhosis listed previously

*table continues*

## ADULT AUTOPSY DESCRIPTION OF GROSS FINDINGS (continued)

Multiple diffuse cysts: polycystic liver disease

Swollen, red-purple liver with tense capsule: hepatic vein (Budd-Chiari syndrome) or inferior vena caval thrombosis/obstruction

Well-demarcated, poorly encapsulated nodules, yellow or slightly lighter than adjacent parenchyma, often with central, gray, stellate scar: focal nodular hyperplasia

Diffuse spherical nodules without parenchymal fibrosis: nodular regenerative hyperplasia

Pale, yellow-tan or bile-stained nodules, generally subcapsular: adenoma

Neoplasms paler than adjacent liver to slightly green: hepatocellular carcinoma (with fibrous bands: fibrolamellar hepatocellular carcinoma)

Gray-white to pale tan, sometimes gelatinous tumor: cholangiocarcinoma

Masses with central necrosis and umbilication: metastatic neoplasms, generally carcinomas

### Gallbladder

Black calculi, usually less than 1.5 cm in diameter: pigment stones (chronic hemolysis, alcoholic cirrhosis, biliary infection, old age)

Round or faceted, pale yellow calculi with granular surfaces; transection reveals crystalline radiations: cholesterol stones (caused by obesity, high-calorie diet, gastrointestinal diseases, oral contraceptives, estrogen therapy, drug therapy, old age)

Central pure cholesterol or bile core surrounded by variegated black (bile) and gray-white (cholesterol) layers: combined stones (inflammatory reaction to initial pure stone)

Calculi variegated throughout: mixed stones (inflammation of gallbladder)

Infiltrating or exophytic tumor: adenocarcinoma

### Pancreas

The pancreas (_____ g) is *gray/other* and located in its *usual position/other* within the duodenal sweep. Its parenchyma has a *firm/lobular/other* architecture with *minimal/abundant* fat in the tail. The pancreatic ducts are *of the usual caliber/other*.

### Pancreas

#### General Observations

Pancreas weight

Inspect color, shape, consistency, lobulation, amount of fat, ducts of Wirsung and Santorini (contents, mucosa, diameter, patency, relationship to ampulla)

#### Specific Findings

Head of pancreas encircling duodenum: annular pancreas

Pancreatic tissue in stomach, small intestines, Meckel diverticulum: ectopic pancreas

Fatty replacement: cystic fibrosis

Fat necrosis (firm, minute, yellow-white deposits becoming chalky white after calcification), parenchymal necrosis (gray-white areas of softening) and hemorrhage (blue-black or dark red areas): acute pancreatitis

Hard parenchyma in lobular distribution with focal areas of calcification; calculi present in pancreatic ducts: chronic pancreatitis

Hard parenchyma in nonlobular distribution, generally involving head of pancreas: obstructive chronic pancreatitis due to obstruction of the sphincter of Oddi (cholelithiasis, neoplasia)

Cystic tumors: cystadenoma, cystadenocarcinoma, solid cystic tumor

Ill-defined, gray-white to gray-yellow, firm mass anywhere in pancreas: adenocarcinoma

Encapsulated pale tan to red-brown tumors: islet cell tumors

## Urinary System

The kidneys (right, _____ g; left, _____ g) are located in their _usual retroperitoneal position/other_ and have capsules that strip with the _usual ease/less difficulty than usual/greater difficulty than usual_ to reveal _smooth/granular/other_ surfaces. The parenchyma is _red-brown/other_ with _clearly demarcated/ill-defined_ corticomedullary junctions. A _minimal/moderate/large_ amount of peripelvic fat is present. The collecting systems are _not dilated/dilated/other_. The pelves and ureter are _patent and not dilated/other_. Their mucosa is _smooth/other_. The urinary bladder contains _____ mL of _clear/turbid/other_ urine. The bladder mucosa is _intact/other_.

## Urinary System

### General Observations

Kidney weights

Inspect kidney position and symmetry, capsule (strips easily or not), cortical surfaces (color, scars, cysts), cut parenchymal surfaces (color, thickness of cortex and medulla, corticomedullary junction, cortical markings, masses), calyces and pelvis (contents, mucosa, dilation), renal arteries and veins (intima, lumens), peripelvic fat; inspect ureters (size, position, contents, mucosa, circumference); probe ureteropelvic and ureterovesical junction for stenosis; inspect bladder (contracted or distended; contents; mucosa; wall thickness and character); inspect urethra (mucosa, patency, diverticula)

### Specific Findings

Kidneys

Fusion of upper or lower poles of kidney: horseshoe kidney

Bilateral massively enlarged kidneys with multiple dilated cysts (up to 4 cm) filled with clear, turbid, or hemorrhagic fluid: autosomal dominant adult polycystic kidney disease

Cortical and medullary cysts (0.5 to 2 cm) containing clear fluid in patients undergoing dialysis: acquired cystic disease

Single or multiple thin-walled translucent cortical cysts (1 to >10 cm) filled with clear fluid: simple cysts

Abscesses in cortex; ulceration of ureteral mucosa; purulent material in ureteral lumen: acute pyelonephritis

Extension of suppurative areas through renal capsule into perinephric fat: perinephric abscess

Suppurative exudate within obstructed renal pelvis, calyces, and ureter: pyelonephrosis

Gray-white to yellow discoloration of distal pyramids: papillary necrosis

Brownish necrotic papillae: analgesic nephropathy

Coarse or irregular cortical scars, primarily in upper or lower poles; dilation and blunting of calyces; dilation and thickening of ureters: chronic pyelonephritis

Chronic pyelonephritis with nodular yellow-orange lesions: xanthogranulomatous pyelonephritis

Normal size or reduced weights; fine, even granular surfaces, cortical narrowing: benign nephrosclerosis due to hypertension; diabetic nephropathy

Small petechial-type hemorrhages on cortical surface ("flea-bitten"): malignant nephrosclerosis

Wedge-shaped, sharply demarcated pale yellow–white areas with hyperemic borders: acute infarcts

Wedge-shaped depressions with underlying pale gray–white scars: remote infarcts

Diffuse, pale, ischemic necrosis limited to the cortex: diffuse cortical necrosis

Blunting of apices of pyramids (early) to transformation of kidney into thin-walled cystic structure with parenchymal atrophy, obliteration of pyramids (late): obstructive uropathy

Small (typically <5 mm), pale gray–yellow, encapsulated nodule: papillary adenoma

Small (typically <1 cm), firm, gray-white lesions in pyramids: renal fibroma

Spherical masses, yellow to gray-white, with foci of hemorrhage, softening, and discoloration: renal cell carcinoma

_table continues_

## ADULT AUTOPSY DESCRIPTION OF GROSS FINDINGS *(continued)*

### Bladder
Pouchlike eversions of bladder wall: diverticula

Mucosal hyperemia and ulcerations, suppurative exudates: acute cystitis

Red, friable, granular, sometimes ulcerated epithelium: chronic cystitis

Cystitis with soft, yellow, flat mucosal plaques: cystitis with malacoplakia

Thickening of bladder wall, enlargement of individual muscle bundles into trabeculations, crypts, diverticula: urethral obstruction

Papillary, flat, nodular or mixed-pattern tumor: transitional cell carcinoma

### Reproductive System (Male)
The prostate (_____ × _____ × _____ cm or _____ g) is *firm/other* with *lobular gray-white/other* parenchyma. The testes have *smooth white/other* capsules and *tan/other* parenchyma. Tubules *string out in the usual manner/do not string out.*

### Reproductive System (Male)
#### General Observations
Prostate size in three dimensions (or weight)

Inspect prostate (shape, capsule, variations in lobes); inspect seminal vesicles (symmetry, size, contents, lining, wall); weigh and inspect testes (position, tunica vaginalis, epididymis, tunica albuginea, parenchyma); perform tubule pluck test

#### Specific Findings
Prostate

Soft, spongy gland enlargement, small or coalescing abscesses: acute prostatitis

Gland enlargement due to nodules of variable color and consistency, white to yellow or yellow-pink, and soft to firm depending on amount of fibrous tissue: nodular hyperplasia

Single nodule or multifocal areas of gritty, firm yellow or gray-white tissue arising in peripheral zone, often difficult to distinguish from surrounding normal prostate: adenocarcinoma

Testes

Decreased weight, thickened tunica albuginea: atrophy, liver disease, genetic disorders

Enlarged testes (macroorchidism): fragile X syndrome; pituitary gonadotrophinomas

Epididymal and testicular edema, congestion, abscess formation and/or necrosis: acute epididymitis and orchitis

Firm, gray to white with decreased stringing of tubules: healed (scarred) orchitis

Homogeneous gray-white lobulated tumor: may be seminoma

Pale gray, soft, friable tumor: may be spermatocytic seminoma

Variegated, focally hemorrhagic and necrotic, poorly demarcated tumor: may be embryonal carcinoma

Homogeneous, yellow-white, mucinous and poorly demarcated tumor: may be yolk sac tumor

Small solid tumors with hemorrhage and necrosis: may be choriocarcinoma

Large, heterogeneous solid or cystic; may have admixed embryonal and/or choriocarcinoma: teratoma

### Reproductive System (Female)
The uterus, tubes, and ovaries are in their *usual/other* relative positions within the pelvis and appear appropriate for age. The cervical os is *round/elongated/other*. The endometrial cavity (_____ × _____ cm) is *empty/other*. The endometrium is *pale/other* and measures _____ cm in thickness. The fallopian tubes are *narrow/other* and *without/other* adhesions. The ovaries (right, _____ × _____ × _____ cm or _____ g; left, _____ × _____ × _____ cm or _____ g) are *gray/other* and *convoluted/smooth/other* with *firm gray parenchyma containing a few scattered cortical corpora lutea and albicantia/homogeneous parenchyma/other.*

### Reproductive System (Female)
#### General Observations
Inspect vagina (mucosa, contents) and uterus (size, shape, position)—if indicated, measure in three dimensions or weigh; inspect exocervix, cervical os, endocervix, endometrium, myometrium; measure endometrial cavity in two dimensions and endometrial thickness; inspect fallopian tubes (serosa, adhesions, cysts, diameter, contents if dilated, condition of fimbria); measure (in three dimensions) or weigh ovaries; inspect ovaries (color, surface, parenchyma)

*Specific Findings*

Uterus

Hyperemia, erosions of cervix: cervicitis

Small, soft, sessile, mucoid polyps: endocervical and endometrial polyps

Fungating, ulcerating, infiltrating tumors of cervix: predominately squamous cell carcinoma

Endometrial hemorrhage, nonmenstrual blood in uterine cavity: endometrial hemorrhage due to systemic shock (uterine apoplexy), disseminated intravascular coagulation, coagulopathies

Red-blue to yellow-brown nodules implanted on serosal surfaces: endometriosis; may cause severe scarring

Enlargement and irregular thickening of uterine wall: adenomyosis

Sharply circumscribed, round, firm, gray-white masses that may be intramural, subserosal or submucosal: leiomyomas

Fallopian Tubes

Small, thin-walled fallopian tube cysts containing serous fluid: paratubal cysts

Larger, thin-walled fallopian tube cysts near fimbriated end or in the broad ligament: hydatids of Morgagni

Ovaries

Cysts, usually multiple, with gray, glistening lining and containing clear serous fluid: follicular cysts

Cysts lined by bright yellow luteal tissue: luteal cysts

Large ovaries with numerous subcortical cysts (0.5 to 1.5 cm in diameter): polycystic ovaries

Cystic masses with variable solid components: serous cystadenoma, serous cystadenocarcinoma, mucinous cystadenoma, mucinous cystadenocarcinoma, endometrioid carcinoma

Unilocular cystic tumors containing hair and sebaceous material: benign teratomas

Large solid tumors with necrosis, hemorrhage, hair, grumous material, bone, cartilage: immature malignant teratomas

Various solid tumors: germ cell tumors and sex-cord stromal tumors

## Lymphoreticular System

The thymic tissue is *ill defined; its parenchyma largely replaced by fat/other*. The spleen (____ g) has a *smooth, intact/other* capsule. Splenic parenchyma is *dark red/other*. The follicles are *small/other,* and trabeculae are *delicate/other*. There is *no/other* lymphadenopathy. The mediastinal lymph nodes are *soft and black/other*. Other lymph nodes are *small and gray/other*. Rib and vertebral marrow is *red, moist, and ample/other*.

## Lymphoreticular System

*General Observations*

Inspect thymus (location, size, color, consistency); weigh thymus if abnormal; weigh spleen; inspect spleen (size, capsule, exterior color, parenchymal color, red and white pulp, trabeculae, vessels); inspect superficial, mediastinal, abdominal (including mesenteric), and retroperitoneal lymph nodes (size, parenchyma); inspect bone marrow of ribs, vertebrae, sternum (color, consistency); always sample femoral bone marrow in hematopoietic disorders

*Specific Findings*

Thymus

Atrophy and fibrofatty replacement: normal involution with aging versus stress involution

Hyperplasia (thymic follicular hyperplasia): myasthenia gravis, chronic inflammatory and immunologic states (Graves' disease, systemic lupus erythematosus, scleroderma, rheumatoid arthritis, other autoimmune diseases)

Lobulated, firm, gray-white masses sometimes with cystic necrosis and calcification: thymomas

Spleen

Accessory masses of splenic tissue (splenunculi): found in 10% to 15% of autopsies

Enlargement (200 to 400 g), very soft, rarely abscess formation: acute splenitis

*table continues*

## ADULT AUTOPSY DESCRIPTION OF GROSS FINDINGS *(continued)*

Marked enlargement (1000 to 5000 g), thick and fibrous capsule, firm parenchyma, gray-red to dark red depending on parenchymal fibrosis, follicles indistinct: congestive splenomegaly

Other splenomegaly: infections, lymphoproliferative disorders, immunologic diseases, storage diseases, amyloidosis, neoplasms

Pale red, wedge-shaped lesions with fibrin on overlying capsule: acute ischemic infarcts

Pale yellow, wedge-shaped lesions becoming depressed scars: healing infarcts

Suppurative, soft, wedge-shaped infarcts: septic infarcts

### Lymph Nodes
Swollen, gray-red: acute lymphadenitis

Enlarged, gray-tan: chronic lymphadenitis

Enlarged, gray-white: lymphomas

### Bone Marrow
Pale (fatty) yellow: bone marrow failure from various causes (dose-related and idiosyncratic drug effects, radiation, viral infections, idiopathic, Fanconi anemia)

### Endocrine System

The pituitary (_____ g) *fills the sella turcica/other*. The thyroid gland is *symmetrical, red-brown, and firm/other*. The adrenal glands have *uniform yellow cortices/other* separated from the medullary *gray/other* by a thin, red line.

### Endocrine System
#### General Observations
Weigh (or measure) pituitary; inspect pituitary (shape, symmetry, color); inspect sella turcica; weigh thyroid; inspect thyroid (color, symmetry, consistency, external parenchyma, pyramidal lobe); identify parathyroids (confirm on microscopic examination); if enlarged, weigh accurately; weigh adrenal glands after removing investing fat; if friable, clean and weigh after fixation; inspect adrenals (color, shape, thickness and regularity of cortex and medulla)

#### Specific Findings
##### Pituitary
Soft, pale, and hemorrhagic (early) and fibrous atrophy (late): anterior lobe ischemic necrosis (Sheehan syndrome, disseminated intravascular necrosis, sickle cell anemia, increased intracranial pressure, trauma, shock)

Soft, well-circumscribed masses of anterior pituitary that when large compress the optic chiasm and adjacent structures and erode the sella turcica and clinoid processes: adenomas

Solid, encapsulated, or cystic and multiloculated masses arising in posterior pituitary (Rathke pouch remnants): craniopharyngioma

##### Thyroid
Diffusely enlarged, firm, pale, gray-tan, slightly nodular with intact capsule: Hashimoto thyroiditis

Unilaterally or diffusely enlarged, firm, yellow-white with intact capsule that may adhere to adjacent tissues: subacute (granulomatous, de Quervain) thyroiditis

Normal or slight symmetrical enlargement: subacute lymphocytic thyroiditis

Firm, white, hyalinized tissue with effacement of the lobules and involvement of adjacent neck tissues: fibrous (Riedel) thyroiditis

Symmetrical enlargement; smooth, soft, red parenchyma with intact capsule: Graves disease

Diffuse, symmetrical enlargement: hyperplastic stage of diffuse goiter

Enlarged, brown, translucent, glassy parenchyma: colloid involution stage of diffuse goiter

Asymmetrically enlarged, multilobulated parenchyma with variable amounts of brown gelatinous parenchyma, hemorrhage, calcification, and cysts: multinodular goiter

Solitary, spherical, encapsulated, gray-white to red-brown masses: adenomas

Solitary to multifocal granular masses varying from well-circumscribed or encapsulated to infiltrating: papillary carcinoma

Single, well-circumscribed or infiltrating, gray, tan, or pale red masses sometimes with translucent brown colloid, central scarring, or calcification: follicular carcinoma

Solitary or multiple, firm, gray-tan, unencapsulated masses with variable hemorrhage and necrosis in larger lesions: medullary carcinoma

Parathyroid

Enlargement of all four glands, though one or two may be spared: parathyroid hyperplasia

Single, soft, tan, encapsulated masses: parathyroid adenomas

Circumscribed or infiltrative gray-white, irregular masses: parathyroid carcinomas

Adrenals

Diffusely thickened, yellow cortex contributing to slight or marked bilateral enlargement: diffuse hyperplasia producing Cushing syndrome (hypercortisolism)

Yellow nodules (0.5 to 2.0 cm) scattered throughout cortex bilaterally: nodular hyperplasia producing Cushing syndrome

Small (generally solitary and <2 cm), bright yellow, encapsulated masses, more often on left than right, without overall gland enlargement: aldosterone-producing adenomas (Conn's syndrome)

Bilateral dark red parenchyma: massive bilateral adrenal hemorrhage (Waterhouse-Friderichsen syndrome)

Irregularly atrophied glands difficult to find within the suprarenal fat: primary autoimmune adrenalitis with chronic adrenocortical insufficiency (Addison disease)

Effacement of adrenal glands by caseous necrosis or tumor: tuberculous or fungal infection and metastatic carcinoma may also cause chronic adrenocortical insufficiency

Small, flattened atrophic adrenals with thickened capsule, very thin cortex, and normal medulla: secondary hypoadrenalism

Yellow to yellow-brown cortical masses, some with hemorrhage, cystic degeneration, and calcification: with adjacent cortex appearing normal, nonfunctioning adrenocortical adenomas; with atrophy of adjacent normal cortex, functioning adrenocortical adenomas

Large yellow masses with hemorrhagic, cystic, and necrotic regions: adrenocortical carcinomas

Yellow-tan to gray-pink masses with foci of hemorrhage, necrosis, and cystic degeneration in larger lesions: pheochromocytoma

## Musculoskeletal System

Cartilage is firm/other. The bone is hard/other. The vertebrae, ribs, pelvis, and long bones are intact without gross evidence of fracture or deformity/other. Skeletal muscles are red-brown, firm and appropriate mass for the decedent's age and sex/other.

## Musculoskeletal System
### General Observations

Inspect external configuration of skeleton; inspect bones and joints (deformities of bones, swellings or deformities of joints, hardness of bones, character of synovial surfaces; collect and characterize any joint effusions); in all cases of suggested bone disease, be sure to consider skeletal X-rays (consult with radiologist as required); sample bones that show radiologic evidence of disease as consent allows; inspect accessible skeletal muscles (color, symmetry, consistency)

*table continues*

## ADULT AUTOPSY DESCRIPTION OF GROSS FINDINGS *(continued)*

*Specific Findings*
Bones
   Softer than usual bones, vertebral compression fractures: osteoporosis
   Bulbous, misshapen, and brittle long bones: osteopetrosis
   Marked thickening and porosity of cut surface: Paget's disease
   Tumor masses filling bone medulla and invading cortex and adjacent soft tissues: may be osteogenic sarcoma, fibrosarcoma, chondrosarcoma
   Multiple destructive ("punched-out") lesions filled with soft red gelatinous tumor: multiple myeloma
   Soft, gray-white to pale yellow, rounded masses causing fusiform swelling: osteolytic metastasis
   Dense, hard tumor obliterating marrow spaces: osteoblastic metastasis
Joints
   Granular articular surfaces, softer than normal (early); ulceration of articular surfaces, fractures articulating bone, dislodgment of cartilage and loose bodies, progressive joint destruction with loculated synovial fluid collections (intermediate); fibrous walled cysts, osteophytes, bone eburnation (later): osteoarthritis
   Synovial swelling with soft, red villous tags (early); granulation tissue, subchondral cysts, osteoporosis (intermediate); cartilage erosions, pannus formation with fibrous adhesions, bony (late): rheumatoid arthritis
   White deposits in synovium: chronic tophaceous arthritis (gout)
   Blood within joint space (acute), synovial adhesions and yellow-brown discoloration (late): hemarthrosis: hemophilia, joint trauma
   Swollen joint containing pus within joint space, sometimes overlying cellulitis: suppurative arthritis
   Red-brown to orange-yellow proliferations or nodules: pigmented villonodular synovitis: giant cell tumor of tendon sheath
Muscles
   Soft, friable, and gray to liquefied, dark red with crepitus: gangrenous necrosis due to gas-forming organisms
   Soft, friable, swollen, gray or yellow-red muscle: dermatomyositis
   Soft, yellow-red mass, relatively well circumscribed, sometimes with hemorrhagic necrosis: rhabdomyosarcoma

### Head and Central Nervous System

Reflection of the scalp reveals *no evidence of subgaleal hemorrhage/other*. The underlying calvarium is *intact and normal in thickness/other*. The dura is *intact/other* and its inner surface *smooth and glistening/other*. The dural sinuses are *patent/other*. Cerebrospinal fluid is *clear/other*.

   The brain weighs _____ g. The leptomeninges are *thin and transparent with no vascular congestion, subarachnoid hemorrhage, or exudate/other*. The circle of Willis and other basal vasculature are *intact and normally formed/other*. The vessels are *patent and thin walled/other*. The cranial nerves are *intact and normally distributed/other*. The dorsal convexities of the brain are *symmetrical with a well-developed gyral pattern/other*. The brainstem and cerebellum show the *usual/other* external configuration. There is *no* localized external softening or contusion of the brain.

   There is *no displacement of the cingulate gyrus, medial temporal lobe, or cerebellar tonsils/other*.

### Head and Central Nervous System
*General Observations*
Initial Examination:
Inspect scalp, thickness of calvarium; note cerebrospinal fluid (characteristics, pressure if unusual); inspect dura of brain and spinal cord (thickness, color, transparency, calcification); examine epidural and subdural space; examine vascular sinuses; strip dura and examine base of skull; inspect leptomeninges (clarity, color, thickness, adhesions); examine cranial nerves; do preliminary examination of convolutions (flattening or narrowing of gyri, width of sulci, lesions); palpate brain gently for softening or tumor; inspect major fissures, falx cerebri, and tentorium; inspect cerebellum and brainstem, circle of pressure effects on cingulated gyrus, cerebellar tonsils, and brainstem; weigh fresh brain
Examination after Fixation:
Weigh fixed brain; reexamine cortical surface, gyri, sulci, and external aspects of cerebellum and brainstem; cut brain and spinal cord; examine cortex (uniform thickness, variation in

Multiple coronal sections of the cerebrum show an intact cortical ribbon of *appropriate thickness/other*. The internal architecture shows the *usual pattern/other without focal lesions or hemorrhage/other*. The ventricular system is of *appropriate configuration and size/other*. Transverse sections of the brainstem show *a well-pigmented substantia nigra and locus caeruleus/other*. The pons shows *well-defined pyramids and inferior olivary nuclei/other*. Sections of the cerebellum show *prominent inferior olivary nuclei/other*; the hemispheres show *the usual foliar pattern and appearance of the dentate nuclei/other*.

The spinal cord dura is *intact/other,* and its inner surface *smooth and shiny/other*. The spinal leptomeninges are *thin and translucent/other*. Anterior and posterior roots are comparable in size. Transverse sections of cord show *no abnormalities/other*. The cauda equina is *unremarkable/other*.

color, focal lesions); examine white matter (swelling, cysts, softening, vascular prominence); examine basal ganglia (symmetry, atrophy, cysts, softening); examine mamillary bodies (atrophy, petechiae); examine ventricles (symmetry, size, blunting, compression, ependymal surface, choroid plexus, aqueduct of Sylvius); examine cerebral peduncles (atrophy, swelling, softening, color of substantia nigra); examine cerebellum; examine pineal (size, cysts, calcifications); examine spinal cord gray matter (outline, lesions, cysts, softenings) and white matter (demyelination of tracts); examine spinal cord nerve roots, cauda equina, and filum terminale

### Specific Observations

Softer than usual brain with flattened gyri, narrowed sulci, and compressed ventricles: edema

Herniations

   Displacement of cingulate gyrus under the falx cerebri: subfalcine herniation

   Displacement of medial temporal lobe against the tentorium cerebelli: transtentorial (uncal) herniation

   Displacement of cerebellar tonsils through the foramen magnum: tonsillar herniation

   Expansion of ventricles: hydrocephalus

   Expansion of ventricles secondary to loss of brain parenchyma: hydrocephalus ex vacuo

Atrophy

   Variable amount of cortical atrophy most pronounced in frontal, temporal, and parietal lobes and hydrocephalus ex vacuo: Alzheimer's disease

   Asymmetrical atrophy of frontal and temporal lobes with sparing of the posterior superior temporal gyrus: Pick disease

   Atrophy of substantia nigra with uneven pigment loss: Parkinson disease

   Atrophy mainly of motor and premotor cortex and anterior parietal lobes: corticobasal degeneration

   Atrophy of caudate nucleus and putamen: striatonigral degeneration

   Atrophy of basis pontis: olivopontocerebellar atrophy

   Atrophy of caudate nucleus (marked), putamen, globus pallidus (secondarily), often frontal lobe, sometimes parietal lobe or entire cortex: Huntington chorea

   Extravasated blood with compression of adjacent structures: intraparenchymal hemorrhage

   Cavitary destruction with rim of brownish discoloration: old intraparenchymal hemorrhage

Nonhemorrhagic Infarcts

   12 to 24 hours: soft, pale

   24 to 48 hours: swollen, darker with indistinct junction between gray and white matter

   2 to 10 days: area yellows, boundaries become definite, generally triangular or wedge-shaped; progressive breakdown of tissue into gelatinous center and friable periphery

   10 days to 3 weeks: liquefied tissue reverting to cavity lined by dark gray tissue

   3 weeks to months: formation of irregular cavity containing clear, pale yellow fluid

Hemorrhagic Infarcts

   Immediate: confluent, wedge-shaped, either diffusely red or red at the periphery with pale center interspersed with petechial hemorrhages

*table continues*

## ADULT AUTOPSY DESCRIPTION OF GROSS FINDINGS *(continued)*

Evolution: similar to nonhemorrhagic infarcts except that there is resorption of hemorrhage and hemosiderin formation, which yield yellow-brown discoloration of cystic fluid and peripheral walls

Linear areas of cortical necrosis: laminar and pseudolamellar necrosis due to global transient ischemia

Wedge-shaped infarcts, sickle-shaped band of necrosis over cerebral convexity just lateral to the interhemispheric fissure: border zone (watershed) infarcts

Small (<15 mm) spaces in lenticular nucleus, thalamus, internal capsule, deep white matter, caudate nucleus, and pons: lacunar infarcts

Tangled vascular channels extending into brain from subarachnoid space or entirely within the brain: arteriovenous malformations

Distended, poorly organized vascular channels often associated with foci of previous hemorrhage, calcification, or even infarction: cavernous hemangioma

Cloudy or purulent cerebrospinal fluid, exudates on leptomeninges, engorged meningeal blood vessels: acute meningitis

Discrete liquefactive lesions with surrounding fibrous response and edema, most commonly in frontal lobe, parietal lobe, and cerebellum: brain abscess

Gelatinous or fibrinous exudates, sometimes with white granules on leptomeninges: chronic tuberculous meningoencephalitis

Well-circumscribed mass with central caseous necrosis, calcification in old lesions: tuberculoma

Necrotizing and hemorrhagic lesions of the inferior and medial temporal lobe and orbital gyri of frontal lobes: may be herpes simplex virus type 1 encephalitis

Irregular, ill-defined white matter lesions of the cerebrum, brainstem, cerebellum, and spinal cord: progressive multifocal leukoencephalopathy

Opacity and thickening of the basal leptomeninges with hydrocephalus and gelatinous material within the subarachnoid space and small cysts within the parenchyma, especially the basal ganglia in the distribution of the lenticulostriate arteries: cryptococcal infection

Septic vascular thrombosis with abscesses: fungi, especially *Mucor* and *Aspergillus* species

Multiple cortical abscesses near gray-white junction and deep gray nuclei: toxoplasmosis

Multiple, well-demarcated areas in the centrum semiovale, peduncles, pons, midbrain, spinal cord, and optic nerves; soft and translucent or slightly pink when recent; gray-tan, glassy, firm, and slightly depressed when older: multiple sclerosis

Grayish discoloration around white matter vessels: acute disseminated encephalomyelitis

Grayish discoloration around white matter vessels with necrosis and acute hemorrhage of gray and white matter: acute necrotizing hemorrhagic encephalomyelitis

Wedge- or diamond-shaped cystic zone in center region of basis pontis: central pontine myelinolysis

Hemorrhage and necrosis in mamillary bodies, adjacent to third and fourth ventricles: Wernicke's encephalopathy

Thin anterior roots of spinal cord: amyotrophic lateral sclerosis

Poorly defined, infiltrative gray masses, variable color and consistency, variable tissue necrosis, cystic degeneration, and hemorrhage: diffuse astrocytoma and glioblastoma multiforme

Well-circumscribed, soft, gray to gray-pink gelatinous tumor that may have areas of hemorrhage, foci of calcification, and cysts: oligodendroglioma

Solid or papillary masses, variable color and consistency, most often arising near ventricles: ependymomas

Well-defined masses often at junction of gray and white matter: metastatic neoplasms

Somewhat defined, often multiple gray-white masses with central necrosis: may be lymphoma

## PEDIATRIC AUTOPSY DESCRIPTION OF GROSS FINDINGS

### External Examination

For fetuses: The body (_____ cm; normal, _____ cm; _____ g; normal g) is that of a *well-developed/other, nonmacerated/macerated male/female* fetus.

For infants/children: The body (_____ cm; normal, _____ cm; _____ kg; normal, _____ kg) is that of *well-nourished/poorly nourished/cachectic, well-developed/other mature/premature/postmature boy/girl* infant/child.

Skin color is *white/tan/yellow/brown*. The skin shows *no irregularity/other*. (For fetuses/infants: The head is *normocephalic/dolichocephalic/asymmetrical/brachycephalic/other*. The anterior fontanel is *open and measures _____ cm/closed*. The posterior fontanel is *open and measures _____ cm/closed*. The fontanels are *flat/depressed/bulging*.) (For child: The head is *symmetrical/other*.) The face is *normal, features present and symmetrical/other*. The irides are *(color)*, and the pupils are *equal/unequal*. The conjunctivae appear *pink/abnormal*, and the sclerae are *clear/icteric/blue*. Ear positions are *normal/low set*. The shape of the ears is *normal/other*. (For fetus/infant: Their development is *mature/immature*.) The external auditory canals are *patent/imperforate on right/imperforate on left*. The choanae are *patent/imperforate on right/imperforate on left*. The configuration of the mouth appears *normal/other*. The chin is *well developed/small*. The palate is *normal/high and arched but complete/incomplete*. The neck is *normal/stiff/other*. The trachea is *straight and in the midline/deviated to the right/deviated to the left*.

The thorax is *symmetrical/asymmetrical, being larger on right/asymmetrical, being larger on left*. The nipples are *appropriately spaced/widely spaced*. (For female child: Breast development is *absent/Tanner stage 1/2/3/4/5*.) The abdomen appears *flat/distended* and is *palpably soft/other*. The liver edge is *not palpable/palpable* below the right costal margin. The spleen tip is *not palpable/palpable* below the left costal margin. (For fetus and neonate: The umbilicus *contains a stump of umbilical cord showing three vessels/contains a stump of umbilical cord showing two vessels/other*.) The external genitalia are *normal/other* for a *boy/girl*. The urinary meatus is *patent/nonpatent/other*. The rectum and anus are *patent/nonpatent*. The spine appears *straight/scoliotic/kyphotic/lordotic* and *complete/other*. The extremities are *symmetrical and well developed/other*. The digits and palmar markings appear *normal/other*. (For child: There *is no/is* palpable cervical, axillary, or inguinal lymphadenopathy.) (For fetus/infant: The following additional measurements are made: crown-rump, _____ cm; head circumference, _____ cm; outer canthal distance, _____ cm; inner canthal distance, _____ cm; palpebral fissure length, _____ cm; philtral length, _____ cm; chest circumference, _____ cm; abdominal circumference, _____ cm; foot length, _____ cm.)

### Body as a Whole
#### General Observations

Give general measurements (weight/length)

Give impression on nutrition, development

For stillborn fetuses, describe degree of maceration

Mild: tone flabby, fluid accumulates beneath epidermis, red-brown discolaration of umbilical stump (6 hours); desquamation $\geq$1 cm (6 hours); desquamation in a few areas (12 hours), desquamation $\geq$25% of body or two more body areas (18 hours)

Moderate: skin red-brown color (24 hours), desquamation >50% (48 hours), >75% (72 hours), sclera red and globes soft, joints loose; cranial bones loose and overlapping (4 to 5 days)

Severe: widely open mouth (1 week); mummification (2 weeks)

#### Specific Findings

Weight <10th percentile for gestational age: small for gestational age

Weight >90th percentile for gestational age: large for gestational age

### Skin
#### General Observations

Elasticity and turgor, color (note if cyanosis is localized—state if it involves nail beds, lips, head only, one limb, and so forth; icterus—state if slight, marked), localized edema (indicate site, state if dependent areas, dorsum of feet in premature infants), generalized edema (state if moderate, severe), pigmentation, nails (state if cyanotic, yellow, malformed), dermatoses (include all types of rashes), tumors (including hemangiomas), hemorrhages (describe: focal, patchy, diffuse, area of discoloration), wounds/scars (describe in detail), describe needle puncture marks in detail—may be a clue to bloody effusions in body cavities

#### Specific Findings

Loose skin that wrinkles when pushed with finger: sign of weight loss

Cyanosis of head only: may indicate umbilical cord around neck

Yellow or discolored skin that does not rub off: may be old meconium staining

Edema in subcutaneous tissues, umbilical cord, placenta with fluid in body cavities (fetuses and neonates): hydrops fetalis (numerous causes)

Edema of fetal scalp during labor: caput succedaneum

Irregular, round to oval, light brown macules: café au lait spots (six or more lesions >1.5 cm suggests neurofibromatosis type 1)

Gray-blue area over sacrum in Asian and dark-skinned children: Mongolian spot (do not confuse with contusion)

*table continues*

## PEDIATRIC AUTOPSY DESCRIPTION OF GROSS FINDINGS (continued)

*Scars and Identifying Marks*
Describe scars and identifying marks.

*Evidence of Therapeutic Intervention*
The following medical paraphernalia are in place: (Describe intravenous or intraarterial lines, Foley catheters, endotracheal tubes, recent surgical incisions, and so forth.)

*Evidence of External Trauma*
See Trauma Template, later.
Note: Specific observations described in the adult autopsy section are not necessarily repeated here.

Flat and smooth to nodular and rough, dark brown to black lesions with variable amount of hair: giant pigmented nevi

Bullae: may be inherited epidermolysis bullosa (multiple types described), infections, other

Vesicular bullous or vesicular pustular lesions: erythema multiforme, infections (staphylococcal scalded skin syndrome, impetigo, other), acne vulgaris, histiocytosis, others

Vesicular lesions: varicella, herpes zoster

Thick, fissured skin; scaling; desquamation: desquamative erythroderma (Leiner disease), seborrheic dermatitis, ichthyosis syndromes ("collodion babies," "harlequin fetus," others)

Maculopapular eruptions, desquamation of palms, soles, rhagades (linear scars at angles of nose, mouth, and inner angles of eyes): congenital syphilis

Single or multiple, sharply demarcated flat areas of nonpitting, woody induration developing on back, cheeks, arms, thighs, buttocks, calves, and shoulders of infants days to a few weeks after delivery: subcutaneous fat necrosis (from birth trauma)

Widespread smooth, hard, dry, cool, waxy induration of skin (except palms, soles, and scrotum) developing in premature infants several days to 3 to 4 weeks after birth: sclerema neonatorum (do not confuse with hardening of subcutaneous fat after refrigeration)

Swollen, doughy, pitting induration in premature or term infants: scleredema

Thick ridges and irregular depressions or convolutions, most commonly on vertex of skull: gyrate skin

Strands connecting fetus and amnion: amniotic bands

Flat, irregular, red-purple lesions: capillary hemangiomas, port-wine stain

Raised or verrucous, red-purple lesions: cavernous hemangiomas

### Head and Neck
*General Observations*
Head size and shape (molding, macrocephaly, microcephaly), fontanels (open, closed, depressed, bulging), facial anomalies, eyelids, orbit, eyes (size, symmetry of pupils; color; cornea; lens; size of globes, coloboma), ears (patency of auditory canals, shape, position of external ears), nares (patency), choana (patency, atresia), mouth (contents, gingiva), teeth (present or absent, condition), tongue (size, coating), palate (anomalies), neck (shape, length, position of trachea and thyroid, midline or lateral sinuses, masses)

*Specific Findings*
Fusion of cranial sutures: craniosynostosis (associated with >50 syndromes)

Coronal suture fusion: brachycephaly (wide, basally short skull)

Sagittal suture fusion: dolichocephaly (elongated skull)

Unilateral coronal or lambdoidal suture fusion: plagiocephaly (twisted skull)

Coronal and sagittal suture fusion: turricephaly (towerlike skull)

Fusion of all sutures: acrocephaly or oxycephaly (tall, pointed skull)

Microphthalmia (small globe and orbital ridge); anophthalmia (absent eye—may be dimple at normal site of globe)

Hypotelorism (eyes spaced too closely); hypertelorism (eyes too wide set)

Ear malformations (major—abnormal outer helix, antihelix or tragus; minor—ear pits, preauricular tags, helical clefts, folds or hypoplasia). External ear malformations should initiate evaluation for other anomalies

Microtia: small ears (Treacher-Collins syndrome)

Cleft lip: generally paramedian following ridge at either side of philtrum (may be isolated anomaly or component of numerous malformation syndromes); midline clefts are rare and generally seen in malformation syndromes

Cleft palate: may be extension of cleft lip; midline cleft hard palate is more severe manifestation of high arched palate

Micrognathia (mandibular underdevelopment) leading to microstomia (small mouth): may be genetic (e.g., DiGeorge syndrome, otocephaly) or acquired due to abnormalities that restrict swallowing (e.g., prolonged oligohydramnios)

Characteristic head and facial anomalies associated with various syndromes and anomalies (some examples):

Microcephaly, sloping forehead, microphthalmos, iris coloboma, low-set dysplastic ears, cleft lip/palate, posterior scalp lesions, capillary hemangioma on forehead: trisomy 13

Prominent occiput, narrow bifrontal diameter, short palpebral fissures, low-set dysplastic ears, small mouth, short upper lip, micrognathia: trisomy 18

Brachycephaly, flat face, protruding tongue, epicanthal folds, small low-set ears, fissured tongue, ears with overlapping helix, prominent antihelix, and small ear lobes: trisomy 21

Cranial bone anomalies, iris coloboma, hypertelorism, microphthalmia, low-set malformed ears, micrognathia: triploidy

Heart-shaped face, epicanthal folds, prominent ears, depressed corners of mouth, micrognathia, redundant skin of posterior neck, low posterior hairline: Turner syndrome

Broad forehead, hypertelorism, epicanthal folds, downward palpebral slant, flat nasal bridge, short neck, pterygium colli: Noonan's syndrome

Microcephaly, short palpebral fissures, epicanthal folds, posterior rotation of ears, short upturned nose, hypoplastic philtrum, retrognathia: fetal alcohol syndrome

Facial asymmetry, downward slant of palpebral fissures, coloboma of outer portion of lower eyelids, deformed dysplastic ears, ear tags, large-appearing nose with narrow nares, micrognathia: Treacher Collins syndrome

Skin fold from inner canthus to upper cheek, blunt nose, creased chin, large low-set ears with posterior rotation, wrinkled facial skin: Potter facies due to oligohydramnios

Webbing or redundant skin folds of neck: Turner syndrome, Klippel-Feil syndrome, Meckel-Gruber syndrome

Enlargement of subcutaneous tissue of anterior or posterior neck compartments by soft, fluid-filled cystic spaces: cystic hygroma

## Chest

### General Observations

Inspect chest symmetry and shape (narrow, short, shield-shaped, pectus deformities); palpate bony thorax (trauma, rib spacing); inspect breasts (development, shape, masses); inspect nipples (size, spacing, discharge); palpate axilla for lymphadenopathy

### Specific Findings

Abnormal shape of thorax

Broad, overexpanded thorax: eventration of the diaphragm

Narrow thorax: thanatophoric dwarfism, achondrogenesis syndromes, homozygous achondroplasia, short-rib polydactyly syndrome, camptomelic syndrome, chondroectodermal dysplasia (Ellis–van Creveld syndrome), asphyxiating thoracic dystrophy (Jeune's syndrome), abnormality affecting the cervical spinal cord

Breast development (sexual maturity [Tanner stage][1])

*table continues*

## PEDIATRIC AUTOPSY DESCRIPTION OF GROSS FINDINGS *(continued)*

1: Preadolescent

2: Breast and papilla elevated as small mounds, areolar diameter increased

3: Breast and areola enlarged; no contour separation

4: Areola and papilla form secondary mound

5: Mature, nipple projects, areola part of general breast contour

Small, widely spaced nipples: Turner's syndrome

### Abdomen
#### General Observations
Contour, discoloration, distension, organomegaly (liver, spleen), masses, umbilicus (for fetus: patency of umbilical veins; for neonates: umbilical cord stump)

#### Specific Findings
Thick ridges and irregular depressions or convolutions involving abdomen, associated with absence or hypoplasia of anterior abdominal muscle, megalocystis, and megaloureter: prune-belly syndrome

Defect in abdominal wall covered by translucent membrane of amnion and peritoneum with umbilical cord arising from dome: omphalocele

Paraumbilical (usually to the right) defect of anterior abdominal wall with eviscerated loops of bowel: gastroschisis

Fistula between urinary bladder and umbilicus: patent urachus

Variably sized defect in abdominal wall below umbilicus communicating with urinary bladder: bladder exstrophy

### External Genitalia
#### General Observations
Development, pubic hair, edema, lesions, trauma, circumcision; palpate scrotum for testes, masses; inspect introitus; vaginal speculum examination for sexual trauma/specimen collection; describe abnormalities in sex differentiation in detail; inspect penis, clitoris (size, shape); identify urethral meatus (location); palpate scrotum for testes, masses; inspect introitus

Determination of gender based on external genitalia before about 20 weeks may be unreliable; normal male genitalia show labioscrotal fusion; normal femal genitalia have probe patent vaginal canal between labial folds; ambiguous genitalia show partial development or overlapping features

#### Specific Findings
Urethra opens on upper surface of penis in males; in females, distal urethra is variably deficient and clitoris is duplicated: epispadias (usually associated with bladder exstrophy)

Urethra opens on underside of penis or through perineum: hypospadias

Absence of external genitalia: seen in sirenomelia

Clitoromegaly seen in viriizing conditions, such as congenital adrenal hyperplasia

### Back
#### General Observations
Inspect anus (position, patency); anus may be located anterior or posterior to external sphincter; if gross variation is present, measure distance from anus to vulva or scrotum; if imperforate, check carefully for fistula; define type of atresia; inspect/palpate back (symmetry, deformities)

#### Specific Findings
Curvature of spinal column: kyphosis, lordosis, scoliosis (radiography suggested)

Pigmented area, tuft of hair, dimple, fistula: spina bifida occulta

Skin or membranous tissue separating perineum from internal structures: imperforate anus (internal examination required to classify anorectal and cloacal anomalies)

Solid cystic mass attached to sacrum, coccyx, or soft tissues of the pelvis: sacrococcygeal teratoma

## Extremities

### General Observations

Inspect upper and lower extremities (development, position, deformities, length); inspect hands and fingers (position, length, abnormalities, palmar creases, fingernails); inspect feet and toes; check deformities of articulations, bones, and muscles (radiographs may be useful)

Hypoplastic muscles in amyoplasia (arthrogryposis) and spinal cord anomalies are easily overlooked; in testing mobility of joints, avoid errors due to rigor or refrigeration; palpate inguinal region for lymphadenopathy

### Specific Findings

Joint contractures or decreased range of motion: occurs in many congenital malformation syndromes but also occurs as secondary effect of neuromuscular disorders or oligohydramnios

Short limb skeletal dysplasia

Rhizomeli/meromelic: proximal segment (humerus, femur)

Mesomelic: middle segment (radius/ulna, tibia/fibula)

Acromelic (distal to trunk): hands/feet

Lethal short-limb chondrodysplasias: thanatophoric dwarfism, achondrogenesis syndromes, homozygous achondroplasia, short-rib polydactyly syndrome, camptomelic syndrome, chondroectodermal dysplasia, asphyxiating thoracic dystrophy

Phocomelia: attenuated limb

Amelia: absent extremity

Longitudinal ray hypoplasia or aplasia: hypoplastic and missing long bones

Transverse ray defect: truncated extremity perpendular to long axis

Enlargement of ends of long bones, bowed legs: rickets

Fingers/toes

Polydactyly (extra digits): range from polypoid skin tags to true extra digits

Brachydactyly (short digits): usually hypoplastic or absent phalanges

Clinodactyly (medial bending): usually fifth digit of hand

Ectrodactyly ("lobster claw") absence of central digit(s) with metatarsal clefting

Syndactyly (fusion of soft tissues between digits): may be partial or complete

Hypoplasia or aplasia (small or absent digits): longitudinal ray defects and not amputations due to amniotic bands

Feet

Equinovarus (clubbed feet or lateral dislocation of lower leg over the foot due to prolonged intrauterine mechanical stress): compare position of leg relative to foot because all fetuses and infants have some degree of medial/plantar flexion

Rocker bottom feet (prominent calcaneus and convex sole—subjective and often over called): trisomy 18; triploidy

Sandal gap (wide gap between first and second toes with base of gap "squared"): may indicate trisomy 21

## Scars and Identifying Marks

Describe characteristics of scars (site, healing, surgical, traumatic); measure scars; describe identifying marks such as tattoos, body piercings

*table continues*

## PEDIATRIC AUTOPSY DESCRIPTION OF GROSS FINDINGS (continued)

### Thoracic Cavity

The thymus (_____ g; normal, _____ g) occupies its *usual position/is not identifiable grossly*. (For infant/child: The parenchyma is *pale gray and lobulated/other*.) The parietal pleural surfaces are *glistening and smooth/other*. The right hemithorax contains *(amount and type of fluid)*; the left contains *(amount and type of fluid)*. The lungs appear to occupy a *normal/small* volume in the thoracic cavity. The mediastinum is *unremarkable/other*. The pericardial sac contains *(amount and type of fluid)*. Its surfaces are *smooth and glistening/other*. The heart is located in its *usual anatomic position in the midline (fetus/neonate)/in its usual position in the left chest (older infant/child)/in the right chest* with its apex pointing to the *left/right*. (For infant/child: Hilar and mediastinal lymph nodes are *small and gray*.)

### Evidence of Therapeutic Intervention

Inspect for evidence of recent medical therapy; describe needle puncture marks in reasonable detail (may be a clue to blood effusions in body cavities); describe remote wounds/scars; note endotracheal tube, nasogastric tube, indwelling peripheral and central intravascular catheters, urethral catheters, feeding tubes; do not remove devices until proper placement is ascertained

### Thoracic Cavity
#### General Observations

Inspect ribs, sternum for trauma, abnormalities; prior to cutting anterior ribs, note height (expressed as rib or intercostal space number) of each hemidiaphragm and check for pneumothorax (see Chapter 6); inspect mediastinum for displacement, blood; identify and inspect thymus (size); remove and weigh thymus; carefully search for thymic tissue, if thymus is not obvious—it may weigh less than 1 g in cases of thymic dysplasia; if not present or hypoplastic, look for parathyroids; inspect mediastinum (emphysema, masses); inspect great arteries (does pulmonary root cross anterior to aortic root or are the arteries "untwisted"—more parallel than usual?); inspect superior caval vein (dilation, dilated tributaries) and inferior caval vein (appropriately connected to right-sided atrium); make diagram or photograph of any vascular anomalies found (see also Cardiovascular System, later); inspect pericardial sac for size, type, and character of fluid, fibrin, adhesions; inspect pleural cavities for type, character of fluid; inspect pleura (dullness, fibrin, type and location of adhesions, other lesions); inspect esophagus, thoracic duct (if indicated); inspect mediastinal and hilar lymph nodes

#### Specific Findings

Absence of thymus: DiGeorge syndrome; associated with absence of parathyroids and cardiovascular anomalies of aortic arch and conotruncal region

Small thymus: stress reaction, immunodeficiency syndromes (lymph nodes may be absent or abnormal histologically)

Petechial hemorrhages of thymic cortex: acute anoxic death

Defects of the diaphragm with herniation of abdominal contents into pleural cavity (usually the left, through foramen of Bochdalek) retrosternally or, rarely, bilaterally: congenital diaphragmatic hernia (associated with hypoplasia of the lung on the affected side and sometimes mediastinal shift and hypoplasia of the contralateral lung)

Hemidiaphragm lacks muscle, consisting only of thin membrane that herniates into thoracic cavity: eventration of the diaphragm

Absence of pericardium: may be total or partial

Cysts or diverticula of pericardium: most common at cardiophrenic angle

Situs of Heart
  Normal heart with left atrium on left side: situs solitus
  Heart with morphologically left atrium on right side and morphologically right atrium on left side: situs inversus
  Heart with bilateral morphologically right atria: situs ambiguous with dextroisomerism
  Heart with bilateral morphologically left atria: situs ambiguous with levoisomerism

## Cardiovascular System

On examining the external surfaces of the heart (_____ g; normal, _____ g), the atrial appendages are *in their normal positions/ other*. The great vessels are *normally related/other*. The epicardial surface is *glistening and smooth/other*. The coronary arteries *course in the usual fashion/other* over the surface of the heart. The superior and inferior venae cavae and coronary sinus connect with the right atrium in the *usual fashion/other*. The diameter of the coronary sinus is *normal/large/small*. The interatrial septum is *intact with/without a patent oval foramen/has an atrial septal defect*. The right atrioventricular connection is *present, and the leaflets of the tricuspid valve are thin and delicate/other*. The right ventricular cavity is *normal in size/dilated*. The wall is of *normal thickness/other,* and its myocardium has *a homogeneous red color/other*. The interventricular septum is *intact/has a perimembranous ventricular septal defect/has a muscular ventricular septal defect*. The right ventricular outflow tract is *unremarkable/ narrowed*. The pulmonary valve contains *three thin and delicate semilunar leaflets/other*. The pulmonary artery is of *normal caliber and configuration/other*. Its intimal surface is *glistening and smooth/other*. The ductus arteriosus is *patent/ stenotic/closed*. Four pulmonary veins connect with the left atrium *in the usual manner/other*. The chamber size is *normal/ large/small*. The left atrioventricular connection is *normal with thin and delicate mitral valve leaflets/other*. The tendinous cords appear *normal/thickened and fused/abnormally long and thin*. The left ventricular cavity is *of normal size/dilated*. The wall is of *normal thickness/hypertrophied/other,* and its myocardium has *a homogeneous red color/other*. The left ventricular outflow tract *appears normal/appears stenotic/ shows the ventricular defect just inferior to the aortic valve*. The aortic valve contains *three thin and delicate semilunar leaflets/ other*. The ascending aorta is *of normal caliber/small/dilated* and arches over the *left main bronchus/right main bronchus* before descending along the *left/right* side of the vertebral column. The major arteries come off the aorta in the *usual configuration/other*. The descending aorta *gives off the usual branches/other,* and its intimal surface is *glistening, smooth, and intact/other*.

## Situs of Lungs

Lobation is not accurate determinant

Morphologically right lung: eparterial bronchus

Morphologically left lung: hyparterial bronchus

In situs ambiguous there are bilateral morphologically right or left lungs

## Cardiovascular System
### General Observations

Inspect heart in situ (location, size, shape, situs, distribution of coronary arteries over surface of heart); inspect great vessels, relationship of great vessels, superior and inferior vena in situ (anomalous great vessels; e.g., a right subclavian vein taking off distally on the arch is easily recognized if all great vessels are examined in the neck before removal of thoracic organs); inspect pulmonary venous return (two veins from each lung should connect with the left atrium); look for vascular rings; keep heart attached to other thoracic organs until dissection is completed; in cases of malformations of great vessels or cardiac defects, the heart and lungs should be left en bloc permanently; inspect dissected heart (chambers, atrioventricular connections, septal walls, valves, myocardium); measure thickness of ventricles (midway between apex and atrioventricular junction, excluding trabeculae carneae); if measuring valves, always record greatest circumference; check aorta and inferior vena cava and their branches for thrombi or emboli, laceration, compression, fatty streaks, atherosclerosis; inspect arterial duct (examine for patency before opening); examine coronary arteries (anomalous takeoff, fatty streaks, atherosclerosis); inspect umbilical vessels (patency, look for intimal injury if catheterizations performed); weigh heart (or heart and lungs combined)

### Specific Observations

The following relationships in fetuses and neonates are normal

Fossa ovalis diameter:inferior vena cava diameter = 1

Ductus arteriosus circumference:largest neck vessel circumference = 1.20

Aortic isthmus circumference:aortic valve circumference = 0.6

Left innominate vein does not cross the midline to the superior vena cava but rather joins a left vertical vein that typically empties into coronary sinus: persistent left superior vena cava

Defects of Atrial Septum

Adjacent to the atrioventricular valve: primum atrial septal defect

Due to deficient fossa ovalis: secundum atrial septal defect

Near entrance of superior vena cava: sinus venosus atrial septal defect

Defects of Ventricular Septum

Defect in membranous portion of ventricular septum: membranous ventricular septal defect

Defect inferior to pulmonary valve: infundibular ventricular defect

Defects within muscular septum: muscular ventricular septal defects

Atrioventricular Septal Defects

Primum atrial septal defect associated with cleft in the anterior mitral valve leaflet: partial atrioventricular septal defect

Combined primum atrial septal and ventricular septal defects with common atrioventricular valve: complete atrioventricular septal defect (common atrioventricular canal)

*table continues*

## PEDIATRIC AUTOPSY DESCRIPTION OF GROSS FINDINGS *(continued)*

### Other Congenital Heart Defects

Aorta located anteriorly and arising from right ventricle, pulmonary artery located posteriorly and arising from left ventricle: D-transposition of the great arteries

Aorta located anteriorly and arising from a right-sided but morphologic left ventricle, pulmonary artery located posteriorly arising from a left-sided but morphologic right ventricle: L-transposition of the great arteries

Aorta and pulmonary artery are side by side and arise primarily from the right ventricle, generally with an associated ventricular septal defect: double-outlet right ventricle

Double-inlet ventricles with single ventricle or dominant ventricle and rudimentary outlet chambers: univentricular heart (single ventricle, double-inlet left ventricle, double-inlet right ventricle)

Single great artery receiving blood from both ventricles with ventricular septal defect: truncus arteriosus

Complete occlusion of tricuspid or mitral valve, generally with associated hypoplasia of the associated ventricle: tricuspid or mitral valve atresia

Inferior displacement of the free portions of the tricuspid valve leaflets into the right ventricle: Ebstein's malformation

Narrowing or complete obstruction of pulmonary valve: pulmonary stenosis/atresia; may be associated with ventricular septal defect and overriding aorta (tetralogy of Fallot) or transposition of the great arteries

Pulmonary veins not connected to left atrium: anomalous pulmonary venous return (connection)

Narrowing or complete obstruction of aortic valve: aortic stenosis/atresia; if severe, leads to hypoplasia of left ventricle and ascending aorta (hypoplastic left heart syndrome)

Hypoplasia and tubular narrowing of aortic arch proximal to a patent ductus arteriosus: coarctation of aorta, infantile type

Infolding of aorta opposite closed ductus arteriosus: coarctation of aorta, adult type

Mottled, flabby myocardium: myocarditis (freeze piece of myocardium)

### Respiratory System

The larynx is *unremarkable/other*. The trachea is of *normal/other* caliber and courses in the *usual/other* fashion. The lungs (right, _____ g; left, _____ g; normal combined weight, _____ g) *contain the usual lobes and fissures/show abnormal lobation*, and the visceral pleural surfaces are *glistening and smooth/other*. The parenchyma is *soft and pale red/other*. The bronchi and vessels appear patent and of *normal caliber/other*.

### Respiratory System

#### General Observations

Inspect larynx and trachea (location, size, shape, luminal contents, mucosa)—the opened larynx and trachea may reveal iatrogenic lesions from intubation; most noniatrogenic lesions are supraglottic (hemangioma, lymphangioma); weigh lungs; for fetus and infant, leave thyroid on the trachea, but look for masses and other pathologic changes by sectioning each lobe; inspect lungs for anomalies, including lobation (complete, incomplete, abnormal, though this is difficult to determine at early gestation); inspect visceral pleural surfaces; palpate lung parenchyma for consistency, crepitation; examine bronchi, vessels, parenchyma, lymphatics (prominent, air-filled), lymph nodes

#### Specific Findings

Soft laryngeal cartilages, excess folding of epiglottis, short aryepiglottic folds: laryngomalacia

Flaccid and elongated epiglottis and narrow larynx: cri du chat syndrome

Laryngeal webs: supraglottic, glottic, subglottic

Atresia of larynx: may be subglottic, infraglottic, or glottic

Papillary masses of larynx and/or trachea: laryngotracheal papillomatosis associated with human papilloma virus type 6

Fistulas between trachea and esophagus with or without esophageal atresia: tracheoesophageal atresia; may be associated with other malformations (VACTERL or CHARGE associations, DiGeorge sequence, trisomy 21, trisomy 18, others)

Bronchiectasis: congenital bronchiectasis (Williams-Campbell syndrome, cystic fibrosis, ciliary dyskinesia, Kartagener's syndrome, immunodeficiency diseases, yellow nail syndrome, postinfection)

Markedly distended lobe (usually upper) with compression of ipsilateral lung, mediastinal shift, and atelectasis of contralateral lung: congenital or infantile lobar overinflation

Hypoplasia of lungs: decreased intrathoracic space (abnormalities of thoracic cage or diaphragm, severe polyhydramnios resulting in pleural effusions), obstructive lesions of the respiratory tract, pulmonary vascular anomalies, urinary system anomalies and other anomalies causing oligohydramnios, central nervous system anomalies (anencephaly, iniencephaly), congenital neurologic or neuromuscular disorders

Solid, airless, dark red to purple, heavy lungs: neonatal respiratory distress syndrome (hyaline membrane disease)

Firm, solid parenchyma with irregular pleural surfaces: bronchopulmonary dysplasia

Cleftlike subpleural spaces or blebs: pulmonary interstitial emphysema

Generally solitary cyst near hilum of lung or elsewhere in mediastinum: may be bronchogenic cyst

Mixed cystic and solid masses with variable sizes: congenital cystic adenomatoid malformation

Chylous pleural effusions, firm hypoplastic lungs with irregular bosselated surfaces, dilated subpleural lymphatics: congenital pulmonary lymphangiectasis

Abnormal pulmonary tissue without normal tracheobronchial tree communications and anomalous systemic artery supply: bronchopulmonary sequestration (intralobar and extralobar types)

## Peritoneal Cavity

The peritoneal surfaces are *glistening and intact/other*. There is *(amount and character of peritoneal fluid)*. There *is no/is* mesenteric or periaortic lymphadenopathy.

## Peritoneal Cavity

### General Observations

Confirm normal development of abdominal muscles; measure subcutaneous fat in obese children; inspect peritoneal membranes (thickness, exudates); position/relationship of viscera; position, thickness, color of omentum; adhesions; fluid (indicate if estimated rather than measured); amount/color of subcutaneous fat; lesser peritoneal cavity; bladder distension; collect urine if indicated; identify position, mobility of appendix; inspect mesentery, if abnormal measure (measure length of mesentery from ligament of Treitz to ileocecal valve; measure radius of mesentery from midline of root to mesenteric attachment); in young male fetus, locate testes in abdominal cavity or inguinal canal; inspect abdominal lymph nodes

### Specific Findings

Situs of Abdominal Organs

Reversal of normal sidedness: situs inversus

Central liver and absent spleen: generally associated with situs ambiguous of right lung type

*table continues*

## PEDIATRIC AUTOPSY DESCRIPTION OF GROSS FINDINGS *(continued)*

Central liver and polysplenia: situs ambiguous of bilateral left lung type

Malrotation: may be complete or incomplete; incomplete rotation is associated with unfixed mesentery and volvulus

Very short mesenteric root: usually common mesentery

If spleen is long and narrow and reaches pelvis: may be splenogonadal fusion

### Liver and Biliary System

The liver (_____ g; normal _____ g) is normally positioned in the *upper right/other,* the stomach on the left midline and symmetrical in the *left upper quadrant/other.* The shape of the liver is *normal/other*; its surface is smooth and *glistening/other.* Cut sections show *normal/congested/other* parenchyma. On the inferior aspect, the vascular pattern is *normal/other.*

The gallbladder is *present/absent.* The biliary tree is patent into the *duodenum/other.*

### Liver and Biliary System
#### General Observations

Liver weight (weigh immediately on removal to avoid excessive loss of blood); inspect liver (location, size, shape); inspect capsule (tears, hematomas), portal vein (presence, patency), ductus venosus (probe patency of portal end, measure maximal circumference); inspect gallbladder (location, size, shape); check patency of cystic and common bile ducts by pressing on gallbladder and expressing bile through the ampulla of Vater

Liver on left side with left lobe larger than right: situs inversus

Two-tone liver: difference in the colors of the right and left lobes due to congestion from incomplete diaphragm in diaphragmatic hernia, also associated with parenchymal groove

Enlargement of fetal liver: terminal anoxic congestion, erythroblastosis fetalis, congenital infections (cytomegalovirus, rubella, syphilis), rarely inborn errors of metabolism

Enlargement of liver of infant or child: may be inborn error of metabolism

Fatty liver: perinatal anoxia, inborn errors of metabolism, familial steatosis, Reye syndrome

Perinatal hepatic necrosis: cardiovascular collapse in utero, hypoplastic left-sided heart syndrome, coarctation of aorta, infections

Congenital cirrhosis: infantile polycystic disease

Stricture and obstruction of extrahepatic biliary tree: extrahepatic biliary atresia

Firm, encapsulated, multinodular, tan-brown masses with hemorrhage, necrosis, and cystic degeneration: may be hepatoblastoma

### Pancreas

The pancreas (_____ g; normal _____ g) is located normally, within the *duodenal sweep/other.* Its surface and parenchyma appear gray-white and *normally lobulated/other.*

### Pancreas
#### General Observations

Inspect pancreas (location, size, shape, parenchymal consistency, fat, ducts); weigh pancreas

#### Specific Findings

Ring of pancreatic tissue around duodenum: annular pancreas

Replacement of normal pancreatic tissue by fibrofatty tissue: cystic fibrosis

### Spleen

The splenic tissue (_____ g; normal, _____ g) consists of *a solitary spleen of normal shape/two small spleens/several spleens of varying sizes.* (For infant/fetus: Cut sections are *unremarkable/other.*) (For child: Splenic parenchyma is *dark red/other.* The follicles are *small/other* and trabeculae are *delicate/other.*)

### Spleen
#### General Observations

Inspect spleen (location, size, shape, parenchyma); do not confuse multilobular spleen with multiple accessory spleens; weigh spleen

#### Specific Findings

Multiple splenunculi present instead of normal spleen: polysplenia

Splenomegaly in infants and children: may be due to intrauterine infection, blood group incompatibility, inborn error of metabolism, leukemia, histiocytosis

## Gastrointestinal System

The tongue is *papillated/smooth*. The esophagus courses *normally to enter the stomach/other*. (For child: Its mucosal surface appears *intact/other*.) The shape of the stomach is *normal/other*. The gastric mucosa is *unremarkable/other*. The pyloric canal is *patent/obstructed*. The duodenum *courses in the usual fashion/abnormally* and is of *normal/other* caliber. The jejunum and ileum are of *normal caliber/other*. (For child: The mucosal surfaces are *unremarkable/other*.) The cecum and appendix *are/are not* fixed in the right lower quadrant and have the *usual/other* configuration. The colon is of *generous/other* caliber, and courses *normally/other*. (For child: Its mucosal surface is unremarkable.) The rectum is *patent/imperforate*.

## Genitourinary System

The kidneys (right, _____ g; left, _____ g; normal combined weight, _____ g) are located *in their usual retroperitoneal position/other*. The surface of each kidney is *normal/shows normal fetal lobulations/other*. On hemisection there are *clearly demarcated corticomedullary junctions/other*, *normal pyramids and collecting system/other*. The ureters are *patent/other* and connected to the bladder *in the usual fashion/other*. The urinary bladder appears *normal/other*. The urethra is *patent/other*.

**For Males:**
The prostate is *small, firm and unremarkable/other.* The testes (right, _____ g; left, _____ g; normal combined weight, _____ g) are located within the scrotal sac *bilaterally/within the inguinal canal/within the abdomen.*

**For Females:**
The uterus, tubes, and ovaries are in their *usual relative position within the pelvis/other*. The vagina and cervix appear *normal/other*. The uterus is *normal/other* in shape. The ovaries (right, _____ g; left, _____ g; normal combined weight, _____ g) appear *normal/other*.

## Gastrointestinal System
### General Observations

Inspect oral cavity and pharynx (contents, mucosa, teeth, gingiva, tongue, mucosa); inspect esophagus (position, contents, mucosa); look for tracheoesophageal fistula; inspect stomach, small intestines, large intestines (size, length, position, contents, mucosa, serosa); identify and note size, position, mobility of appendix

### Specific Findings

Stenosis and atresia of gastrointestinal tract: may have diaphragm across segments, interruption of gut continuity with intervening fibrous cord, and complete interruption associated with defect in mesentery at site of atresia

Esophageal atresia: most common type consists of dilated, thick-walled blind esophageal pouch superiorly and segment with fistulous communication to trachea inferiorly

Pyloric stenosis

Duodenal atresia

Atresia of large bowel (rare)

Anorectal agenesis

Ectopic tissues: generally pancreatic but may be gastric mucosa

Long, saccular structures: duplications

Dilation and hypertrophy of rectum and variable amount of proximal colon: Hirschsprung disease

Obstruction of ileum with hard gray meconium, proximal ileum dilated and containing thick green meconium, colon collapsed and empty: meconium ileus

Edema, hemorrhage, and necrosis of terminal ileum, ascending colon, and sometimes entire small and large intestines: neonatal necrotizing enterocolitis

## Genitourinary System
### Urinary Tract
### General Observations

Inspect kidneys (location, size, shape); weigh kidneys; in preterm infants, do not strip the renal capsule so as not to tear the renal cortex; inspect renal vessels (patency); cut kidneys and inspect parenchyma; inspect ureters (location, size, shape, patency); probe ureteropelvic and ureterovesical junction for stenosis; inspect bladder (size, contents, mucosa, wall thickening); inspect urethra (mucosa, patency, diverticula); if urethral pathology is suspected (stenosis, diverticulum), dissect carefully and open (use dissecting microscope, if necessary); fistulas between bladder and urethra, as well as between rectum and vagina, may have to be demonstrated by injection study

### Specific Findings

Absent kidneys and ureters, small tubular bladder: bilateral renal agenesis (Potter syndrome)

Absence of one kidney and ureter: unilateral renal agenesis (associated with agenesis of ipsilateral fallopian tube)

Renal ectopia, malrotation, fusion

Rounded, discoid, or lobulated kidneys located at pelvic brim or cavity with anteriorly positioned collecting system: pelvic kidney (may be associated with anorectal anomalies)

Kidneys located close to midline

Both kidneys and ureters on same side of body: crossed ectopia (kidneys may be fused—fused crossed ectopia)

*table continues*

## PEDIATRIC AUTOPSY DESCRIPTION OF GROSS FINDINGS *(continued)*

Fusion of kidneys at lower poles but retention of separate pelves and ureters: horseshoe kidney (fusion may be at superior pole or at both poles—ring or doughnut kidney)

Small cystic kidneys: renal hypoplasia with cystic dysplastic change

Markedly enlarged kidneys of normal form but with parenchyma with dilated collecting tubules, producing appearance of multiple small radially oriented cysts or spongelike appearance: autosomal recessive polycystic kidney disease

Enlarged, irregular, and multicystic, with cysts ranging from microscopic to several centimeters in diameter associated with ureteropelvic obstruction, ureteral agenesis, or other obstructive anomalies of lower urinary tract: renal obstructive dysplasia

Enlarged kidneys with small, rounded cysts and small, poorly demarcated medullary pyramids: diffuse cystic dysplasia (associated with several autosomal malformation syndromes)

Dilation of medullary papillary ducts with cyst formation: medullary sponge kidney

Small kidneys with contracted granular surfaces and cortical and medullary cysts, though cysts are most prominent at corticomedullary junction: nephronophthisis—uremic medullary cystic disease complex

Accentuation of posterior urethral mucosal folds resulting in obstruction of urethra: posterior urethral valve obstruction (associated with cystic renal dysplasia and dilation of the urinary tract)

Soft, homogenous tan to gray, solitary mass that may have foci of hemorrhage, cysts, or necrosis: Wilms' tumor

### Male Reproductive Organs
*General Observations*

Determine position of testes (abdominal cavity, inguinal canal, scrotum); inspect testes (development, size, shape); weigh testes; always sample both gonads (they may be different histologically); consider need to obtain gonadal tissue for karyotype; inspect prostate

*Specific Findings*

Descent of testes

Orifice of inguinal canal: 6 months' gestation

Inguinal canal: 6 to 7 months' gestation

Final intrascrotal position: by end of 8th gestational month

Undescended testis: 80% inguinal canal; 20% intraabdominal

Absence of male gonads and female pattern of external genitalia: gonadal agenesis with XY karyotype

Ectopic testis: superficial inguinal region, base of penis, femoral area, subcutaneous, transverse in superior scrotum, perineal in subcutaneous tissues

### Female Reproductive Organs
*General Observations*

Inspect vagina and uterus (location, size, shape, development); inspect ovaries and fallopian tubes (location, size, shape); weigh ovaries; always sample both gonads (they may be different histologically); consider need to obtain gonadal tissue for karyotype

*Specific Findings*

Atresia of female reproductive organs

Absence of uterus: blind fallopian tubes generally still present

Partial or complete absence of fallopian tubes

Unilateral absence of ovary

Agenesis of distal cervix

Atresia of vagina
Absence or hypoplasia of uterus, fallopian tubes, and upper
    vagina: müllerian aplasia
Some uterine fusion anomalies
    Partial or complete fusion of lower part of müllerian ducts:
        uterus didelphys, bicervical uterus bicornis, unicervical
        uterus bicornis
    Partial or total atresia of lower part of one or both müllerian
        ducts: uterus bicornis bicollis (rudimentary horn), cervical
        atresia, vaginal atresia
    Persistent uterovaginal septum after fusion of müllerian ducts:
        complete bilocular uterus, unicervical bilocular uterus,
        bilocular bicervical uterus

## Endocrine System

The pituitary (_____ g; normal, _____ g) *fills the sella/other.*
(For child: The thyroid (_____ g; normal, _____ g) is *symmetrical,
red-brown, and firm/other. Four/other* parathyroid glands of *usual
size/other* are identified grossly.) The adrenal glands (right, _____
g; left, _____ g; normal combined weight, _____ g) are *of normal
size and shape/other.* (For infant/child: They have *uniform
yellow cortices separated from the medullary gray by a thin red
line/other.*)

## Endocrine System

### General Observations

Weigh (or measure) pituitary; inspect pituitary (shape, symmetry,
    color); inspect sella turcica; weigh thyroid; inspect thyroid
    (color, symmetry, consistency, external parenchyma,
    pyramidal lobe); identify parathyroids (confirm on
    microscopic examination)—if enlarged, weigh accurately;
    weigh adrenal glands after removing investing fat; if friable,
    clean and weigh after fixation; inspect adrenals (color, shape,
    thickness, and regularity of cortex and medulla)

### Specific Findings

Absence of pituitary gland: rare familial cases
Absence or hypoplasia of pituitary gland: alobar
    holoprosencephaly
Absence of posterior lobe, variable-sized anterior lobe of
    pituitary: anencephaly
Congenital hypothyroidism: 60% show aplasia or failure of
    descent of thyroid (cryptothyroidism); 14% normal or enlarged
    thyroid glands; 25% ectopic thyroid glands
Enlarged, firm, congested thyroid in neonate: may be neonatal
    thyrotoxicosis
Absence of parathyroid glands: DiGeorge syndrome
Ectopic parathyroid tissue: mediastinal, thymic, pericardial,
    paratracheal, retropharyngeal, retroesophageal, wall of
    thymic duct cyst
Bilateral adrenal hyperplasia with thick, brown, nodular cortex:
    congenital adrenal hyperplasia, pigmented micronodular
    adrenal disease
Small to very large, soft, gray adrenal masses; large tumors with
    necrosis, cystic degeneration, and hemorrhage:
    neuroblastoma (also found along sympathetic chain, posterior
    mediastinum, lower abdominal paravertebral region, pelvis,
    neck, other)

## Musculoskeletal System

Skeletal muscles are *red-brown and firm/other.* The cartilage and
bone are *firm and normal/other.* The bone marrow appears *red,
moist and ample/pale.*

## Musculoskeletal System

### General Observations

Inspect muscle (color, consistency, symmetry, mass); sample
    muscle and nerve appropriately to evaluate neuromuscular
    disorders (see Chapter 8); inspect external configuration of
    skeleton; inspect bones and joints; bisect portions of two ribs
    and the vertebral column; inspect the marrow; check firmness
    of cartilage and bone; check the bone marrow for color and
    consistency; in all cases of suggested bone involvement, be
    sure to obtain
X-rays and consult with a radiologist, then sample bones that
    show radiologic evidence of disease

*table continues*

## PEDIATRIC AUTOPSY DESCRIPTION OF GROSS FINDINGS *(continued)*

### Specific Findings

Hypotonia: spinal muscular atrophy, congenital myopathies, neuromuscular disorders

Muscle wasting, limb distortion (arthrogryposis): congenital muscular dystrophy

Subperiosteal hemorrhage limited to surface of one cranial bone, generally after bone trauma: cephalhematoma

Lethal short-limb chondrodysplasias: thanatophoric dwarfism, achondrogenesis syndromes, homozygous achondroplasia, short-rib polydactyly syndrome, camptomelic syndrome, chondroectodermal dysplasia, asphyxiating thoracic dystrophy

Segmentation defects (hemivertebrae; fused ribs): best detected by x-ray on anteroposterior view seen in VACTERL association or OEIS complex (Omphalocele-exstrophy-imperforate anus-spinal defects)

Neural tube defects (anencephaly, rachischisis, myelomeningocele, encephalocele): see Head and Central Nervous System

Fragile bones with old and recent fractures, curved legs, multiple small bones making up calvarium: osteogenesis imperfecta congenita

Increased bone density: osteopetrosis

Soft calvarium, short bowed limbs, prominent laterally displaced costochondral junctions, short ribs, soft long bones with fractures: hypophosphatasia

Frontal bossing, expanded costochondral junctions (rachitic rosary), soft ribs, pigeon breast deformity, lumbar lordosis, bowed legs: rickets

### Head and Central Nervous System

Reflection of the scalp reveals *no evidence of subgaleal hemorrhage/other*. The underlying calvarium is *intact and normal in thickness/other*. The dura is *intact/other,* and its inner surface *smooth and glistening/other*. The dural sinuses are *patent/other*. Cerebrospinal fluid is *clear/other*.

The brain weighs _____ g. The leptomeninges are *thin and transparent with no vascular congestion, subarachnoid hemorrhage, or exudate/other*. The circle of Willis and other basal vasculature are *intact and normally formed/other*. The vessels are *patent and thin-walled/other*. The cranial nerves are *intact and normally distributed/other*. The dorsal convexities of the brain are *symmetrical with a well-developed gyral pattern/other*. The brainstem and cerebellum show the *usual* external configuration. There is *no* localized external softening or contusion of the brain. There is *no displacement of the cingulate gyrus, medial temporal lobe, or cerebellar tonsils/other*.

Multiple coronal sections of the cerebrum show *an intact cortical ribbon of appropriate thickness/other*. The internal architecture shows *the usual pattern/other without focal lesions or hemorrhage/other*. The ventricular system is of *appropriate configuration and size/other*. Transverse sections of the brainstem show *a well-pigmented substantia nigra and locus caeruleus/other*. The pons shows *well-defined pyramids and inferior olivary nuclei/other*. Sections of the cerebellum show *prominent inferior olivary nuclei/other*; the hemispheres show *the usual foliar pattern and appearance of the dentate nuclei/other*.

The spinal cord dura is *intact/other,* and its inner surface *smooth and shiny/other*. The spinal leptomeninges are *thin and translucent/other*. Anterior and posterior roots are comparable in size. Transverse sections of cord show *no abnormalities/other*. The cauda equina is *unremarkable/other*.

### Head and Central Nervous System
### General Observations
#### Initial Examination:

Inspect scalp (hemorrhage), calvarium (intactness, thickness); note characteristics of cerebrospinal fluid (color, clarity); before removal of the brain determine whether there are tears or hemorrhages in the falx and tentorium; inspect dura of brain and spinal cord (thickness, color, transparency, calcification); examine epidural and subdural space; examine vascular sinuses; strip dura and examine base of skull; inspect leptomeninges (clarity, color, thickness, adhesions); examine cranial nerves; perform preliminary examination of convolutions (flattening or narrowing of gyri, width of sulci, lesions); inspect major fissures; inspect cerebellum, brainstem, and circle of Willis; check for pressure effects on cingulated gyrus, cerebellar tonsils, and brainstem; weigh fresh brain if possible

#### Examination after Fixation:

Weigh fixed brain; reexamine cortical surface, gyri, sulci, and external aspects of cerebellum and brainstem; cut brain and spinal cord; examine cortex, white matter, basal ganglia, mamillary bodies, cerebral peduncles, brainstem, cerebellum; examine ventricles (hemorrhage, symmetry, size, blunting, compression, ependymal surface, choroid plexus, aqueduct of Sylvius; examine spinal cord gray and white matter; examine spinal cord nerve roots, cauda equina, and filum terminale

### Specific Findings

Top of head flat, crowned by mass of red vascular and remnant brain tissue without overlying skin and bone: anencephaly

Posterior continuation of anencephalic defect along spine: craniorachischisis

Diverticulum of malformed central nervous system tissue through defects in occipital (most common), parietal, or frontal bone: seen with occipital, interparietal or frontonasal encephalocele

Defect in spinal column with extension of central nervous system tissue and meninges through defect in spinal column: myelomeningocele or, if extension of meninges only, meningocele

Abnormal occipital skull and cervical vertebrae, absence of neck, spinal retroflexion, sometimes with occipital encephalocele: iniencephaly

Variable degrees of incomplete separation of cerebral hemispheres: holoprosencephaly

Small posterior fossa with downward extension of cerebellar vermis through foramen magnum, hydrocephalus, lumbar myelomeningocele: Chiari type II malformation

Small posterior fossa with downward extension of cerebellar vermis through occipital encephalocele, hydrocephalus, lumbar myelomeningocele: Chiari type III malformation

Small posterior fossa with downward extension of cerebellar tonsils through foramen magnum: chronic cerebellar herniation (Chiari type I malformation)

Hydrocephalus and enlarged posterior fossa with absent or rudimentary cerebellar vermis, midline cyst contiguous with enlarged fourth ventricle, elevated transverse sinuses and tentorium, and sometimes obstruction of foramina of the fourth ventricle: Dandy-Walker syndrome

Smoothening of cortex due to decreased number or complete lack of gyri and sulci with thickened cortex, narrow cerebral mantle, and enlarged ventricles: agyria or pachygyria

Cortical surface consists of numerous small convolutions yielding a cobblestone appearance (may be complete or partial): polymicrogyria (microscopic confirmation required)

Microcephalic, megaloencephalic, or normal-sized brain with hard, potato-shaped hamartomas (tubers) over the cortical surface and similar-appearing subependymal nodules ("candle-gutterings"): tuberous sclerosis

Bilirubin staining of deep gray-matter nuclei of brain and brainstem: kernicterus

Aberrant arterial branches from posterior or middle cerebral vein to dilated vein of Galen: aneurysm of the vein of Galen

Abnormal dilated veins typically involving parietooccipital cortex: Sturge-Weber syndrome

Acoustic schwannomas, multiple meningiomas, gliomas, ependymomas of spinal cord: neurofibromatosis type 2

Capillary hemangioblastomas of cerebellum, retina, brainstem, and spinal cord: von Hippel–Lindau disease

## Placenta

The placenta (_____ g; _____ cm *average diameter; _ cm average thickness*) is *intact/other*. Attached *centrally/eccentrically/other* to the placenta is a _ -cm segment of *white/other* umbilical cord averaging _____ cm in diameter. Sections through the cord reveal vessels. The placental membranes are *thin, delicate, and translucent/other*. The fetal surface is *smooth and glistening/other*. The maternal surface is *dark red/other* and consists of *intact/other* cotyledons. The parenchyma is *dark red and spongy/other*.

## Placenta[2]

### General Observations

Measure (average diameter and thickness) and weigh; inspect fetal surface; note point of rupture in reference to edge of placenta if possible; inspect membranes (color, translucency); trim membranes and prepare membrane roll for histologic analysis; measure umbilical cord (length, diameter); inspect cord (color, character, location, and type of insertion); section cord short and note number of vessels; inspect maternal surface (color, consistency, pallor, adherent blood, cotyledons); inspect sectioned parenchyma

### Specific Findings

Weight
<10th percentile for gestational age: chronic insufficiency, chromosomal anomalies, maternal tobacco use, congenital infection

*table continues*

## PEDIATRIC AUTOPSY DESCRIPTION OF GROSS FINDINGS *(continued)*

>95th percentile for gestational age: hydrops fetalis; macrosomia, infant of diabetic mother; Beckwith-Weidemann syndrome; triploidy

Shape

Accessory lobe (succenturiate lobe): may present as placenta previa

Bilobate placenta: associated with multiparity, older maternal age, assisted reproduction

Circummarginate placenta: chorion laeve inserts inside the rim of the placenta with flat transition; no associated clinical complications

Circumvallate placenta: chorion laeve inserts inside the rim of the placenta, with membranes folded back to create raised transition; associated with membrane rupture and antepartum hemorrhage

Firm, gray-white, waxy peripheral lesions that may be seen throughout placenta: perivillous fibrin deposition (associated with intrauterine growth retardation)

Placental infarcts: triangular

Acute: red, palpably firmer than adjacent parenchyma

Subacute: brown to tan

Old: Pale tan to off-white

Hematomas separating basal plate of placenta from uterine wall: retroplacental hematoma

Hemorrhage into decidua with separation and compression of central part of placenta: placental abruption

White to yellow or yellow-green, opaque membranes; may have exudates of frank pus: acute chorioamnionitis

Green discoloration of cord and membranes: meconium staining

Acute chorioamnionitis with white to yellow nodules: may be due to *Candida albicans*

Insertion of umbilical vessels into membranes: velamentous insertion

Umbilical cord lesions

True knots: may be associated with fetal distress if tightened before or during labor; grooving of cord and constriction of umbilical vessels in longstanding cases, congestion or thrombosis in acute cases

False knots: local dilation of umbilical vessels

Local dilation of umbilical

## FRAMENTED FETUS TEMPLATE*

### Gross Description

The specimen is received fresh and consists of multiple fragments of fetal and placental tissues, decidua, and blood (__×__×__cm in aggregate). *Four/other* extremities are present (__cm foot length), *without abnormalities/other*. There are __ *normal-appearing fingers/toes on the hands/feet/other*. Palmar creases are *normal/ other*. The cranium and face are *identified/other*. The ear(s) are *present, well formed, and are not low set/other*. Both eyes are *present and in normal anatomic configuration/other*. The nose is *normal and the nares are probe patent/other*. The mouth is *normally formed, without cleft lip, cleft palate or high palatal arch/other*. The neck shows *no nuchal thickening or cystic hygroma/other*. The external genitalia are those of a *phenotypically normal [male/female] fetus at this gestational age/other*. Portions of grossly unremarkable fetal organs are present: heart, gastrointestinal tract, kidneys, skin, etc.

Placental tissues include a __cm, *2/3* vessel cord, fragmented chorionic villi, and extraplacental membranes. *No gross abnormalities are noted/other*.

*Add-ins for more intact specimens (no anomalies, or see general observations and specific findings in pediatric autopsy description earlier). Weigh intact viscera. In many instances, weights and corresponding normative values may not be possible due to fragmentation.*

### Cardiovascular System

All four cardiac chambers and the great vessels are *symmetric in size and in normal anatomic configuration/other*. Atrioventricular and semilunar valves are *normally formed; no atrial or ventricular septal defects are identified/other*. The foramen ovale and ductus arteriosus are *patent/other*.

## Respiratory System

The left and right lungs have *2 and 3 lobes, respectively/other*. Visceral pleural surfaces are *smooth and parenchyma is soft and pale red/other*.

## Gastrointestinal System

The stomach is present and *does not show atresia into the duodenum/other*. The small and large intestines are *present/other*. The vermiform appendix *is/is not* identified. *No atresia or abnormal dilated intestinal segments are seen/other*.

## Hepatobiliary System

The liver has *an attached gallbladder and umbilical vein that leads into the portal sinus through a patent ductus venosus/other*.

## Genitourinary System

The kidneys are *symmetrical in size and exhibit the expected fetal lobulations/other*. On cut surface they are *noncystic, and the ureters are nondilated/other*. The urinary bladder is appears *normal/other*. The urethra is *patent/other*.

### For Males

The prostate is *present and unremarkable/other*. The gonads *are/are not* identified.
   —or—
*One testicle/both testes* are identified and appear normally *formed/other*.

### For Females

The uterus is *normal in shape/other*. The fallopian tubes are *present/other*. The gonads *are/are not* identified.
   —or—
*One/both ovary(ies) is/are* identified and appear(s) *normal/other*.

## Endocrine System

The pituitary is present in the *sella/other*. The thyroid is identified and *symmetrical/other*. The adrenal glands are *identified at the superior poles of the kidneys/other*; they appear of *expected triangular shape and on cut surface are composed predominantly of fetal cortex/other*.

## Lymphoproliferative System

The thymus is identified and consists of *soft, lobulated parenchyma/other*. A single spleen is *identified/other*.

## Diagnosis

* Phenotypically (*male/female*) fetus, ___weeks' gestation ( __cm foot length; mean for __ weeks __ ± __ cm)
* No gross anomalies identified, but examination limited by fragmentation

—or—

* Multiple anomalies include: (*List anomalies*)
* Organs examined microscopically (e.g., kidney, liver, lung) appear unremarkable for gestational age

—or—

* The following organs are abnormal microscopically: (*List anomalies*)
* Ancillary testing: karyotype, radiographs, cultures
* Placenta: Immature chorionic villi, umbilical cord, extraplacental membranes, chorionic plate; decidua and implantation site noted

\*Modified with permission from Jonathan L. Hecht, MD, PhD, Departments of Pathology, Beth Israel Deaconess Medical Center and Harvard Medical School, Boston.

## TRAUMA TEMPLATE

Numbering of wounds is arbitrary and used for reference purposes only. It is not meant to imply the sequence in which the injuries were sustained. All measurements are taken with the body in the standard anatomic position.

### Gunshot Wounds

Entrance. Describe location, dimensions, abrasions, contusions, soot, stippling, or muzzle mark; satellite injuries; bone beveling.
   This wound is centered _____ cm from the top of the head and _____ cm to the *left/right* of the *anterior/posterior* midline.
   Exit. Describe location, description, dimensions, abrasions, contusions.
   This wound is centered cm from the top of the head and cm to the *right/left* of the *anterior/posterior* midline.
   Path of projectile. Highlight path of projectile through body.
   Recovery of projectile. A *projectile/projectile fragment* is recovered from the _____ and is labeled "No. _____." This fragment is a *deformed, copper-colored, lead-cored slug/other*. There *is no radiographic evidence of metal fragments or retained projectile/other*.
   —or—
   Recovery of projectile. No projectile is recovered (perforating wound).

Direction of wound. The projectile traveled from (*right to left, front to back, and downward/other*).
   Summary. In summary, this is a (*perforating/penetrating*) (*gunshot/shotgun*) wound _____ of range that entered the body _____, (*highlights of path*), and exited the body _____. The direction of the wound track is _____. *A/No* projectile is recovered.

### Sharp-Force Injuries
#### Stab Wound

Describe location, dimensions, orientation, wound edges, contusions, abrasions.
   The wound is centered ___ cm from the top of the head and cm to the *left/right* of the *anterior/posterior* midline.
   Wound track. This incised wound penetrates at a depth of ___cm (describe internal injuries).
   Direction of wound. This wound tracks from (*right to left, front to back, and downward/other*).

#### Incised Wound

Describe location, dimensions, orientation.
   The wound is centered _____ inches from the top of the head and _ inches to the (*left/right*) of (*anterior/posterior*) midline.

*table continues*

## TRAUMA TEMPLATE *(continued)*

### Blunt-Force Injuries

Hemorrhages. Describe location, color, size, characteristics.

Lacerations. Describe location, size, characteristics.

Fractures. Describe site, characteristics (focal, crush, penetrating, traction, angulation, rotation, compression, combinations).

Abrasions/contusions. Describe location, color, size, characteristics.

### Injuries from Hanging and Strangulation

Ligature marks. *Completely/partially* encircling the neck is a ligature mark measuring cm in length by cm in width with a furrow depth of cm. The ligature mark is centered across the *anterior/posterior/lateral/right/left* neck at the level of the _____. One end is located _____cm from the top of the head and _____cm to the right of the *anterior/posterior* midline; the other is _____ cm from the top of the head and _____cm to the left of *anterior/posterior* midline. The angulation of the ligature mark is _____.

Describe any wound patterns, margins, point of suspension, and excoriations of the skin above or below the mark.

Ligatures. Accompanying the body is a ligature consisting of (*type of material/associated pattern/length of ligature/diameter*). Describe knot if present. The pattern/texture of the ligature is *compatible with the pattern of the mark on the decedent's neck/ other*.

### REFERENCES

1. Tanner JM: *Growth at adolescence*, ed 2, Oxford, UK, Blackwell Scientific Publications, 1962.
2. Roberts DJ: Placental pathology, a survival guide, *Arch Pathol Lab Med* 132:641-651, 2008.

# Appendix B

# Measures, Weights, and Assessment of Growth and Development

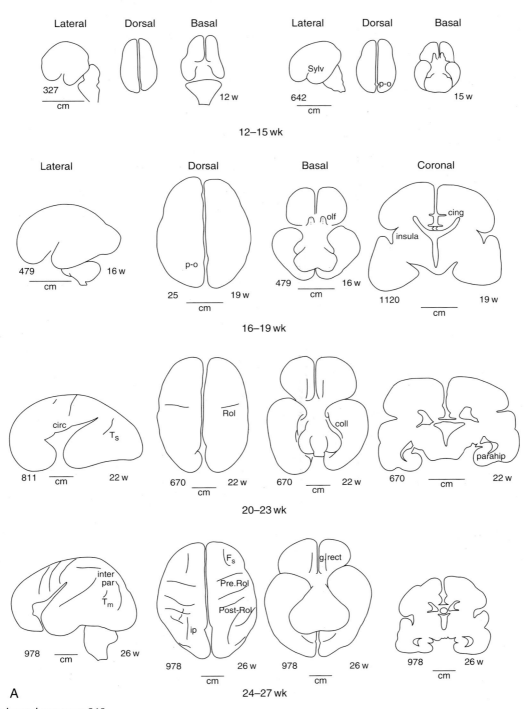

A

**Figure B-1** For legend see page 318.

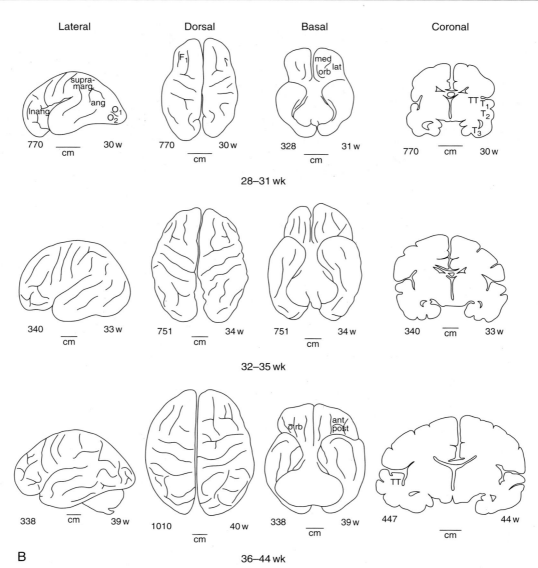

**Figure B-1** Progressive development of sulci and gyri in the fetal brain, 12 to 44 weeks. *Ang,* angular gyrus; *ant/post,* anterior and posterior orbital gyri; *cc,* corpus callosum; *cing,* cingulated sulcus; *circ,* circular sulcus; *coll,* collateral sulcus; $F_1$, superior frontal gyrus; $F_s$, superior frontal sulcus; *g. rect,* gyrus rectus; *interpar* or *ip,* interparietal sulcus; *med/lat orb,* medial and lateral orbital gyri; $O_1$, superior occipital gyrus; $O_2$, inferior occipital gyrus; *olf,* olfactory sulcus (dotted lines to indicate sulci are underneath the olfactory bulbs); *parahip,* parahippocampal gyrus; *p-o,* parietooccipital fissure; *post-Rol,* postrolandic sulcus; *pre-Rol,* prerolandic sulcus; *Rol,* rolandic (central) sulcus; $T_1$, superior temporal gyrus; $T_2$, middle temporal gyrus; $T_3$, inferior temporal gyrus; $T_m$, middle temporal sulcus; *triang,* triangular gyrus; $T_s$, superior temporal sulcus; *TT,* transverse temporal gyrus. Reprinted with permission of John Wiley & Sons, Inc.
(From Chi JG, Dooling EG, Gilles FH: Gyral development of the human brain, *Ann Neurol* 1:86-93, 1977.)

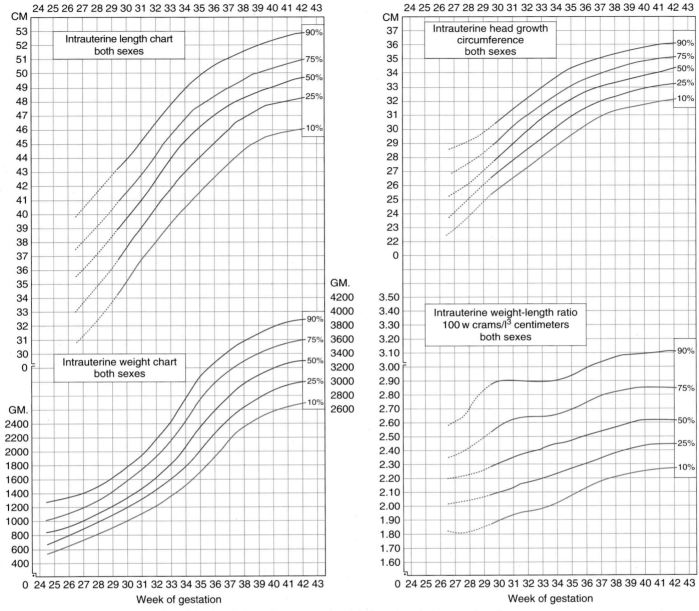

**Figure B-2** Intrauterine length, weight, head circumference, and weight-length ratio by gestational age.
(From Lubchenco LO, Hansman C, Boyd E: Intrauterine growth in length and head circumference as estimated from live births at gestational ages from 26 to 42 weeks, *Pediatrics* 37:403-408, 1966.)

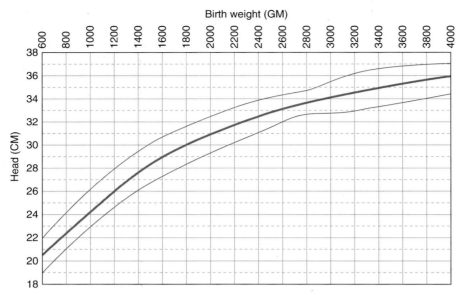

**Figure B-3** Mean head circumference ± 2 standard deviations by birth weight.
(From Usher R, McClean F: Intrauterine growth of live-born Caucasian infants at sea level: Standards obtained from measurements in 7 dimensions of infants born between 25 and 44 weeks of gestation, *J Pediatr* 74:901-910, 1969.)

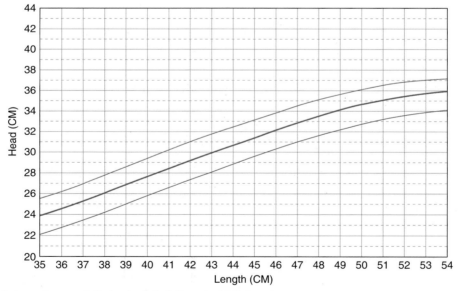

**Figure B-4** Mean head circumference ± 2 standard deviations by birth length.
(From Usher R, McClean F: Intrauterine growth of live-born Caucasian infants at sea level: Standards obtained from measurements in 7 dimensions of infants born between 25 and 44 weeks of gestation, *J Pediatr* 74:901-910, 1969.)

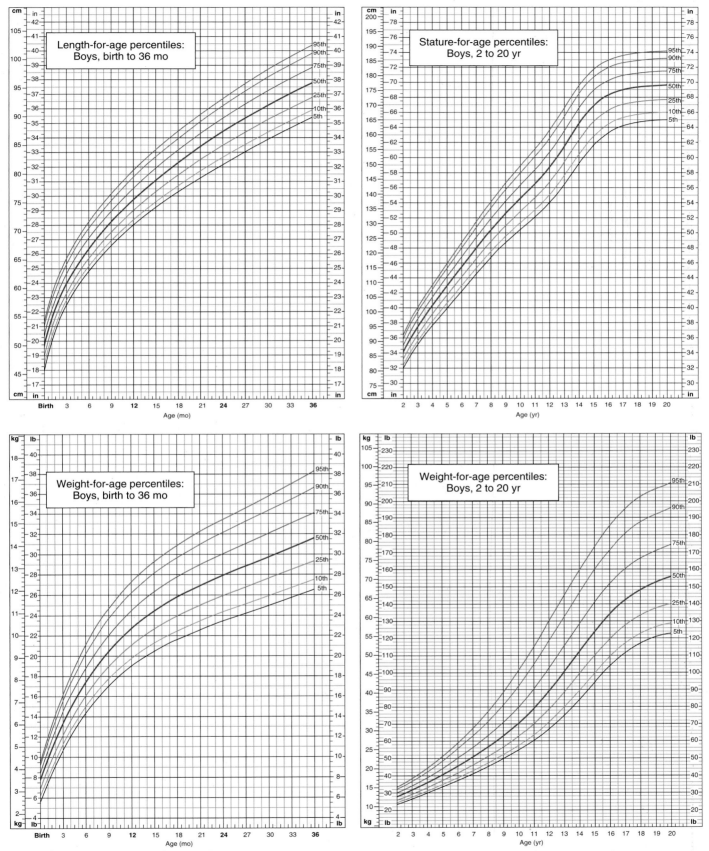

**Figure B-5** Males. Weight and length (or stature) curves for infants and young children *(left)* and for older children *(right).* (Redrawn from Hamill PVV, Drizd TA, Johnson CL, et al: Physical growth: National Center for Health Statistics percentiles, *Am J Clin Nutr* 32:607-629, 1979.)

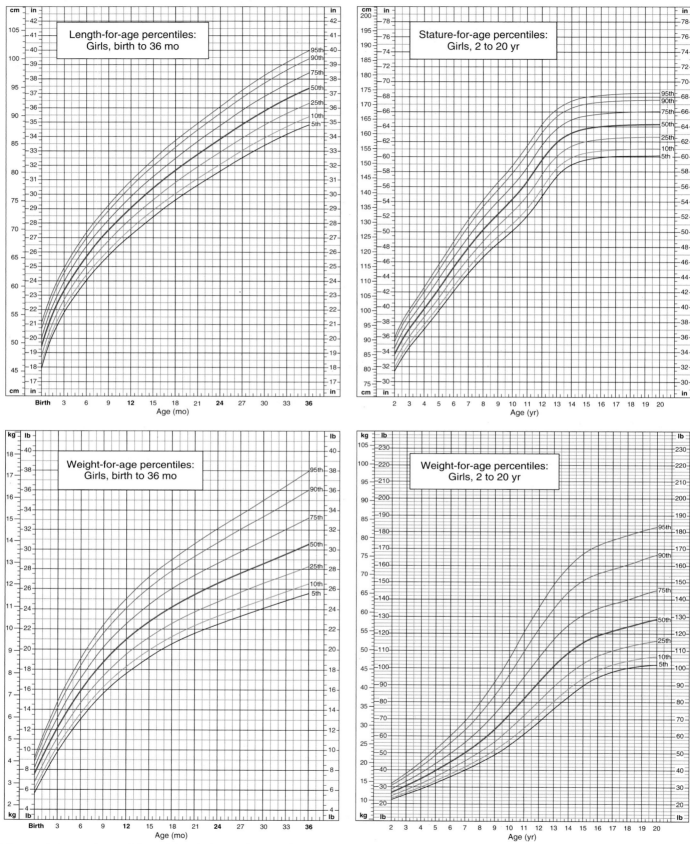

**Figure B-6** Females. Weight and length (or stature) curves for infants and young children *(left)* and for older children *(right).*
(From Hamill PVV, Drizd TA, Johnson CL, et al: Physical growth: National Center for Health Statistics percentiles, *Am J Clin Nutr* 32:607-629, 1979.)

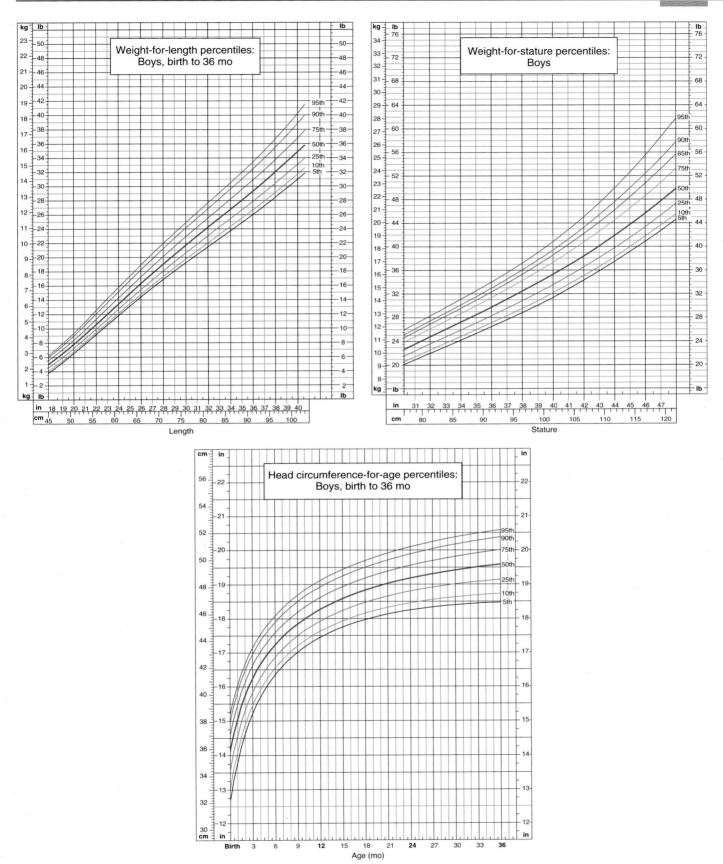

**Figure B-7**  Males. Weight for length (or stature) by age (upper curves) and head circumference by age (lower curves) for age newborn to 36 months. Each curve corresponds to the indicated percentile levels.
(From Hamill PVV, Drizd TA, Johnson CL, et al: Physical growth: National Center for Health Statistics percentiles, *Am J Clin Nutr* 32:607-629, 1979.)

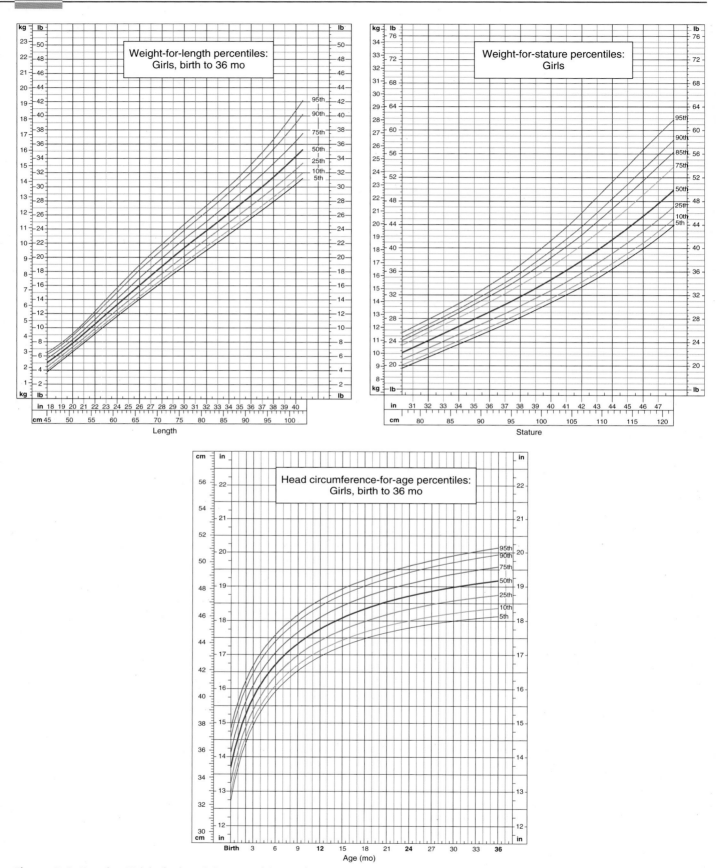

**Figure B-8** Females. Weight for length (or stature) by age (upper curves) and head circumference by age (lower curves) for age newborn to 36 months. Each curve corresponds to the indicated percentile levels.

(From Hamill PVV, Drizd TA, Johnson CL, et al: Physical growth: National Center for Health Statistics percentiles, *Am J Clin Nutr* 32:607-629, 1979.)

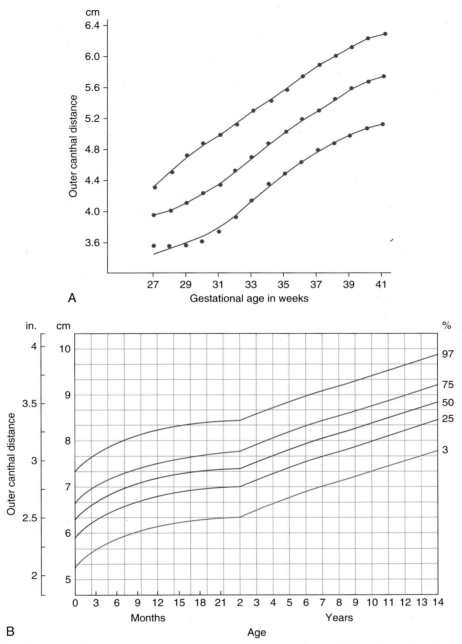

**Figure B-9** Outer canthal distance. **A,** Fetus. Points represent mean value ± 2 standard deviations from the mean for each age group.
**B,** Infant and child.
(**A,** From Sivan Y, Merlob P, Reisner SH: Eye measurements in preterm and term newborn infants, *J Craniofac Genet Dev Biol* 2:239-242, 1982. **B,** From Feingold M, Bossert WH: Normal values for selected physical parameters: An aid to syndrome delineation. In Bergsma D, editor: *Birth defects X(13),* White Plains, NY, The National Foundation—March of Dimes, 1974.)

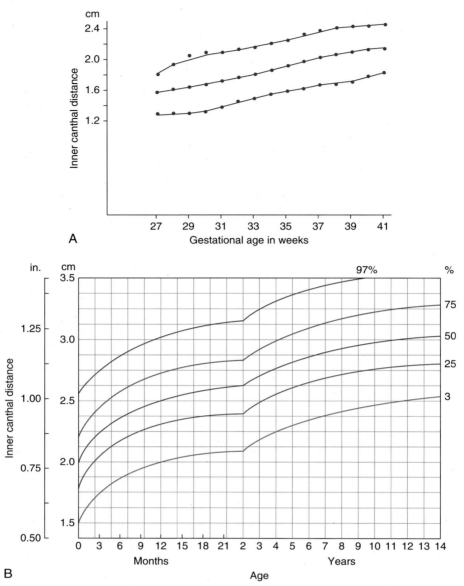

**Figure B-10** Inner canthal distance. **A,** Fetus. Points represent mean value ± 2 standard deviations from the mean for each age group. **B,** Infant and child.

(**A,** From Sivan Y, Merlob P, Reisner SH: Eye measurements in preterm and term newborn infants, *J Craniofac Genet Dev Biol* 2:239-242, 1982. **B,** From Feingold M, Bossert WH: Normal values for selected physical parameters: An aid to syndrome delineation. In Bergsma D, editor: *Birth defects X(13)*, White Plains, NY, The National Foundation—March of Dimes, 1974.)

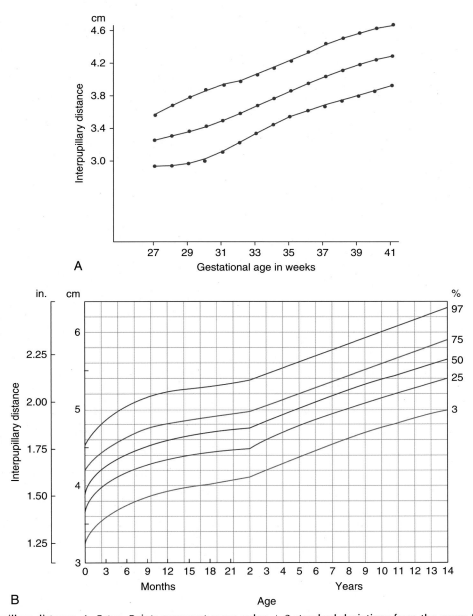

**Figure B-11** Interpupillary distance. **A,** Fetus. Points represent mean value ± 2 standard deviations from the mean for each age group. **B,** Infant and child.

(**A,** From Sivan Y, Merlob P, Reisner SH: Eye measurements in preterm and term newborn infants, *J Craniofac Genet Dev Biol* 2:239-242, 1982. **B,** From Feingold M, Bossert WH: Normal values for selected physical parameters: An aid to syndrome delineation. In Bergsma D, editor: *Birth defects X(13),* White Plains, NY, The National Foundation—March of Dimes, 1974.)

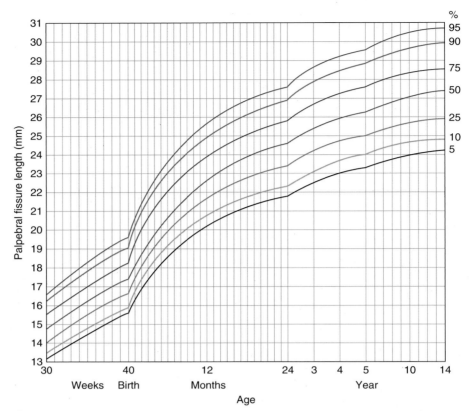

**Figure B-12** Palpebral fissure length.
(From Thomas IT, Gaitantzis YA, Frias JL: Palpebral fissure length from 29 weeks gestation to 14 years, *J Pediatr* 111:267-268, 1987.)

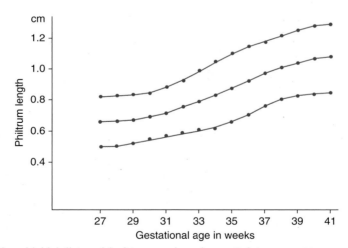

**Figure B-13** Length of philtrum (nasal-labial distance) in fetuses and newborns. Points represent mean value ± 2 standard deviations from the mean for each age group.
(From Sivan Y, Merlob P, Reisner SH: Philtrum length and intercommissural distance in newborn infants, *J Med Genet* 20:130-131, 1982.)

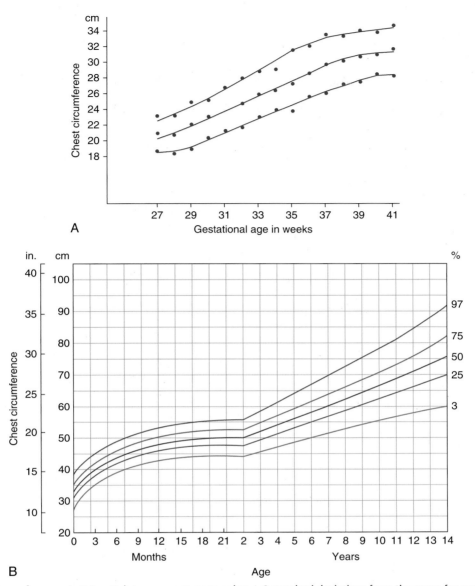

**Figure B-14**  Chest circumference. **A,** Fetus. Points represent mean value ± 2 standard deviations from the mean for each age group. **B,** Infant and child.

(**A,** From Merlob P, Sivan Y, Reisner SH: Anthropometric measurements of the newborn infant [27 to 41 gestational weeks]. In Paul NW, editor: *Birth defects 20[7],* White Plains, NY, 1984, March of Dimes Birth Defects Foundation. **B,** From Feingold M, Bossert WH: Normal values for selected physical parameters: An aid to syndrome delineation. In Bergsma D, editor: *Birth defects X[13],* White Plains, NY, The National Foundation—March of Dimes, 1974.)

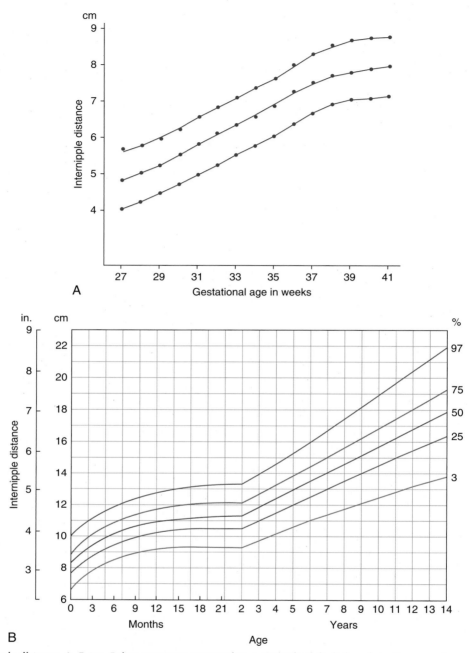

**Figure B-15** Internipple distance. **A,** Fetus. Points represent mean value ± 2 standard deviations from the mean for each age group. **B,** Infant and child.

(**A,** From Silvan Y, Merlob P, Reisner SH: Sternum length, torso length, and inter-nipple distance in newborn infants, *Pediatrics* 72:523-525, 1983. **B,** From Feingold M, Bossert WH: Normal values for selected physical parameters: An aid to syndrome delineation. In Bergsma D, editor: *Birth defects X[13],* White Plains, NY, The National Foundation—March of Dimes, 1974.)

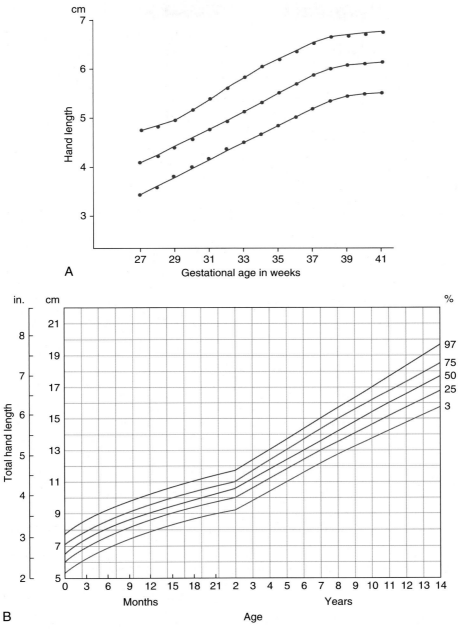

**Figure B-16**  Total hand length. **A,** Fetus. Points represent mean value ± 2 standard deviations from the mean for each age group. **B,** Infant and child.

(**A,** From Silvan Y, Merlob P, Reisner SH: Upper limb standards in newborns, *Am J Dis Child* 137:829-832, 1983. **B,** From Feingold M, Bossert WH: Normal values for selected physical parameters: An aid to syndrome delineation. In Bergsma D, editor: *Birth defects X[13]*, White Plains, NY, The National Foundation—March of Dimes, 1974.)

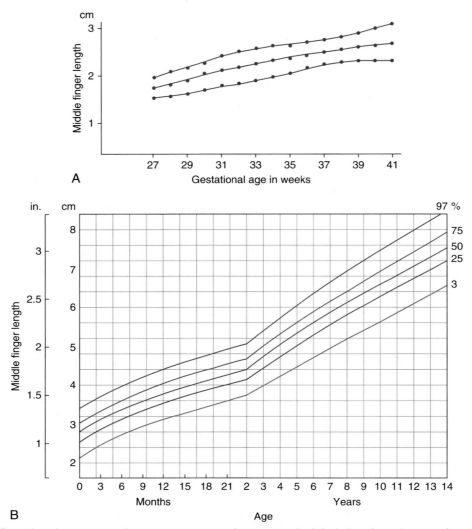

**Figure B-17** Middle finger length. **A,** Fetus. Points represent mean value ± 2 standard deviations from the mean for each age group. **B,** Infant and child.

(**A,** From Silvan Y, Merlob P, Reisner SH: Upper limb standards in newborns, *Am J Dis Child* 137:829-832, 1983. **B,** From Feingold M, Bossert WH: Normal values for selected physical parameters: An aid to syndrome delineation, In Bergsma D, editor: *Birth defects X[13],* White Plains, NY, The National Foundation—March of Dimes, 1974.)

| Table B-1 | Weights and measures of organs of adults |
|---|---|

| Organ/structure | Weight (g) | Mean percent change with formalin fixation | Measurement (cm) | Comment |
|---|---|---|---|---|
| *Cardiovascular system* | | | | |
| Heart | | −5.8%[1] | | See also Table B-2 |
| Male | 300 (270-360)[2] | | | |
| Female | 250 (200-280)[2] | | | |
| Ventricles only (right ventricle [RV]; left ventricle [LV]; septum [S]) | <250[3] | | | LV + S/RV 2.3-3.3 : 1[3] |
| Right ventricle | <65 (RV free wall)[3] | | 0.2-0.4 (wall thickness measured 2 cm proximal to pulmonary valve)[2,4] | Right ventricular hypertrophy if LV + S/R < 2:1 or RV > 80g[3] |
| Left ventricle | <190 (LV + S)[3] | | 1.5 (wall thickness measured 2 cm distal to mitral valve)[2] | LV + S > 225g[3] |
| Atria | | | 0.2 (thickness)[2] | |
| Aorta | | | | |
| Ascending | | | 8.5 (circumference)[5] | |
| Thoracic | | | 4.5-7.0 (circumference)[5] | |
| Abdominal | | | 3.5-4.5 (circumference)[5] | |
| *Respiratory system* | | | | |
| Lungs | | | | |
| Right | 450 (360-570)[2] | | | Male = 455; female = 402[6] |
| Left | 375 (325-480)[2] | | | Male = 402; female = 345[6] |
| *Gastrointestinal system* | | | | |
| Esophagus | | | 25 (length)[2] | |
| Stomach | | | 25-30 (length) | |
| Duodenum | | | 30 (length)[2] | |
| Small intestine | | | 550-650 (length)[2] | |
| Colon | | | 150-170 (length)[2] | |
| Liver | 1650 (1500-1800)[2] | −4%[1] | 25-30 × 19-21 × 6-9[2] | |
| Gallbladder | | | 7.5 × 2.8 × 2.8[2] | Average volume 50 mL[2] |
| Pancreas | | | 23 × 4-5 × 3.8[2] | |
| Male | 143 (103-186)[7] | | | |
| Female | 122 (86-179)[7] | | | |
| Omentum | | | 23-43 × 16-34[8] | |
| *Urinary system* | | | | |
| Kidneys | | +1.9%[1] | 9-12 × 5-6 × 3-4[2] | Maximal weight 3rd-4th decade[9] |
| Male (combined) | 313 (230-440)[2] | | | |
| Female (combined) | 288 (240-350)[2] | | | |
| Cortex | | | 0.6-0.7 cm (thickness)[10] | |
| Medulla | | | 1.3-1.7 cm (thickness)[10] | |
| Ureters | | | 0.2-1.0 (luminal diameter)[11] | |

*table continues*

**Table B-1** Weights and measures of organs of adults *(continued)*

| Organ/structure | Weight (g) | Mean percent change with formalin fixation | Measurement (cm) | Comment |
|---|---|---|---|---|
| *Endocrine system* | | | | |
| Adrenals (each) | | 0%[12] | 4.5 × 2.5-3.5 × 0.5[2] | |
|   Male | 9.7[12] | | | |
|   Female | 8.3[12] | | | |
|   Parathyroids | 0.12-0.18 (combined)[2] | | 0.3-0.6 × 0.2-0.4 × 0.05-0.2[2] | |
| Pituitary | | | 2.1 × 1.4 × 0.5[2] | |
|   10–20 years | 0.56[2] | | | |
|   >20 years | 0.61[2] | | | |
| In pregnancy | 0.95 (0.84-1.06)[2] | | | |
| Thyroid | 40 (30-70)[2] | +14.8%[1] | 5-7 × 3-4 × 1.5-2.5[2] | |
| Male | 25[7] | | | |
| Female | 18[7] | | | |
| *Reproductive system* | | | | |
| Testis (each) | 25 (20-27)[2] | +3.2%[1] | 4-5 × 2.5-3.5 × 2-2.7[2] | |
| Seminal vesicles | | | 4.1-4.5 × 1.6-1.8 × 0.9[2] | |
| Prostate | | | 3.6 × 2.8 × 1.9[13] | |
|   20-30 years | 15[13] | | | |
|   31-50 years | 20[13] | | | |
|   51-80 years | 40[13] | | | |
| Uterus | | | | |
|   Nullipara | 35 (33-41)[2] | | 7.8-8.1 × 3.4-4.5 × 1.8-2.7[2] | |
|   After pregnancy | 110 (102-117)[2] | | 8.7-9.4 × 5.4-6.1 × 3.2-3.6[2] | |
| Cervix | | | 2.9-3.4 × 2.5 × 1.6-2.0[2] | |
| Ovaries (each) | 5-8[14] | | 3.0-5.0 × 1.5-3.0 × 0.6-1.5[14] | |
| *Lymphoreticular system* | | | | |
| Thymus | | | | |
|   6–25 years | 25[2] | | | |
|   26–35 years | 20[2] | | | |
|   36–65 years | 16[2] | | | |
|   >65 years | 6[2] | | | |
| Spleen | <250[15] | +2.1%[1] | 12-14 × 19-21 × 6-9[2] | |
|   16–20 years | 170 (150-200)[2] | | | |
|   20–65 years | 155[2] | | | |
|   >80 years | 100[2] | | | |
| *Central nervous system* | | | | |
| Brain | | +8.8%[1] | | See also Table B-3 |
|   Male | 1400[16] | | | |
|   Female | 1275[16] | | | |
| Pineal | 0.2[2] | | | |
| Spinal cord | 27[2] | | 45 cm (length)[2] | |
| Cerebrospinal fluid | | | | Average volume 150 mL[17] |

**Table B-2**  Adult normal heart weight in relation to body length

| Body length (cm) | Heart weight (g) | | Body length (cm) | Heart weight (g) | |
|---|---|---|---|---|---|
| | Males SD ± 40 g | Females SD ± 30 g | | Males SD ± 40 g | Females SD ± 30 g |
| 135 | 254 | 219 | 168 | 317 | 277 |
| 136 | 256 | 220 | 169 | 319 | 279 |
| 137 | 258 | 222 | 170 | 321 | 281 |
| 138 | 260 | 224 | 171 | 323 | 283 |
| 139 | 262 | 226 | 172 | 325 | 284 |
| 140 | 264 | 227 | 173 | 327 | 286 |
| 141 | 266 | 229 | 174 | 329 | 288 |
| 142 | 268 | 231 | 175 | 330 | 290 |
| 143 | 270 | 233 | 176 | 332 | 291 |
| 144 | 272 | 235 | 177 | 334 | 293 |
| 145 | 273 | 236 | 178 | 336 | 295 |
| 146 | 275 | 238 | 179 | 338 | 297 |
| 147 | 277 | 240 | 180 | 340 | 299 |
| 148 | 279 | 242 | 181 | 342 | 300 |
| 149 | 281 | 243 | 182 | 344 | 302 |
| 150 | 283 | 245 | 183 | 346 | 304 |
| 151 | 285 | 247 | 184 | 348 | 306 |
| 152 | 287 | 249 | 185 | 349 | 307 |
| 153 | 289 | 251 | 186 | 351 | 309 |
| 154 | 291 | 252 | 187 | 353 | 311 |
| 155 | 292 | 254 | 188 | 355 | 313 |
| 156 | 294 | 256 | 189 | 357 | 315 |
| 157 | 296 | 258 | 190 | 359 | 316 |
| 158 | 298 | 259 | 191 | 361 | 318 |
| 159 | 300 | 261 | 192 | 362 | 320 |
| 160 | 302 | 263 | 193 | 365 | 322 |
| 161 | 304 | 265 | 194 | 367 | 323 |
| 162 | 306 | 267 | 195 | 368 | 325 |
| 163 | 308 | 268 | 196 | 370 | 327 |
| 164 | 310 | 270 | 197 | 372 | 329 |
| 165 | 311 | 272 | 198 | 374 | 331 |
| 166 | 313 | 274 | 199 | 376 | 332 |
| 167 | 315 | 275 | 200 | 378 | 334 |

Data from Zeek PM: Heart weight, *Arch Pathol* 34:820-832, 1942.

| Table B-3 | Brain weight in males and females by age | | | | |
|---|---|---|---|---|---|
| | **Brain weight (g) males** | | | **Brain weight (g) females** | |
| Age (years) | Mean | Standard deviation | | Mean | Standard deviation |
| 0 (0-10 days) | 380 | 90 | | 360 | 80 |
| 0.5 (4-8 months) | 640 | 160 | | 580 | 120 |
| 1 (9-18 months) | 970 | 160 | | 940 | 120 |
| 2 (19-30 months) | 1120 | 200 | | 1040 | 130 |
| 3 (31-43 months) | 1270 | 210 | | 1090 | 230 |
| 4-5 | 1300 | 20 | | 1150 | 70 |
| 6-7 | 1330 | 10 | | 1210 | 30 |
| 8-9 | 1370 | 20 | | 1180 | 30 |
| 10-12 | 1440 | 10 | | 1260 | 40 |
| 13-15 | 1410 | 10 | | 1280 | 40 |
| 16-18 | 1440 | 30 | | 1340 | 40 |
| 19-21 | 1450 | 20 | | 1310 | 50 |
| 22-30 | 1440 | 20 | | 1300 | 10 |
| 31-40 | 1440 | 20 | | 1290 | 30 |
| 41-50 | 1430 | 20 | | 1290 | 20 |
| 51-55 | 1410 | 10 | | 1280 | 20 |
| 56-60 | 1370 | 20 | | 1250 | 20 |
| 61-65 | 1370 | 10 | | 1240 | 20 |
| 66-70 | 1360 | 10 | | 1240 | 20 |
| 71-75 | 1350 | 20 | | 1230 | 20 |
| 76-80 | 1330 | 20 | | 1190 | 10 |
| 81-85 | 1310 | 10 | | 1170 | 30 |
| 86+ | 1290 | 130 | | 1140 | 100 |

Data from Dekaban AS, Sadowsky D: Changes in brain weights during the span of human life: Relation of brain weights to body heights and body weights, *Ann Neurol* 4:345-356, 1978.

| Table B-4 | Weight, length, and organ weights in fetuses from 9 to 20 weeks of development | | | | | | | |
|---|---|---|---|---|---|---|---|---|---|
| Developmental age (days) | Weight (g) | Crown-rump length (cm) | Heart (g) | Lungs (g) | Liver (g) | Kidneys (g) | Adrenals (g) | Brain (g) | No. of cases |
| 63 | 11 | 3 | 0.1 | 0.1 | 0.2 | 0.1 | 0.1 | 1.2 | 30 |
| 67 | 13 | 4 | 0.2 | 0.3 | 0.7 | 0.1 | 0.1 | 1.5 | 27 |
| 71 | 15 | 6 | 0.2 | 0.4 | 0.8 | 0.1 | 0.1 | 2.6 | 15 |
| 73 | 20 | 7 | 0.3 | 0.4 | 1.1 | 0.2 | 0.1 | 4.3 | 21 |
| 76 | 25 | 7 | 0.4 | 0.7 | 1.1 | 0.2 | 0.2 | 4.8 | 14 |
| 79 | 30 | 8 | 0.4 | 1.0 | 1.3 | 0.2 | 0.2 | 5.4 | 15 |
| 84 | 35 | 9 | 0.5 | 1.4 | 2.0 | 0.3 | 0.2 | 6.2 | 14 |

| | | | | | | | | | |
|---|---|---|---|---|---|---|---|---|---|
| 89 | 45 | 9 | 0.5 | 1.9 | 2.5 | 0.4 | 0.4 | 7.4 | 22 |
| 90 | 50 | 10 | 0.5 | 1.9 | 3.0 | 0.5 | 0.5 | 8.5 | 23 |
| 91 | 60 | 10 | 0.5 | 2.5 | 3.4 | 0.6 | 0.6 | 10 | 21 |
| 92 | 70 | 11 | 0.6 | 3.0 | 3.6 | 0.8 | 0.6 | 11 | 24 |
| 96 | 80 | 11 | 0.7 | 3.0 | 4.3 | 0.8 | 0.6 | 12 | 7 |
| 100 | 90 | 12 | 0.9 | 3.0 | 4.7 | 0.9 | 0.7 | 14 | 15 |
| 105 | 100 | 12 | 1.1 | 3.9 | 5.6 | 1.4 | 0.7 | 17 | 28 |
| 109 | 125 | 13 | 1.3 | 4.1 | 7.4 | 1.4 | 0.7 | 23 | 21 |
| 115 | 150 | 14 | 1.4 | 5.3 | 9.2 | 1.4 | 0.8 | 23 | 20 |
| 117 | 175 | 14 | 1.4 | 5.6 | 11 | 1.8 | 0.8 | 23 | 27 |
| 118 | 200 | 15 | 1.7 | 7.2 | 12 | 2.2 | 1.1 | 33 | 39 |
| 124 | 250 | 16 | 2.2 | 9.1 | 15 | 2.7 | 1.2 | 39 | 37 |
| 130 | 300 | 17 | 2.4 | 10 | 17 | 3.1 | 1.5 | 46 | 43 |
| 133 | 350 | 18 | 2.9 | 11 | 21 | 3.8 | 2.0 | 54 | 31 |
| 143 | 400 | 18 | 3.4 | 11 | 23 | 4.2 | 2.2 | 61 | 32 |

Data from Valdés-Dapena M, Kalousek DK, Huff DS: Perinatal, fetal and embryonic autopsy. In Gilbert-Barness E, editor: *Potter's pathology of the fetus and infant,* St. Louis, 1997, Mosby, pp 483-524.

**Table B-5** Mean weights and measurements of fetuses of 8 to 26 weeks' gestation

| Gestation (wk) | Weight (g) | Crown-heel length (cm) | Crown-rump length (cm) | Foot length (cm) |
|---|---|---|---|---|
| 8 | 10 | 2 | — | — |
| 9 | 11 | 3 | — | — |
| 10 | 14 | 4 | — | — |
| 11 | 18 | 6 | 4 | 0.9 |
| 12 | 25 | 7 | 6 | 1.1 |
| 13 | 27 | 9 | 7 | 1.4 |
| 14 | 38 | 10 | 8 | 1.7 |
| 15 | 53 | 13 | 9 | 2.1 |
| 16 | 73 | 14 | 10 | 2.2 |
| 17 | 122 | 17 | 12 | 2.4 |
| 18 | 161 | 19 | 13 | 2.6 |
| 19 | 188 | 20 | 14 | 2.9 |
| 20 | 227 | 21 | 15 | 3.2 |
| 21 | 303 | 24 | 16 | 3.4 |
| 22 | 384 | 26 | 18 | 3.8 |
| 24 | 389 | 27 | 19 | 4.1 |
| 26 | 394 | 28 | 20 | 4.5 |

**Table B-6**    Expected weights ± standard deviations at various postmenstrual gestational ages

| Age (wk) | Body (g) | Brain (g) | Thymus (g) | Lungs, combined (g) | Heart (g) | Liver (g) | Spleen (g) | Adrenals, combined (g) | Pancreas (g) | Kidneys (g) |
|---|---|---|---|---|---|---|---|---|---|---|
| 12 | 20.9 ± 6.6 | 3.20 ± 1.44 | 0.01 ± 0.01 | 0.50 ± 0.28 | 0.15 ± 0.02 | 1.01 ± 0.38 | 0.01 ± 0.01 | 0.10 ± 0.03 | — | 0.16 ± 0.04 |
| 13 | 31.2 ± 10.1 | 5.19 ± 1.95 | 0.03 ± 0.01 | 1.08 ± 0.45 | 0.20 ± 0.06 | 1.38 ± 0.57 | 0.01 ± 0.01 | 0.15 ± 0.05 | — | 0.22 ± 0.07 |
| 14 | 49.1 ± 14.5 | 8.14 ± 2.58 | 0.05 ± 0.02 | 1.79 ± 0.67 | 0.31 ± 0.11 | 2.18 ± 0.84 | 0.03 ± 0.02 | 0.23 ± 0.08 | — | 0.36 ± 0.13 |
| 15 | 74.7 ± 19.8 | 12.0 ± 3.3 | 0.09 ± 0.04 | 2.64 ± 0.92 | 0.50 ± 0.17 | 3.41 ± 1.18 | 0.05 ± 0.03 | 0.33 ± 0.12 | — | 0.59 ± 0.19 |
| 16 | 108 ± 26 | 16.9 ± 4.2 | 0.14 ± 0.06 | 3.61 ± 1.21 | 0.76 ± 0.24 | 5.06 ± 1.60 | 0.09 ± 0.05 | 0.47 ± 0.16 | — | 0.90 ± 0.28 |
| 17 | 149 ± 33 | 22.8 ± 5.2 | 0.20 ± 0.08 | 4.70 ± 1.55 | 1.10 ± 0.31 | 7.14 ± 2.10 | 0.15 ± 0.07 | 0.64 ± 0.22 | — | 1.30 ± 0.39 |
| 18 | 197 ± 42 | 29.7 ± 6.3 | 0.28 ± 0.12 | 5.92 ± 1.92 | 1.50 ± 0.40 | 9.65 ± 2.66 | 0.21 ± 0.10 | 0.84 ± 0.30 | — | 1.79 ± 0.51 |
| 19 | 255 ± 51 | 37.2 ± 7.6 | 0.41 ± 0.17 | 7.30 ± 2.34 | 1.88 ± 0.49 | 12.8 ± 3.3 | 0.30 ± 0.14 | 1.03 ± 0.34 | — | 2.36 ± 0.65 |
| 20 | 319 ± 61 | 45.7 ± 8.9 | 0.54 ± 0.23 | 8.84 ± 2.80 | 2.41 ± 0.59 | 16.5 ± 4.0 | 0.41 ± 0.18 | 1.29 ± 0.41 | 0.50 ± 0.14 | 3.00 ± 0.81 |
| 21 | 389 ± 72 | 54.6 ± 10.4 | 0.72 ± 0.29 | 10.4 ± 3.3 | 2.89 ± 0.71 | 19.9 ± 4.8 | 0.54 ± 0.22 | 1.51 ± 0.49 | 0.54 ± 0.21 | 3.63 ± 0.99 |
| 22 | 452 ± 84 | 63.7 ± 12.0 | 0.92 ± 0.37 | 12.0 ± 3.8 | 3.38 ± 0.82 | 22.7 ± 5.7 | 0.66 ± 0.28 | 1.73 ± 0.57 | 0.60 ± 0.26 | 4.23 ± 1.18 |
| 23 | 510 ± 97 | 72.3 ± 13.8 | 1.15 ± 0.46 | 13.5 ± 4.4 | 3.81 ± 0.96 | 24.3 ± 6.5 | 0.75 ± 0.32 | 1.88 ± 0.66 | 0.68 ± 0.31 | 4.77 ± 1.39 |
| 24 | 579 ± 115 | 82.8 ± 15.6 | 1.38 ± 0.58 | 15.0 ± 5.0 | 4.23 ± 1.12 | 26.4 ± 7.1 | 0.91 ± 0.36 | 2.00 ± 0.074 | 0.77 ± 0.34 | 5.65 ± 1.63 |
| 25 | 660 ± 134 | 93.4 ± 17.4 | 1.63 ± 0.71 | 16.8 ± 5.6 | 4.80 ± 1.31 | 29.4 ± 7.8 | 1.11 ± 0.44 | 2.16 ± 0.82 | 0.85 ± 0.36 | 6.55 ± 1.91 |
| 26 | 744 ± 163 | 105 ± 19 | 1.96 ± 0.86 | 18.7 ± 6.2 | 5.50 ± 1.57 | 33.2 ± 8.8 | 1.38 ± 0.55 | 2.36 ± 0.90 | 0.92 ± 0.38 | 7.46 ± 2.21 |
| 27 | 839 ± 199 | 118 ± 21 | 2.37 ± 1.02 | 20.6 ± 6.8 | 6.28 ± 1.84 | 37.8 ± 9.9 | 1.78 ± 0.71 | 2.58 ± 0.99 | 1.10 ± 0.38 | 8.53 ± 2.53 |
| 28 | 946 ± 239 | 135 ± 24 | 2.85 ± 1.22 | 22.7 ± 7.3 | 7.13 ± 2.11 | 42.6 ± 11.5 | 2.26 ± 0.96 | 2.83 ± 1.10 | 1.08 ± 0.37 | 9.75 ± 2.85 |
| 29 | 1,064 ± 286 | 154 ± 26 | 3.44 ± 1.49 | 25.1 ± 7.9 | 7.95 ± 2.44 | 46.9 ± 13.3 | 2.73 ± 1.19 | 3.09 ± 1.21 | 1.14 ± 0.37 | 11.1 ± 3.2 |
| 30 | 1,211 ± 330 | 172 ± 30 | 4.02 ± 1.85 | 27.4 ± 8.4 | 8.84 ± 2.71 | 51.3 ± 14.8 | 3.20 ± 1.36 | 3.36 ± 1.34 | 1.27 ± 0.39 | 12.5 ± 3.7 |

| 31 | 1,351 ± 373 | 191 ± 33 | 4.52 ± 2.17 | 29.2 ± 8.8 | 9.83 ± 2.86 | 55.9 ± 15.8 | 3.74 ± 1.58 | 3.71 ± 1.42 | 1.46 ± 0.42 | 13.8 ± 4.0 |
|---|---|---|---|---|---|---|---|---|---|---|
| 32 | 1,492 ± 406 | 206 ± 35 | 4.91 ± 2.43 | 31.2 ± 9.0 | 10.8 ± 3.0 | 61.2 ± 17.0 | 4.37 ± 1.87 | 4.07 ± 1.50 | 1.77 ± 0.47 | 15.0 ± 4.4 |
| 33 | 1,650 ± 433 | 222 ± 36 | 5.40 ± 2.63 | 34.1 ± 9.4 | 11.9 ± 3.2 | 66.3 ± 18.8 | 5.06 ± 2.18 | 4.42 ± 1.56 | 1.95 ± 0.55 | 16.5 ± 4.9 |
| 34 | 1,832 ± 457 | 242 ± 37 | 6.03 ± 2.84 | 37.5 ± 10.1 | 13.1 ± 3.5 | 72.8 ± 20.9 | 5.76 ± 2.51 | 4.77 ± 1.63 | 2.11 ± 0.63 | 18.0 ± 5.3 |
| 35 | 2,040 ± 487 | 265 ± 39 | 6.87 ± 3.06 | 41.7 ± 11.0 | 14.5 ± 3.7 | 81.8 ± 22.3 | 6.47 ± 2.79 | 5.19 ± 1.76 | 2.36 ± 0.69 | 19.6 ± 5.7 |
| 36 | 2,246 ± 511 | 292 ± 42 | 7.85 ± 3.22 | 45.1 ± 12.2 | 16.0 ± 4.0 | 92.8 ± 22.9 | 7.21 ± 3.07 | 5.74 ± 1.92 | 2.61 ± 0.77 | 21.3 ± 6.0 |
| 37 | 2,424 ± 535 | 319 ± 44 | 8.95 ± 3.41 | 47.0 ± 13.2 | 17.6 ± 4.3 | 104 ± 23 | 8.11 ± 3.30 | 6.46 ± 2.10 | 2.84 ± 0.85 | 22.5 ± 6.4 |
| 38 | 2,603 ± 559 | 340 ± 46 | 9.61 ± 3.60 | 48.4 ± 14.0 | 18.6 ± 4.5 | 116 ± 26 | 9.15 ± 3.53 | 7.01 ± 2.31 | 3.04 ± 0.94 | 23.9 ± 6.8 |
| 39 | 2,787 ± 582 | 355 ± 49 | 9.98 ± 3.78 | 49.4 ± 14.8 | 19.4 ± 4.8 | 124 ± 29 | 9.83 ± 3.73 | 7.44 ± 2.55 | 3.33 ± 1.04 | 24.9 ± 7.1 |
| 40 | 2,942 ± 603 | 368 ± 51 | 10.2 ± 3.9 | 50.8 ± 15.5 | 20.3 ± 5.0 | 130 ± 32 | 10.2 ± 3.9 | 7.75 ± 2.82 | 3.65 ± 1.15 | 25.7 ± 7.5 |
| 41 | 3,098 ± 623 | 382 ± 53 | 10.2 ± 4.1 | 52.3 ± 16.1 | 21.3 ± 5.2 | 136 ± 36 | 10.5 ± 4.0 | 7.99 ± 3.11 | 4.01 ± 1.26 | 26.4 ± 7.8 |
| 42 | 3,267 ± 641 | 395 ± 55 | 10.1 ± 4.3 | 54.0 ± 16.5 | 22.4 ± 5.3 | 141 ± 40 | 10.8 ± 4.0 | 8.14 ± 3.44 | 4.40 ± 1.39 | 27.0 ± 8.2 |
| 43 | 3,444 ± 657 | 408 ± 57 | 9.83 ± 4.46 | 55.9 ± 16.8 | 23.6 ± 5.4 | 145 ± 45 | 10.9 ± 4.0 | 8.21 ± 3.79 | — | 27.6 ± 8.5 |
| 44 | 3,633 ± 6761 | 421 ± 59 | 9.44 ± 4.64 | 57.8 ± 16.9 | 24.8 ± 5.5 | 149 ± 50 | 11.1 ± 4.0 | 8.22 ± 4.17 | — | 28.3 ± 8.8 |

Data from Archie JG, Collins JS, Lebel RR: Quantitative standards for fetal and neonatal autopsy, *Am J Clin Pathol* 126:256-265, 2006.

**Table B-7** Expected linear measurements ± standard deviations at various postmenstrual gestational ages

| Age (wk) | CHL (mm) | CRL (mm) | HC (mm) | BPD (mm) | OCD (mm) | ICD (mm) | PL (mm) | CC (mm) | IND (mm) | AC (mm) | HL (mm) | FL (mm) | SIL (mm) | LIL (mm) |
|---|---|---|---|---|---|---|---|---|---|---|---|---|---|---|
| 12 | 93.0 ± 9.7 | 76.1 ± 6.7 | 67.7 ± 11.6 | 19.5 ± 3.5 | 14.0 ± 4.0 | 6.04 ± 1.55 | — | — | 14.1 ± 3.4 | — | — | 9.74 ± 1.11 | 194 | 20 |
| 13 | 114 ± 11 | 86.7 ± 7.8 | 82.1 ± 11.7 | 23.2 ± 3.6 | 16.7 ± 4.0 | 6.93 ± 1.56 | 2.80 | 76.7 | 16.3 ± 3.5 | 59.8 | 11.3 | 12.3 ± 1.1 | 282 | 39 |
| 14 | 134 ± 12 | 97.7 ± 8.8 | 96.2 ± 11.9 | 26.8 ± 3.6 | 19.3 ± 4.0 | 7.80 ± 1.57 | 3.09 | 86.1 | 18.5 ± 3.7 | 68.9 | 13.7 | 15.1 ± 1.1 | 370 | 58 |
| 15 | 154 ± 14 | 109 ± 10 | 110 ± 12 | 30.4 ± 2.7 | 21.9 ± 4.0 | 8.64 ± 1.58 | 3.39 | 95.4 | 20.7 ± 3.9 | 78.0 | 16.1 | 17.9 ± 1.1 | 458 | 77 |
| 16 | 174 ± 15 | 121 ± 11 | 123 ± 12 | 33.9 ± 3.8 | 24.4 ± 4.0 | 9.45 ± 1.59 | 3.68 | 105 | 22.9 ± 4.1 | 87.2 | 18.6 | 20.9 ± 1.2 | 547 | 96 |
| 17 | 193 ± 16 | 133 ± 11 | 136 ± 12 | 37.3 ± 3.8 | 26.8 ± 4.0 | 10.2 ± 1.6 | 3.98 | 114 | 25.0 ± 4.3 | 96.3 | 21.0 | 24.0 ± 1.2 | 635 | 115 |
| 18 | 212 ± 17 | 145 ± 12 | 149 ± 13 | 40.7 ± 3.9 | 29.2 ± 4.0 | 11.0 ± 1.6 | 4.27 | 124 | 27.2 ± 4.4 | 105 | 23.4 | 27.2 ± 1.4 | 723 | 134 |
| 19 | 230 ± 18 | 158 ± 13 | 161 ± 13 | 43.9 ± 4.0 | 31.5 ± 4.1 | 11.7 ± 1.6 | 4.57 | 133 | 29.4 ± 4.6 | 115 | 25.8 | 30.5 ± 1.5 | 811 | 152 |
| 20 | 247 ± 19 | 171 ± 14 | 173 ± 13 | 47.1 ± 4.1 | 33.8 ± 4.1 | 12.5 ± 1.6 | 4.86 | 142 | 31.6 ± 4.8 | 124 | 28.2 | 33.9 ± 1.7 | 900 | 171 |
| 21 | 264 ± 19 | 184 ± 14 | 185 ± 13 | 50.2 ± 4.1 | 35.9 ± 4.1 | 13.1 ± 1.7 | 5.16 | 152 | 33.8 ± 5.0 | 133 | 30.6 | 37.12 ± 1.9 | 988 | 190 |
| 22 | 278 ± 20 | 195 ± 15 | 196 ± 13 | 53.3 ± 4.2 | 38.1 ± 4.1 | 13.8 ± 1.7 | 5.45 | 161 | 36.0 ± 5.1 | 142 | 32.9 | 40.0 ± 2.1 | 1,076 | 209 |
| 23 | 291 ± 20 | 204 ± 15 | 207 ± 14 | 56.2 ± 4.3 | 40.1 ± 4.1 | 14.4 ± 1.7 | 5.75 | 170 | 38.2 ± 5.3 | 151 | 35.3 | 41.7 ± 2.4 | 1,164 | 228 |
| 24 | 303 ± 21 | 213 ± 16 | 218 ± 14 | 59.1 ± 4.3 | 42.1 ± 4.1 | 15.0 ± 1.7 | 6.04 | 180 | 40.4 ± 5.5 | 160 | 37.8 | 43.8 ± 2.6 | 1,253 | 247 |
| 25 | 316 ± 22 | 223 ± 17 | 228 ± 14 | 61.9 ± 4.4 | 44.0 ± 4.1 | 15.6 ± 1.7 | 6.33 | 189 | 42.6 ± 5.7 | 169 | 40.4 | 46.0 ± 3.0 | 1,341 | 266 |
| 26 | 328 ± 23 | 232 ± 18 | 238 ± 14 | 64.7 ± 4.5 | 45.9 ± 4.1 | 16.2 ± 1.7 | 6.63 | 199 | 44.8 ± 5.8 | 179 | 43.0 | 48.0 ± 3.5 | — | — |
| 27 | 340 ± 26 | 242 ± 19 | 248 ± 14 | 67.3 ± 4.5 | 47.7 ± 4.2 | 16.7 ± 1.7 | — | 208 | 47.0 ± 6.0 | — | 45.7 | 50.0 ± 3.9 | — | — |
| 28 | 351 ± 30 | 250 ± 21 | 257 ± 14 | 69.9 ± 4.6 | 49.4 ± 4.2 | 17.2 ± 1.7 | — | 217 | 49.2 ± 6.2 | — | 48.4 | 52.0 ± 4.3 | — | — |

| | | | | | | | | | | | | | | |
|---|---|---|---|---|---|---|---|---|---|---|---|---|---|---|
| 29 | 362 ± 33 | 259 ± 24 | 266 ± 15 | 72.4 ± 4.7 | 51.1 ± 4.2 | 17.7 ± 1.7 | — | 227 | 51.4 6.4 | — | 51.0 | 54.1 ± 4.9 | — | — |
| 30 | 374 ± 35 | 267 ± 27 | 275 ± 15 | 74.8 ± 4.8 | 52.7 ± 4.2 | 18.1 ± 1.8 | — | 236 | 53.5 ± 6.6 | — | 53.4 | 56.2 ± 5.4 | — | — |
| 31 | 386 ± 37 | 276 ± 30 | 283 ± 15 | 77.2 ± 4.8 | 54.2 ± 4.2 | 18.6 ± 1.8 | — | 245 | 55.7 ± 6.7 | — | 55.6 | 58.2 ± 6.0 | — | — |
| 32 | 397 ± 38 | 284 ± 32 | 291 ± 15 | 79.4 ± 4.9 | 55.7 ± 4.2 | 19.0 ± 1.8 | — | 255 | 57.9 ± 6.9 | — | 57.6 ± 2.1 | 60.4 ± 6.3 | — | — |
| 33 | 408 ± 40 | 292 ± 33 | 298 ± 15 | 81.6 ± 5.0 | 57.1 ± 4.2 | 19.3 ± 1.8 | — | 264 | 60.1 ± 7.1 | — | 59.2 ± 2.9 | 62.5 ± 6.4 | — | — |
| 34 | 419 ± 41 | 301 ± 33 | 306 ± 16 | 83.7 ± 5.0 | 58.5 ± 4.2 | 19.7 ± 1.8 | — | 274 | 62.3 ± 7.3 | — | 60.5 ± 4.1 | 64.7 ± 6.6 | — | — |
| 35 | 432 ± 43 | 310 ± 33 | 312 ± 16 | 85.8 ± 5.1 | 59.8 ± 4.2 | 20.0 ± 1.8 | — | 283 | 64.5 ± 7.4 | — | 61.9 ± 4.8 | 66.9 ± 6.7 | — | — |
| 36 | 444 ± 44 | 318 ± 33 | 319 ± 16 | 86.8 ± 5.2 | 61.0 ± 4.3 | 20.3 ± 1.8 | — | 292 | 66.7 ± 7.6 | — | 63.2 ± 5.1 | 69.2 ± 6.7 | — | — |
| 37 | 457 ± 44 | 327 ± 32 | 325 ± 16 | 89.6 ± 5.2 | 62.2 ± 4.3 | 20.6 ± 1.8 | — | 302 | 68.9 ± 7,8 | — | 64.4 ± 5.4 | 71.3 ± 6.7 | — | — |
| 38 | 470 ± 44 | 336 ± 32 | 331 ± 16 | 91.5 ± 5.3 | 63.3 ± 4.3 | 20.8 ± 1.9 | — | 311 | 71.1 ± 8.0 | — | 65.4 ± 5.5 | 73.4 ± 6.7 | — | — |
| 39 | 482 ± 44 | 344 ± 30 | 336 ± 17 | 93.2 ± 5.4 | 64.3 ± 4.3 | 21.0 ± 1.9 | — | 321 | 73.3 ± 8.1 | — | 66.3 ± 5.5 | 75.6 ± 6.7 | — | — |
| 40 | 493 ± 42 | 352 ± 29 | 342 ± 17 | 94.9 ± 5.5 | 65.3 ± 4.3 | 21.2 ± 1.9 | — | 330 | 75.5 ± 8.3 | — | 67.0 ± 5.3 | 77.8 ± 6.6 | — | — |
| 41 | 505 ± 41 | 360 ± 27 | 346 ± 17 | 96.4 ± 5.5 | 66.2 ± 4.3 | 21.4 ± 1.9 | — | — | 77.7 ± 8.5 | — | 67.6 ± 4.9 | 80.1 ± 6.4 | — | — |
| 42 | 516 ± 38 | 367 ± 25 | 351 ± 17 | 97.6 ± 5.6 | 67.0 ± 4.3 | 21.5 ± 1.9 | — | — | 79.9 ± 8.7 | — | 68.0 ± 4.2 | 82.5 ± 6.3 | — | — |

AC, Abdominal circumference; BPD, biparietal diameter; CC, chest circumference; CHL, crown-heel length; CRL, crown-rump length; FL, foot length; HC, head circumference; HL, hand length; ICD, inner canthal distance; IND, internipple distance; LIL, large intestine length; OCD, outer canthal distance; PL, philtrum length; SIL, small intestine length.

Data from Archie JG, Collins JS, Lebel RR: Quantitative standards for fetal and neonatal autopsy, Am J Clin Pathol 126:256-265, 2006.

**Table B-8** Means and standard deviations of body measurements and organ weights of stillborn infants, 20 to 42 weeks gestation

| Gestation (wk) | Body weight (g) | Crown-rump (cm) | Crown-heel (cm) | Toe-heel (cm) | Heart (g) | Lungs (g) | Liver (g) | Pancreas (g) | Kidneys (g) | Adrenals (g) | Thymus (g) | Spleen (g) | Brain (g) |
|---|---|---|---|---|---|---|---|---|---|---|---|---|---|
| 20 | 313 ± 139 | 18.0 ± 2.0 | 24.9 ± 2.3 | 3.3 ± 0.6 | 2.4 ± 1.0 | 7.1 ± 3.0 | 17 ± 9 | 0.5 ± 0.1 | 2.7 ± 2.9 | 1.3 ± 0.6 | 0.4 ± 0.3 | 0.3 ± 1.0 | 41 ± 24 |
| 21 | 353 ± 125 | 18.9 ± 4.8 | 26.2 ± 3.6 | 3.5 ± 0.6 | 2.6 ± 0.9 | 7.9 ± 3.8 | 18 ± 7 | 0.5 ± 0.4 | 3.1 ± 1.3 | 1.4 ± 0.7 | 0.5 ± 0.3 | 0.4 ± 0.6 | 48 ± 18 |
| 22 | 398 ± 117 | 19.8 ± 9.6 | 27.4 ± 2.5 | 3.8 ± 0.4 | 2.8 ± 0.9 | 8.7 ± 3.1 | 19 ± 10 | 0.6 ± 0.5 | 3.5 ± 0.8 | 1.4 ± 0.6 | 0.6 ± 0.4 | 0.5 ± 0.4 | 55 ± 15 |
| 23 | 450 ± 118 | 20.6 ± 2.3 | 28.7 ± 3.3 | 4 ± 0.5 | 3 ± 1.4 | 9.5 ± 5.7 | 21 ± 7 | 0.7 ± 0.3 | 4.1 ± 1.7 | 1.5 ± 0.8 | 0.8 ± 0.5 | 0.7 ± 0.5 | 64 ± 18 |
| 24 | 510 ± 179 | 21.5 ± 3.1 | 29.9 ± 4.3 | 4.2 ± 0.8 | 3.3 ± 1.8 | 10.5 ± 5.6 | 22 ± 8 | 0.7 ± 0.3 | 4.6 ± 2.4 | 1.5 ± 0.8 | 0.9 ± 0.7 | 0.9 ± 0.7 | 74 ± 25 |
| 25 | 581 ± 178 | 22.3 ± 4.0 | 31.1 ± 6.5 | 4.4 ± 0.8 | 3.7 ± 1.3 | 11.6 ± 4.9 | 24 ± 35 | 0.8 ± 0.7 | 5.3 ± 2.4 | 1.6 ± 0.8 | 1.1 ± 0.8 | 1.2 ± 0.4 | 85 ± 31 |
| 26 | 663 ± 227 | 23.2 ± 4.1 | 32.4 ± 5.3 | 4.7 ± 0.9 | 4.2 ± 2.2 | 12.9 ± 8.7 | 26 ± 16 | 0.8 ± 0.7 | 6.1 ± 3.6 | 1.7 ± 0.9 | 1.4 ± 1.4 | 1.5 ± 1.1 | 98 ± 37 |
| 27 | 758 ± 227 | 24.1 ± 2.9 | 33.6 ± 3.2 | 4.9 ± 1.4 | 4.8 ± 3.6 | 14.4 ± 9.7 | 29 ± 24 | 0.9 ± 0.3 | 7 ± 3.1 | 1.9 ± 1.5 | 1.7 ± 1.1 | 1.9 ± 1.0 | 112 ± 37 |
| 28 | 864 ± 247 | 24.9 ± 2.2 | 34.9 ± 5.6 | 5.1 ± 1.2 | 5.4 ± 2.6 | 16.1 ± 7.0 | 32 ± 32 | 1 ± 0.3 | 7.9 ± 2.5 | 2.1 ± 1.6 | 2 ± 2.1 | 2.3 ± 1.1 | 127 ± 39 |
| 29 | 984 ± 511 | 25.8 ± 4.1 | 36.1 ± 5.9 | 5.3 ± 1.2 | 6.2 ± 2.4 | 18 ± 13.6 | 36 ± 23 | 1.1 ± 1.2 | 9 ± 4.5 | 2.4 ± 1.2 | 2.4 ± 2.6 | 2.7 ± 2.0 | 143 ± 57 |
| 30 | 1115 ± 329 | 26.6 ± 2.4 | 37.3 ± 3.6 | 5.6 ± 0.7 | 7 ± 2.8 | 20.1 ± 8.6 | 40 ± 22 | 1.2 ± 0.2 | 10.1 ± 6.0 | 2.7 ± 1.3 | 2.8 ± 4.1 | 3.1 ± 1.5 | 160 ± 72 |
| 31 | 1259 ± 588 | 27.5 ± 3.0 | 38.6 ± 2.7 | 5.8 ± 0.7 | 8 ± 3.1 | 22.5 ± 10.1 | 46 ± 38 | 1.4 ± 1.4 | 11.3 ± 4.1 | 3 ± 1.8 | 3.2 ± 1.9 | 3.6 ± 4.0 | 178 ± 32 |
| 32 | 1413 ± 623 | 28.4 ± 2.8 | 39.8 ± 5.4 | 6 ± 0.6 | 9.1 ± 4.1 | 25 ± 10.7 | 52 ± 32 | 1.6 ± 0.6 | 12.6 ± 8.0 | 3.5 ± 1.8 | 3.7 ± 2.2 | 4.2 ± 2.4 | 196 ± 92 |
| 33 | 1578 ± 254 | 29.2 ± 3.5 | 41.1 ± 3.1 | 6.2 ± 0.4 | 10.2 ± 2.0 | 27.8 ± 5.8 | 58 ± 17 | 1.8 ± 0.8 | 13.9 ± 3.5 | 3.9 ± 1.4 | 4.3 ± 1.5 | 4.7 ± 2.3 | 216 ± 51 |
| 34 | 1750 ± 494 | 30.1 ± 3.5 | 42.3 ± 4.3 | 6.5 ± 0.8 | 11.4 ± 3.2 | 30.7 ± 15.2 | 66 ± 22 | 2 ± 0.5 | 15.3 ± 5.1 | 4.4 ± 1.3 | 4.8 ± 5.6 | 5.3 ± 2.5 | 236 ± 42 |
| 35 | 1930 ± 865 | 30.9 ± 3.9 | 43.5 ± 5.8 | 6.7 ± 0.9 | 12.6 ± 5.3 | 33.7 ± 14.3 | 74 ± 46 | 2.3 ± 0.7 | 16.7 ± 7.1 | 4.9 ± 1.9 | 5.4 ± 3.4 | 5.9 ± 6.8 | 256 ± 70 |
| 36 | 2114 ± 616 | 31.8 ± 4.0 | 44.8 ± 7.2 | 6.9 ± 0.8 | 13.9 ± 5.8 | 36.7 ± 16.8 | 82 ± 36 | 2.6 ± 2.6 | 18.1 ± 6.3 | 5.4 ± 2.4 | 6.1 ± 4.1 | 6.5 ± 2.9 | 277 ± 94 |
| 37 | 2300 ± 647 | 32.7 ± 5.1 | 46 ± 7.9 | 7.2 ± 0.9 | 15.1 ± 9.9 | 39.8 ± 11.1 | 91 ± 57 | 2.9 ± 3.1 | 19.4 ± 9.7 | 5.8 ± 6.2 | 6.7 ± 3.9 | 7.2 ± 6.3 | 297 ± 69 |
| 38 | 2485 ± 579 | 33.5 ± 2.6 | 47.3 ± 3.9 | 7.4 ± 0.8 | 16.4 ± 4.4 | 42.9 ± 15.7 | 100 ± 44 | 3.2 ± 1.6 | 20.8 ± 6.0 | 6.3 ± 2.1 | 7.4 ± 6.1 | 7.8 ± 5.9 | 317 ± 83 |
| 39 | 2667 ± 596 | 34.4 ± 3.7 | 48.5 ± 4.9 | 7.6 ± 0.5 | 17.5 ± 3.9 | 45.8 ± 15.2 | 109 ± 53 | 3.5 ± 1.9 | 22 ± 5.8 | 6.7 ± 5.3 | 8.1 ± 4.7 | 8.5 ± 4.5 | 337 ± 132 |
| 40 | 2842 ± 482 | 35.2 ± 6.4 | 49.7 ± 3.2 | 7.8 ± 0.7 | 18.6 ± 12.9 | 48.6 ± 19.4 | 118 ± 49 | 3.9 ± 1.7 | 23.1 ± 8.6 | 7 ± 2.9 | 8.9 ± 4.3 | 9.2 ± 4.1 | 355 ± 57 |
| 41 | 3006 ± 761 | 36.1 ± 3.7 | 51 ± 5.4 | 8.1 ± 0.8 | 19.5 ± 4.9 | 51.1 ± 17.0 | 126 ± 53 | 4.2 | 24.1 ± 10.5 | 7.1 ± 3.0 | 9.6 ± 5.6 | 9.9 ± 4.5 | 373 ± 141 |
| 42 | 3156 ± 678 | 36.9 ± 2.0 | 52.2 ± 3.0 | 8.3 ± 0.5 | 20.3 ± 4.5 | 53.2 ± 10.1 | 135 ± 54 | 4.5 ± 2.3 | 24.9 ± 8.1 | 7.2 ± 2.9 | 10.4 ± 5.0 | 10.6 ± 3.7 | 389 ± 36 |

Compiled October 1, 1988, by Sung CJ, Singer DB, with 1975-1984 data from Women and Infants' Hospital, Providence, RI.

**Table B-9** Means and standard deviations of measurements and organ weights of live-born infants, 20 to 42 weeks gestation

| Gestation (wk) | Body Weight (g) | Crown-Rump (cm) | Crown-Heel (cm) | Toe-Heel (cm) | Heart (g) | Lungs (g) | Liver (g) | Pancreas (g) | Kidneys (g) | Adrenals (g) | Thymus (g) | Spleen (g) | Brain (g) |
|---|---|---|---|---|---|---|---|---|---|---|---|---|---|
| 20 | 381 ± 104 | 18.3 ± 2.2 | 25.6 ± 2.2 | 3.6 ± 0.7 | 2.8 ± 1.0 | 11.5 ± 2.9 | 22.4 ± 8.0 | 0.5 ± 0.5 | 3.7 ± 1.3 | 1.8 ± 1.0 | 0.8 ± 2.3 | 0.7 ± 0.3 | 49 ± 15 |
| 21 | 426 ± 66 | 19.1 ± 1.2 | 26.7 ± 1.7 | 3.8 ± 0.1 | 3.2 ± 0.4 | 12.9 ± 2.8 | 24.1 ± 4.2 | 0.5 | 4.2 ± 0.7 | 2 ± 0.5 | 1 ± 0.3 | 0.7 ± 0.2 | 57 ± 8 |
| 22 | 473 ± 63 | 20 ± 1.3 | 27.8 ± 1.6 | 4 ± 0.4 | 3.5 ± 0.6 | 14.4 ± 4.3 | 25.4 ± 5.2 | 0.6 ± 0.3 | 4.7 ± 1.5 | 2 ± 0.6 | 1.2 ± 0.3 | 0.8 ± 0.4 | 65 ± 13 |
| 23 | 524 ± 116 | 20.8 ± 1.9 | 28.9 ± 3.0 | 4.2 ± 0.5 | 3.9 ± 1.3 | 15.9 ± 4.9 | 26.6 ± 8.0 | 0.7 ± 0.4 | 5.3 ± 1.8 | 2.1 ± 0.8 | 1.4 ± 0.7 | 0.8 ± 0.4 | 74 ± 11 |
| 24 | 584 ± 92 | 21.6 ± 1.4 | 30 ± 1.7 | 4.4 ± 0.3 | 4.2 ± 1.0 | 17.4 ± 5.9 | 28 ± 7.1 | 0.8 ± 0.5 | 6 ± 1.8 | 2.2 ± 0.8 | 1.5 ± 0.7 | 0.9 ± 0.5 | 83 ± 15 |
| 25 | 655 ± 106 | 22.5 ± 1.6 | 31.1 ± 2.0 | 4.6 ± 0.4 | 4.7 ± 1.2 | 19 ± 5.3 | 29.7 ± 9.8 | 0.9 ± 0.3 | 6.8 ± 1.9 | 2.2 ± 1.4 | 1.8 ± 1.2 | 1.1 ± 1.6 | 94 ± 25 |
| 26 | 739 ± 181 | 23.3 ± 1.9 | 32.2 ± 2.4 | 4.8 ± 0.7 | 5.2 ± 1.3 | 20.6 ± 6.3 | 32.1 ± 10.9 | 1 ± 0.5 | 7.6 ± 2.5 | 2.4 ± 1.1 | 2 ± 1.1 | 1.3 ± 0.7 | 105 ± 21 |
| 27 | 836 ± 197 | 24.2 ± 2.5 | 33.4 ± 3.5 | 5 ± 0.5 | 5.8 ± 1.9 | 22.1 ± 9.7 | 35.1 ± 13.3 | 1.2 ± 0.5 | 8.6 ± 3.0 | 2.5 ± 1.1 | 2.3 ± 1.2 | 1.7 ± 1.0 | 118 ± 21 |
| 28 | 949 ± 190 | 25 ± 1.7 | 34.5 ± 2.3 | 5.2 ± 0.6 | 6.5 ± 1.9 | 23.7 ± 10.0 | 38.9 ± 12.6 | 1.4 ± 0.5 | 9.7 ± 12.0 | 2.7 ± 1.2 | 2.6 ± 1.5 | 2.1 ± 0.8 | 132 ± 29 |
| 29 | 1077 ± 449 | 25.9 ± 2.8 | 35.6 ± 4.4 | 5.4 ± 0.8 | 7.2 ± 2.7 | 25.3 ± 12.6 | 43.5 ± 15.8 | 1.5 ± 1.0 | 10.9 ± 4.4 | 3 ± 1.2 | 3 ± 1.9 | 2.6 ± 0.9 | 147 ± 49 |
| 30 | 1219 ± 431 | 26.7 ± 3.3 | 36.7 ± 4.2 | 5.7 ± 0.7 | 8.1 ± 2.6 | 26.9 ± 20.3 | 49.1 ± 18.8 | 1.7 ± 1.0 | 12.3 ± 8.5 | 3.3 ± 2.7 | 3.5 ± 2.6 | 3.3 ± 2.0 | 163 ± 38 |
| 31 | 1375 ± 281 | 27.6 ± 3.8 | 37.8 ± 3.1 | 5.9 ± 0.7 | 9 ± 2.8 | 28.5 ± 13.2 | 55.4 ± 17.3 | 1.8 ± 0.6 | 13.7 ± 5.2 | 3.7 ± 1.3 | 4 ± 3.4 | 4 ± 1.2 | 180 ± 34 |
| 32 | 1543 ± 519 | 28.4 ± 9.5 | 38.9 ± 5.7 | 6.1 ± 1.1 | 10.1 ± 4.4 | 30.2 ± 19.0 | 62.5 ± 30.0 | 2 ± 0.8 | 15.2 ± 7.4 | 4.1 ± 1.7 | 4.7 ± 3.6 | 4.7 ± 5.4 | 198 ± 48 |
| 33 | 1720 ± 580 | 29.3 ± 3.3 | 40 ± 3.5 | 6.3 ± 0.7 | 11.2 ± 4.0 | 31.8 ± 13.5 | 70.3 ± 25.4 | 2.1 ± 0.8 | 16.8 ± 7.7 | 4.6 ± 1.5 | 5.4 ± 3.2 | 5.5 ± 3.5 | 217 ± 49 |
| 34 | 1905 ± 625 | 30.1 ± 4.3 | 41.1 ± 4.0 | 6.5 ± 0.6 | 12.4 ± 2.8 | 33.5 ± 16.5 | 78.7 ± 30.2 | 2.3 ± 1.1 | 18.5 ± 9.3 | 5.1 ± 2.2 | 6.1 ± 3.8 | 6.4 ± 3.0 | 237 ± 53 |
| 35 | 2093 ± 309 | 30.9 ± 2.0 | 42.3 ± 2.9 | 6.7 ± 0.4 | 13.7 ± 3.6 | 35.2 ± 20.5 | 87.4 ± 30.6 | 2.5 ± 0.6 | 20.1 ± 10.9 | 5.6 ± 2.8 | 6.9 ± 4.5 | 7.2 ± 5.2 | 257 ± 45 |
| 36 | 2280 ± 615 | 31.8 ± 3.9 | 43.4 ± 5.9 | 6.9 ± 1.1 | 15 ± 5.1 | 36.9 ± 17.5 | 96.3 ± 33.7 | 2.6 ± 0.7 | 21.7 ± 6.8 | 6.1 ± 3.1 | 7.7 ± 5.0 | 8.1 ± 3.1 | 278 ± 96 |
| 37 | 2462 ± 821 | 32.6 ± 5.0 | 44.5 ± 7.0 | 7.1 ± 1.2 | 16.4 ± 5.7 | 38.7 ± 22.9 | 105.1 ± 33.7 | 2.8 ± 0.9 | 23.3 ± 9.9 | 6.6 ± 3.3 | 8.4 ± 5.6 | 8.8 ± 6.4 | 298 ± 70 |
| 38 | 2634 ± 534 | 33.5 ± 3.2 | 45.6 ± 5.1 | 7.3 ± 0.8 | 17.7 ± 5.4 | 40.6 ± 17.1 | 113.5 ± 34.7 | 3 ± 1.1 | 24.8 ± 7.2 | 7.1 ± 2.9 | 9 ± 2.8 | 9.5 ± 3.5 | 318 ± 106 |
| 39 | 2789 ± 520 | 34.3 ± 1.9 | 46.7 ± 4.4 | 7.5 ± 0.5 | 19.1 ± 2.8 | 42.6 ± 14.9 | 121.3 ± 39.2 | 3.3 ± 0.5 | 26.1 ± 4.9 | 7.4 ± 2.5 | 9.4 ± 2.5 | 10.1 ± 3.5 | 337 ± 91 |
| 40 | 2922 ± 450 | 35.2 ± 2.8 | 47.8 ± 4.2 | 7.7 ± 0.8 | 20.4 ± 5.6 | 44.6 ± 22.7 | 127.9 ± 35.8 | 3.6 ± 1.3 | 27.3 ± 11.5 | 7.7 ± 3.0 | 9.5 ± 5.0 | 10.4 ± 3.3 | 356 ± 79 |
| 41 | 3025 ± 600 | 36 ± 3.1 | 48.9 ± 5.4 | 7.9 ± 0.8 | 21.7 ± 10.9 | 46.8 ± 26.2 | 133.1 ± 55.7 | 3.9 ± 1.5 | 28.1 ± 12.7 | 7.8 ± 2.8 | 9.1 ± 4.8 | 10.5 ± 4.5 | 372 ± 65 |
| 42 | 3091 ± 617 | 36.9 ± 2.4 | 50 ± 3.8 | 8.1 ± 1.1 | 22.9 ± 6.2 | 49.1 ± 14.6 | 136.4 ± 38.9 | 4.3 ± 1.9 | 28.7 ± 9.7 | 7.8 ± 3.2 | 8.1 ± 3.8 | 10.3 ± 3.6 | 387 ± 61 |

Compiled October 1, 1988, by Sung CJ, Singer DB, with 1975-1984 data from Women and Infants' Hospital, Providence, RI.

| Table B-10 | Organ weight (g) in relation to total body weight (g) | | | | | | | | |
|---|---|---|---|---|---|---|---|---|---|
| | **Total Body Weight** | | | | | | | | |
| | **500-999** | **1000-1499** | **1500-1999** | **2000-2499** | **2500-2999** | **3000-3499** | **3500-3999** | **4000-4499** | **≥4500** |
| Thyroid | 0.8 | 0.8 | 0.9 | 1.1 | 1.3 | 1.6 | 1.7 | 1.9 | 2.4 |
| Thymus | 2.1 | 4.3 | 6.6 | 8.2 | 9.3 | 11.0 | 12.6 | 14.3 | 17.3 |
| Both lungs | 18.2 | 27.1 | 37.9 | 43.6 | 48.9 | 54.9 | 58.0 | 65.8 | 74.0 |
| Heart | 5.8 | 9.4 | 12.7 | 15.5 | 19.0 | 21.2 | 23.4 | 28.0 | 36.0 |
| Spleen | 1.7 | 3.4 | 4.9 | 7.0 | 9.1 | 10.4 | 12.0 | 13.6 | 16.7 |
| Pancreas | 1.0 | 1.4 | 2.0 | 2.3 | 3.0 | 3.5 | 4.0 | 4.6 | 6.2 |
| Both kidneys | 7.1 | 12.2 | 16.2 | 19.9 | 23.0 | 25.3 | 28.5 | 31.0 | 33.2 |
| Both adrenals | 3.1 | 3.9 | 5.0 | 6.3 | 8.2 | 9.8 | 10.7 | 12.5 | 15.1 |
| Brain | 108.7 | 179.5 | 255.6 | 307.6 | 358.7 | 403.3 | 420.6 | 424.1 | 406.2 |
| Liver | 38.8 | 59.8 | 76.3 | 98.1 | 127.4 | 155.1 | 178.1 | 215.2 | 275.6 |

Data from Valdés-Dapena M, Kalousek DK, Huff DS: Perinatal, fetal and embryonic autopsy. In Gilbert-Barness E, editor: *Potter's pathology of the fetus and infant,* St. Louis, Mosby, 1997, pp 483-524.

| Table B-11 | Means and standard deviations of body length and weights of organs of male infants, 1 to 12 months | | | | | | | | | | |
|---|---|---|---|---|---|---|---|---|---|---|---|
| Age (mo) | Body length (cm) | Heart (g) | Lungs, combined (g) | Liver (g) | Pancreas (g) | Kidneys, combined (g) | Adrenal glands, combined (g) | Thymus (g) | Spleen (g) | Brain (g) | No. of cases |
| 1 | 51.4 ± 3.2 | 23 ± 7 | 64 ± 21 | 140 ± 40 | 6.2 ± 3.6 | 34 ± 9 | 5.1 ± 1.7 | 7.8 ± 5.3 | 12 ± 4 | 460 ± 47 | 56 |
| 2 | 54.0 ± 2.9 | 27 ± 7 | 74 ± 26 | 100 ± 46 | 7.2 ± 4.4 | 39 ± 9 | 5.0 ± 1.6 | 9.4 ± 4.4 | 15 ± 5 | 506 ± 67 | 53 |
| 3 | 57.7 ± 2.9 | 30 ± 7 | 89 ± 23 | 179 ± 41 | 7.7 ± 3.1 | 45 ± 10 | 5.0 ± 1.3 | 10 ± 5 | 16 ± 5 | 567 ± 81 | 43 |
| 4 | 60.4 ± 4.1 | 31 ± 7 | 96 ± 27 | 195 ± 41 | 11 ± 5 | 47 ± 12 | 4.9 ± 2.0 | 10 ± 6 | 17 ± 5 | 620 ± 71 | 42 |
| 5 | 62.0 ± 3.1 | 35 ± 5 | 93 ± 18 | 228 ± 47 | 11 ± 4 | 54 ± 11 | 5.3 ± 1.9 | 12 ± 7 | 18 ± 7 | 746 ± 91 | 40 |
| 6 | 64.2 ± 3.9 | 40 ± 8 | 115 ± 31 | 259 ± 58 | 11 ± 5 | 62 ± 14 | 5.2 ± 2.0 | 10 ± 6 | 20 ± 7 | 762 ± 73 | 47 |
| 7 | 66.7 ± 5.0 | 43 ± 8 | 118 ± 33 | 276 ± 54 | 12 ± 6 | 69 ± 14 | 5.5 ± 2.1 | 12 ± 9 | 23 ± 10 | 767 ± 32 | 27 |
| 8 | 68.2 ± 3.4 | 44 ± 8 | 104 ± 32 | 285 ± 57 | 13 ± 7 | 66 ± 14 | 5.4 ± 2.3 | 10 ± 6 | 20 ± 7 | 774 ± 95 | 27 |
| 9 | 69.4 ± 4.2 | 45 ± 7 | 109 ± 33 | 288 ± 47 | 16 ± 7 | 67 ± 16 | 5.4 ± 2.0 | 10 ± 4 | 22 ± 5 | 820 ± 49 | 25 |
| 10 | 69.7 ± 5.9 | 46 ± 6 | 110 ± 34 | 300 ± 69 | 14 ± 6 | 72 ± 17 | 5.7 ± 2.1 | 9 ± 5 | 24 ± 11 | 850 ± 96 | 20 |
| 11 | 70.5 ± 4.3 | 48 ± 7 | 130 ± 31 | 305 ± 81 | 16 ± 3 | 76 ± 19 | 6.1 ± 1.8 | 19 ± 4 | 28 ± 10 | 875 ± 89 | 16 |
| 12 | 73.8 ± 4.1 | 50 ± 6 | 116 ± 23 | 325 ± 39 | 14 ± 6 | 76 ± 13 | 6.3 ± 2.2 | 12 ± 5 | 28 ± 7 | 954 ± 35 | 19 |

Data from Schulz DM, Giordano DA, Schulz DH: Weights of organs of fetuses and infants, *Arch Pathol* 74:244–250, 1962.

**Table B-12**    Means and standard deviations of body length and weights of organs of female infants, 1 to 12 months

| Age (mo) | Body length (cm) | Heart (g) | Lungs, combined (g) | Liver (g) | Pancreas (g) | Kidneys, combined (g) | Adrenal glands, combined (g) | Thymus (g) | Spleen (g) | Brain (g) | No. of cases |
|---|---|---|---|---|---|---|---|---|---|---|---|
| 1 | 51.9 ± 4.5 | 21 ± 5 | 64 ± 27 | 139 ± 31 | 5.0 ± 1.8 | 31 ± 8 | 4.8 ± 1.9 | 6.6 ± 4.9 | 11 ± 4 | 433 ± 59 | 28 |
| 2 | 54.0 ± 3.7 | 26 ± 6 | 74 ± 23 | 159 ± 31 | 7.1 ± 2.9 | 36 ± 10 | 4.7 ± 1.4 | 5.8 ± 4.7 | 14 ± 5 | 490 ± 51 | 39 |
| 3 | 57.0 ± 3.7 | 28 ± 4 | 81 ± 14 | 183 ± 39 | 8.5 ± 3.2 | 42 ± 12 | 4.8 ± 1.4 | 9.7 ± 6.9 | 15 ± 5 | 525 ± 89 | 36 |
| 4 | 59.0 ± 3.7 | 30 ± 6 | 91 ± 24 | 204 ± 49 | 9.0 ± 3.0 | 50 ± 11 | 4.6 ± 2.1 | 9.0 ± 7.3 | 17 ± 5 | 595 ± 80 | 29 |
| 5 | 62.2 ± 3.3 | 36 ± 5 | 102 ± 22 | 227 ± 38 | 11 ± 3 | 52 ± 13 | 4.8 ± 2.2 | 13 ± 5 | 19 ± 5 | 725 ± 62 | 24 |
| 6 | 63.0 ± 3.0 | 37 ± 7 | 111 ± 30 | 242 ± 58 | 11 ± 4 | 58 ± 20 | 4.6 ± 1.6 | 10 ± 6 | 18 ± 8 | 730 ± 85 | 23 |
| 7 | 65.4 ± 4.2 | 40 ± 9 | 111 ± 38 | 272 ± 51 | 10 ± 3 | 65 ± 14 | 5.5 ± 2.2 | 10 ± 8 | 22 ± 8 | 750 ± 92 | 21 |
| 8 | 60.5 ± 4.5 | 41 ± 7 | 109 ± 35 | 276 ± 54 | 11 ± 5 | 60 ± 13 | 5.3 ± 2.3 | 8 ± 5 | 20 ± 9 | 770 ± 96 | 24 |
| 9 | 68.3 ± 4.7 | 41 ± 5 | 105 ± 28 | 288 ± 67 | 14 ± 5 | 62 ± 10 | 5.4 ± 1.5 | 9 ± 5 | 18 ± 6 | 810 ± 82 | 15 |
| 10 | 67.5 ± 4.2 | 43 ± 7 | 105 ± 21 | 284 ± 48 | 13 ± 6 | 66 ± 10 | 0.7 ± 1.7 | 12 ± 7 | 25 ± 11 | 830 ± 117 | 14 |
| 11 | 70.5 ± 3.1 | 44 ± 8 | 125 ± 31 | 292 ± 36 | 14 ± 7 | 68 ± 14 | 6.2 ± 2.0 | 15 ± 8 | 23 ± 9 | 875 ± 64 | 18 |
| 12 | 71.5 ± 4.7 | 49 ± 6 | 115 ± 34 | 315 ± 38 | 15 ± 8 | 72 ± 19 | 6.0 ± 1.4 | 11 ± 8 | 27 ± 9 | 886 ± 64 | 15 |

Data from Schulz DM, Giordano DA, Schulz DH: Weights of organs of fetuses and infants, *Arch Pathol* 74:244-250, 1962.

**Table B-13**    Lung weight/body weight (± standard deviations) during gestation

| Age (wks) | Lung weight/body weight (%) |
|---|---|
| 16-19 | 3.14 ± 0.84 |
| 20-23 | 2.98 ± 0.73 |
| 24-27 | 3.15 ± 0.47 |
| 28-36 | 2.55 ± 0.27 |
| 37-41 | 1.79 ± 0.44 |

Data from De Paepe ME, Friedman RM, Gundogan F, Pinar H: Postmortem lung weight/body weight standards for term and preterm infants, *Pediatr Pulmonol* 40:445-448, 2005.

**Table B-14**  Organ weights of children

| Age | Body length (cm) | Heart (g) | Lungs Right (g) | Lungs Left (g) | Liver (g) | Kidneys Right (g) | Kidneys Left (g) | Prostate (g)* | Testes, combined (g)* | Uterus (g)* | Ovaries, combined (g)* | Spleen (g) | Brain (g) |
|---|---|---|---|---|---|---|---|---|---|---|---|---|---|
| Birth-3 days | 49 | 17 | 21 | 18 | 78 | 13 | 14 | 0.9 | 0.4 | 4.6 | 0.4 | 8 | 335 |
| 3-7 days | 49 | 18 | 24 | 22 | 96 | 14 | 14 | | | | | 9 | 358 |
| 1-3 weeks | 52 | 19 | 29 | 26 | 123 | 15 | 15 | | | | | 10 | 382 |
| 3-5 weeks | 52 | 20 | 31 | 27 | 127 | 16 | 16 | | | | | 12 | 413 |
| 5-7 weeks | 53 | 21 | 32 | 28 | 133 | 19 | 18 | | | | | 13 | 422 |
| 7-9 weeks | 55 | 23 | 32 | 29 | 136 | 19 | 18 | | | | | 13 | 489 |
| 9-12 weeks | 56 | 23 | 35 | 30 | 140 | 20 | 19 | | | | | 14 | 516 |
| 4 months | 59 | 27 | 37 | 33 | 160 | 22 | 21 | | | | | 16 | 540 |
| 5 months | 61 | 29 | 38 | 35 | 188 | 25 | 25 | | | | | 16 | 644 |
| 6 months | 62 | 31 | 42 | 39 | 200 | 26 | 25 | | | | | 17 | 660 |
| 7 months | 65 | 34 | 49 | 41 | 227 | 30 | 30 | | | | | 19 | 691 |
| 8 months | 65 | 37 | 52 | 45 | 254 | 31 | 30 | | | | | 20 | 714 |
| 9 months | 67 | 37 | 53 | 47 | 260 | 31 | 30 | | | | | 20 | 750 |
| 10 months | 69 | 39 | 54 | 51 | 274 | 32 | 31 | | | | | 22 | 809 |
| 11 months | 70 | 40 | 59 | 53 | 277 | 34 | 33 | | | | | 25 | 852 |
| 12 months | 73 | 44 | 64 | 57 | 288 | 36 | 35 | 1.2 | 1.4 | 2.3 | 1.0 | 26 | 925 |
| 14 months | 74 | 45 | 66 | 60 | 304 | 36 | 35 | | | | | 26 | 944 |
| 16 months | 77 | 48 | 72 | 64 | 331 | 39 | 39 | | | | | 28 | 1010 |
| 18 months | 78 | 52 | 72 | 65 | 345 | 40 | 43 | | | | | 30 | 1042 |

| | | | | | | | | | | | | | |
|---|---|---|---|---|---|---|---|---|---|---|---|---|---|
| 20 months | 79 | 56 | 83 | 74 | 370 | 43 | 44 | | | | | 30 | 1050 |
| 22 months | 82 | 56 | 80 | 75 | 380 | 44 | 44 | | | | | 33 | 1059 |
| 2 years | 84 | 56 | 88 | 76 | 394 | 47 | 46 | | | 1.9 | 1.0 | 33 | 1064 |
| 3 years | 88 | 59 | 89 | 77 | 418 | 48 | 49 | 1.1 | 1.8 | 2.5 | 0.9 | 37 | 1141 |
| 4 years | 99 | 73 | 90 | 85 | 516 | 58 | 56 | | | | 1.4 | 39 | 1191 |
| 5 years | 106 | 85 | 107 | 104 | 596 | 65 | 64 | 1.2 | 1.8 | 2.9 | 2.1 | 47 | 1237 |
| 6 years | 109 | 94 | 121 | 122 | 642 | 68 | 67 | | | 2.9 | 2.2 | 58 | 1243 |
| 7 years | 113 | 100 | 130 | 123 | 680 | 69 | 70 | | | 2.6 | 2.6 | 66 | 1263 |
| 8 years | 119 | 110 | 150 | 140 | 736 | 74 | 75 | 1.3 | 1.6 | 2.6 | 3.1 | 69 | 1273 |
| 9 years | 125 | 115 | 174 | 152 | 756 | 82 | 83 | 1.4 | 1.6 | 3.4 | 3.1 | 73 | 1275 |
| 10 years | 130 | 116 | 177 | 166 | 852 | 92 | 95 | 1.6 | 1.6 | 3.4 | 3.1 | 85 | 1290 |
| 11 years | 135 | 122 | 201 | 190 | 909 | 94 | 95 | 2.3 | 2.5 | 5.3 | 4.3 | 87 | 1320 |
| 12 years | 139 | 124 | — | — | 936 | 95 | 96 | 2.8 | 3.0 | 5.3 | 4.3 | 93 | 1351 |

Data from Coppolette JM, Wolbach SB: Body length and organ weights of infants and children, *Am J Pathol* 9:55–70, 1933; except *from Weissenberg S: *Das Wachstrum des Menschen*, Stuttgart, Strecker and Schroder, 1911.

**Table B-15**   Organ weights of males, 13 to 18 years

| Age (years) | Heart (g) | Lungs | | Liver (g) | Kidneys | | Prostate* (g) | Testes, combined* (g) | Spleen (g) |
| --- | --- | --- | --- | --- | --- | --- | --- | --- | --- |
| | | Right (g) | Left (g) | | Right (g) | Left (g) | | | |
| 13 | 196 (173-218) | 376 (272-479) | 329 (245-410) | 1201 (1063-1340) | 98 (87-109) | 103 (91-116) | 3.7 | | 139 (84-194) |
| 14 | 213 (189-237) | 376 (285-466) | 361 (289-434) | 1204 (1095-1313) | 113 (102-125) | 117 (104-130) | 3.5 | 13.6 | 151 (111-191) |
| 15 | 232 (204-260) | 448 (348-548) | 420 (310-530) | 1361 (1247-1474) | 131 (114-146) | 131 (116-146) | 5.1 | 13.6 | 155 (119-191) |
| 16 | 259 (240-278) | 407 (317-496) | 366 (292-439) | 1647 (1506-1787) | 134 (123-145) | 134 (121-146) | 6.1 | | 165 (135-195) |
| 17 | 278 (262-295) | 527 (451-604) | 488 (411-564) | 1589 (1486-1692) | 140 (130-151) | 151 (141-166) | 11.4 | | 213 (164-261) |
| 18 | 279 (262-296) | 460 (370-549) | 403 (323-483) | 1706 (1610-1802) | 153 (141-166) | 157 (145-168) | | | 181 (156-206) |

Data from Kayser K: Height and weight in human beings: autopsy report, München, 1987, Verlag für angedwandte Wissenschaften; except *from Weissenberg S: *Das Wachstrum des Menschen,* Stuttgart, Strecker and Schroder, 1911.

**Table B-16    Organ weights of females, 13 to 18 years**

| Age (years) | Heart (g) | Lungs | | Liver (g) | Kidneys | | Uterus* (g) | Ovaries, combined* (g) | Spleen (g) |
| | | Right (g) | Left (g) | | Right (g) | Left (g) | | | |
|---|---|---|---|---|---|---|---|---|---|
| 13 | 177 (158-196) | 346 (286-405) | 297 (253-341) | 1050 (913-1187) | 102 (90-113) | 108 (97-120) | 15.9 | | 129 (98-160) |
| 14 | 208 (179-236) | 264 (178-349) | 237 (151-323) | 1194 (1082-1308) | 105 (97-113) | 114 (104-124) | | | 163 (111-215) |
| 15 | 190 (172-208) | 363 (300-426) | 283 (237-328) | 1308 (1197-1418) | 113 (101-126) | 118 (108-129) | | | 129 (97-161) |
| 16 | 229 (200-258) | 464 (233-695) | 431 (194-668) | 1348 (1134-1561) | 122 (105-140) | 128 (111-144) | 43.0 | 4.0 | 219 (160-278) |
| 17 | 230 (210-250) | 474 (360-590) | 391 (305-478) | 1398 (1250-1546) | 129 (120-139) | 135 (123-146) | | | 158 (141-175) |
| 18 | 235 (216-254) | 415 (288-542) | 326 (227-425) | 1504 (1351-1658) | 124 (116-131) | 129 (121-138) | | | 146 (121-172) |

Data from Kayser K: Height and weight in human beings: Autopsy report, München, Verlag für Angedwandte Wissenschaften, 1987; except *from Weissenberg S: Das Wachstrum des Menschen, Stuttgart, Strecker and Schroder, 1911.

## Table B-17 Fetal and placental measurements

| Weeks' gestation, postmenstrual | Fetal crown-rump length (cm) | Fetal weight (g) | Placental weight (g) | Placental diameter (cm) | Placental thickness (cm) | Fetal/placental ratio | Cord length (cm) |
|---|---|---|---|---|---|---|---|
| 8 | 1.4 | 1.7 | 5 | 3.0 | 0.75 | 0.34 | 7 |
| 10 | 4.0 | 5 | 14 | 5.0 | | 0.36 | 10 |
| 12 | 6.0 | 14 | 26 | 6.0 | 1.20 | 0.65 | 6-13 |
| 14 | 8.7 | 45 | 42 | 6.5 | | 0.71 | 16 |
| 16 | 12.0 | 110 | 65 | 7.5 | 1.60 | 0.90 | 15-19 |
| 18 | 14.0 | 200 | 90 | 8.0 | | 1.67 | 23 |
| 20 | 16.0 | 320 | 123 | 9.0 | 2.00 | 2.60 | 22-32 |
| 22 | 19.0 | 460 | 150 | 10.0 | | 3.10 | 36 |
| 24 | 21.0 | 630 | 182 | 12.5 | 2.40 | 3.40 | 28-40 |
| 26 | 23.2 | 820 | 210 | 13.5 | | 3.90 | 43 |
| 28 | 25.2 | 1045 | 250 | 15.0 | 2.80 | 4.20 | 28-45 |
| 30 | 26.5 | 1323 | 285 | 16.0 | | 4.60 | 48 |
| 32 | 28.0 | 1700 | 323 | 17.0 | 2.80 | 5.20 | 42-50 |
| 34 | 30.0 | 2100 | 362 | 18.0 | | 5.80 | 53 |
| 36 | 32.0 | 2478 | 404 | 20.0 | 3.00 | 6.10 | 46-56 |
| 38 | 34.0 | 2900 | 443 | 21.0 | | 6.50 | 57 |
| 40 | 36.0 | 3400 | 482 | 22.0 | 3.00 | 7.00 | 35-60 |
| 42 | 37.2 | 3513 | 487 | — | | 7.20 | 61 |
| >42 | 39.1 | 4077 | 738 | — | 5.84 | 5.50 | |

Data from Popek EJ: Normal anatomy and histology of the placenta. In Lewis SH, Perrin E, editors: *Pathology of the placenta,* ed 2, New York, Churchill Livingstone, pp 49-88, 1999.

## Table B-18 Fetal foot length based on regression model using "best estimates" records

| Gestational duration (wk)* | Foot length (mm)† | Foot length range (mm)‡ | Foot length range ± 1 SD (mm) |
|---|---|---|---|
| 10 to <11 | 4 | 2-5 | 0-6 |
| 11 to <12 | 7 | 5-8 | 4-10 |
| 12 to <13 | 10 | 8-11 | 7-13 |
| 13 to <14 | 13 | 12-14 | 10-16 |
| 14 to <15 | 16 | 15-17 | 13-19 |
| 15 to <16 | 20 | 18-21 | 16-23 |
| 16 to <17 | 23 | 21-24 | 19-26 |
| 17 to <18 | 26 | 24-27 | 22-29 |
| 18 to <19 | 29 | 27-30 | 25-32 |
| 19 to <20 | 32 | 31-33 | 29-36 |
| 20 to <21 | 35 | 34-37 | 32-39 |
| 21 to <22 | 39 | 37-40 | 35-42 |
| 22 to <23 | 42 | 40-43 | 38-45 |
| 23 to <24 | 45 | 43-46 | 41-49 |
| 24 to <25 | 48 | 47-49 | 44-52 |

*Weeks of gestational duration as measured by the "best estimate" (i.e., gestational duration by last menstrual period confirmed by ultrasonography within 1 standard deviation of last menstrual period).
†Foot length calculated by the model at the midpoint of the week (e.g., midpoint of 10 to <11 = 10 weeks, 3.5 days).
‡Range represents the foot length values from the beginning to the end of the week (e.g., range of 10 to <11 = values from 70 to 76 days).
Data from Drey EA, Kang M-S, McFarland W, Darney PD: Improving the accuracy of fetal foot length to confirm gestations duration, *Obstet Gynecol* 105:773-778, 2005.

**Table B-19    Criteria for estimating fetal age**

| Age (wk) | Crown-rump length (mm) | Foot length (mm) | Fetal weight (g) | Main external characteristics | Microscopic appearance |
|---|---|---|---|---|---|
| | | | | *Previable fetuses* | |
| 9 | 50 | 7 | 8 | Eyes closing or closed, head more rounded, external genitalia still not distinguishable as male or female, intestines are in umbilical cord | |
| 10 | 61 | 9 | 14 | Intestine in abdomen, early fingernail development | Cartilage in trachea |
| →12 | 87 | 14 | 45 | Sex distinguishable externally, well-defined neck | Bronchial glands and goblet cells evident |
| 14 | 120 | 20 | 110 | Head erect, lower limbs well developed | Prominent duct system in lung |
| →16 | 140 | 27 | 200 | Ears stand out from head | Cartilage in segmental bronchi |
| 18 | 160 | 33 | 320 | Vernix caseosa present, early toenail development | |
| 20 | 190 | 39 | 460 | Head and body hair (lanugo) visible | Lymphatics present in lung, periarteriolar lymphocytes in spleen, thymic cortex equal to medulla in thickness |
| 22 | 210 | 45 | 630 | Skin wrinkled and red | |
| →24 | 230 | 50 | 820 | Fingernails present, lean body | |
| | | | | *Viable fetuses* | |
| 26 | 250 | 55 | 1000 | Eyes partially open, eyelashes present | |
| →28 | 270 | 59 | 1300 | Eyes open, good head of hair, skin slightly wrinkled | |
| 30 | 280 | 63 | 1700 | Toenails present, body filling out, testes descending | |
| →32 | 300 | 68 | 2100 | Fingernails reach fingertips, skin pink and smooth | |
| 36 | 340 | 79 | 2900 | Body usually plump, lanugo hairs almost absent, toenails reach toe tips | |
| →38 | 360 | 83 | 3400 | Prominent chest, breasts protrude, testes in scrotum or palpable in inguinal canals, fingernails extend beyond fingertips | |

→, important landmarks.
Data from Valdés-Dapena M, Kalousek DK, Huff DS: Perinatal, fetal and embryonic autopsy. In Gilbert-Barness E, editor: *Potter's pathology of the fetus and infant,* St. Louis, 1997, Mosby, pp 483-524.

# REFERENCES

1. Schremmer C-N: Gewichtsänderungen verschiedener Gewebe nach Fomalinfixierung, *Frankfurt Z Pathol* 77:299-304, 1967.
2. Sunderman WF, Boerner F: *Normal values in clinical medicine,* Philadelphia, WB Saunders, 1949.
3. Fulton RM, Hutchinson EC, Jones AM: Ventricular weight in cardiac hypertrophy, *Br Heart J* 14:413-420, 1952.
4. Armed Forces Institute of Pathology: *The autopsy,* Washington, DC, Armed Forces Institute of Pathology, 1951.
5. Faulkner WR, King JW, Damm HC: *Handbook of clinical laboratory data,* ed 2, Cleveland, CRC Press, 1968.
6. Whimster WF, MacFarlane AJ: Normal lung weights in a white population, *Am Rev Respir Dis* 110:478-483, 1974.
7. de la Grandmaison GL, Clairand I, Durigon M: Organ weight in 684 adult autopsies: New tables for a Caucasoid population, *Forensic Sci Int* 119:149-154, 2001.
8. Das SK: Assessment of the size of the human omentum, *Acta Anat* 110:108-112, 1981.
9. Wald H: The weight of normal adult human kidneys and its variability, *Arch Pathol* 23:493-500, 1937.
10. Coppoletta JM, Wolbach SB: Body length and organ weights of infants and children: A study of the body length and normal weights of the more important vital organs of the body between birth and twelve years of age, *Am J Pathol* 9:55-70, 1933.
11. Eisendrath DN, Rolnick HC: *Urology,* Philadelphia, JB Lippincott, 1938.

12. Bloodworth JMB Jr: The adrenal. In Sommers SC, editor: *Pathology annual:* New York, 1966, Appleton-Century-Crofts, pp 172-192, 1996.

13. Moore RA: The evolution and involution of the prostate gland, *Am J Pathol* 12:599-624, 1936.

14. Clement PB: Ovary. In Sternberg SS, editor: *Histology for pathologists*, New York, 1992, Raven Press, pp 765-795, 1992.

15. Myers J, Segal RJ: Weight of the spleen. I. Range of normal in a nonhospital population, *Arch Pathol* 98:33-35, 1974.

16. Saphir O: *Autopsy diagnosis and technic*, ed 4, New York, Hoeber-Harper, 1958.

17. McComb JG: Cerebrospinal fluid, hydrocephalus, and cerebral edema. In Davis RL, Robertson DM, editors: *Textbook of neuropathology*, Baltimore, Williams & Wilkins, pp 225-251, 1997.

# Index

Note: Page numbers followed by "*f*" indicate figures, "*t*" indicate tables and "*b*" indicate boxes.